Communication Sciences and Disorders Across the Lifespan

Communication Sciences and Disorders Across the Lifespan

Patricia A. Prelock, PhD, CCC-SLP, BCS-CL, F-ASHA, FNAP-SLP
Ashley Brien, PhD, CCC-SLP

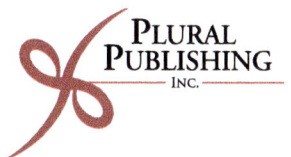

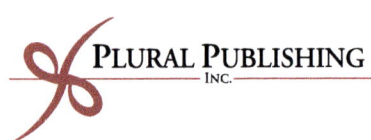

9177 Aero Drive, Suite B
San Diego, CA 92123

email: information@pluralpublishing.com
website: https://www.pluralpublishing.com

Copyright © 2026 by Plural Publishing, Inc.

Typeset in 11/15 Times New Roman by Flanagan's Publishing Services, Inc.
Printed in the United States of America by Bradford & Bigelow

All rights, including that of translation, reserved. No part of this publication may be reproduced, stored in a retrieval system, or transmitted in any form or by any means, electronic, mechanical, recording, or otherwise, including photocopying, recording, taping, web distribution, or information storage and retrieval systems without the prior written consent of the publisher.

For permission to use material from this text, contact us by
Telephone: (866) 758-7251
Fax: (888) 758-7255
email: permissions@pluralpublishing.com

Every attempt has been made to contact the copyright holders for material originally printed in another source. If any have been inadvertently overlooked, the publisher will gladly make the necessary arrangements at the first opportunity.

NOTICE TO THE READER
Care has been taken to confirm the accuracy of the indications, procedures, drug dosages, and diagnosis and remediation protocols presented in this book and to ensure that they conform to the practices of the general medical and health services communities. However, the authors, editors, and publisher are not responsible for errors or omissions or for any consequences from application of the information in this book and make no warranty, expressed or implied, with respect to the currency, completeness, or accuracy of the contents of the publication. The diagnostic and remediation protocols and the medications described do not necessarily have specific approval by the Food and Drug administration for use in the disorders and/or diseases and dosages for which they are recommended. Application of this information in a particular situation remains the professional responsibility of the practitioner. Because standards of practice and usage change, it is the responsibility of the practitioner to keep abreast of revised recommendations, dosages and procedures.

Library of Congress Cataloging-in-Publication Data
Names: Prelock, Patricia A., author. | Brien, Ashley R., author.
Title: Communication sciences and disorders across the lifespan / Patricia
　A. Prelock, Ashley Brien.
Description: San Diego, CA : Plural Publishing, Inc., [2026] | Includes
　bibliographical references and index.
Identifiers: LCCN 2024035635 (print) | LCCN 2024035636 (ebook) | ISBN
　9781635504538 (paperback) | ISBN 1635504538 (paperback) | ISBN
　9781635504361 (ebook)
Subjects: MESH: Communication Disorders | Neurologic Manifestations
Classification: LCC RC425 (print) | LCC RC425 (ebook) | NLM WL 340.2 |
　DDC 616.85/5—dc23/eng/20240903
LC record available at https://lccn.loc.gov/2024035635
LC ebook record available at https://lccn.loc.gov/2024035636

Contents

Preface	xv
Acknowledgments	xvii
About the Authors	xix
Contributor	xxiii
Reviewers	xxv
Using This Textbook	xxvii

Chapter 1. **An Introduction to Communication Disorders and the Professions of Speech-Language Pathology and Audiology** — 1

Learning Objectives	2
Key Terms	2
Introduction	2
What We Know About This Topic	3
What Is a Communication Disorder?	3
Cultural Considerations	4
What Are the Career Pathways for Audiologists and Speech-Language Pathologists?	4
Audiologists	5
Speech-Language Pathologists	7
Career Pathways for Audiology or Speech-Language Pathology Assistants	9
Research Innovations in Communication Sciences and Disorders	10
Why Is This Topic Important?	12
Overview of the Book Chapters	12
Chapter Summary	13
Key Takeaways	14
Chapter Review Questions	14
Learning Activities	15
Additional Resources	15
References	15

Chapter 2. **Disability Across the Lifespan** — 17

Learning Objectives	17
Key Terms	18
Introduction	18
Language Used in This Chapter	18

What Is Disability?	19
History of Disability	20
Models of Disability	23
Stigmatization	25
Disability and Illness	27
Ableism and Accessibility	27
The Intersectionalities of Disability	28
Disability and Race	29
Disability and Gender	30
Disability and Age	32
Disability and Socioeconomic Status	32
Disability Rights in the United States	34
Why Is This Topic Important?	36
Chapter Summary	36
Chapter Review Questions	37
Learning Activities	38
Suggested Reading	39
Suggested Films	39
References	41

Chapter 3. Understanding Speech and Language Development — 45

Learning Objectives	45
Key Terms	46
Introduction	46
Early Speech Development	47
Early Language Development	50
Receptive and Expressive Language	53
Phonology	53
Semantics	53
Morphology and Syntax	55
Pragmatics	56
Late Talkers	58
Assessment	60
Intervention	61
Why Is It Important to Understand Speech and Language Development?	62
Chapter Summary	63
Chapter Review Questions	63
Learning Activities	64
Suggested Reading	65
Additional Resources	66
References	66

Chapter 4. Anatomy and Physiology of the Speech Mechanism — 71

Learning Objectives	71
Key Terms	72
Introduction	72
Respiratory System	73
Phonatory System	74
Characteristics of Voice Production: Pitch and Loudness	76
Articulatory System	77
Resonatory System	79
Chapter Summary	81
Chapter Review Questions	81
Learning Activities	82
References	82

Chapter 5. Developmental Speech Sound Disorders — 85

Learning Objectives	85
Key Terms	86
Introduction	86
What We Know About This Topic	87
Risk Factors for Functional Speech Sound Disorders	88
Incidence/Prevalence of Childhood Speech Sound Disorders	88
Characteristics of Speech Sound Disorders	89
Cultural Considerations in Speech Production	89
What Can We Do to Address This Communication Challenge?	91
Assessment	91
Cultural Considerations for Assessing Bilingual Children	94
Intervention for Childhood Speech Disorders	94
Intervention Considerations for Culturally and Linguistically Diverse Populations	97
Why Is This Topic Important?	99
Application to a Child	100
Chapter Summary	101
Chapter Review Questions	102
Learning Activities	102
Suggested Reading	102
Additional Resources	103
References	103

Chapter 6. Motor Speech Disorders — 107

Learning Objectives	107
Key Terms	108

Introduction	108
The Brain	109
Motor Speech Disorders	109
Dysarthria	110
Apraxia of Speech	115
Cerebral Palsy	115
Impact of Motor Speech Disorders Across the Lifespan	116
Cross-Cultural Information	118
Assessment	119
Assessment for Adult Populations	119
Assessment Considerations for Pediatric Populations	121
Cross-Cultural Considerations in Assessment	122
Treatment	125
Treatment for Adult Populations	125
Treatment Considerations for Pediatric Populations	128
Why Is This Topic Important?	130
Application to a Child	132
Application to an Adult	133
Chapter Summary	134
Chapter Review Questions	135
Learning Activities	136
Suggested Reading	137
References	139

Chapter 7. Childhood Language Disorders   145

Learning Objectives	145
Key Terms	146
Introduction	146
What We Know About This Topic	146
Signs and Symptoms of Language Disorders	148
Incidence and Prevalence of Language Disorders	150
Causes of Language Disorders	150
Other Disorders That Share Characteristics of a Language Disorder	151
What Do We Do to Address This Communication Challenge?	158
Assessment of Childhood Language Disorders	158
Cultural Considerations	163
Intervention for Childhood Language Disorders	164
Intervention Applications in Cultural Groups	168
Additional Intervention Approaches	168
Service Delivery Options	170
Why Is This Topic Important?	170
Application to a Child	172
Chapter Summary	173

	Chapter Review Questions	174
	Learning Activities	174
	Suggested Reading	174
	Additional Resource	176
	References	176

Chapter 8. Specific Learning Disorders and Literacy Impairments — 185

	Learning Objectives	186
	Key Terms	186
	Introduction	186
	What Is a Specific Learning Disorder?	187
	What We Know About This Topic	188
	Incidence and Prevalence of Learning Disorders	189
	Signs of Learning Disorders	190
	Causes of Learning Disorders	191
	Co-Occurring Disorders	191
	Reading Disorders	191
	Written Language Disorders	193
	Math Disorders	194
	Nonverbal Learning Disability	194
	What Do We Do to Address This Communication Challenge?	196
	Assessment	196
	Intervention	198
	Why Is This Topic Important?	208
	Application to a Child	208
	Application to an Adolescent	209
	Chapter Summary	211
	Chapter Review Questions	212
	Learning Activities	212
	Suggested Reading	213
	Additional Resources	214
	References	214

Chapter 9. Adult Language and Cognitive Communication Disorders — 221

	Learning Objectives	221
	Key Terms	222
	Introduction	222
	The Brain	223
	Aphasia	226
	Fluent Aphasia	227

Nonfluent Aphasia	228
Causes	229
Impact of Aphasia Across the Lifespan	229
Right Hemisphere Disorder	230
Causes	232
Impact of Right Hemisphere Brain Injury Across the Lifespan	232
Traumatic Brain Injury	232
Causes	234
Impact of Traumatic Brain Injury Across the Lifespan	234
Dementia	234
Causes	235
Alzheimer's Disease	235
Impact of Dementia Across the Lifespan	236
Assessment	236
Aphasia	237
Right Hemisphere Disorder	238
Traumatic Brain Injury	238
Dementia	238
Cultural Considerations	239
Intervention	239
Aphasia	240
Right Hemisphere Disorder	241
Traumatic Brain Injury	242
Dementia	243
Cultural Considerations	244
Why Is This Topic Important?	244
Application to an Adult	246
Chapter Summary	247
Chapter Review Questions	248
Learning Activities	248
Suggested Reading	249
References	251

Chapter 10. Fluency Disorders   257

Learning Objectives	257
Key Terms	258
Introduction	258
What We Know About This Topic	261
Incidence and Prevalence	261
Characteristics of Stuttering	262
Characteristics of Cluttering	263
Causes of Stuttering	263
Causes of Cluttering	264

Assessment	264
Results of an Assessment	265
Cultural and Linguistic Considerations for Assessment	266
What Do We Do to Address This Communication Challenge?	267
Interventions for Stuttering	267
Interventions for Cluttering	270
Cultural and Linguistic Considerations for Stuttering Intervention	271
Why Is This Topic Important?	271
Application to a Child	272
Application to an Adolescent or Adult	273
Chapter Summary	274
Chapter Review Questions	274
Learning Activities	275
Suggested Reading	276
Additional Resources	277
References	277

Chapter 11. Voice Disorders   283

Learning Objectives	283
Key Terms	284
Introduction	284
What We Know About This Topic	285
Voice Disruption in Voice Disorders	288
Causes of Voice Disruption	289
What Do We Do to Address This Communication Challenge?	290
Assessment of Voice Disorders	291
Intervention for Voice Disorders	293
Why Is This Topic Important?	298
Application to a Child	298
Application to an Adolescent or Adult	299
Chapter Summary	300
Chapter Review Questions	301
Learning Activities	301
Suggested Reading	302
Additional Resources	304
References	304

Chapter 12. Feeding and Swallowing Disorders   311

Learning Objectives	312
Key Terms	312
Introduction	312
What We Know About This Topic	313

Preoral Phase	314
Oral Preparatory/Oral Phase	314
Pharyngeal Phase	315
Esophageal Phase	316
Characteristics of Dysphagia	316
Impact of the Disorder Across the Lifespan	319
Cross-Cultural Information	320
Assessment	321
Assessment Considerations for Adult Populations	321
Assessment Considerations for Pediatric Populations	324
Treatment	325
Treatment Considerations for Adult Populations	325
Treatment Considerations for Pediatric Populations	328
Why Is This Topic Important?	330
Application to a Child	331
Application to an Adolescent or Adult	334
Chapter Summary	335
Chapter Review Questions	336
Learning Activities	337
Suggested Reading	337
References	339

Chapter 13. Hearing Disorders and Their Impact on Communication — 343

Learning Objectives	343
Key Terms	344
Introduction	344
What We Know About This Topic	346
Anatomy of the Hearing Mechanism	346
Normal Hearing Development	348
What Does Hearing Impairment Look Like?	351
What Do We Do to Address This Communication Challenge?	356
Hearing Assessment	357
Hearing Assessment in Children	361
Treatment Planning, Management, and Options for Individuals With Hearing Loss 362	
Cultural and Linguistic Considerations	367
Why Is This Topic Important?	368
Application to a Child	369
Application to an Adolescent or Adult	370
Chapter Summary	371
Chapter Review Questions	372
Learning Activities	372

Suggested Reading	373
Additional Resources	374
References	375

Chapter 14. Augmentative and Alternative Communication — 387

Learning Objectives	387
Key Terms	388
Introduction	388
Characteristics of AAC	388
Unaided AAC	389
Aided AAC	389
No-Tech/Low-Tech AAC	389
High-Tech AAC	390
Access	391
Symbols and Vocabulary	393
Importance of AAC	393
AAC Users	394
AAC Assessment	394
AAC Intervention	396
AAC Intervention for Developmental Conditions	396
AAC Intervention for Acquired Conditions	397
Considerations for AAC	398
AAC Abandonment	399
Multimodal Communication	399
Bilingual AAC Users	400
Myths of AAC	400
Application to a Child	401
Application to an Adult	403
Chapter Summary	405
Chapter Review Questions	406
Learning Activities	407
Suggested Reading	407
References	409

Chapter 15. Understanding Research and Evidence-Based Practice — 413

Learning Objectives	413
Key Terms	414
Introduction	414
Types of Research	415
Quantitative Research	417
Qualitative Research	420

Importance of Research for Clinical Practice	423
Chapter Summary	426
Chapter Review Questions	426
Learning Activities	427
Suggested Reading	427
References	429
Appendix 15–1. Tips for Reading a Primary Source	431
Glossary	*435*
Index	*461*

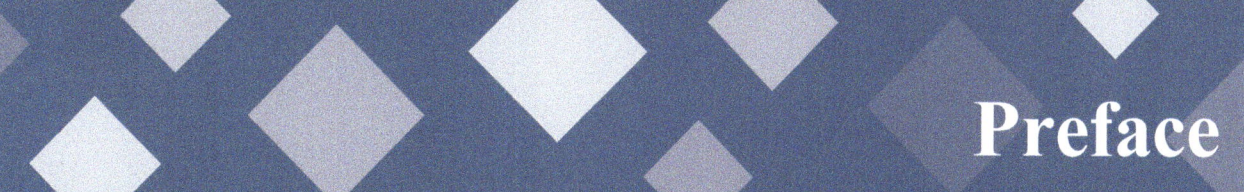

Preface

We have written this book to provide students in introductory communication sciences and disorders courses an opportunity to understand the power of communication and the role that speech-language pathologists and audiologists have in recognizing and supporting communication challenges in children and adults. We have tried to provide information that is current and follows best practice, and we have included several resources for students to expand their learning as well as case studies to facilitate the application of learning. There are many learning tools included throughout the chapters, such as suggested readings, video links, study guide questions, and more. There is also a comprehensive glossary of terms.

Together, we have more than 50 years of experience as speech-language pathologists. We have practiced in multiple settings from the schools to clinics and hospitals to institutions of higher education. We have taught several introductory and advanced courses in communication sciences and disorders and appreciate the opportunity to share our excitement about the professions of speech-language pathology and audiology. Our research expertise spans language and cognitive development of children with specific language disorders to children and adults with autism. We are both American Speech-Language-Hearing Association–certified speech-language pathologists, and Dr. Prelock is a board-certified specialist in child language.

We hope that you find the content of this book and the accompanying learning tools helpful to your understanding of the discipline. This will be the first of many opportunities for you to learn about communication and communication disorders in children and adults.

—*Patricia A. Prelock, PhD, CCC-SLP, BCS-CL, F-ASHA, FNAP-SLP*
—*Ashley Brien, PhD, CCC-SLP*

Acknowledgments

A huge thank you to everyone who contributed to the creation of this book. Special thanks to Claudia Abbiati, Dorothy Yang, Sophie Knox, and Alyssa Thornburg, who contributed ideas, feedback, edits, and moral support. Thanks to Alissa Tryforos and Crystal Rubio-Martinez for their work in helping put together the chapter summary, study guide questions, and glossary terms for Chapter 14 and Chapter 2, respectively. I am also grateful to Patty for entrusting me to complete this task alongside her.

—*Ashley Brien*

Special thanks to Caitlin Allan, who did a great deal of the literature searches for the content included in this book, supported the development of suggested readings, and prepared PowerPoints to align with the content of each chapter. I acknowledge the outstanding work of my colleague and friend, Ashley Brien, for her partnership in this endeavor.

—*Patricia A. Prelock*

About the Authors

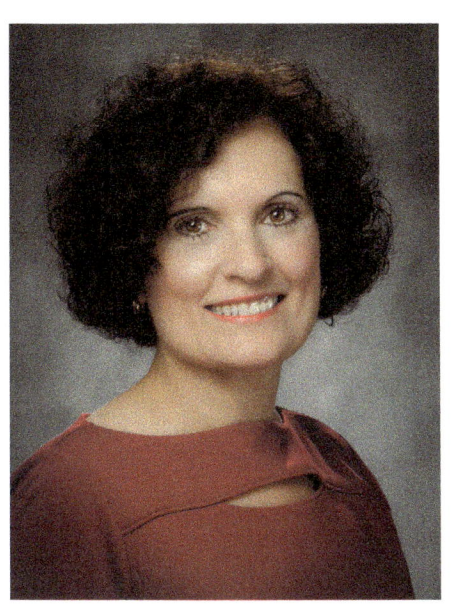

Patricia A. Prelock, PhD, CCC-SLP, BCS-CL, F-ASHA, FNAP-SLP, is the Interim President, University of Vermont. Formerly, she was Provost and Senior Vice President for 5 years, and the Dean of the College of Nursing and Health Sciences at the University of Vermont for 10 years. She is also a Professor of Communication Sciences and Disorders, and Professor of Pediatrics in the College of Medicine at the University of Vermont. Dr. Prelock received her PhD in speech-language pathology from the University of Pittsburgh. She is a recognized expert in the nature and treatment of autism spectrum disorders (ASD) and has been awarded nearly $25 million dollars in university, state, and federal funding as a PI or Co-PI to develop innovations in interdisciplinary training supporting children and youth with neurodevelopmental disabilities and their families, to facilitate training in speech-language pathology, and to support her intervention work in ASD. She has over 220 publications including 20 books and 598 peer-reviewed and invited presentations/keynotes in the areas of autism and other neurodevelopmental disabilities, collaboration, IPE, leadership, and language learning disabilities. In 2019, she was named Associate Editor for the *Journal of Autism and Developmental Disorders*. Dr. Prelock received the University of Vermont's Kroepsch-Maurice Excellence in Teaching Award in 2000, was named an ASHA Fellow in 2000, and a University of Vermont Scholar in 2003. Dr. Prelock was named a Distinguished Alumna of the University of Pittsburgh. In 2016, she received the ASHA Honors of the Association and in 2017 she was named a Distinguished Alumna of Cardinal Mooney High School. Dr. Prelock also received the 2018 Jackie M. Gribbons Leadership Award from Vermont Women in Higher Education. Dr. Prelock is a Board-Certified Specialist in Child Language and was named a Fellow in the National Academies of Practice (NAP) in speech-language pathology in 2018. She was the 2013 President for the American Speech-Language-Hearing Association and was President of the ASHFoundation in 2020 and 2021.

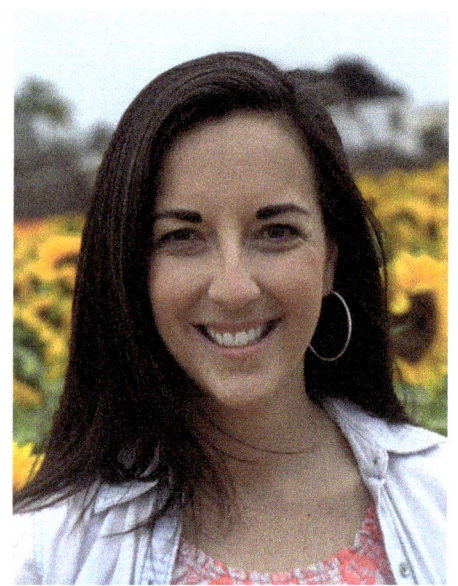

Ashley Brien, PhD, CCC-SLP, is an ASHA certified speech-language pathologist. She received her MS in Communication Sciences and Disorders and her PhD in Interprofessional Health Sciences from the University of Vermont. She has instructed many courses at the undergraduate and graduate levels in the areas of autism, social cognition, augmentative and alternative communication, disability, and research methods. Additionally, she provides intervention in speech, language, AAC, and social communication to children and adolescents and their families. Dr. Brien's research focuses on the development, implementation, and social validity of family-centered interventions to support social learning and episodic memory in individuals with autism. She has also designed intervention materials to support social cognition and communication in a variety of populations with social learning challenges. She has written about her work in several peer-reviewed articles and presented her findings nationally and internationally. She is also co-author of the book *Supporting Social Learning in Autism: An Autobiographical Memory Program to Promote Communication and Connection.*

This book is dedicated to the undergraduate students who we have had the pleasure of learning from, teaching, and mentoring and to the children, adolescents, and adults with communication disorders we have had the honor of supporting.

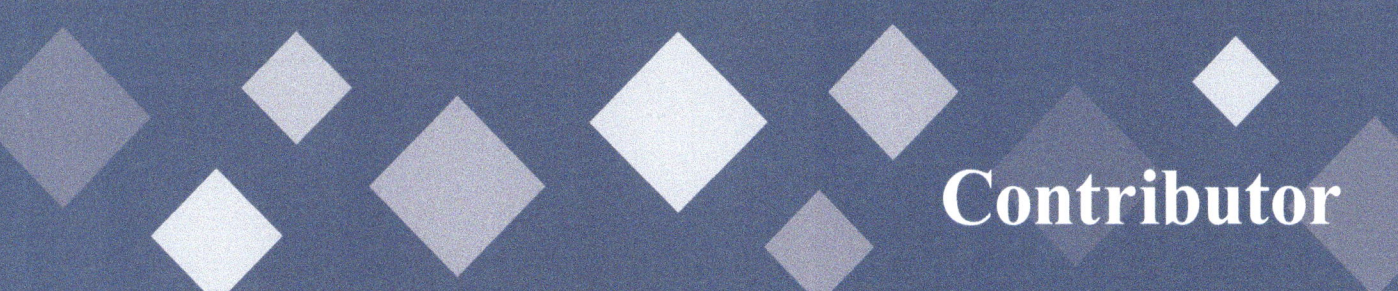

Contributor

Dorothy Yang, PhD, CCC-SLP
Speech-Language Pathologist
Jennifer Moreno Department of Veterans Affairs Medical Center
San Diego, California
Chapters 6 and 12

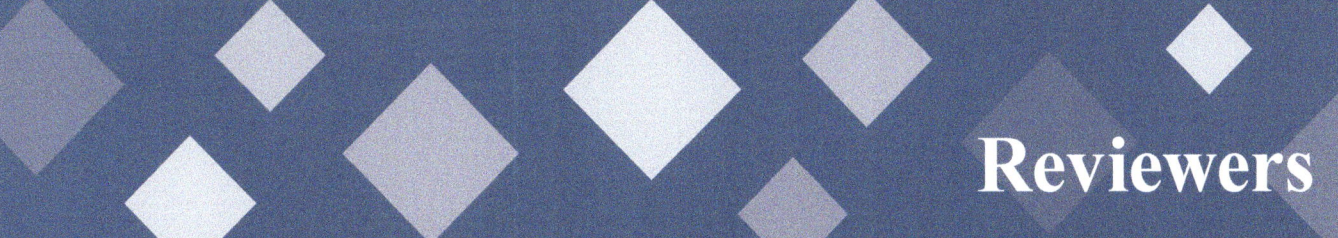

Reviewers

Plural Publishing and the authors thank the following reviewers for taking the time to provide their valuable feedback during the manuscript development process. Additional anonymous feedback was provided by other expert reviewers.

Natalie Armstrong, DEd, CCC-SLP
Pennsylvania Western University
Clarion, Pennsylvania

An Dinh, PhD
The University of Toledo
Toledo, Ohio

Ruth Renee Hannibal, PhD, CCC-SLP
Valdosta State University
Valdosta, Georgia

Susana L. Keller, MS, MBA, CScD
DeSales University
Center Valley, Pennsylvania

Nicole Lewis, MS, CCC-SLP
Gannon University
Erie, Pennsylvania

Emily Weston, MS, CCC-SLP
Arkansas State University
Jonesboro, Arkansas

Using This Textbook

This textbook offers the following pedagogical features to enhance your learning and comprehension.

Chapters begin with:

Learning Objectives and a list of **Key Terms** to provide a guide on how to navigate the depth and breadth of the chapter content.

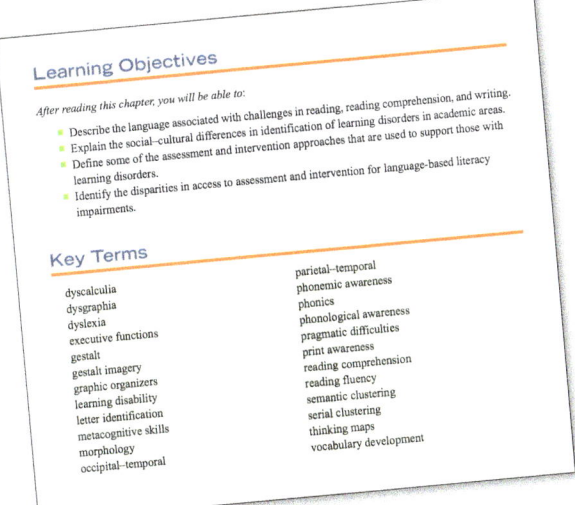

As you delve into the chapters, you will find:

Bolded key terms and a comprehensive **Glossary** that help improve retention of the material and help you easily find definitions.

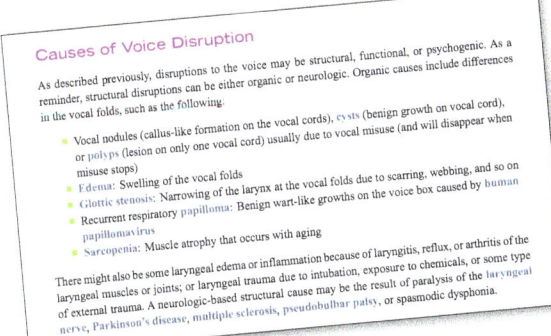
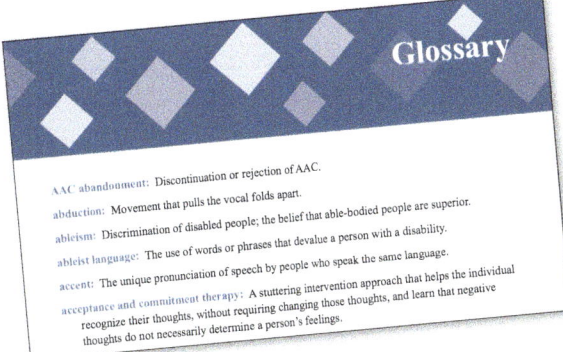

Detailed color **Figures**, **Tables**, and **Photos** aid in understanding complex concepts.

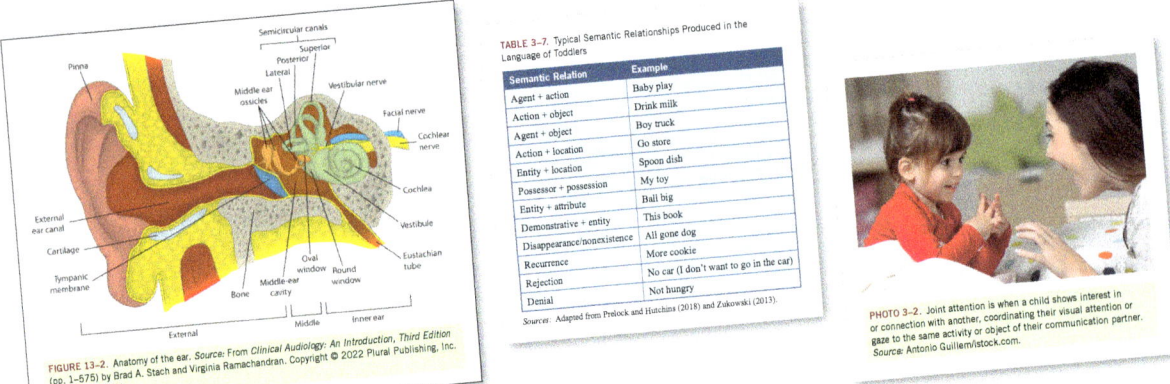

Pause and Ponder **Boxes** offer thought-provoking discussion topics to encourage critical thinking and class participation.

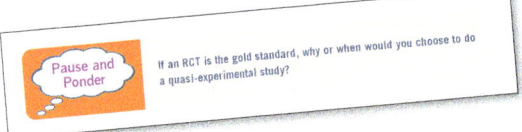

QR Codes help readers get to websites and videos easily from the text.

Real-world **Case Studies** are integrated to illustrate the application of theoretical concepts in clinical settings.

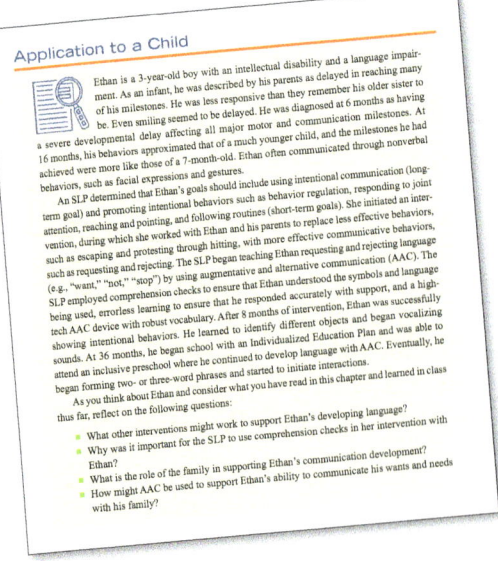

Chapters end with:

Chapter Summaries: Each chapter concludes with a summary recapping the key points covered. This helps reinforce learning and provides a quick review for studying.

Chapter Review Questions reinforce key concepts and provide an opportunity for self-assessment.

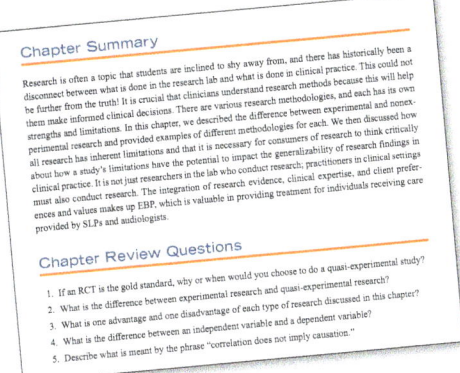

Learning Activities focus on bridging the gap between research and practice.

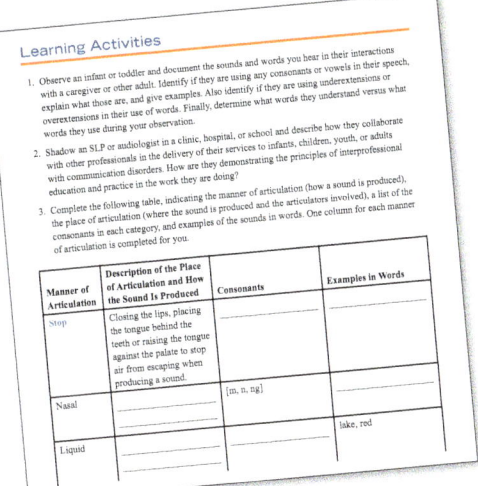

Additional Resources and a comprehensive list of **References** showcase the evidence base and encourage you to delve deeper into the literature.

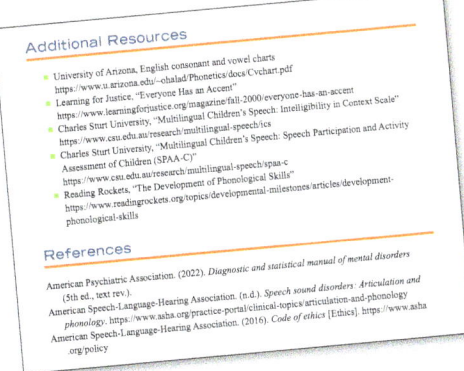

This textbook also comes with ancillary resources accessible on a **PluralPlus companion website**, including **practice quizzes** and **study guides**. See instructions on how to access the student materials on the inside front cover of the book.

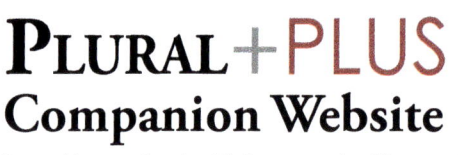

Chapter 1

An Introduction to Communication Disorders and the Professions of Speech-Language Pathology and Audiology

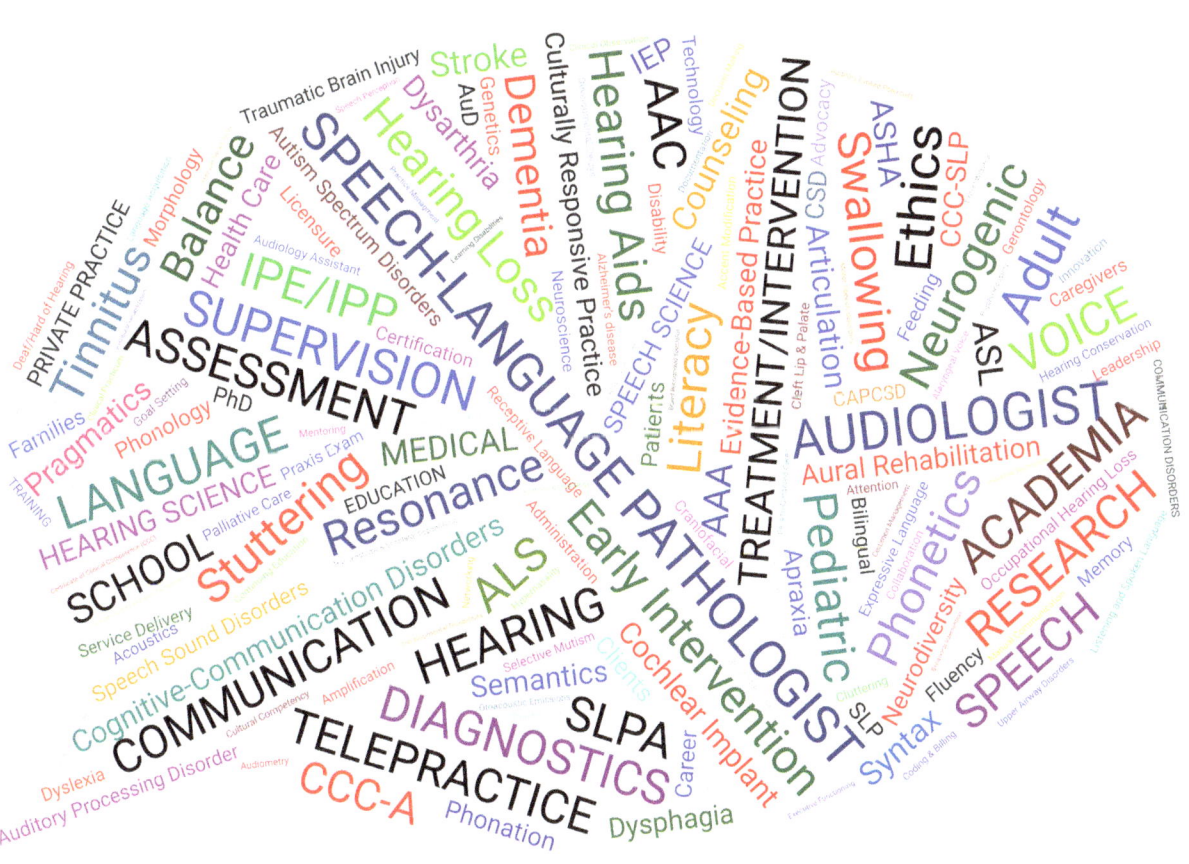

Learning Objectives

After reading this chapter, you will be able to:

- Explain communication disorders and what speech-language pathologists and audiologists do to support those with communication disorders.
- Describe the career pathways for speech-language pathologists and audiologists.
- Describe the career pathways for speech-language pathology and audiology assistants.
- Identify some of the innovations that have occurred in the professions to ensure communication is achievable for all.

Key Terms

Alzheimer disease	morphology
amyotrophic lateral sclerosis	neurodiverse
aphasia	oral dysphagia
apraxia of speech	pharyngeal or oropharyngeal dysphagia
articulation	phonological disorder
cochlear implant	phonology
communication difference	pragmatics
communication disorder	receptive language
disability	semantics
dysarthria of speech	stroke
dysphagia	syntax
esophageal dysphagia	vocal cord paralysis
expressive language	vocal nodules
hair cells	

Introduction

Have you ever thought about not being able to share your thoughts, ideas, feelings, or needs with your parents, your peers, or other people with whom you interact. Our ability to communicate is something most of us never have to think about, but for those with a communication disorder, the experience of communicating may be very different. Some individuals may not be able to find the right word to share their idea, others may struggle to formulate sounds and words we can understand, and still others may not be able to hear what is being said to them. Any one of these challenges is disruptive to our ability to share meaning with one another, whether we are decoding what someone has said or encoding a response to share our thoughts.

Communication is the ability to exchange information between individuals or groups of individuals that is critical to our social existence. Language is what we use to communicate the thoughts, ideas, and beliefs we have and allows us to share these with others. It includes the ability to use gestures, spoken speech, signs, and other symbol systems to communicate with our parents, siblings, friends, and co-workers. Imagine if you could not share an idea you had, struggled to have your message understood by others, or could not tell someone how you felt. It would be an isolating and frustrating experience.

This chapter introduces what communication disorders are and the terms typically used to describe communication disorders, and it provides a brief description of the communication disorders you are most likely to hear about. The chapter also discusses the career pathways that are available for those interested in the discipline and some of the innovations in research that have implications for practice in the field. In addition, an outline of content for each of the chapters that follows is presented. Importantly, communication disorders exist across the lifespan, so this book highlights communication disorders in both children and adults.

What We Know About This Topic

The presence of a **communication disorder** takes many forms. A person can be born with a congenital condition (e.g., deafness, cerebral palsy, Down syndrome) that affects their ability to communicate, or they can acquire a communication problem after birth (e.g., traumatic brain injury, **stroke**) (Gillam & Marquardt, 2016; Prelock & Hutchins, 2018). A communication disorder may also be organic, indicating there may be a functional, physical, or unknown cause.

Approximately 1 in 12 children (7.7%) aged 3 to 17 years have a speech, language, voice, or swallowing disorder in the United States, and many have multiple communication disorders (Black et al., 2015). Overall, 46 million people have some difficulty speaking or hearing that impacts their daily functioning (National Institute on Deafness and Other Communication Disorders, 2015a, 2015b).

What Is a Communication Disorder?

Communication is intentional or unintentional verbal or nonverbal behavior that influences the ideas, thoughts, or behaviors of another person (American Psychiatric Association, 2022). A communication disorder suggests an individual has a deficit in speech, language, and/or communication. Communication disorders are also seen in conditions such as Down syndrome, autism, traumatic brain injury, stroke, cleft palate, learning disorders, and other acquired, organic, or genetic disorders that impact speech, language, and/or hearing.

Speech refers to sound production and includes **articulation** or the way we form sounds to produce words. You will learn more about speech sound disorders in Chapters 5 and 6. Language includes the form (**syntax** or grammar, **morphology**, and **phonology**), function (**semantics** or word meaning), and use (**pragmatics** or use of language in social contexts) of symbol systems, including spoken and written words, sign language, and pictures that are rule governed (American Psychiatric Association, 2022). You will learn more about a variety of language disorders in Chapters 7, 8, and 9.

There are several terms used to describe a person with a communication disorder. The words you will hear most often are impairment, disorder, disability, difference, and **neurodiverse**. **Impairment** typically refers to a loss of function or some difference in structure that impedes behavior, in this case communication (World Health Organization, 2011). For example, someone with a hearing loss may have difficulty hearing but will still be able to function, such as going to school, having a job, developing friendships, and so on. **Disorder** suggests the inability to function in a way we would expect in daily activities. In the case of someone who is hard of hearing, they may not have sufficient hearing to talk on the phone even when they wear hearing aids. The term **disability** suggests the need to understand how much support would be needed for a person to engage in daily life activities (Prelock & Hutchins, 2018). Again, in the case of someone who is deaf or hard of hearing, they may require a notetaker in the classroom or interpreter services during health care visits.

You will most often hear the term communication disorder used by speech-language pathologists (SLPs) and audiologists, and it is sometimes used synonymously with impairment and disability. We think of it as a limitation in communication structure or function (Gillam & Marquardt, 2016).

A **communication difference** suggests that a child communicates in a way that is different than you might expect in English. For example, second language learners may exhibit typical development in their native language (e.g., Italian), yet their English might not be as fluid, an accent might interfere with intelligibility, and word selection might not always be accurate. Learning English as a second language, however, is not considered a communication disorder.

Many of these terms suggest a medical model approach to understanding communication, identifying a deficit or impairment in function. A more recent neurodiversity movement has suggested that we should acknowledge that we are made up of diverse neurotypes with unique strengths and challenges (Dwyer, 2022). This has been an area of particular focus in the autistic population. We talk more about this in Chapter 2.

Cultural Considerations

There appears to be a greater incidence of communication disorders in children identified as males versus females, although it remains unclear if symptom recognition may look different across genders, creating greater ease and access to diagnosis, or if, in fact, there is a true gender difference. This is an important question for researchers and clinicians to continue to examine. Interestingly, however, there are also higher incidences of communication disorders for Black versus White children and slightly less for Hispanic children, although these percentages are also higher than the percentage for females alone. Most important, however, is the access to services for those with communication disorders. For example, although the percentage of communication disorders is greater among Black than White children, the percentage of services they receive is less. This is also true for Hispanic children, and it suggests the existence of health disparities in the delivery of services for diverse populations, which is an issue that needs to be addressed.

What Are the Career Pathways for Audiologists and Speech-Language Pathologists?

The professional organization for audiologists and SLPs is the American Speech-Language-Hearing Association (ASHA). ASHA has a public website on which you can access specific information about a career in communication sciences and disorders.

⊘ www

Careers in Communication Sciences and Disorders

You might ask, why should I choose a career in this field? There are several reasons to consider, and answering the following questions might help you think about the opportunities:

- *Do I have the skill set to be successful in this career?*
  - If you like science, enjoy working with others and solving problems, and are curious about how people think, communicate, and learn, then this career is worth your consideration.
- *Does this career offer a competitive salary?*
  - Yes, and salaries continue to increase for both SLPs and audiologists as per the U.S. Bureau of Labor Statistics

Bureau of Labor Statistics

- *Would I have job security?*
  - The need for SLPs and audiologists is strong and continues to grow. Those who can speak more than one language are in demand.
- *How will I serve my community and make a difference in this career?*
  - In this career, you will have an opportunity to improve the quality of life of those with whom you work who have communication disorders. We want individuals to pursue this career who are passionate about ensuring communication for all.
- *Is there flexibility in the kind of job I would do?*
  - Yes, as a certified SLP, audiologist, or speech and hearing scientist, you could work across several different environments—schools, hospitals, clinics, private practice, industry, colleges/universities, and so on. You can choose the environment that will give you the greatest flexibility in terms of hours to fit your lifestyle.

Audiologists

The median salary for audiologists in 2021 was $78,950, with a professional doctorate and state license required. The job outlook is strong, with an expected growth of 10% between 2021 and 2031. There are approximately 800 openings for audiologists each year (U.S. Bureau of Labor Statistics, 2023).

See the "Audiology Service Delivery Areas" section of the **ASHA Scope of Practice in Audiology** and ASHA's **Hearing and Speech Careers** website for more information on a career in audiology.

What Do Audiologists Do?

Using science and the latest technology, audiologists prevent, identify, diagnose, and treat hearing, balance, and other auditory disorders. Audiologists work with several populations including, but not limited to, the following:

- Patients with **cochlear implants**
- Musicians to prevent hearing loss
- Patients experiencing hearing loss as a result of drugs used to treat cancer
- Children and adults who are deaf or hard of hearing and require ongoing assessment and support with hearing aids
- Patients with genetic disorders that impact hearing
- Veterans who were exposed to explosions and gunfire

Audiologists provide education to patients and their families about available options for communication when a hearing loss exists. They assess, treat, and research hearing and balance disorders. Importantly, audiologists work with patients across the lifespan to help prevent hearing loss, assess hearing, and support hearing health including the use of hearing aids.

Where Do Audiologists Work?

Audiologists work with a variety of health care and educational professionals, including SLPs, physicians (e.g., otolaryngologists or ENTs—ear, nose, and throat doctors), teachers, engineers, and scientists. Their work settings vary from health care settings to schools and colleges to private practice.

Health Care Settings. A significant percentage of audiologists work in health care settings, including resident and nonresidential health care facilities and hospitals. In these settings, they may screen newborns' hearing, educate patients on the use and care of hearing aids, design rehabilitation programs to increase sound recognition, or work with patients who have experienced a traumatic brain injury.

Early Intervention and Schools. Audiologists might also serve infant and toddler programs providing family support, education, and programming for cochlear implants or provide hearing screenings for preschools. For school-age children, they help promote self-advocacy for those with hearing loss, educate school personnel on ways to support students with hearing loss, and collaborate with teachers to provide rehabilitation services for children who are deaf or hard of hearing.

Colleges and Universities. Audiologists may also wish to teach or engage in hearing research at a college or university. In this capacity, they often work with patients in a university or affiliate clinical facility; mentor students; serve as hearing experts; and engage in creating new knowledge about hearing development, hearing and balance disorders, and hearing health.

Private Practice. Many audiologists may choose to go into private practice where they own a clinic with employees in which they provide a range of audiological services. Private practice audiologists might also provide consultation and/or hearing services for other agencies, clinics, schools, and so on.

1 ◆ An Introduction to Communication Disorders and the Professions

See the American Academy of Audiology's **(AAA) Scope of Practice** and the **"Become an Audiologist"** section of the AAA website for more information on what audiologist do.

Speech-Language Pathologists

The median salary for SLPs in 2021 was $79,050 with a master's degree and state license. The job outlook is strong, with an expected growth of 21% between 2021 and 2031. In fact, growth in this field is much faster than the average for all occupations. There are approximately 14,000 openings for SLPs each year (U.S. Bureau of Labor Statistics, 2023).

See the "Speech-Language Pathology Service Delivery Areas" section of the **ASHA Scope of Practice in Speech-Language Pathology** and ASHA's Hearing and Speech Careers website for more information on a career in speech-language pathology.

What Do Speech-Language Pathologists Do?

Speech-language pathologists serve individuals with communication disorders throughout their lifespan. They assess and treat speech, language, and swallowing disorders. There are several disorder areas that SLPs address, including the following:

- Speech disorders: Stuttering, articulation, and voice difficulties
- Language disorders: **Receptive** (what a person understands)/**expressive** (what a person says) **language**, spoken and written language, and **social/pragmatic language** (how language is used for social purposes)
- Gender affirming voice services: Work with transgender youth and adults
- Swallowing disorders (also known as **dysphagia**): Feeding challenges for both pediatric and adult patients whether it is **oral dysphagia** (difficulties with tongue movement), **pharyngeal or oropharyngeal dysphagia** (food has difficulty passing through the throat), or **esophageal dysphagia** (food cannot move through the esophagus)
- Cognitive disorders: This includes those with intellectual disabilities or those with dementia such as **Alzheimer disease**

Table 1–1 provides a summary of the nine knowledge outcomes expected for SLPs as determined by the Council on Academic Accreditation for Speech-Language Pathology.

TABLE 1–1. Knowledge Outcomes Expected for Speech-Language Pathologists (as Outlined by the Council on Academic Accreditation for Speech-Language Pathology, 2023)

Demonstrated Knowledge	Including
Speech sound production	Articulation, motor planning and execution, phonology, and accent modification
Fluency and fluency disorders	
Voice and resonance	Respiration and phonation
Receptive and expressive language	Phonology; morphology; syntax; semantics; pragmatics (language use and social aspects of communication); prelinguistic communication; paralinguistic communication (e.g., gestures, signs, body language); and literacy in speaking, listening, reading, and writing
Hearing	Impact on speech and language
Swallowing/feeding	Structure and function of orofacial myology and oral, pharyngeal, laryngeal, pulmonary, esophageal, gastrointestinal, and related functions across the life span
Cognitive aspects of communication	Attention, memory, sequencing, problem-solving, and executive functioning
Social aspects of communication	Challenging behavior, ineffective social skills, and lack of communication opportunities
Augmentative and alternative communication modalities	

Where Do Speech-Language Pathologists Work?

Speech-language pathologists work in a variety of health care and educational settings, as well as universities and in private practice.

Health Care Settings. More than 30% of SLPs work in health care settings, including resident and nonresidential health care facilities and hospitals. They serve patients across the lifespan, from supporting premature babies to facilitate their ability to safely drink milk to diagnosing cognitive, language, and swallowing problems that require treatment. This might include working with families on ways to create structure for patients with Alzheimer disease, finding alternative communication strategies for those with **amyotrophic lateral sclerosis**, or guiding the communication recovery of patients who have had a stroke.

Early Intervention and Schools. More than 50% of SLPs work in educational settings, including infant–toddler programs, preschools, and elementary and high schools. In early intervention, SLPs might provide parent training to support early language development or address feeding problems in infants and toddlers. They also might consult with day care centers to educate professionals on the receptive and **expressive language** needs of preschool children. In elementary school and high school, SLPs help children understand and produce sounds, words, sentences, and discourse. They collaborate with teachers to support language and literacy development, including understanding letter–sound relationships and vocabulary development. They work with a variety of populations who typically have communication disorders, such as those with autism, cerebral palsy, Down syndrome, and other genetic disorders.

Colleges and Universities. Speech-language pathologists with doctoral degrees may also wish to teach or engage in research at a college or university. In this capacity, they often work with patients in a university or affiliate clinical facility, they mentor students, and they engage in creating new knowledge about speech and language development and a variety of communication disorders. SLPs with a master's degree and clinical certification may be hired to serve as clinical supervisors for graduate students who are gaining practical experience in university clinics.

Private Practice. Some SLPs may choose to go into private practice where they are owners of a clinic with employees who provide a range of speech and language services. Private practice SLPs might also provide consultation and/or contract services for other agencies, clinics, schools, and so on.

Career Pathways for Audiology or Speech-Language Pathology Assistants

An audiology or speech-language pathology assistant is someone educated to support the work of certified audiologists and SLPs. Assistants have varied experience and educational backgrounds governed by state regulations for the use of support personnel. Specific information about each state's regulations can be found in the ASHA State-by-State requirements and contact information resource by clicking on "Support Personnel" for the state in which you are interested. Importantly, not all states have regulations for or use SLP assistants (SLPAs) or audiology assistants.

ASHA State-by-State

SLPAs and audiology assistants work under the supervision of licensed SLPs and audiologists. They learn to maintain materials and equipment used for assessment and intervention, as well as documentation processes and implementing routine clinical services. Some SLPAs or audiology assistants may go on to apply to graduate school to become licensed professionals, whereas others will choose to make this their final career. Students who have graduated from an undergraduate program in communication sciences and disorders are able to work as assistants and often do so before applying to or being accepted into a graduate program.

See the **ASHA Scope of Practice for the Speech-Language Pathology Assistant (SLPA)** and the **ASHA Audiology Assistants Practice Portal** for more information on a career as an SLPA or audiology assistant.

Responsibilities of Audiology Assistants

Audiology assistants typically have on-the-job training, obtain training while in the military, or are trained to be hearing conservationists. Audiology assistants are supervised by a certified or licensed audiologist and are typically assigned the following tasks:

- Pure-tone hearing screening and universal newborn hearing screening tests
- Hearing and tympanometric screening for older children and adults without interpretation
- Assistance in treatment programs
- Translators, interpreter, and/or cultural brokers

Responsibilities of Speech-Language Pathology Assistants

Speech-language pathology assistants perform tasks assigned by a certified SLP, such as the following:

- Speech, language, and hearing screenings without providing interpretation
- Telepractice treatment support for clients selected by the supervising SLP as appropriate
- Interpreter support for clients and families unable to speak English
- Advocacy through community awareness about health literacy and education

Research Innovations in Communication Sciences and Disorders

In addition to the educational and clinical pathways for speech-language pathology and audiology, the professions contribute significantly to research. The people in the discipline are innovative researchers who are forging new frontiers for the study of communication sciences and disorders and have made some remarkable findings during the past 10 years. The next few paragraphs share just a few highlights of the discoveries our colleagues have made through funded research. This is just a small slice of the creativity that contributes to and informs our practice, from the use of computer games to increase attention to auditory input to identifying the impact of specific language impairment and understanding how the brain adjusts during stroke recovery.

Researchers at the Virginia Merrill Bloedel Hearing Research Center at the University of Washington are examining the tiny **hair cells** that are in the inner ear. Their goal is to prevent the death of the hair cells to help preserve hearing loss in adults. To do this, they are using zebra fish to learn about hair cell loss due to medicinal or environmental toxins. Interestingly, zebra fish use "hair cells" to detect water currents just like humans do to detect sounds (Cutter, 2014a).

Another innovation related to hearing loss is demonstrated by researchers at the Medical University of South Carolina who are involved in a longitudinal study of hearing. They are looking at older adults using new approaches, such as genetics and neuroimaging, to examine age-related hearing loss, which you will learn more about in Chapter 13. Age-related hearing loss is one of the most frequent health concerns that affects the ability to communicate and often affects the quality of life for the millions of adult affected (Cutter, 2014b).

At Washington University School of Medicine, audiologists are collaborating with researchers across disciplines to create auditory training exercises that are motivating and help individuals make sense of the speech they hear. They are doing this using computer games and establishing meaning-based, engaging activities that help clients build a paragraph or solve a murder mystery after listening to sentences or clues presented auditorily. The computer games are designed to support listening for meaning at several levels (e.g., words, sentences, comprehension). Thus, for those who use hearing aids, audiologists not only can provide the hardware to increase auditory input but also can implement motivating technology to increase the ability to listen and understand information presented auditorily (Polovoy, 2014d).

For those interested in supporting the speech and language of children, researchers at the University of Kansas and the University of Nebraska followed children from age 4 years through age 18 years and examined their genetic and family history as well as the duration of intervention services. Questions remain for researchers about whether children diagnosed with specific language impairment who receive services early on really catch up to where we expect them to be as they get older. These researchers are seeing remaining language lags around third grade even though services had been previously discontinued because of progress made. With these findings, researchers are challenging clinicians to expand how, when, and how long they implement intervention for children with language delays to ensure their growth through adolescence (Murray-Law, 2014a).

Researchers at MIT and Boston University are examining grammar and phonological working memory in children aged 5 to 17 years with autism who also have language-learning problems to determine where there might be breakdowns in language. They are using functional magnetic resonance imaging to examine the responses of children's brains to two tasks—hearing sentences with different grammatical structure and hearing and repeating nonwords. There appear to be differences in the way children with autism and those with specific language impairment process language, and this has implications for intervention (Murray-Law, 2014b).

At the University of Wisconsin–Madison, researchers are studying the language function of children with language impairment and children with autism and the possibility that language impairment can disrupt a child's executive functioning or present a self-regulation challenge. Such a disruption can impact a child's ability to navigate their academic and social worlds (Murray-Law, 2014a).

There is also funded research occurring at the Autism Center of Excellence at Boston University, where researchers are testing new ways to support the communication skills of autistic children who do not speak verbally or who have minimal verbal output. They are collaborating with researchers at Harvard Medical School, Northeastern University, and the Albert Einstein School of Medicine to examine brain differences in children with autism who do not speak. It is unclear if the inability to speak is related to a child's ability to process the auditory input they receive or their ability to connect the motor speech system to produce speech output (Polovoy, 2014a). A better understanding of the gaps in brain connections will help facilitate researchers to target and improve intervention. The intervention being tested involves the imitation of sounds, words, and phrases using a melodic tone while also following a drum rhythm. Because both our music and motor systems are near language areas in the brain, such an intervention could act as a catalyst for speech and language development (Polovoy, 2014a).

Recovery from stroke with the help of an SLP is an important role for the profession. Those who have a stroke often lose language or are diagnosed with **aphasia** (loss of the ability to speak). Those affected by stroke and aphasia want to know if their ability to speak will return and how quickly that will happen. Researchers at Northwestern University are investigating factors that affect the ability to speak and/or understand language so that the most effective intervention plan can be initiated. They are collaborating with researchers from Boston University, Harvard University, and Johns Hopkins University. They are examining more than 200 brains post-stroke, implementing the same brain imaging to identify what might impact recovery, whether it be the size of the insult to the brain or the location within the brain. Ultimately, this will help researchers guide clinicians on what to focus on in intervention to activate targeted brain networks (Polovoy, 2014b).

Stuttering is another area of practice interest for clinicians and researchers as 80% of children who stutter recover whether or not they have treatment, but the puzzle is the 20% for whom stuttering persists. At Purdue University, researchers are studying what might predict stuttering persistence from a behavioral (e.g., temperament questionnaires) and physiological perspective (e.g., electroencephalogram) and the impact on language processing. These researchers hope to provide SLPs with measures they can use to determine risk of a child's stuttering persisting without intervention (Murray-Law, 2014c).

Researchers at Case Western Reserve University are studying the impact of speech sound disorders on a child's behavior, social–emotional, and academic development. They believe there is a genetic basis to speech sound disorders, and with new technologies and a longitudinal study of individuals from preschool age through adulthood, researchers have identified genes and some rare gene variants that are connected to not only speech sound difficulties but also other language problems, learning challenges, reading difficulties, and attention disorders especially if the speech sound impairments persist beyond age 8 years. Such findings also suggest that children with speech sound difficulties might be at risk for other neurodevelopmental problems (Polovoy, 2014c).

A multisite study by researchers at City University of New York, University of Cincinnati, Haskins Laboratories, New York University, and University of Syracuse is focused on translating research to practice to support the production of the /r/ sound for children who have difficulty producing the sound correctly. The researchers are using ultrasound feedback or images of children's tongue movements when producing the /r/ sound to help them improve their pronunciation (Cutter, 2014c).

These are just some of the innovations that are occurring in the discipline of speech-language pathology and audiology. Research is an important pathway for creating new knowledge for the professions. Ultimately, the research being performed both increases our knowledge of the nature of communication disorders and informs potential treatment approaches to increase an individual's access to communication.

Why Is This Topic Important?

Exploring career pathways is an exciting part of your college experience. Understanding the options for jobs is an important part of that exploration. Speech-language pathology and audiology offer multiple opportunities to increase an individual's access to listening, hearing, speech, language, and communication. Without the capacity and ability to communicate, quality of life is impacted, including the ability to learn; communicate one's needs, wants, and desires; and socialize with different people in different environments. Whether you choose to pursue a career as an SLP or audiologist, what you learn will help you communicate with others and better understand the communication difficulties of those with impairments.

Overview of the Book Chapters

In this final section of the chapter, we introduce you to the content you will be reading about and learning. This chapter introduced you to what a communication disorder is, the professions of SLP and audiology, the career pathways available in the discipline, and innovations that have occurred in the discipline to support achieving communication for all. In Chapter 2, you will explore the history of disability—how the concept of disability came to be, including a discussion of strengths-based approaches and family/

client-centered care. Chapter 3 focuses on the development and understanding of speech and language, and Chapter 4 describes the anatomy and physiology of the speech mechanism and associated processes.

The next nine chapters focus on both child and adult speech and language disorders. Developmental speech sound disorders are the focus of Chapter 5. This chapter describes the development of speech sounds with an emphasis on **articulation** and **phonological disorders**. Social–cultural differences in identification and disparities in access to assessment and intervention of speech disorders will again be highlighted. Chapter 6 focuses on motor speech disorders including **dysarthria** and **apraxia of speech** from childhood through adulthood.

In Chapter 7, we examine childhood language disorders. This chapter describes the language impairments typically associated with specific language impairment, social communication disorder, intellectual disability, autism, and selected genetic disorders. Social–cultural differences in identification and disparities in access to assessment and intervention are highlighted. Chapter 8 highlights learning disorders and literacy impairments. Specifically, you will learn about the role of language in reading, reading comprehension, and writing. Again, social–cultural differences in identification and disparities in access to assessment and intervention are highlighted. Adult language disorders are the focus of Chapter 9 as you will learn about disorders typically experienced in adulthood, including aphasia, traumatic brain injury, and dementia.

Fluency disorders are the focus of Chapter 10, in which you will learn about the onset and development of stuttering as well as strategies to address stuttering in preschool children through adults. In Chapter 11, voice disorders are described, highlighting the array of voice disorders affecting children and adults, from **vocal nodules** to **vocal cord paralysis**, as well as carcinoma and gender transition. Swallowing disorders are the focus of Chapter 12. This chapter describes the role of the SLP in the management of swallowing disorders in children and adults. In Chapter 13, we explore hearing disorders. In this chapter, we discuss the tools typically used to assess hearing, the types of hearing loss experienced across the lifespan, and approaches to addressing the needs of those who are deaf and hard of hearing. Social–cultural differences in identification and disparities in access to testing and management are highlighted for those impacted by hearing loss.

The final two chapters focus on practice and research considerations in communication disorders. Chapter 14 describes augmentative and alternative communication (AAC), defining what it is and identifying options for supporting communication using AAC across the lifespan. Finally, Chapter 15 pushes you to consider the ways we move from knowledge creation to evidence-based practice. This chapter emphasizes how research informs practice and why it is critical to the work done by SLPs, audiologists, and speech and hearing scientists.

There is much to learn about communication disorders and the impact on one's ability to speak, hear, understand, and learn. Please take this opportunity to not only learn the content presented but also explore the resources, websites, and activities so you can get a sense of the discipline and how becoming an SLP or audiologist, a speech and hearing scientist, or an SLPA or audiology assistant can provide you an interesting career path to consider.

Chapter Summary

Communication is the ability to exchange information between individuals or groups of individuals, and language is what we use to communicate the thoughts, ideas, and beliefs we wish to share with others. A communication disorder is a condition that interferes with our ability to communicate with others, and it may be the result of a congenital condition (e.g., Down syndrome) or a condition acquired after birth (e.g., stroke). More than 46 million people have difficulty speaking or hearing, which impacts their ability to function in their day-to-day lives. SLPs and audiologists are health professionals who address communication disorders. There are multiple career pathways across the two disciplines, from working with infants and toddlers to supporting elderly patients across multiple settings (clinics, hospitals, schools, private practice, etc.). In addition to the educational and clinical pathways for speech-language pathology and audiology, there are also numerous contributions that the professions make to research.

Key Takeaways

- Communication disorders take many forms, from congenital conditions (e.g., deafness, cerebral palsy, Down syndrome) to acquired communication problems after birth (e.g., traumatic brain injury, stroke).
- In the United States, approximately 1 in 12 children (7.7%) aged 3 to 17 years have a speech, language, voice, or swallowing disorder, and many have multiple communication disorders.
- In the United States, 46 million people have some difficulty speaking or hearing that impacts their daily functioning.
- Audiologists use science and the latest technology to prevent, identify, diagnose, and treat hearing, balance, and other auditory disorders.
- Speech-language pathologists assess and treat speech, language, and swallowing disorders across the lifespan.
- An audiology or SLP assistant is someone educated to support the work of certified audiologists and SLPs.
- Speech-language pathologists, audiologists, and speech and hearing scientists are innovative researchers who are studying the nature of communications disorders and developing new assessments of and treatments for these disorders.

Chapter Review Questions

1. How would you define communication?
2. What is a congenital communication disorder?
3. What is an acquired communication disorder?
4. Does a communication difference require intervention?
5. What is involved in the scope of practice for an SLP?
6. What is involved in the scope of practice for an audiologist?
7. What are some of the activities an SLP might engage in when serving in an early intervention or preschool setting?
8. What are some of the strategies an audiologist will use to support an individual with a cochlear implant?
9. What is the role of an SLPA?
10. What is the role of an audiology assistant?

Learning Activities

1. Take a quiz to discover your potential career path on ASHA's Hearing and Speech Careers website.

Hearing and Speech Careers Quiz

2. Interview an SLP, audiologist, SLPA, or audiology assistant and ask them how they made their decision to enter their profession and what their passion is in their job.
3. After reviewing information in the "About Speech, Language, and Hearing Scientist Careers" section on the ASHA website, describe what speech, language, and hearing scientists do.

About Speech, Language, and Hearing Scientist Careers

Additional Resources

- ASHA Speech-Language Pathology Assistants Practice Portal
  https://www.asha.org/practice-portal/professional-issues/speech-language-pathology-assistants
- Technical Training Program for Speech-Language Pathology Assistants
  https://www.asha.org/assistants-certification-program/slpa-technical-training-programs

References

American Psychiatric Association. (2022). *Diagnostic and statistical manual of mental disorders* (5th ed., text rev.).

Black, L. I., Vahratian, A., & Hoffman, H. J. (2015). Communication disorders and use of intervention services among children aged 3–17 years: United States, 2012. *NCHS Data Brief* (205), 1–8.

Council on Academic Accreditation in Audiology and Speech-Language Pathology. (2023). *Standards for accreditation of graduate education programs in audiology and speech-language pathology* (2017). https://caa.asha.org/siteassets/files/accreditation-standards-for-graduate-programs.pdf

Cutter, M. (2014a, October). Chicks, zebra fish—and a cure for hearing loss. *The ASHA Leader*, *19*(10).

Cutter, M. (2014b, October). Reversing age-related hearing loss. *The ASHA Leader*, *19*(10).

Cutter, M. (2014c, October). Correcting speech by 'seeing' the sound. *The Asha Leader*, *19* (10).

Dwyer, P. (2022). The neurodiversity approach(es): What are they and what do they mean for researchers? *Human Development, 66*, 73–92.

Gillam, R. B., & Marquardt, T. P. (2016). *Communication sciences and disorders: From science to clinical practice*. Jones & Bartlett Learning.

Murray-Law, B. M. (2014a, October). The forgotten group: Older children with SLI. *The ASHA Leader, 19*(10).

Murray-Law, B. M. (2014b, October). Probing the language breakdowns of ASD. *The ASHA Leader, 19*(10).

Murray-Law, B. M. (2014c, October). Why stuttering sticks for some—and how to help. *The ASHA Leader, 19*(10).

National Institute on Deafness and Other Communication Disorders. (2015a). *Health information.* http://www.nidcd.nih.gov/health/Pages/Default.aspx

National Institute on Deafness and Other Communication Disorders. (2015b). *Statistics on voice, speech and language.* https://www.nidcd.nih.gov/about/nearly-1-12-children-ages-3-17-has-disorder-related-voice-speech-language-or-swallowing-text-version

Polovoy, C. (2014a, October). Seeking an elusive goal in severe autism: Spoken language. *The ASHA Leader, 19*(10).

Polovoy, C. (2014b, October). Attacking aphasia with more targeted diagnosis and treatment. *The ASHA Leader, 19*(10).

Polovoy, C. (2014c, October). It's all in the genes. *The ASHA Leader, 19*(10).

Polovoy, C. (2014d, October). Auditory playing? *The ASHA Leader, 19*(10).

Prelock, P. A., & Hutchins, T. L. (2018). *Clinical guide to assessment and treatment of communication disorders*. Springer.

U.S. Bureau of Labor Statistics. (n.d.). *Occupational outlook handbook*: Audiologists. Retrieved August 21, 2023, from https://www.bls.gov/ooh/healthcare/audiologists.htm

World Health Organization. (2011). *World report on disability.* http://www.who.int/disabilities/world_report/2011/en

Chapter 2

Disability Across the Lifespan

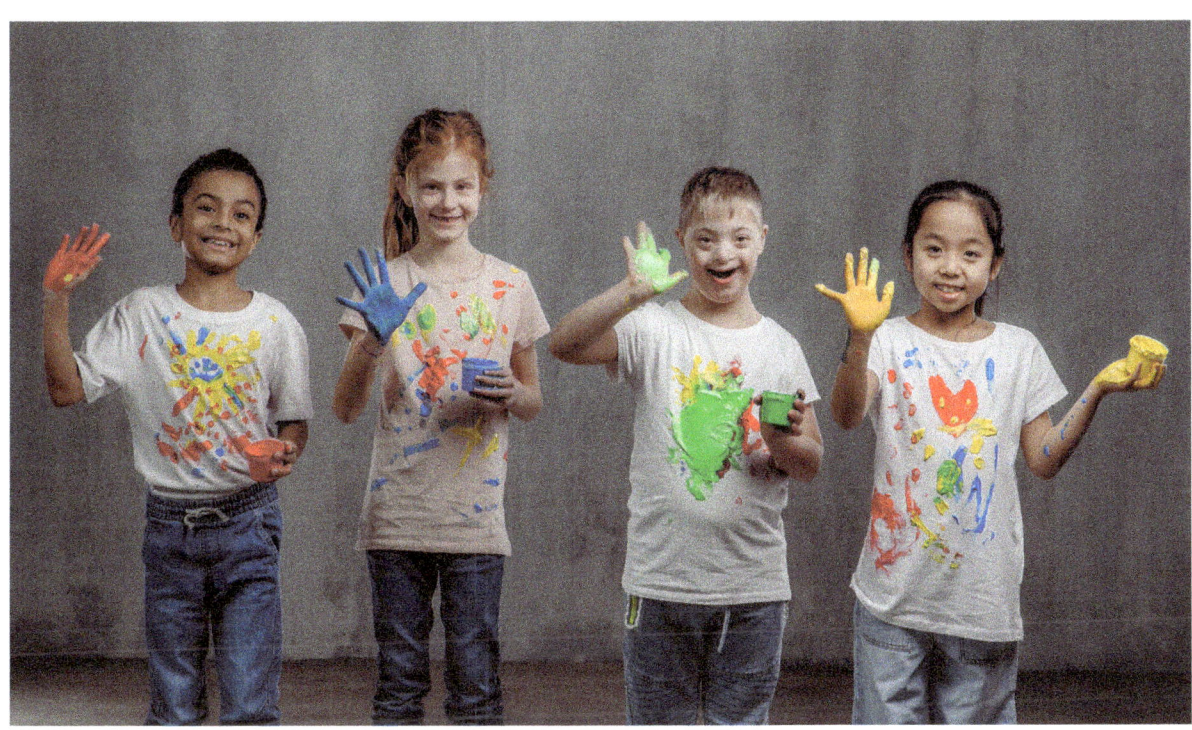

Learning Objectives

After reading this chapter, you will be able to:

- Summarize the World Health Organization's *International Classification of Functioning, Disability and Health* and the domains of functioning.
- Evaluate the various models and constructs of disability.
- Interpret the literature on the intersectionality between disability and race, gender, age, and socioeconomic status from a global lens.
- Summarize the disability rights movement, including the Individuals With Disabilities Education Act, Section 504 of the Rehabilitation Act, and the Americans With Disabilities Act.

Key Terms

- ableism
- aging with disability
- Americans With Disabilities Act (ADA)
- curb cut phenomenon
- deinstitutionalization movement
- differential exposure hypothesis
- differential vulnerability hypothesis
- dignity of risk
- disability
- disability–poverty cycle
- disability rights movement
- disability with aging
- identity-first language
- independent living movement
- Individuals With Disabilities Education Act (IDEA)
- internalized ableism
- *International Classification of Functioning, Disability and Health* model
- medical model of disability
- minority group model
- person-first language
- Section 504 of the Rehabilitation Act
- social model of disability
- social referencing
- sterilization
- universal model

Introduction

"Disability is not a brave struggle or courage in the face of adversity. Disability is an art. It's an ingenious way to live."—Neil Marcus

This book focuses on supporting the communication and quality of life of individuals with various communication disorders across the lifespan along with their families. To effectively understand these conditions and how best to support them, it is important to have a general understanding of what disability is, where it comes from, and how it (and our views of it) has shifted over time. Moreover, to be culturally responsive clinicians, we must shine a light onto the complex intersectionalities of disability, including race, gender, age, and socioeconomic status, while understanding that people with disabilities are not monolithic but, instead, are a diverse group of people, each with a unique culture, background, and lived experience.

Language Used in This Chapter

Throughout this chapter, we use both person-first and identity-first language. When using **person-first language**, the individual is mentioned before the disability (e.g., person with a disability, child with autism). This type of language emphasizes that individuals are people first and are not defined by their disabilities. Because of the history of disability (described later in this chapter), person-first language was adopted to remove some of the stigma associated with disabilities and allow society to see the humanity and personhood of individuals who were historically viewed as less than human. This was essential for the advancement of the disability rights movements (discussed later). Nowadays, however, many (although not all) people with disabilities prefer identity-first language to person-first language. When using identity-first language, the person's disability is mentioned before the individual (e.g., disabled person, autistic adult). This language signifies that a person is who they are because of their disability; disability is part of their identity. Individuals with disabilities are not a monolithic group, and no two people have the same experiences. For this reason, there is no right answer when determining whether to use person-first or identity-first language. So then what should you do—what do you think?

It depends! Ask the person what they prefer.

What Is Disability?

Take a moment to think about what disability means to you. What, if any, are your experiences with disability? Do you have any current existing knowledge or biases about disability? If so, where does this knowledge come from? Take a minute to jot your thoughts down.

According to Merriam-Webster (2024b), disability is defined as "a physical, mental, cognitive, or developmental condition that impairs, interferes with, or limits a person's ability to engage in certain tasks or actions or participate in typical daily activities and interactions." The Americans With Disabilities Act (ADA; U.S. Department of Justice, n.d.-b) defines disability in a similar way as "a physical or mental impairment that substantially limits one or more major life activities of an individual; a record of such impairment; being regarded as having such impairment." Although these definitions attempt to define the disability, they do not offer a full description of the term as it is beginning to be understood today. Disability is more complex and multifaceted than these definitions imply, and the American Psychological Association (APA; 2023) define it as "a broad concept used to describe the interaction of physical, psychological, intellectual, and socioeconomical differences with personal and environmental factors including attitudes, cultural beliefs, legal and economic policies, transportation, buildings, etc." (para. 1). This definition highlights how various factors can contribute to and shape disability, as opposed to merely focusing on the impairments that often come with such conditions.

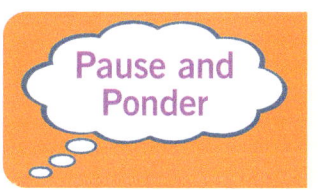 **What do these three definitions have in common? How do they differ?**

To further understand the complexities involved in defining disability, we can explore how individuals with disabilities define the term (excerpts quoted from Ladau, 2021, pp. 9–10):

Disability isn't static. It evolves, both physically and emotionally.—Ellen Ladau

Disability, to me, is a social identity, but it's also about having functional limitations.—Cara Liebowitz

Once upon a time, disability was just a diagnosis. Thankfully through time, the notion has evolved to embrace broader concepts, like constituency, identity, and culture.—Lawrence Carter-Long

Disability is a holistic experience, so it must have a holistic definition. Disability is not just a physical diagnosis, but a lived experience in which parameters and barriers are placed upon our lives because of that diagnosis. —Imani Barbarin

Disability means that there's something people can't do. I believe that there's something everyone can't do as well as they would like, except that people with disabilities have a label. But I am very proud of my disability, because that's who I am. —Liz Weintraub

These definitions underscore the intricacies inherent in disabilities, along with the humanness of having a disability. In fact, almost everyone in their lifetime will experience some sort of disability, whether it be a permanent disability or a temporary one (APA, 2023). That's because disabilities come in many shapes and sizes.

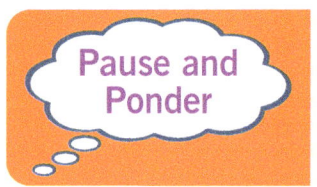

What are some types of disabilities that you know about?

Some types of disabilities include communication disorders, developmental disabilities, mental health disorders, neurological disabilities, physical disabilities, sensory disabilities (hearing/vision), and chronic illnesses. Sometimes disabilities are apparent or visible, and other times they are invisible; just because you can't see the person's disability does not mean that it doesn't exist. Moreover, even within disabilities, there is not a one-size-fits-all. People can have multiple disabilities, and the way that these disabilities present and interact will be different for each person. As such, disability exists in infinite forms, and there is not one singular disability experience. We will keep this in mind as we explore the various intersectionalities that exist within disability throughout this chapter.

History of Disability

Kim Nielsen, a historian of disability, meticulously and thoughtfully describes what has been left out of most historical textbooks: the history of the United States from a disability lens. Her reframing of historical experiences places those with disabilities at the forefront of American history, giving her reader a more comprehensive view of where the concept of *disability* comes from and why it carries so much social stigma. In this section, we highlight some of Nielsen's (2012) accounts.

In the United States, the concept of disability has been around for about as long as Europeans set foot on the soil in the 15th century. Prior to this, Indigenous people of North America recognized that some people had physical impairments, but this was not considered to be the same thing as disability. Disability only occurred when a person was unable to contribute and engage in the greater community. For example, a person could have a physical or cognitive impairment and still contribute meaningfully to society by gathering fruit and nuts for their community. The Indigenous people acknowledged that each person had unique abilities and skills that were well-suited to accomplish the assortment of tasks required for community living. Another common practice among Indigenous peoples was communicating through sign. This allowed multiple groups of Indigenous people (whether they were hearing or deaf) to communicate with one another even if they did not speak the same verbal language. Signed communication resulted in social connectedness and engagement across communities.

In the 15th through 18th centuries, the nature of life changed for Indigenous people when Europeans made their way to what we now consider to be North America. This encounter has informed how we understand disability in the United States today. When the European men encountered the signed communication used within and across Indigenous nations, they discarded it as a form of social connectedness and declared that it was a sign of cognitive impairment. Moreover, many of the diseases that the Europeans carried were spread to Indigenous people who had no previous exposure to these ailments, which resulted in various disabilities and death. The diseases, such as smallpox and scarlet fever, disproportionately affected the weaker members of the community, resulting in more responsibilities for the physically stronger members, as well as physical impairments such as vision loss, hearing loss, and deaf blindness. A person's value came to be inherent in their ability to engage in physical labor and support themselves financially, which came to be synonymous with "able-bodied." Anyone who did not meet this definition of an able-bodied person and who did not have familial financial support came to be viewed as less valuable to society. This thought process continued, and in the late 18th century, individuals with cognitive disabilities were sent to institutions and asylums.

Let's pause our discussion on the history of disability for just a moment as we consider how the definition of "able-bodied" came to be one of the characteristics that was desirable. The idea of "normalcy" is a relatively new concept. According to Merriam-Webster (2024c), *normal* is defined as "conforming to a type, standard, or regular pattern; characterized by that which is considered usual, typical, or routine." According to Davis (2013), this word was introduced in the English language in the mid-1800s after a statistician introduced "averages" for humans (e.g., average weight, average weight). From here, the thinking came to be that populations could be "normed" and "ranked," and anyone who was below the average range was to be considered "abnormal." Placing people on a continuum of norms and ranks allowed for a clear view of desirable and undesirable traits. To be considered a strong nation, it was necessary that the United States foster the ideal citizen, one who was strong and fit himself. "Normality" allowed for people to desire "good" traits that were in the normal or above average rank on the continuum, such as intelligence, and disfavor "bad" traits that were outliers on the below average side of the continuum, such as birth defects. This desire to increase "good" traits and decrease "bad" traits led to forced sterilization of disabled people (discussed momentarily).

As we continue our discussion of the history of disability, we move into the late 1800s and early 1900s, during which the ideal American citizen is becoming more and more specific and narrow in scope, particularly in terms of physical abilities. Individuals who did not fit the definition of "normalcy" began being banned from being visible in public under the "ugly laws" of the late 1800s and early 1900s. These ugly laws prohibited people who were "diseased, maimed, mutilated, or in any way deformed so as to be an unsightly or disgusting object" from being in public spaces (Burgdorf & Burgdorf, 1975, p. 863). At approximately the same time, individuals whose bodies deviated significantly from the norm were often put on display at circuses, fairs, and "freak shows" for the public, who would pay money to witness these individuals. Being a "performer" in these shows offered people with disabilities small paychecks at the expense of displaying their bodies for able-bodied people to marvel at. One well-known woman with dwarfism, Lavinia Warren, shared her experiences in an autobiography, noting that as an exhibit, she "belonged to the public" for much of her life (Umansky, 2009, p. 950).

▶ video

Check out the YouTube video **"Why Was It Illegal to Be 'Ugly'?"** to learn more about the ugly laws.

The concept of normalcy not only impacted American citizens but also played a role in the immigration laws of the early 1900s. It was also around this time that the idea of physical disabilities was viewed as linked, or equivalent, to cognitive deficits. American immigration officers were instructed to deny anyone entry into the United States who appeared to have any mental disorders or "defects, derangements, symptoms of disease" (Nielsen, 2012, p. 104) because these individuals were perceived to be unable to work. This desire for a specific type of American citizen led to many potential immigrants being rejected and further bolstered the idea that able-bodied people were superior, what is now referred to as **ableism**.

Because turning away existing American citizens who didn't fit the able-bodied bill was not possible, common practice at the time was to force individuals who had certain traits into **sterilization** (Hubbard, 2013). Note here that a person's characteristics and traits were dichotomized into "good" and "bad"; however, many traits that were considered hereditary at the time would not be considered hereditary today. Some "good" hereditary traits included leadership, responsibility, and appropriate displays of one's assigned gender; "bad" hereditary traits, on the other hand, included criminality, "feeble-mindedness," and immorality (Davis, 2013; Nielsen, 2012). In addition to these "bad" traits, prominent doctors in the 1900s claimed that there was a steady increase in the number of American citizens who fell into the "socially inadequate class," which included, but was not limited to, criminals, orphans, prostitutes, poor people, those with epilepsy, and "most of the insane" (Nielsen, 2012, pp. 113–115). To strengthen the number of U.S. citizens who had more good traits than bad, and reduce the number of "degenerates," more than 65,000 Americans endured forced sterilization by the 1960s, most of whom were women (Reilly, 1987). This forced sterilization was legal, and during the Supreme Court case of *Buck v. Bell*, U.S. Supreme Court Justice Oliver Wendell Holmes was quoted as saying that

> it is better for all the world if, instead of waiting to execute degenerate offspring for crime or to let them starve for their imbecility, society can prevent those who are manifestly unfit from continuing their kind. . . . Three generations of imbeciles are enough. (*Buck v. Bell*, 1927)

This ruling, which was not considered a violation of constitutional rights, allowed for the forced sterilization of many women who were perceived to have cognitive deficits, and it has yet to be overturned.

Along with undergoing procedures for forced sterilization, in the mid-1900s, many individuals with cognitive impairments were sent away to live in institutions. Parents were urged to take this route by physicians, as well as to pretend that their children who were institutionalized no longer existed. Once institutionalized, patients were treated as less than human and were often abused, neglected, and forced to endure terrible living conditions.

Explore and Find Out!

Check out *A Disability History of the United States* by Kim E. Nielsen and *The Encyclopedia of American Disability History* by Susan Burch for a more in-depth discussion of the history of disability.

▶ video

Check out the documentary *Unforgotten: Twenty-Five Years After Willowbrook* for a glimpse at some of the living conditions for institutionalized patients.

Around the 1950s, parents began joining forces to advocate for those who had been sent away to live in institutions, and it is through these parent advocacy groups that national attention was brought to the horrendous conditions of institutional life, as well as the limited resources available for families and individuals with disabilities. It was also during this time and through these parent advocacy groups that people began to discard the negative beliefs that had thus far been associated with cognitive impairments. Moreover, advocacy groups (now consisting of parents and individuals with disabilities) highlighted the lack of resources that people with disabilities and their families had regarding educational and living options, which paved the way for many of the changes that took place regarding education and living support for persons with disabilities. This process included exposing the inner workings of the horrible living conditions of institutions to the public.

Models of Disability

As society's understanding of disability has shifted over time, so too have the models of disability. There are currently three primary models that attempt to describe disability: the medical model, the social model, and the functional model.

The **medical model of disability** describes disability as something that has occurred because of a particular health condition or disease. Under this model, a person with a disability has limited functioning in either physical or cognitive capacities, and it is the person's impairment that has caused this disruption in functioning and has impacted their ability to participate in society. The **social model of disability** considers functioning and disability from a different perspective. Here, the person who has a disability is not limited from participating in activities due to their impairments but instead due to the inaccessibility of the environment. Whereas the medical model describes the person's impairment as the primary barrier that is preventing the person from participating in societal activities, the social model notes that barriers to access are a product of society (Haegele & Hodge, 2016). Figure 2–1 shows an example of how disability may be perceived from the medical and the social model.

The *International Classification of Functioning, Disability and Health* **model** (ICF; World Health Organization, 2001) is a functional model of disability that combines aspects of the medical and social models (Shakespeare, 2013) and considers how the person's health condition interacts with the environment to either support or hinder participation in various life activities. The ICF model highlights the importance of the interaction between a person's physical abilities, the environment, and factors associated with the individual person. Because of this, a person's ability to function in any given activity is a result of a combination of factors that is unique to that person and the environment in which they live. See Figure 2–2 for a visual depiction of the ICF model.

The ICF model can be particularly useful in considering the person with a disability from a holistic lens. Consider the ICF framework for a child (Jacob) who has Down syndrome (Figure 2–3). To get a better sense of how Jacob's disability interacts with various environmental and personal factors to support

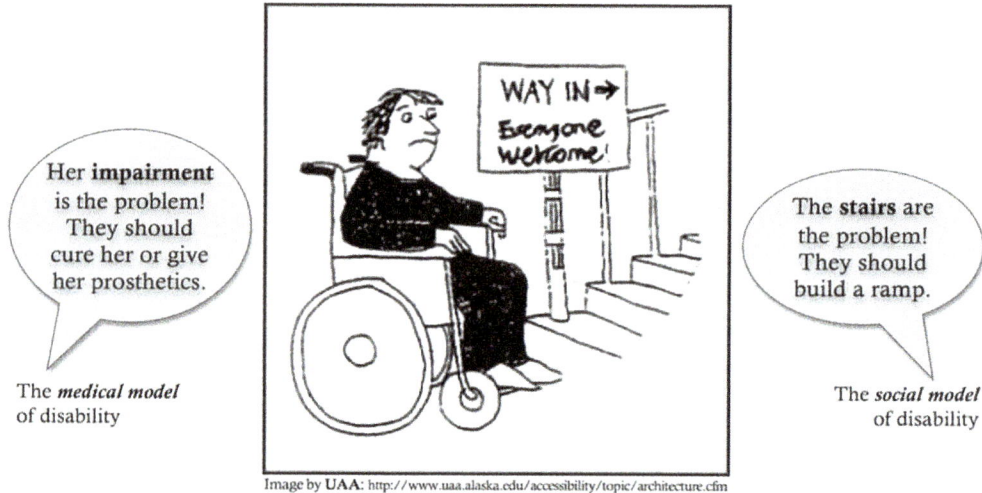

FIGURE 2–1. Depiction of the medical versus social models of disability. *Source:* University of Alaska Anchorage.

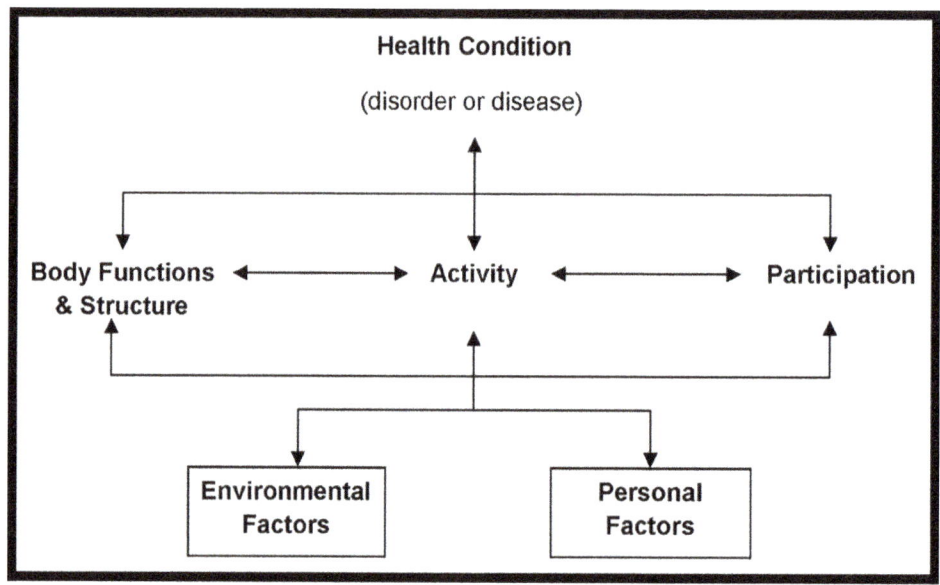

FIGURE 2–2. World Health Organization's International Classification of Functioning, Disability, and Health. *Source:* World Health Organization (2002).

or hinder his participation in activities throughout his day, let's look at a completed ICF diagram. Here, we want to know about Jacob's ability to participate in a common activity at school: show and tell. We consider the factors that are both supportive of and barriers to his participation in this activity. Several factors contribute to Jacob's ability to engage in show and tell. Although quite communicative, Jacob is nonspeaking, which is a physical/structural part of his disability that has the potential to influence how he engages in show and tell (body functions and structure). Having access to his augmentative and alternative communication (AAC; see Chapter 14) device, however, supports his expressive language and thus his participation in this activity. Environmental factors that may impact his participation in this activity

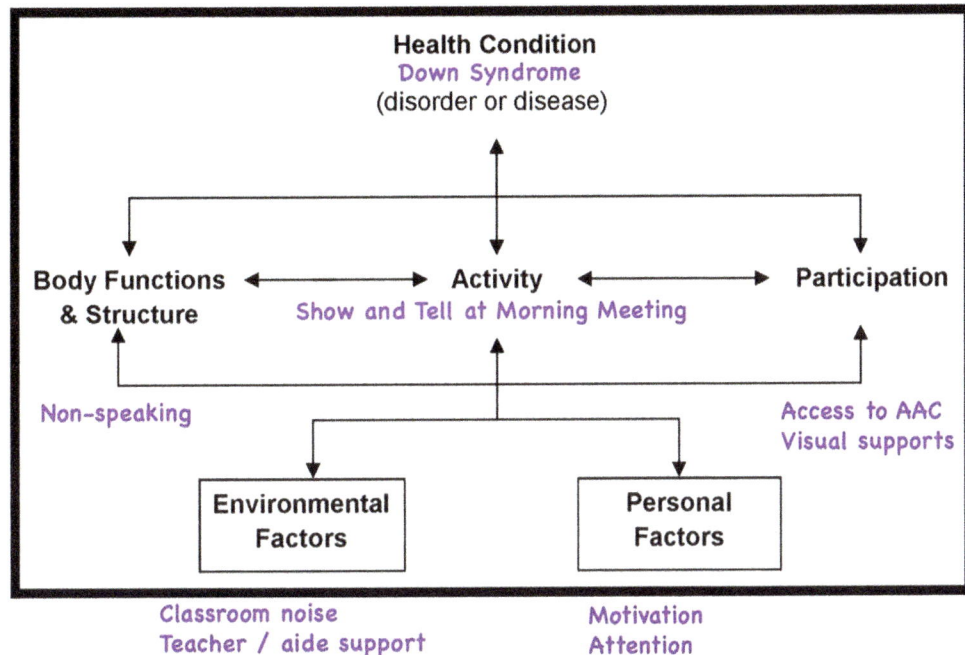

FIGURE 2–3. ICF model example. AAC, augmentative and alternative communication. *Source:* Adapted from the World Health Organization (2002).

include the level of noise in the classroom and whether Jacob receives any support from his teacher or aide. If the classroom is too loud, the voice output from Jacob's AAC device might not be loud enough for other students to hear him. Moreover, because Jacob is still learning language and how to use his AAC device, as well as the sequence for how show and tell works, he requires more teacher support than other students in his class. In addition, some personal factors also impact Jacob's level of participation in show and tell, including (but not limited to) his internal motivation to share his toys with his peers, as well as his ability to tend to the entirety of the task.

Stigmatization

When you think about the word "stigma," what do you think of? Defined by Merriam-Webster (2024d) as "a mark of shame or discredit; an identifying mark or characteristic," stigmas are bound up with social contexts. Each human being is unique in their attributes, characteristics, physical stature, and so on, and essentially any of these attributes can be stigmatized. Because there are infinite ways that people differ from one another, what is stigmatized in one social context is often valued in another (Brown, 2013). Stigmas are often determined by the dominant people in power in any given group, and so it is not difficult to understand why disability, viewed historically as inferior to being able-bodied, is associated with stigmatization. So where does stigmatization come from? As children, we make use of our caregivers' reactions to novel objects and people to learn about the world and understand how we are supposed to react to certain stimuli. This is referred to as **social referencing**. So, when a child encounters a strange object that they have never seen before, they will likely look to their caregiver to help them decide if they should touch and explore the object or get as far away from it as possible.

▶ video

Check out the YouTube video **"An Experiment by Joseph Campos: The Visual Cliff"** to learn more about social referencing in young children.

Consider how social referencing can play a role in the perpetuation of stigmatization. If a child (for example) has never been exposed to individuals with disabilities and encounters a person in a wheelchair, they may look to their caregiver to help them figure out how to react. If the caregiver reacts in ways that subtly or obviously deter the child from looking at or engaging with the person in the wheelchair, the child may learn to associate negative or "bad" feelings with disabled people. Whereas children may be at first curious about objects or people who are different than them, it is the perceived fear of the "other" that leads to stigma and stereotypes. Moreover, when people stigmatize others, it can lead to "a sense of fundamental inferiority to stigmatized people [as a result of] social rejection or social isolation and lowered expectations" (Brown, 2013, p. 154). These stigmas can become pervasive, and those who are stigmatized may come to believe the stereotypes and lower sense of self-worth that exist about themselves and those with similar traits (Brown, 2013).

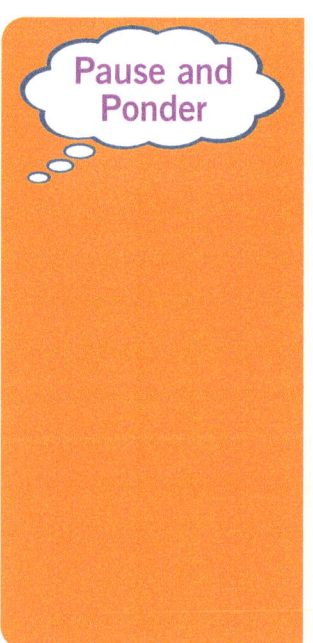

Pause and Ponder

Consider the following thought questions posed by Brown (2013, p. 153):

1. When and under what conditions does an attribute become a stigmatized one?
2. Can a person experience stigmatization without knowing that a trait is devalued in a specific social context?
3. Does a person feel stigmatized even though in a particular social context the attribute is not stigmatized or the stigma is not physically or behaviorally apparent?
4. Can a person refuse to be stigmatized or destigmatize an attribute by ignoring the prevailing norms that define it as a stigma?
5. Would stigma persist if stigmatized people did not feel stigmatized or inferior?

▶ video

Check out the TED Talk where **Adam Pearson** talks about his experiences with disability.

Disability and Illness

As we have talked about disability, it is likely that you have been primarily considering individuals with physical, cognitive, or neurodevelopmental disabilities. What about people who have chronic illness? Although the terms *illness* and *disability* are not synonymous, it is the case that some illnesses are caused by disabilities, some disabilities are caused by illness, and some people with disabilities have co-occurring illnesses that are unrelated to their disability. Scholars have distinguished between individuals with disabilities who are healthy and those who are unhealthy. **Healthy disabled** people are defined as those whose abilities and limitations are "relatively stable and predictable for the foreseeable future" (Wendell, 2001, p. 19) and generally include those who were born with a disability or acquired one later in life and who do not require much more medical assistance than a nondisabled person. **Unhealthy disabled** people, on the other hand, tend to have chronic illnesses that cannot be reliably cured and persist over time or acute diseases that result in death. These illnesses are also usually accompanied by a sense of fatigue and/or pain that results in loss of functioning (Wendell, 2001). Often, individuals with chronic illness have invisible disabilities, which leads to judgments about their overall health and well-being. These suspicions include how ill the person really is, if they are doing everything that they can to get healthier, and if current lifestyle choices are contributing to their illness. It is often the case that those with chronic illness are not visibly disabled enough to pass as having a disability, but they are not functioning well enough to pass as being nondisabled (Young, 2000).

Disability advocacy, as evidenced by the social model of disability, has primarily focused on removing barriers to participation in society so that disabled people can access those environments. When considering individuals who experience chronic illness, removing said barriers does not always lead to successful participation in society. For example, for someone with a chronic illness who experiences fatigue, accommodations for the workplace might include increased flexibility for working hours. Incorporating the viewpoints of individuals with unhealthy disabilities into disability advocacy discussions can help ensure that disability rights and advocacy are inclusive of all persons with disabilities. It is also important to consider what accommodations are appropriate for any given job and if those accommodations interfere (or not) with a person's ability to successfully complete the task. That is, do a person's accommodations inhibit the completion of a task? Or do the accommodations support the completion of a task (albeit in an unconventional manner)?

Ableism and Accessibility

Because of the deep-rooted history of disability, along with the beliefs that those with disabilities are less capable of performing everyday activities and leading meaningful lives, many disabled people encounter both subtle and overt ableism. *Ableism* is defined as "discrimination or prejudice against individuals with disabilities" (Merriam-Webster, 2024a) and can take many forms. Often, ableism is so subtly engrained in our society that nondisabled people (and even disabled people) don't think about it. And what's more is that something that is obvious ableism to one person with a disability may be a form of subtle ableism to another person with a disability. Some examples of ableism include lack of access to public transportation, websites that are inaccessible to blind people, the small size of airplane bathrooms, as well as sheltered workshops where disabled people are "employed" and paid a small amount to do menial and redundant tasks. Ableist thinking can have a profound effect on individuals with disabilities, such that they may come to believe that they are a burden to society. This is known as **internalized ableism** and can lead to further discrimination and feelings of low self-worth (Dunn, 2019).

How, then, do we begin to rid society of ableist thinking? One way to do this is by becoming aware of and removing barriers to access for all. By doing so, we are providing everyone with the opportunity to participate in life as fully as possible. And the best way to ensure that spaces and environments are accessible is to ask groups of people what they need to best access that environment. Although nondisabled people often have good intentions when designing spaces for disabled individuals, they do not have the life experiences to know exactly what disabled people need to actively participate. For this reason, it is paramount that disabled individuals have a seat at the table when decisions are being made about them. Having disabled people as members of the team is a necessary step to creating a society that is inclusive.

In addition, when thinking about disability through the lens of the social model, a variety of environmental accommodations have been put forth. The **curb cut phenomenon** occurs when physical structures or systems are modified so that they are accessible to disabled people, which results in benefits for nondisabled people as well (Mate, 2022). Examples of this are listed in Table 2–1.

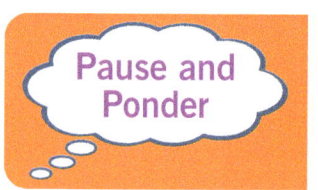

Pause and Ponder Can you think of other adaptations that benefit society as a whole?

The Intersectionalities of Disability

Individuals with disabilities are more than just individuals with disabilities. Each person has their own unique life experiences and intersecting identities that contribute to who they are and their sense of self. Simply because two people may be disabled does not mean that their experiences of having that disability

TABLE 2–1. Examples of Adaptations Designed for Those With Disabilities That Benefit Other Members of Society

Adaptation	Who It Was Designed For	Who Else Benefits
Texting	Deaf or hard of hearing	Everyone
Closed captions on films/videos	Deaf or hard of hearing	People watching foreign films, people watching films/videos in a loud environment or with the sound turned off
Curb cuts and ramps	Individuals with wheelchairs	People pushing a stroller or shopping cart, cyclists, skateboarders
Elevators	Individuals with wheelchairs or mobility challenges	Everyone

are the same. For instance, a male child who has Down syndrome will have different life experiences than a female adult with Down syndrome. Now imagine that these two individuals are from different cultures, come from differing socioeconomic classes, and are of different races. In this section, we dive into the intersections of disability and race, age, gender, and socioeconomic status.

Consider the following barriers and disadvantages that individuals with disabilities often face (World Health Organization, 2011):

Barriers

- Inadequate policies and standards
- Negative attitudes
- Lack of services (e.g., health care)
- Challenges with service delivery
- Inadequate funding
- Lack of accessibility
- Lack of involvement in decision making

Disadvantages

- Poor health outcomes
- Lower educational achievements
- Less economically active
- Higher rates of poverty
- Cannot always live independently or participate fully in community activities

As we discuss the varying intersectionalities in this section, keep these barriers and disadvantages in mind and consider how these factors might impact a person who has more than one of these identities.

Disability and Race

The prevalence of disability in the United States varies between races (Centers for Disease Control and Prevention, 2020; Table 2–2). Despite disability existing in all races, most of the research on the intersections of disability and race focuses on Black individuals. Because disability came to be defined as the inability to economically support oneself through physical labor tasks, many people who were

TABLE 2-2. Adults With Disabilities in the United States, 2017

Race	No. of People With a Disability
American Indian/Alaska Native	3 in 10
Asian	1 in 10
Black	1 in 4
Hispanic	1 in 6
Native Hawaiian/Pacific Islander	1 in 6
White	1 in 5

not legally permitted to work became linked with the term *disabled*. This included women and slaves (Nielsen, 2012). This, in turn, led to the idea that African American individuals were both physically and mentally disabled, which justified the concept of slavery (Nielsen, 2012). The idea that slave owners used a person's perceived disability to justify slavery was not acceptable to all. Activists and abolitionists viewed disability and slavery in the opposite lens: that slavery was causing disabilities. After the Civil War, when slavery had ended, public portrayals and media representations of Black people became more apparent; yet it was portrayals of mentally and physically healthy Black people (not disabled people) that dominated the American culture precisely to demonstrate that Black people as a whole fit into the label of able-bodied American citizens. Moreover, many members of the Black community equated being Black with being disabled: "Many African-Americans consider being black as having a disability, and so they didn't really identify with disability as a disability but just as one other kind of inequity that black people had to deal with" (Lacy, 1960, as cited in Lukin, 2013, p. 309). Disabled Black people, however, conceptualized being Black and being disabled as two separate identities that presented with unique lived experiences. It was from this perspective that Black, disabled people identified with the Black movement, but Black nondisabled individuals did not identify with the disability movement (Lukin, 2013). According to Johnnie Lacy (as cited in Lukin, 2013), a Black disabled activist,

> African Americans see disability in the same way that everybody else sees it—[perceiving people with disabilities as] worthless, mindless—without realizing that this is the same attitude held by others toward African Americans. This belief in effect cancels out the black identity they share with a disabled black person, both socially and culturally, because the disability experience is not viewed in the same context as if one were only black, and not disabled. Because of this myopic view, I as a black disabled person could not share in the intellectual dialogue viewed as exclusive to black folk. In other words, I could be one or the other but not both. (p. 309)

The impacts of race and disability can be seen in the current educational system. According to the Office of Special Education Programs (U.S. Department of Education, 2021), discrepancies exist among children who receive special education services under the **Individuals With Disabilities Education Act (IDEA)** in terms of their race and which disabilities they have. That is, of students with disabilities, Asian students are more likely to have autism or hearing impairment, Black students are more likely to have intellectual disability or emotional disturbances, Hispanic students are more likely to have hearing impairment or specific learning disability, and White students are more likely to have specific learning disability or intellectual disability compared to all students with disabilities. Moreover, these data suggest that Black students with disabilities are more likely to be removed from school compared to all students with disabilities, resulting in less instructional time overall.

Disability and Gender

Similar to how Black disabled people were originally not included in Black activist groups, disabled women were historically left out of feminist groups in the 1970s. This was due to the fact that women were historically marginalized because of their gender and they were not considered capable of performing various types of work, including manual labor. To counter these notions, able-bodied women distanced themselves from disabled women during the women's movement of the 1970s to show the world that women were strong and independent (Thomas, 2006). Consequently, disabled women were left unseen and considered "dependent burdens" at the time (Thomas, 2006, p. 183). Although this line of thinking has since shifted, consider how the history of women, and specifically disabled women, has shaped the way that broader society has come to view and understand this population of people.

Most of the statistics on the intersection of disability and gender capture the data of binary gender roles: men and women. For that reason, this section focuses primarily on those two genders; although we will touch on some data on nonbinary, transgendered populations as well. According to the World Health Organization (2011) and Lee and colleagues (2021), the global prevalence of disability is higher in women than in men, and these data report on individuals between the ages of 45 and 75 years or older. Because, on average, women tend to live longer than men (Baum et al., 2021), it makes sense that rates of disability are higher in women. Moreover, two different theories have been put forth that attempt to explain why women tend to present with disabilities more so than men: the differential exposure hypothesis of health and the differential vulnerability hypothesis. The **differential exposure hypothesis** posits that compared to men, women worldwide are exposed to more risk factors (including living in poverty and being exposed to stress) and have access to fewer resources that protect against certain disabilities. The **differential vulnerability hypothesis**, on the other hand, suggests that women and men have exposure to the same risk factors that result in disability; yet women present with greater challenges and disabilities as a result (McDonough & Walters, 2001; Wheaton & Crimmins, 2016). Regardless of which theory may hold more merit, the data show that compared to men, women (a) have higher rates of disability, (b) experience worse physical functioning, and (c) report greater challenges completing tasks associated with daily living (Wheaton & Crimmins, 2016). Compared to men with disabilities, women with disabilities worldwide also experience greater challenges, including reduced access to health care, transportation, education, employment, and independent living (Thomas, 2006). Similarly, poor outcomes are reported for women with disabilities compared to women without disabilities on a global level. Those with disabilities are more likely to be diagnosed with cancer, chronic illness, mental health disorders, and substance abuse disorders; experience violence and divorce; and have reduced access to health care and preventative screenings (Chevarley et al., 2006; Ramjan et al., 2016; Wisdom et al., 2010). Moreover, disabled girls are less likely to have access to education and are reported to have lower literacy rates than their male counterparts. Women with disabilities are offered fewer employment opportunities than males, often obliged to work solely in the home; however, those who do work outside of the home earn significantly smaller paychecks than males with disabilities (Women Enabled International, n.d., World Health Organization, 2011). In addition to these findings related to reduced access, women and girls with disabilities also face increased exposure to violence (including intimate partner violence and sexual abuse; Breiding & Armour, 2015; Schröttle & Glammeier, 2013; Shah et al., 2016) with fewer legal protections, as well as the likelihood of being a victim of human trafficking and forced prostitution (European Women's Lobby, 2011; U.S. Department of State, 2016).

If you are familiar at all with the data on children with developmental and intellectual disabilities, learning that women are more likely to experience disability compared to men may seem surprising. It is often the case that prevalence rates are higher among boys than girls for developmental conditions. For example, boys are diagnosed with autism at a higher rate than girls, at a ratio of four to one (Maenner et al., 2023). To continue with this example, it has been hypothesized that females experience autism at similar rates as males; however, their clinical presentations may look different. Moreover, females may be particularly good at camouflaging or masking their clinical symptoms (Hull et al., 2020). Considering the idea that the diagnostic criteria for many developmental conditions have been based on how those conditions manifest in boys, how might this impact how girls are (or are not) getting diagnosed at young ages?

Check out Cornell University's **"Disability Statistics"** tool to explore disability statistics in the United States. Notice how disability rates change based on age, gender, and disability type.

As mentioned previously, data on nonbinary, transgendered populations are lacking. What we do know, however, is that these individuals experience disability at similar rates as those reported by men and women, but they often indicate (a) that their primary disability is a developmental disability and (b) higher rates of unmet health care needs (Mulcahy et al., 2022). Further exploration of the unmet health care needs includes less access to doctors, dentists, health care specialists, and prescription medications. What factors do you think contribute to this lack of care for transgender, nonbinary populations?

Disability and Age

Another crucial identity that intersects with disability is age. Although disability is present among all ages, older populations are at a higher risk of acquiring a disability, and it is estimated that more than 40% of people older than age 60 years and 97% of individuals older than age 99 years have a disability (Berlau et al., 2009). Several risk factors are associated with acquiring disability with old age, including lower levels of physical activity, cognitive impairment, social interaction, and increased risk of falls (Berlau et al., 2012). Most individuals who acquire disabilities in older age, and lose at least some independent functioning, do so slowly over time (as opposed to from a sudden event).

It is important here to distinguish between individuals who develop disabilities due to older age (**disability with aging**) and those who have disabilities when they are younger and age as a part of life (**aging with disability**). Individuals with developmental disabilities often experience high levels of stress, which can lead to accelerated aging (Hayes et al., 2009; Yegorov et al., 2020). Moreover, evidence suggests that individuals with intellectual and developmental disabilities tend to have lower life expectancies than those without disabilities (Stankiewicz et al., 2018). Some intellectual and developmental disabilities are associated with accelerated aging more so than others, particularly those that impact an individual's respiratory, cardiovascular, and/or immune system. Individuals with disabilities face additional challenges as they age, including aging out of services that supported their functioning and participation in society, losing caregivers (e.g., parents) to old age or death, reduced access to providers who understand the nuances and interactions of aging and having a disability, and being inappropriately treated (or not treated) for other co-occurring conditions.

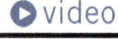

Check out the YouTube video **"Disability With Aging & Aging With Disability"** from the University of California, San Francisco for more information.

Disability and Socioeconomic Status

Disability disproportionally affects individuals from lower socioeconomic classes for a variety of reasons, but it is not just those individuals who are negatively impacted. Caregivers and families of disabled people also experience negative consequences associated with disability. For instance, when a family member becomes disabled, family and caregiver roles may be altered. Children who are used to being cared for may now have to care for disabled parents. Sometimes when this happens, children who are still in school may be forced to drop out of school or adult children may quit their jobs to provide full-time care for their parents. This then hinders their educational, and thus employment, opportunities, which contributes to their poverty and societal poverty.

Moreover, as outlined in Figure 2–4, the relationship between disability and poverty is bidirectional: Disability can lead to poverty, and poverty can lead to disability (Pinilla-Roncancio, 2015).

To illustrate, people who live in poverty have a higher chance of becoming disabled compared to those who do not live in poverty. This is due to several factors, including poor nutrition, less access to health care and clean water, and increased exposure to violence. On the other side of the cycle, people with disabilities are more likely to become poor due to the extra costs that are associated with disability. This includes direct costs such as medical equipment, as well as indirect costs as described previously (family members losing out on education and employment to care for disabled family members). Of course, the way in which the disability–poverty cycle impacts any given person depends on several factors, which include, but are not limited to, the person's age, gender, race, impairment type and severity, geographical location, educational status, and social environment. Moreover, the risk of poverty is higher when a disabled person experiences two or more of the following: identifies as a woman, is of older age, is from a minority racial group, and lives in a rural area. Because of this and the bidirectional nature of disability

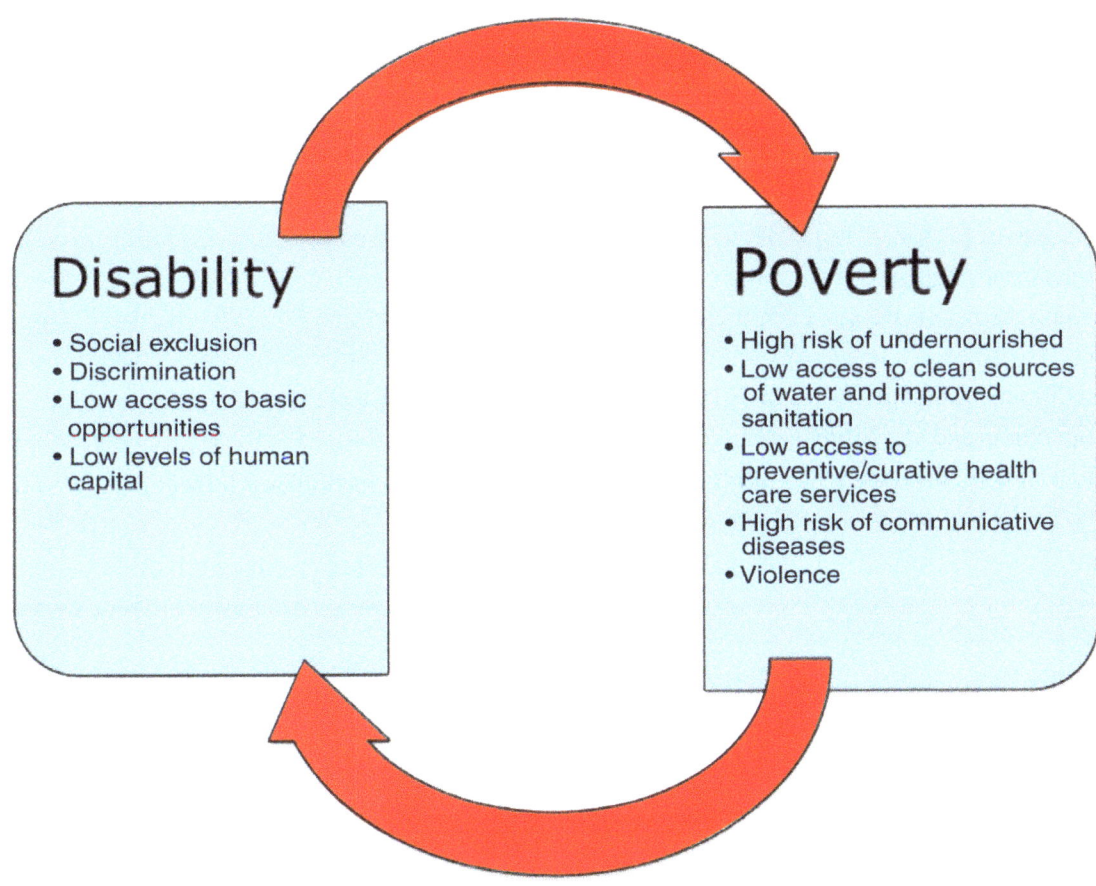

FIGURE 2–4. Disability and poverty vicious circle. *Source:* Pinilla-Roncancio (2015)

and poverty, those who are both disabled and poor are often considered the "poorest of the poor" and more likely to experience chronic poverty.

▶ video

Check out the YouTube video **"The Man Who Lives in a Basket for 40 Years"** and reflect on the various intersecting identities of this family and consider how poverty and disability are bidirectional.

Pinilla-Roncancio (2015) states,

> People with disabilities are *not a homogeneous group*. Their needs vary according to the *type and severity* of their impairment, alongside *personal and social characteristics* which can also affect *their levels of vulnerability*. In fact, depending on the type of impairment, different barriers may limit access to basic opportunities and services, such as education, health, and employment. As a result of this *heterogeneity*, policies and strategies aiming to prevent, mitigate or overcome poverty for people with disabilities *cannot be the same*. There is *not a unique strategy* that will reduce the risk of poverty. (p. 114, italics added)

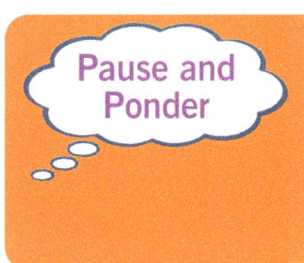

Consider what you have learned so far about disability, as well as how disability and poverty are related. What are some ways that disabled people have less access to basic services as it relates to the following: health care, education, shelter, food, transport, and information?

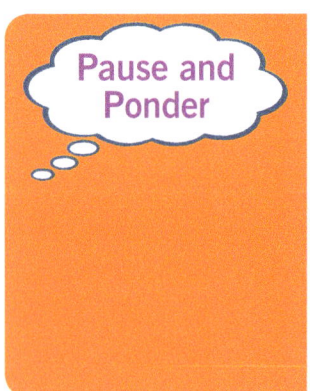

Consider age at time of disability. How do you think these different time frames of becoming disabled could interact with poverty?

- Disabled at birth: Access to education is lower than that of nondisabled peers.
- Disabled at working age: Access to formal jobs is a main limitation for social inclusion.
- Disabled after working age: Access to education or employment is not a major issue, but access to health care is.

Disability Rights in the United States

The understanding of disability has shifted tremendously over time, and despite still having a long way to go, the United States has progressed toward equal access and inclusion for disabled people. This is being accomplished through the **disability rights movement**, which is composed of many social projects that are distinctly different, albeit related and interconnected. These include the independent living movement, the deinstitutionalization movement, the education movement (all in the 1970s), as well as the AIDs movement and the deaf movement of the 1980s. Although each has its own unique call to action, the projects of the disability rights movement had (and continue to have) the same underlying principles: that disabled people (a) should be allowed to make decisions for themselves, (b) should decide for themselves what services would be beneficial for them, and (c) are discriminated against and this discrimination leads to reduced opportunity for community integration. In addition, these projects aimed to move people's thinking about disability away from the medical model of disability and more in line with the social model of disability. We briefly discuss a few of those projects in the following sections, but for a more comprehensive view, we recommend reading *Law and the Contradictions of the Disability Rights Movement* by Samuel Bagenstos (2009).

Check out the **Disability Rights Timeline** from Temple University for more information on the history of disability rights.

The **independent living movement** was among the first projects of the disability rights movement, and it served to support disabled people by providing them with the independence to begin to make their own decisions about medical care and about the services they should receive for themselves. The **deinstitutionalization movement** was also monumental because it was founded on the belief that disabled people were being denied basic human rights and freedoms when they were sentenced to live in institutions. It was believed that the institutions themselves were in fact causing disabilities in their patients, and this included mental, physical, and intellectual disabilities. One of the goals of this movement was to expose these institutions to the public so that society could bear witness to the inhumane treatment of their relatives, friends, community members, and strangers. Out of this movement came the "people first" organization, which highlighted that disabled people are more than just their impairment; they are in fact people! Because many disabled people were living in institutions, this movement was first formed and led by nondisabled activists; however, over time and as more institutions were shut down, disabled people began joining in and forming their own advocacy groups to support the closure of institutions throughout the country.

Another monumental move forward for disability rights came in 1973 when **Section 504 of the Rehabilitation Act** was passed. This act stated that people with disabilities could not be "denied benefits of, or be subjected to discrimination under any program or activity receiving federal financial assistance" (U.S. Department of Labor, n.d.). Although this does not apply to private institutions, Section 504 makes it illegal to discriminate against someone based on their disability status in many settings. Similar to Section 504 of the Rehabilitation Act is **Individuals With Disabilities Education Act (IDEA**; U.S. Department of Education, n.d.), which was originally passed in 1975 but continued to be modified until 2004. This law ensures that all children in the United States have access to a free and appropriate education. IDEA covers children from birth through 21 years, and different sections of the law apply to children aged 0 to 2 years and those between ages 3 and 21 years.

Finally, ADA (U.S. Department of Justice, n.d.-a) is probably the most well-known disability rights law and was passed in 1990. ADA provides disabled people with protection against discrimination in the workplace as well as when accessing many public spaces. Increased access to public spaces reduces discrimination regarding housing, transportation, education, health care, and voting.

Check out the **Disability Rights Education & Defense Fund** website to learn more about Section 504 of the Rehabilitation Act, IDEA, and ADA.

As with most social movements, tensions exist within the disability rights movement, particularly pertaining to how disabled people access services that are rightfully available to them (Bagenstos, 2009). Two models, which are both in line with the social model of disability, are the **minority group model** and the **universal model**. The minority group model highlights that because people are disabled by the barriers constructed by society, as a society, we should be directly responsible for providing resources to disabled people to access and participate in their environment. The universal model, on the other hand, brings attention to the fact that all people are at risk of becoming disabled at any time and that the environment should be structured in a way that is accessible for all. Moreover, tensions exist regarding the role of nondisabled professionals in disability rights. Although disabled people often rely on the support of nondisabled professionals for legal, educational, and health care services, there may be criticism around the involvement of these nondisabled professionals; many disability advocates argue that people with disabilities should not be beholden to nondisabled professionals and should be allowed to decide what is best for themselves. The bottom line, however, is that disabled people value independence, which often equates to having the opportunity to be a part of the community, participate in all life activities, and work for a living. Their strive for independence unites advocates—both disabled and nondisabled—to voice their desires around equality, access, and independence and to promote **dignity of risk**—to feel empowered to make one's own choices in life, assume personal responsibility for one's actions, and consequently succeed or fail.

Why Is This Topic Important?

Understanding the history of disability is important to grasp the stigma and bias that are often associated with disability. As health care professionals working with individuals who have disabilities, we must have knowledge of disability at various levels to best serve our clients. In addition, many of our clients will experience other factors that intersect with their disability, and we must be knowledgeable about how these characteristics impact one another and the person with the disability. Because each person has their own unique experiences, no two people with a disability are alike, regardless of whether their disabilities are the same on paper.

Chapter Summary

The term disability is a complex and multifaceted concept that describes the interactions of physical, psychological, intellectual, and socioeconomic differences that affect a person's ability to function and participate in society. Throughout history, the definition of disability has shifted, and our views of disability today have been shaped based on how individuals with physical and mental differences have been stigmatized and "othered" since as early as the 15th century.

Currently, three primary models attempt to describe disability: the medical model, the social model, and the functional model of disability. The medical model of disability describes disability as something that has occurred due to a particular health condition or disease that limits a person's physical or cognitive functioning. The social model of disability describes that a disabled person is not limited from participating in activities due to their impairments but, rather, it is that the environment is not accessible to them. The ICF model highlights the interactions between a person's physical abilities, the environment, and other personal factors that impact their ability to participate in life activities.

Ableism is a term used to describe the discrimination of disabled people through the belief that able-bodied individuals are naturally superior. Ableism is often present throughout society in various forms, such as access to public transportation, size and availability of restrooms, and lack of ramps and elevators. Individuals with disabilities also face stigmatization.

Several identities interact with disability, including race, gender, age, and socioeconomic status, with disabilities being more prevalent in individuals from historically marginalized racial groups, women, older adults, and those with lower socioeconomic status. IDEA, Section 504 of the Rehabilitation Act, and ADA stand as milestones in advancing rights for disabled individuals, promoting equal opportunities in education and public access. However, tensions persist within the disability rights movement regarding access to services, the role of nondisabled professionals, and the quest for independence and inclusion for all disabled individuals.

Chapter Review Questions

1. What are examples of using identity-first language and person-first language when addressing someone?
2. What were some of the events that happened in history to shape how disabled people came to be viewed as inferior?
3. Why were people being denied entry to the United States in the early 1900s?
4. What is ableism?
5. What are some examples of ableism in the community?
6. What are the three primary models that describe disability today?
7. What is the disability–poverty cycle?
8. What is the difference between the differential vulnerability hypothesis and the differential exposure hypothesis?
9. What is the Individuals With Disabilities Education Act (IDEA)?
10. What is Section 504 of the Rehabilitation Act?
11. What is the Americans With Disabilities Act (ADA)?

Learning Activities

1. Find and choose a disability hashtag or account on social media to follow. Explore the hashtag or account in depth and find a post that speaks to you. Write a 2- or 3-page reflection paper that addresses the following:
   a. Identify the hashtag or social media account.
      i. Who runs the account?
      ii. What is the theme?
      iii. Who is the target audience (if there is one)?
   b. Provide a description of the post that speaks to you.
      i. What is the post about?
      ii. Include a quote or excerpt from the post.
      iii. What are the comments like?
   c. Reflect on the post.
      i. Why did you choose this post?
      ii. What does it mean to you?
      iii. How has this post changed or challenged your thinking about disability?
   d. Social model of disability.
      i. Describe the social model of disability.
      ii. How does the post fit (or not fit) with the social model of disability?

2. Choose any disability to research and write a 4- or 5-page research paper that addresses the following:
   a. The nature of the disability (prevalence, signs/symptoms, characteristics including strengths and challenges).
   b. A description of how that disability presents and intersects with race, gender, age, and/or socio-economic status.
   c. A comparison of how it is viewed in the United States in relationship to one other country of your choosing.
   d. The status of rights, policies, or protections available for people with that disability in the two countries.

3. Based on data collected for the research paper (described previously), develop an advocacy plan for individuals with your chosen disability in one or both countries you discussed. The advocacy plan should be something you come up with and not a plan that already exists. You can use any form of media to create your presentation (e.g., PowerPoint, Prezi, Canva, brochure, flyer, pamphlet). The advocacy plan will address the following:
   a. Details about what the plan entails.
   b. How it will serve people with the disability you chose.
   c. How other members of society will benefit from this advocacy plan.
   d. One or more benefits to the disabled community that are a result of your advocacy plan.

4. Explore the disability rights movement in depth by watching the documentary *Crip Camp* and exploring the freely available educational curriculum at https://www.cripcamp.com.

5. Check out the documentary *The Ugly Face of Disability Hate Crimes*.

The Ugly Face of Disability Hate Crimes

▶ video

Suggested Reading

Ladau, E. (2021). *Demystifying disability: What to know, what to say, and how to be an ally*. Ten Speed Press.

This book was written from the perspective of a disabled woman and is about understanding disability from this perspective. Ladau describes disability, the history of disability, as well as how disabilities are viewed in today's society. She discusses ways in which society can be more inclusive of disabled persons, as well as how we can break down barriers to access for people with disabilities.

Suggested Films

Media representations of disabilities tend to be inaccurate portrayals of the lived experiences of persons with disabilities. The following are a list of films which we recommend watching that relate to various topics and intersectionalities discussed in this chapter, along with associated discussion questions.

- *Ahaan*
  1. Ahaan is an adult male with Down syndrome. Ozzy is an adult man with obsessive–compulsive disorder. Compare and contrast the two disabilities. How does society view each, and how is this depicted in the film?
  2. The film producers chose to cast Ahaan's romantic interest (Onella) as a nondisabled woman. What are your thoughts on this? Discuss how this could impact societal understanding and acceptance of disabilities.
  3. Based on this film, do you think the perception of disabilities is different in India than it is in the United States?

- *Give Me Liberty*
  1. A Black disabled man asks Vic (the van driver), "Why don't you have any ambition?" and Vic responds with "I guess I haven't found my purpose yet." Talk about the irony in this question and response and the underlying message that bringing disabled people to the places they need to go is associated with not having ambition or purpose.
  2. Tracey is a woman, is Black, and is disabled, and she provides for her entire family. Talk about how her intersecting identities have historically been viewed as being unable to work and maintain oneself economically. How do you think exposure to more media such as *Give Me Liberty* would help shift society's thinking about race, gender, and disability?
  3. Vic asks Tracey, "How do you do it?" and she says, "I do what I do just like everybody else." Think about this statement. Do you think it is accurate and appropriate or not? Why?

- *Inside I'm Dancing*

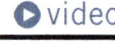

Inside I'm Dancing

1. Michael and Rory are young adults with disabilities. How are they treated in the film? Give examples.
2. Michael clearly likes Shibhon. Do you think Shibhon realizes this? How does she act toward Michael? Would she act this way with someone she didn't like who didn't have a disability?
3. When Rory gets arrested and makes his way back home, he is rude to Shibhon and Michael. Shibhon leaves because she is fed up, but then comes back. Why do you think she came back?
4. Rory insults Michael when Michael says he likes Shibhon. Talk about how this is internalized ableism.

- *Sanctuary*

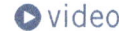

Sanctuary

1. This group of disabled adults are about to be out of work because the factory they work at is shutting down. Talk about the implications this has for them (from their point of view), as well as how the factory work that they are doing is likely tedious and pays very little.
2. Although both adults, Larry and Sophie rely on their group "supervisor" to secretly get them a hotel room so they can spend alone-time together. This is risky to do. Why is this risky, and how does this infringe on people's rights?
3. At the end of the film, Sophie has a seizure. Tom, the group supervisor, tells them not to call the ambulance, but Larry is worried and does it anyway. No matter what choice Larry made, it would have been the wrong one. Why?

- *The Imitation Game*
    1. What skills/traits enabled Alan to get hired to attempt to crack the German Enigma Code?
    2. What skills/traits led to Alan being teased and disliked by his peers? Are these traits the same or different than those that got him hired and allowed him to crack the code?
    3. Despite his brilliance and ability to crack the code, he did not fit the "normal, able-bodied" definition of a man. Discuss the irony of the world simultaneously needing people like Alan and ostracizing them.

- *The Intouchables*

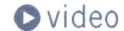

The Intouchables

1. When Phillipe tells Driss about how he became disabled, Driss says, "I would have shot myself." Talk about this message and how it devalues the disabled experience.
2. When Driss finds out that Phillipe has never seen his romantic pen-pal, he is appalled and says, "Maybe she is disabled." He doesn't seem to catch this, and Phillipe doesn't react. How might you react to Driss' comment?
3. This film and *Inside I'm Dancing* both highlight the main character with a disability and his "rebel sidekick." What do you think of the approach as part of the plot? Why do you think the producers chose this approach?
4. Phillipe tells Driss that they should stop working together because Driss "can't be pushing an invalid for the rest of [his] life." Talk about any irony here (based on the relationship they have developed). How does this relate to other films on the list?

Unforgotten: Twenty-Five Years After Willowbrook
1. What was supposed to be the resident-to-staff ratio at Willowbrook? What was the actual ratio?
2. When the narrator talks about individuals with disabilities, what does he mean when he says, "The assembly line works for cars, it does not work for people."
3. During the interview with Bernard, what were some challenges he experienced at Willowbrook? How did he describe the institution?
4. During the discussion with Patty's sisters, how do you think they felt as children when they saw her sister being taken away to Willowbrook? What burdens were placed on the family that they mentioned?
5. Refer to the interview with Luis' brother and mother. Why did Luis' brother feel upset and jealous as a child? What did his brother come to terms with or acknowledge as an adult?

References

American Psychological Association. (2023). *Disabilities.* https://www.apa.org/topics/disabilities#:~:text=Disability%20is%20a%20broad%20concept,also%20part%20of%20being%20human

Bagenstos, S. (2009). *Law and the contradictions of the disability rights movement.* Yale University Press.

Baum, F., Musolino, C., Gesesew, H., & Popay, J. (2021). New perspective on why women live longer than men: An exploration of power, gender, social determinants, and capitals. *International Journal of Environmental Research and Public Health, 18*(2), Article 661.

Berlau, D., Corrada, M., & Kawas, C. (2009). The prevalence of disability in the oldest-old is high and continues to increase with age: Findings from the 90+ study. *International Journal of Geriatric Psychiatry, 24*(11), 1217–1225.

Berlau, D., Corrada, M., Peltz, C., & Kawas, C. (2012). Disability in the oldest-old: Incidence and risk factors in the 90+ study. *American Journal of Geriatric Psychiatry, 20*(2), 159–168.

Breiding, M., & Armour, B. (2015). The association between disability and intimate partner violence in the United States. *Annals of Epidemiology, 25*(6), 455–457.

Brown, L. (2013). Stigma: An enigma demystified. In L. Davis (Ed.), *The disability studies reader* (4th ed., pp. 147–160). Routledge.

Buck v. Bell, 292 U.S. (1927). Retrieved January 12, 2024, from https://www.docsteach.org/documents/document/supreme-court-opinion-buck-v-bell

Burgdorf, M., & Burgdorf, R. (1975). A history of unequal treatment: The qualifications of handicapped persons as a suspect class under the Equal Protections Clause. *Santa Clara Law Review, 15*(4), 855–910.

Centers for Disease Control and Prevention. (2020, September 16). *Adults with disabilities: Ethnicity and race.* https://www.cdc.gov/ncbddd/disabilityandhealth/materials/infographic-disabilities-ethnicity-race.html

Chevarley, F., Thierry, M., Gill, C., Ryerson, A., & Nosek, M. (2006). Health, preventative health care, and health care access among women with disabilities in the 1994–1995 National Health Survey Interview Survey, supplement on disability. *Women's Health Issues, 16*(6), 297–312.

Davis, L. (2013). Introduction: Normalcy, power, and culture. In L. Davis (Ed.), *The disability studies reader* (4th ed., pp. 1–14). Routledge.

Dunn, D. (2019). Outsider privileges can lead to insider disadvantages: Some psychosocial aspects of ableism. *Journal of Social Issues, 75*(3), 665–682.

European Women's Lobby. (2011, May 17). *Women more prone to disability than men, and particularly vulnerable to discrimination and violence.* https://www.womenlobby.org/Women-more-prone-to-disability-than-men-and-particularly-vulnerable-to

Haegele, J., & Hodge, S. (2016). Disability discourse: Overview and critiques of the medical and social models. *Quest, 68*(2), 193–206.

Hayes, K., Wolfe, D., Trujillo, S., & Burkell, J. (2009). On the interaction of disability and ageing: Accelerated degradation models and their influence on projections of future care needs and costs for personal injury litigation. *Disability and Rehabilitation, 32*(5), 424–428.

Hubbard, R. (2013). Abortion and disability: Who should and should not inhabit the world? In L. Davis (Ed.), *The disability studies reader* (4th ed., pp. 74–86). Routledge.

Hull, L., Petrides, K., & Mandy, W. (2020). The female autism phenotype and camouflaging: A narrative review. *Review Journal of Autism and Developmental Disorders, 7*, 306–317.

Ladau, E. (2021). *Demystifying disability: What to know, what to say, and how to be an ally.* Ten Speed Press.

Lee, J., Meijer, E., Phillips, D., & Hu, P. (2021). Disability incidence rates for men and women in 23 countries: Evidence on health effects of gender inequality. *Journal of Gerontology: Series A, 76*(2), 328–338.

Lukin, J. (2013). Disability and Blackness. In L. Davis (Ed.), *The disability studies reader* (4th ed., pp. 308–315). Routledge.

Maenner, M., Warren, Z., Williams, A., Amoakohene, E., Bakian, A. V., Bilder, D. A., . . . Shaw, K. A. (2023). Prevalence and characteristics of autism spectrum disorder among children aged 8 years—Autism and Developmental Disabilities Monitoring Network, 11 sites, United States, 2020. *Surveillance Summaries, 72*(2), 1–14.

Mate, K. (2022). The curb cut. *American Journal of Medical Quality, 37*(2), 272–275.

McDonough, P., & Walters, V. (2001). Gender and health: Reassessing patterns and explanations. *Social Science & Medicine, 52*(4), 547–559.

Merriam-Webster. (2024a). Ableism. In *Merriam-Webster.com dictionary.* Retrieved January 9, 2024, from https://www.merriam-webster.com/dictionary/ableism

Merriam-Webster. (2024b). Disability. In *Merriam-Webster.com dictionary.* Retrieved January 9, 2024, from https://www.merriam-webster.com/dictionary/disability

Merriam-Webster. (2024c). Normal. In *Merriam-Webster.com dictionary.* Retrieved January 9, 2024, from https://www.merriam-webster.com/dictionary/normal

Merriam-Webster. (2024d). Stigma. In *Merriam-Webster.com dictionary.* Retrieved January 9, 2024, from https://www.merriam-webster.com/dictionary/stigma

Mulcahy, A., Streed, C. G., Jr., Wallisch, A. M., Batza, K., Kurth, N., Hall, J. P., & McMaughan, D. J. (2022). Gender identity, disability, and unmet healthcare needs among disabled people living in the community in the United States. *International Journal of Environmental Research and Public Health, 19*(5), Article 2588.

Nielsen, K. (2012). *A disability history of the United States.* Beacon.

Pinilla-Roncancio, M. (2015). Disability and poverty: Two related conditions: A review of the literature. *Revista Facultad de Medicina, 63*(1), 113–123.

Ramjan, L., Cotton, A., Algoso, M., & Peters, K. (2016). Barriers to breast and cervical cancer screening for women with physical disability: A review. *Women & Health, 56*(2), 141–156.

Reilly, P. (1987). Involuntary sterilization in the United States: A surgical solution. *Quarterly Review of Biology, 62*(2), 153–170.

Schröttle, M., & Glammeier, S. (2013). Intimate partner violence against disabled women as a part of widespread victimization and discrimination over the lifetime: Evidence from a German representative study. *International Journal of Conflict & Violence, 7,* 233–248.

Shah, S., Tsitsou, L., & Woodin, S. (2016). Hidden voices: Disabled women's experiences of violence and support over the life course. *Violence Against Women, 22*(10), 1189–1210.

Shakespeare, T. (2013). The social model of disability. In L. Davis (Ed.), *The disability studies reader* (4th ed., pp. 214–221). Routledge.

Stankiewicz, E., Oulette-Kuntz, H., McIsaac, M., Shooshtari, S., & Balogh, R. (2018). Patterns of mortality among adults with intellectual and developmental disabilities in Ontario. *Canadian Journal of Public Health, 109*(5–6), 866–872.

Thomas, C. (2006). Disability and gender: Reflections on theory and research. *Scandinavian Journal of Disability Research, 8*(2–3), 177–185.

Umansky, L. (2009). Lavinia Warren. In S. Burch (Ed.), *Encyclopedia of American disability history* (Vol. 3, p. 209). Facts on File of Library of American History.

U.S. Department of Education. (n.d.). *IDEA: Individuals With Disabilities Education Act.* https://sites.ed.gov/idea

U.S. Department of Education. (2021, August 10). *OSEP releases fast facts on the race and ethnicity of children with disabilities served under the IDEA Part B.* https://sites.ed.gov/osers/2021/08/osep-releases-fast-facts-on-the-race-and-ethnicity-of-children-with-disabilities-served-under-idea-part-b

U.S. Department of Justice, Civil Rights Division. (n.d.-a). *The Americans With Disabilities Act (ADA) protects people with disabilities from discrimination.* https://www.ada.gov

U.S. Department of Justice, Civil Rights Division. (n.d.-b). *Introduction to the Americans With Disabilities Act.* https://www.ada.gov/topics/intro-to-ada

U.S. Department of Labor. (n.d.). *Section 504, Rehabilitation Act of 1973.* https://www.dol.gov/agencies/oasam/centers-offices/civil-rights-center/statutes/section-504-rehabilitation-act-of-1973

U.S. Department of State. (2016). *Trafficking in persons report 2016.* https://2009-2017.state.gov/j/tip/rls/tiprpt/2016/index.htm

Wheaton, F., & Crimmins, E. (2016). Female disability disadvantage: A global perspective on sex differences in physical function and disability. *Ageing Society, 36*(6), 1136–1156.

Wisdom, J. P., McGee, M. G., Horner-Johnson, W., Michael, Y. L., Adams, E., & Berlin, M. (2010). Health disparities between women with and without disabilities: A review of the research. *Social Work in Public Health, 25*(3), 368–386.

Women Enabled International. (n.d.). *The rights to education for women and girls with disabilities* [Fact sheet]. https://www.ungei.org/sites/default/files/2021-03/Right-to-Education-for-Women-and-Girls-with-Disabilities-2021-eng.pdf

World Health Organization. (2001). *International classification of functioning, disability and health.*

World Health Organization. (2002). *Towards a common language for functioning, disability, and health: ICF.* https://cdn.who.int/media/docs/default-source/classification/icf/icfbeginnersguide.pdf

World Health Organization. (2011). *World report on disability 2011.* https://www.who.int/teams/noncommunicable-diseases/sensory-functions-disability-and-rehabilitation/world-report-on-disability

Yegorov, Y., Poznyak, A., Nikiforov, N., Socenin, I., & Orekhov, A. (2020). The link between chronic stress and accelerated aging. *Biomedicines, 8*(7), Article 198.

Young, I. (2000). Disability and the definition of work. In L. Francis & A. Silvers (Eds.), *Americans with disabilities: Exploring implications of the law for individuals and institution*. Routledge.

Chapter 3

Understanding Speech and Language Development

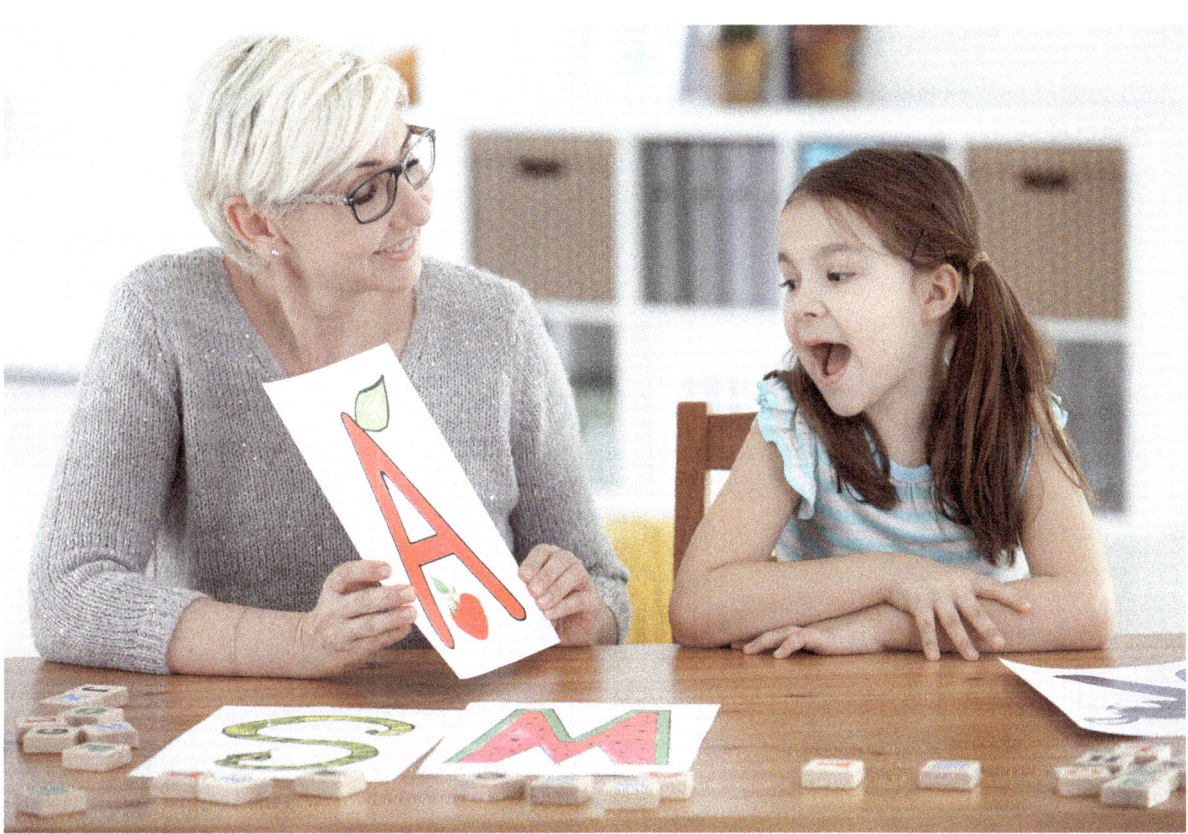

Learning Objectives

After reading this chapter, you will be able to:

- Describe the development of speech and language.
- Identify the mechanisms associated with this development.
- Explain the importance of understanding typical development to identify where challenges in speech and language exist.

Key Terms

- affricates
- alveolar
- alveolo-palatal
- articulators
- closed syllables
- criterion-reference measure
- dental
- expressive language
- fricatives
- glottal
- hard palate
- initiation of joint attention
- intelligibility
- interprofessional education
- interprofessional practice
- labial
- liquid
- morphology
- nasal sounds
- nonsyllabic
- norm-referenced measure
- open syllables
- overextensions
- plosive sounds
- pragmatics
- receptive language
- response to joint attention
- semantics
- stops
- syllabic
- syntax
- underextensions
- voiced
- voiceless

Introduction

In this chapter, you will learn about the development of speech and language. Speech is the production of sounds that can be described as prelinguistic (sounds made by infants before they say words) or linguistic (sounds used to form words and sentences). You will learn about typical speech and language development in children. Prelinguistic speech in infancy is described, followed by language development in toddlerhood, early childhood, and later language learning. A discussion of late talkers is also included.

Speech has many components to it, from the way we use our lips, mouth, and tongue to produce sounds to the way we produce speech in a smooth rhythmic manner. See a brief description and examples of the elements of speech in Table 3–1.

Language is the words we use to share our ideas. It follows a system of shared rules that helps us put words together to make sentences and to use our language in a variety of social contexts. A brief description and examples for each element of language are presented in Table 3–2.

See **"What Is Speech? What Is Language?"** on the American Speech-Language-Hearing Association (ASHA) website to learn more about typical speech and language development.

This chapter focuses on the development of speech and language, whereas fluency, voice, and hearing are described in later chapters. These later chapters will highlight both typical and atypical development in these areas of communication and their associated disorders.

TABLE 3–1. Description of Speech Elements and Examples

Element	Description	Examples
Articulation	How sounds are formulated with our articulators (e.g., lips, mouth, tongue)	/p/ sound is made by putting your lips together and allowing air to blow out from the mouth.
Voice	How we coordinate our breathing with the vibration of our vocal folds to produce sound	This is also known as phonation. Voice is impacted when the vocal folds can't vibrate or come together to make sound.
Fluency	The ability to produce speech smoothly with a typical rhythm.	Stuttering or repeating sounds or syllables and struggling to get words out.

TABLE 3–2. Description of Language Elements and Examples

Element	Description	Examples
Phonology	Knowledge of how consonant and vowel sounds come together to form syllables and words in a specific language	Children speaking American English learn that [b] can come at the beginning of a word like "bee." They also learn that [b] can go with other consonants at the beginning of a word like "blue" or "broom," but that [b] and [t] can't be combined at the beginning of any words in English.

Morphology	How to make new words by adding small units of language	Play
		  play + s
		  play + ing
		  play + ed

Syntax	How to put words together to create sentences that follow a set of rules	"The dog was barking as he played with the little girl" versus "Dog played the girl."
Semantics	What words mean; the vocabulary of language	The word "bark" can mean a sound a dog makes or the part of a tree.
Pragmatics	Use of language in social situations	Knowing how to take turns in conversation, understanding idioms, etc.

Early Speech Development

It is during the prelinguistic period (before language develops) that speech sound development begins. The first sounds to develop are vowels. Consonants follow, but the range is limited as the child enters their babbling phase. Consonant sounds that appear early are **nasal** sounds (e.g., [m]), where the lips are closed and air escapes through the nose, and **plosive sounds** (e.g., [b]), where the air is briefly blocked from flowing out through the mouth and nose. The child's native language most often determines the order of speech sound development, and in English the following sounds usually occur first: [h, d, b, m, t, w]; these are followed by [n, k, p, j (as in "yoyo")] (Bauman-Waengler, 2009). **Open syllables**, those ending with a vowel, are most frequent in the babbling stage (e.g., vowel [a], consonant + vowel [ba], vowel + consonant + vowel [aba], consonant + vowel +consonant + vowel [baba]), whereas **closed syllables**, those ending with a consonant, are less frequent (Prelock & Hutchins, 2018).

As speech and language continue to develop, a toddler's consonant sounds evolve to include the production of more difficult sounds. There are three categories of sounds that create the greatest difficulty: **liquids**, **fricatives**, and **affricates**. A liquid is a consonant sound where the tongue provides partial mouth closure leading to a vowel-like sound (e.g., [l, r]). To make the [l] sound, you raise your tongue and place it behind your teeth, and to produce the [r] sound, you move the tongue so both sides touch the top of the mouth and then you pull the tongue back. A liquid consonant can be **syllabic** as in "mother" or "paddle" (consonant is produced as a syllable) or **nonsyllabic** as in "ram" or "lamb" (consonant is not produced as a syllable). A fricative consonant is produced by narrowing parts of the vocal tract to let air out to make a hissing sound, whereas an affricate begins by occluding air and then allowing the air to escape as in a fricative. There are several types of fricatives that are described by the placement of the **articulators** in the mouth and vocal tract (i.e., **dental**, **alveolar**, **alveolo-palatal**, and **glottal**), as described in Chapter 4. The most common fricatives are **siblants** [s, z, sh, zh]. Some fricatives are produced using the upper teeth and lower lip (**labiodental**, [f, v]), the tip of tongue against the teeth (**dental**, [th]), the tip of the tongue against the gum behind the upper teeth (alveolar, [s, z]), the tongue against the alveolar ridge at the top of the mouth but further behind (alveolo-palatal, [sh, zh]), or the back of the tongue moves up and against the gum line behind the upper teeth (glottal, [h]). Sounds can also be described as **voiced** (produced with the vocal folds vibrating) and **voiceless** (produced without the vocal folds vibrating). Table 3–3 shows the mean age at which we would expect a child to produce sounds in the English language correctly more than incorrectly. Table 3–4 displays the ages of consonant acquisition in the United States and globally.

Intelligibility, or the clarity of a child's speech and the amount of their speech that a listener can understand, is also a skill that develops during this period. It is the most reliable aspect of a child's speech for caregivers to report. Notably, intelligibility is influenced by both the linguistic context (e.g., single words are easier to understand than connected speech) and the communicative partner's experience listening to the child. In typical development, as a child grows older, their intelligibility usually increases. We expect a child to be intelligible (or understood in connected speech) approximately 50% of the time by age 2 years, 75% of the time by age 3 years, and 100% of the time by age 4 years (Coplan & Gleason, 1988; Prelock & Hutchins, 2018). If a child's intelligibility is less than 66% by age 4 years, this would be considered a possible indicator of a speech problem (Gordon-Brannan & Hodson, 2000).

It is important to note that as children learn to produce speech sounds in their native language, those sounds are also placed within larger components of speech, including consonant clusters (or what you might know as blends), syllables, and words. The structure of children's speech development varies across languages, but in English first words are usually single syllables (Prelock & Hutchins, 2018). In other languages, single-syllable words are less common.

TABLE 3–3. Age of Acquisition of Consonants in the United States

Sounds	50% Criterion		75% Criterion		90% Criterion	
	Months	Range (Months)	Months	Range (Months)	Months	Range (Months)
Plosives						
p	30.60	18–36	32.73	24–36	33.25	24–48
b	30.60	18–36	32.73	24–36	31.38	24–48
t	31.20	24–36	33.82	24–36	38.54	24–48
d	30.60	18–36	33.09	24–36	35.69	24–48
k	31.20	24–36	33.82	24–36	37.69	24–48
g	31.20	24–36	33.82	24–36	36.77	24–48
Nasals						
m	30.60	18–36	32.73	24–36	33.23	24–48
n	30.60	18–36	32.73	24–36	33.08	24–48
ŋ	30.00	24–36	36.67	24–36	40.30	24–55
Fricatives						
f	31.20	24–36	33.82	24–36	38.31	24–48
v	32.80	24–36	42.73	30–72	50.83	36–66
θ	46.00	36–60	64.20	60–72	77.00	72–96
ð	41.80	36–48	56.73	48–72	69.00	54–96
s	32.40	24–36	38.55	24–60	51.33	24–84
z	33.40	24–42	44.40	24–84	56.82	30–84
ʃ	32.40	24–36	41.27	24–60	55.00	36–72
ʒ	37.00	28–48	54.00	36–84	70.67	60–84
ʍ	32.00	28–36	48.00	36–60	—	—
h	30.60	18–36	32.73	24–36	35.00	24–48
Approximants/laterals						
ɹ	35.40	24–48	47.64	24–66	66.58	30–96
j	33.00	24–36	39.60	24–48	45.77	30–60
l	33.20	24–36	40.91	24–48	53.75	24–60
w	30.60	18–36	32.73	24–36	35.23	24–48
Affricates						
tʃ	34.20	24–36	41.64	24–54	53.50	36–72
dʒ	34.20	24–36	41.27	24–54	51.00	36–72

Source: Adapted from Crowe and McLeod (2020).

TABLE 3–4. Speech Sound Acquisition in the United States and Globally

Age (Months)	U.S. Sample			Global Sample		
	50%	75%	90%	50%	75–85%	90–100%
24–35	/p, b, t, d, k, g, m, n, ŋ, f, v, s, z, ʃ, ʍ, h, ɹ, j, l, w, tʃ, dʒ/	/p, b, t, d, k, g, m, n, f, h, w/	/p, b, d, m, n, h, w/	/p, b, d, t, k, g, m, n, f, s, ʃ, h, j, w/	/p, b, d, k, g, m, n, ŋ, f, h, w/	/p/
36–47	/θ, o, ʒ/	/ŋ, v, s, z, ʃ, ɹ, j, l, tʃ, dʒ/	/t, k, g, ŋ, f, j/	/ŋ, v, z, ɹ, ʒ, ʍ, ɹ, l, tʃ, dʒ/	/t, s, ʃ, j, l/	/b, t, d, k, g, m, n, ŋ, f, h, j, w/
48–59		/o, ʒ, ʍ/	/v, s, z, ʃ, l, tʃ, dʒ/	/θ/	/v, z, ʒ, ɹ, tʃ, dʒ/	/v, s, z, ʃ, l, tʃ, dʒ/
60–71		/θ/	/o, ʒ, ɹ/		/o/	/o, ʒ, ɹ/
72–83			/θ/		/θ/	/θ/

Source: Adapted from Crowe and McLeod (2020).

Early Language Development

There is a period of prelinguistic development that occurs from birth through approximately age 1 year before language as we know it is exhibited. Infants recognize sounds and voices during this early period, including their mothers' voices and sounds in their native language versus another language. During this time, infants communicate in several ways without using words, and gestures begin to emerge (Prelock &

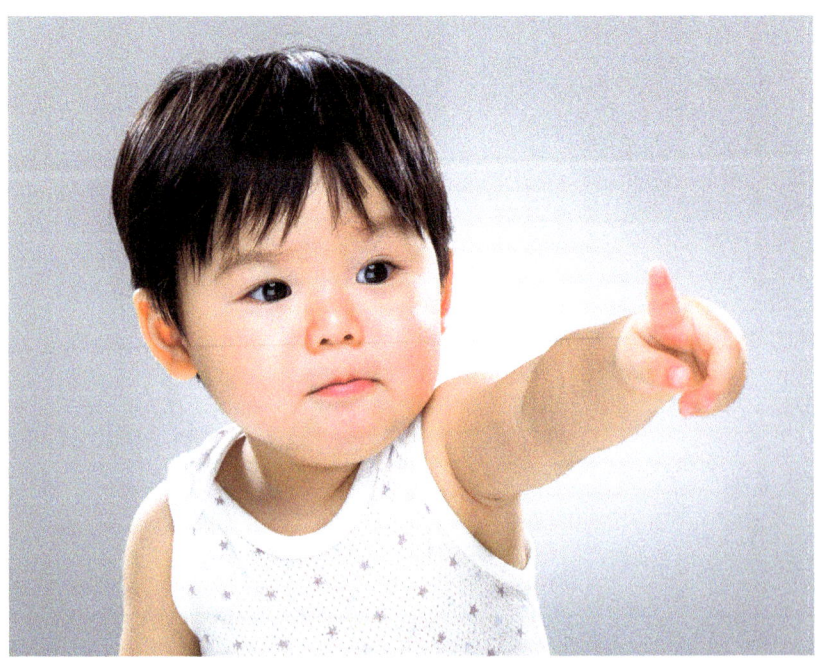

PHOTO 3–1. Infants become more intentional communication partners at approximately 9 months of age when they purposefully try to get the attention of their caregivers using gestures (e.g., reaching, pointing). *Source:* Leung Chopan/istock.com.

Hutchins, 2018). There are several stages that an infant goes through to get ready to speak as their vocalizations begin to take form. They are also in a period of hearing and understanding language. Table 3–5 provides a description of early vocalizations and patterns of speech development in the first 12 months as well as what an infant is typically hearing and understanding.

Early on, infants are moving, looking, smiling, and vocalizing with caregivers, but there is little indication they are showing "intention" in their communication. Infants become more intentional communication partners at approximately age 9 months when they purposefully try to get the attention of their caregivers using gestures (e.g., reaching, pointing) and vocalizations. Several communicative functions

TABLE 3–5. Early Stages of Vocalizations, Listening, and Understanding Between Birth and Age 1 Year

Stage	Vocalizations	Hearing and Understanding
Stage 1: Reflexive vocalizations (birth–2 months)	Crying and vegetative sounds (e.g., coughing) with some vowel-like sounds	Startles at loud sounds Recognizes caregiver's voice Smiles when the caregiver talks
Stage 2: Cooing (2–4 months)	Comfort-like vocalizations (e.g., cooing); laughter appears	Moves eyes in the direction of sounds Responds to differences in voice tones Notices toys with sounds Attends to music
Stage 3: Vocal play (4–6 months)	Loud (e.g., yells) and soft (e.g., whispers) sounds appear as well as trill sounds (e.g., raspberries); more sustained vowel productions	
Stage 4: Canonical babbling (6–12 months)	Rhythmically use consonant–vowel sequences, including **reduplicated babbles** (e.g., da da da) and **variegated syllables** (e.g., ma bi du)	Turns and looks to a sound heard Looks when you point Turns in response to name being called Understands common words (e.g., ball, water, mommy) Responds to simple words and phrases (e.g., more juice, come to mommy) Plays games like peek-a-boo Listens to songs and short stories
Stage 5: Jargon stage (10 months and older)	Syllables produced with different stress and intonation patterns; sounds like conversational speech often accompanied by gestures (e.g., reaching to indicate "up"; waving to say goodbye) Imitates different speech sounds Might say a few words that are unclear at 12 months	Points to objects Shows objects to others

Sources: Adapted from the American Speech-Language-Hearing Association (https://www.asha.org), Prelock and Hutchins (2018), and Stoel-Gammon and Menn (2013).

are exhibited even more so as an infant says their first words—the most common of which are requests and protests. An infant might request social interaction when a caregiver is not attending to them, request an object by pointing to something they can't reach, or request an action by reaching and vocalizing to be picked up. Infants protest with vocalizations or gestures to keep the communication partner from doing something they don't want or like (e.g., pushing a toy away).

With the development of intentional communication, a very important skill develops—the ability to establish joint attention. Joint attention requires that a child show interest in or connection with another, coordinating their visual attention or gaze to the same activity or object of their communication partner. Ultimately, the infant–toddler is demonstrating mutual interest and social engagement—as if they are commenting without words (Carpenter & Tomasello, 2000; Mundy et al., 2003, 2007; Mundy & Stella, 2000). Joint attention is a strong predictor of language ability and is linked to the acquisition of new words (Kasari et al., 2001).

There are two types of joint attention: (a) **response to joint attention** or someone else's bid to connect and (b) **initiation of joint attention** in which you intentionally engage another person's attention to make a social connection. Response to joint attention typically develops between ages 8 and 12 months, although you might see it slightly earlier (~6 months) or later (~13–15 months). Response to joint attention requires the child to be able to "read" the direction of their communication partner's eye gaze. A child will demonstrate this by turning their head and/or pointing to the object that their communication partner is attending to (Sullivan et al., 2007). For example, you might place a picture or object behind a toddler, and you call their name while looking at the picture or object. You are looking for the toddler to respond by turning their head and looking at the picture you are looking at or pointing to. Infants and toddlers who are delayed in establishing response to joint attention will experience missed opportunities for social learning.

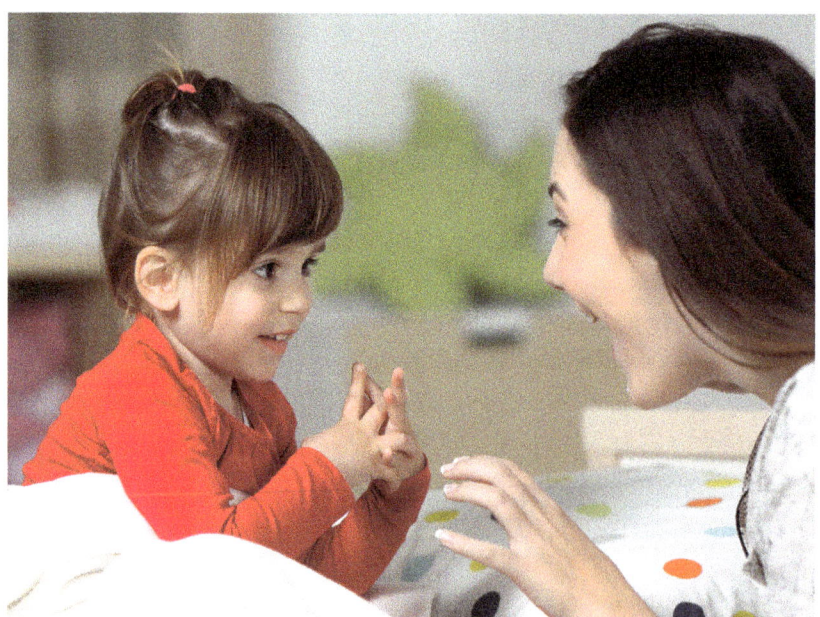

PHOTO 3–2. Joint attention is when a child shows interest in or connection with another, coordinating their visual attention or gaze to the same activity or object of their communication partner. *Source:* Antonio Guillem/istock.com.

Initiating joint attention is intentionally directing another person's attention for social purposes, as in sharing an experience rather than requesting an action or object. Initiation of joint attention usually develops by age 12 months. For example, a toddler may make eye contact with a caregiver while they manipulate a toy and alternate their eye contact between a moving mechanical toy and the caregiver. A toddler might also raise an object toward a caregiver's face while making eye contact and showing the object (Mundy et al., 2007). Infants and toddlers must be able to disengage their attention to an object to initiate joint attention with another. Joint attention usually involves gestural (points to indicate interest, shows an object) and nongestural (smiles at a caregiver while playing with a toy, makes gaze switches from the toy to the caregiver and back to the toy to socially reference the toy or the action the toy is making) (Clifford & Dissanayake, 2008). Joint attention is associated with language ability at age 3 or 4 years, including a greater mean length of utterance, higher language scores, better understanding of language, and greater language gains over time (Bono et al., 2004; Murray et al., 2008; Schietecatte et al., 2012; Toth et al., 2006).

Receptive and Expressive Language

Language is most often described as being composed of receptive skills (what a child understands) and expressive skills (what a child produces). Typically, receptive language skills are developed before expressive skills. Major developmental milestones in speech and language (receptive and expressive) occur between ages 1 and 5 years; some of these are briefly outlined in Table 3–6. This section of the chapter discusses early language sound systems, vocabulary, and grammatical development, including what is known as phonology, semantics, morphology, syntax, and pragmatics.

Phonology

The study of sound patterns or language sounds systems is known as phonology. It is composed of **phonemes**, which are distinct sound units that help distinguish words. Speech sounds help us to differentiate words. For example, if a child says [pa], it is difficult to understand what they mean, but when you add sounds that are phonemes [t, d], then new words that have meaning are formed ("pat," "pad"). A final consonant makes a difference between "boo" and "boot," one a scary sound and the other something you wear on your feet. Adding a consonant blend or cluster also adds meaning as in "play" and "pay." A child might also add a syllable to sounds to form a meaningful word such as "boo" that becomes "boo boo" (Prelock & Hutchins, 2018). Adding phonemes differentiates meaning for words children are producing.

Semantics

The way children learn word meanings is known as **semantics**. Typically, a child will say their first word at age 12 months, although a range of occurrence between ages 8 and 16 months is not unusual. Children's understanding of words, or receptive vocabulary, appears to develop earlier than this and is usually aligned with their development of intentional communication and joint attention, which were discussed previously. Children usually demonstrate the ability to use 50 different words by age 18 months, and then their vocabulary begins to take off, understanding and using more words each day, although the rate of

TABLE 3–6. Speech and Language Development Between Ages 1 and 5 Years

Age (Years)	Speech and Language Development	Examples
1–2	Understands opposites	Open–close
	Follows two-step directions	"Get the ball and put it in the box."
3–4	Uses specific speech sounds	Produces [k, g, f, t, d, n]
	Uses location words	Uses in, on, and under
	Uses two or three words in combination	"Help me"; "Baby play ball"
	Asks questions	Why?
	Responds when called from another room	Mother calls child from bedroom to the kitchen: "JJ come here."
	Understands some color words	Blue, green, red
	Understands some shape words	Square, circle
	Understands words for family	Grandpa, grandma, brother, sister
	Answers simple questions	Responds to who, what, and where
	Produces rhyming words	Fat–bat; pig–big
	Uses pronouns	I, me, you, we, they
	Begins using plural words	Trees, balls, cats
	Asks questions	When? How?
	Puts four words together in a sentence with some mistakes	"I runned to store."
	Talks about what happened during the day	"Played on the swings. Went down the sliding board. We played in the sandbox. We made a sandcastle."
4–5	Understands words that indicate order	First, last
	Understands words that indicate time	Today, yesterday, tomorrow
	Follows longer, three- or four-step directions	"Put your boots in the closet, hang up your coat, and put your book bag on the table."
	Follows teacher's directions for classroom activities	"Put an X on the items on your paper that you can drink."
	Says all speech sounds in words	May make errors on more difficult sounds to produce [l, s, r, v, z, ch, sh, th]
	Names letters and numbers	A, B, C; 1, 2, 3
	Uses sentences that have more than one action word	"I get the ball and throw it."
	Tells a short story	May tell a story about a friend or a story read
	Keeps a conversation going	Takes turns in conversation and makes comments or asks questions to keep it going
	Talks in different ways, depending on the listener and place	Will use short phrases with younger children; talks louder outside than inside

Source: Adapted from the American Speech-Language-Hearing Association (https://www.asha.org).

acquisition varies from 18 months to 2 years (Ganger & Bent, 2004; Prelock & Hutchins, 2018). Although single exposure to a word supports word learning, the more a child is exposed to a word, the greater their semantic development, and this is especially true for more abstract word meanings. In addition, context influences a child's early understanding and use of words such that they may say the word "bear" in response to a favorite stuffed animal but may not use the word when they see a "bear" in a picture book or at the zoo. This is known as **underextension**, which is a typical part of early language development. Over time, children learn to detach specific word meanings from the setting in which they first learned the word. In contrast, there is also a process called **overextension** in which a child overgeneralizes a word based on similar features of the object while ignoring differentiating features (e.g., saying "cow" for both a "cow" and a "horse"). Both underextension and overextension occur frequently in the early language development of toddlers, and they occur less frequently in older children (Prelock & Hutchins, 2018).

Children's early expressive vocabularies are made up of predominately nouns (e.g., names of objects), and this seems to be true across languages (Bornstein et al., 2004). This is likely related to the complexity of words, such that nouns may be less complex than verbs or action words. The types of word classes are also limited early on and tend to consist of words most often used in the child's life (e.g., food, toys).

How children learn new words varies. For some, it may be that children struggle to break down information for understanding (decode), whereas others may struggle to develop a response they can express (encode). It could also be that they have trouble with both decoding or understanding information and encoding or producing a response. Word learning and vocabulary development are impacted by both external (e.g., the type and extent of the language input received) and internal (e.g., attention and memory processes) factors. Gordon et al. (2022) found that word learning is highly influenced by the robustness of the information the child encodes when they are first exposed to words. Word learning requires explicit and repeated instruction to support learning and language development. Common semantic relationships that develop in young children are highlighted in Table 3–7.

Morphology and Syntax

There are rules that exist for building words and enhancing word meaning, which is known as **morphology**. For example, the verb "play" can become "played" (the past tense of play) by adding "ed". Or the noun "dog" can become "dogs" (indicating more than one) by adding "s." The "ed" and "s" are called **morphemes** as they are the smallest units of language that can add meaning to words. Grammar or **syntax** refers to the rules that are followed to build sentences. For example, simple sentences are made up of a noun phrase (e.g., "the dog") and a verb phrase (e.g., "barked loudly"). Because of syntax, children can systematically build and combine words. By age 18 months, when toddlers are beginning to grow their vocabularies, two- (e.g., "big ball") and three-word (e.g., "baby drinks milk") combinations begin to occur. The child begins to understand the doer and receiver of an action based on word position, so they know the difference between "The boy hugged his mom" and "The mom hugged the boy."

The presence of two-word combinations facilitates a child's ability to talk about a variety of topics. Children develop semantic relationships which ties meaning between the words a child uses. At approximately age 2 years, children will also produce three-word utterances, although some words or morphemes may be missing. These include definite (e.g., "the") and indefinite ("a") articles, prepositions (e.g., "in," "on"), and other morphemes such as past tense ("ed") and pluralization ("s"). These missing words make a child's early language appear telegraphic (e.g., "girl play ball" vs. "the girl played ball"), which seems to be common across languages (Hoff, 2001). For English-speaking children aged 2 to 2½ years,

TABLE 3–7. Typical Semantic Relationships Produced in the Language of Toddlers

Semantic Relation	Example
Agent + action	Baby play
Action + object	Drink milk
Agent + object	Boy truck
Action + location	Go store
Entity + location	Spoon dish
Possessor + possession	My toy
Entity + attribute	Ball big
Demonstrative + entity	This book
Disappearance/nonexistence	All gone dog
Recurrence	More cookie
Rejection	No car (I don't want to go in the car)
Denial	Not hungry

Sources: Adapted from Prelock and Hutchins (2018) and Zukowski (2013).

however, telegraphic language appears to be systematic. See Table 3–8 for examples of the 14 common grammatical morphemes.

The early development of sentence types includes declarative or descriptive sentences, as in the example, "The car is fast." Children then begin to ask questions, although they may not have all the words they need to do so (e.g., "My baby?") but use rising intonation to indicate they are asking a question. As morphemes and different sentence forms develop, the number of clauses within a sentence increases.

Pragmatics

The use of language in social contexts or for social purposes is known as **pragmatics** or social communication. Children learn what it means to be a social communicator from their caregivers, peers, and other members in their community, adjusting what and how things are said based on the social circumstance. Every day we use language socially for a variety of purposes, including greeting someone, asking for something, or sharing information. We also change the language that we use depending on who our listener is (e.g., child vs. an adult) or the situation in which we are talking (e.g., at home or at a lecture). Imagine how you might ask a 4-year-old what he had for dinner compared to a 40-year-old! We also use language socially when we engage in conversation with others, and there are general rules for engaging in a conversation (e.g., taking turns, staying on topic), as well as for storytelling (e.g., your proximity to the person you are talking with, recognizing when a person doesn't understand the story you are telling). In addition, different cultures have their own rules, and these rules tend to be unspoken. Despite these "hidden" social rules, children can learn how to interact with others and use language for social purposes based on experiences with their caregivers and other adults in their environment.

TABLE 3–8. Brown's (1973) Acquisition of 14 Grammatical Morphemes

Order of Development of Grammatical Features	Description	Example	Expected Age of Mastery (Months)
1. Present progressive *-ing*	Grammatical tense indicating an action is in progress	Mommy cook<u>ing</u>	19–28
2. In	Location term	Spoon <u>in</u> cup	27–30
3. On	Location term	Book <u>on</u> table	27–33
4. Regular plural *-s*	Nouns representing more than one are indicated by adding "s"	Two tree<u>s</u>	27–33
5. Irregular past tense	Verbs that do not change form in the usual way by adding "d" or "ed"	Billy <u>ran</u>	25–46
6. Possessive *-s*	"s" always comes after a noun or a name showing possession	Patty'<u>s</u> truck	26–40
7. Uncontractible copular	A copula is a verb form of "to be" (e.g., is, are, was, were) that is the main verb in a sentence and is not a contraction.	He <u>is</u> (in response to: who is here?)	28–46
8. Articles	A word that comes before a noun to show whether it is specific (the) or general (a)	She has <u>a</u> bike. She rides <u>the</u> bike.	28–46
9. Regular past tense *-ed*	Simple past tense verbs are formed by adding "ed"	Georgie play<u>ed</u>	26–48
10. Regular third person *-s*	Simple present tense always ends in "s"	Antonia talk<u>s</u>	28–50
11. Irregular third person	Verbs (e.g., to have, to do, to go) that are irregular in the present tense when using third person singular (he, she, it)	JJ <u>has</u> a guitar	28–50
12. Uncontractible auxiliary	Full form of a helping verb that supports the main verb in a sentence and is not a contraction	Tracey <u>might</u> come	29–48
13. Contractible copula	Linking verb that is a contraction or shortened version of a word	She'<u>s</u> sad	29–49
14. Contractible auxiliary	Shortened form of a helping verb that supports the main verb in a sentence	He'<u>d</u> like to play	30–50

Source: Adapted from Prelock and Hutchins (2018).

See **"Your Child's Communication Development: Kindergarten Through Fifth Grade?"** on the ASHA website to learn about later language learning.

See **"Reading and Writing (Literacy)"** on the ASHA website to learn about the development of reading and writing and its relationship to language skills.

See **"Social Communication"** on the ASHA website to learn more about the development of social communication skills.

Late Talkers

You may have heard the term "late bloomers" when talking about a child's language development. A late talker seems to demonstrate appropriate **receptive language** (understanding what people say), but when they are expected to say well over 50 words and begin to put 2 words together, they seem to use fewer words and word combinations than you would expect for their age (Prelock & Hutchins, 2018). Most children appear to close the gap on this delay by age 3 years, but approximately one-fourth of children seem to have persistent **expressive language** delays, which can compromise their educational success (Rescorla, 2011; Shipley & McAfee, 2009).

Typically, late talking suggests that a child is using a limited vocabulary; parents often report a delay in expressive language when all other aspects of development appear to be as expected (Roos & Weismer, 2008). Varying criteria have been used to identify late talkers, but it seems that merely asking families if they have concerns can help improve the speech-language pathologist's (SLP) identification of late talkers (Klee et al., 2000). For example, a 2-year-old might be referred for assessment if they use fewer than 50 words and they have had multiple ear infections or parents report language development as a concern.

Predicting outcomes for late talkers is unclear because a majority appear to outgrow the expressive language delay reported at age 2 years. Those who do outgrow the delay tend to demonstrate the following (Prelock & Hutchins, 2018):

- Frequent use of gestures to communicate
- Higher performance on measures of receptive language
- Better accuracy in their speech sound productions and syllable structures
- Greater number of speech sounds produced with speech error expected for their age

Those who do not outgrow the delay will exhibit the following:

- Simplified syllable structures
- Fewer gestures
- Poorer performance on measures of receptive language
- Fewer verb forms
- Fewer speech sounds produced with a greater number of initial and final consonants deleted
- Poor spontaneous and sentence imitations
- Some behavior challenges
- Less pretend play

Other demographic factors that might be associated with increased risk of a child being a late talker include a family history of speech and language difficulties, premature birth, lower socioeconomic status, male status, lower maternal education, maternal directive interaction style, and identified parent concern (Nelson et al., 2006; Wankoff, 2011). Table 3–9 presents a brief outline of the red flags frequently associated with late talking in the first 3 years of life.

Although many late talkers appear to catch up to their peers, there is some indication that underlying weaknesses exist in vocabulary and grammar (Ellis & Thal, 2008; Ellis Weismer, 2007; Rescorla et al.,

TABLE 3–9. Red Flags for Delays in Early Language Development Ages Birth to 3 Years

Age Range (Months)	Selected Red Flags
0–3	Poor sound awareness Inattention to surroundings Feeding problems
3–6	Poor sound awareness Unaware of environment Difficulty orienting to sound
6–9	Limited babbling Less enjoyment in social interaction
9–18	Limited spontaneous or imitated words produced Fewer gestures (e.g., pointing, reaching) Limited sharing attention with others
18–24	Less than 50 words Absent word combinations Less pretend play
24–36	Behavior problems if cannot be understood Repeats words heard in the moment or previously Few words or multiword utterances

Sources: Adapted from Prelock et al. (2013) and Prelock and Hutchins (2018).

2005; Roos & Weismer, 2008). It is difficult to predict, however, which late talking children will have persistent delays because the early developmental period is highly variable across children (Ellis & Thal, 2008). When to intervene is a question that is often difficult to answer. A "wait and see" approach is supported by some, although not all, pediatricians because many late talkers catch up to their peers and perform in the expected range on language measures. Practically, late talkers might not qualify for services and early intervention support can be expensive, so allocating such resources to those who really need them may be the preferred approach. Another perspective is that although late talkers may perform as expected on early language measures, some demonstrate later language-based deficits such as challenges in grammar, narrative language, and literacy (Prelock & Hutchins, 2018). For this reason, taking the "wait and see" approach would not be the best outcome. Ultimately, it is important to refer late talkers for a comprehensive language assessment so that a determination can be made regarding underlying language challenges so intervention services can be initiated. Consideration should also be given to children with a family history of language delay, minimal gesture use, and delays in both receptive and expressive language. In all cases, especially where services are not available, parent training has been used successfully to support expressive language development (Paul & Norbury, 2012).

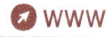

See **"Late Blooming or Language Problem?"** on the ASHA website to learn more about understanding differences between language delays and language problems.

Assessment

Assessment is an important part of our discovery of how individuals understand and communicate their needs, wants, and ideas. There are many formal and informal approaches to gathering information about school-age children's comprehension and spoken language. Valid assessments for infants and toddlers, however, are lacking in the literature, and those that are available are impacted by linguistic and cultural biases (Cycyk et al., 2021). Clinical research continues to evaluate assessment models and tools to ensure that reliable approaches exist so as not to delay diagnosis or intervention that has potential to have long-term impact (Hus & Segal, 2021).

Formal or traditional approaches to assessment are generally static—creating a standard testing environment for all children without giving them feedback or support—leading to a score that compares a child's performance to that of others at a particular point in time (Spicer-Cain et al., 2023). One of the flaws in this approach to assessment is the lack of information an SLP will gather on a child's speech and language in more natural contexts. For the youngest children with or at risk for developmental language disorders (DLDs), most SLPs gather information from observations and from parental report. Others consider a more "dynamic assessment" approach in which clinicians measure children's emerging developmental skills as well as their potential for learning (Bamford et al., 2022). Dynamic assessment focuses on the learning process and an individual child's capacity for learning with scaffolded support (e.g., modeling, cueing/cuing, prompting).

Typically, dynamic assessment uses a test–teach–retest framework in which children experience a static assessment, receive a brief intervention, and then a retest reveals the amount of change that occurred. With dynamic assessment, the "teach" phase typically includes a metacognitive component that facilitates the child's ability to learn a strategy for completing a specific task (Peña et al., 2014). Ultimately, dynamic assessment can be used to inform a clinician about a child's learning potential.

SLPs are expected to follow an evidence base when engaged in the evaluation and assessment of individuals with or at risk for communication disorders (ASHA, 2010; Bawayan & Brown, 2022). This expectation aligns with federal regulations that require SLPs to gather information through a variety of means that yield valid information for determining the educational and service needs for children (Individuals With Disabilities Education Act, 2004). SLPs use multiple approaches to assessment to address variable performance across measures. This is important when making decisions about an individual's communication ability.

The following steps are involved in the assessment process:

- Select assessment materials that will help determine eligibility for services.
- Use assessments that will help develop goals.
- Consider cultural and linguistic diversity in your selection of assessments to help differentiate a language disorder from a language *difference*.
- Include both **norm-** and **criterion-referenced** tests as well as informal assessment measures to ensure accuracy in diagnosis with functionally relevant material to develop an intervention plan (Danahy Ebert & Scott, 2014).

A **norm-referenced measure** compares a child's score to the performance of others. For example, if the expected score for moving to the next-level reading group is 80% and the child receives a score of 85%, they are above the criteria expected to move on. If the student receives a reading quotient of 95 on a norm-referenced reading assessment and the average reading quotient for students their age is 80, then their performance would be considered above average. In contrast, a criterion-reference measure is one that evaluates a student's learning against a predetermined set of criteria without comparing the student's performance to that of others. Criterion-referenced assessments and more informal language assessments such as sampling language in narrative or expository discourse are effective tools for monitoring the progress of culturally and linguistically diverse students who also exhibit language disorders (Danahy Ebert & Scott, 2014; Petersen et al., 2017).

See **"Early Identification of Speech, Language, Swallowing, and Hearing Disorders"** on the ASHA website for more information on assessment.

Intervention

Often, there are delays in the identification of children with speech and language or communication disorders, even though parents report concerns early on. Delays in identification also mean delays in access to early intervention, which is so important to developing communication skills. Difficulty communicating inhibits an individual's ability to fully participate in daily activities and often results in negative outcomes. Moreover, challenges with participation in daily life activities vary depending on the etiology and severity of the communication challenge, as well as various personal and environmental factors (Baylor & Darling-White, 2020).

It is important, therefore, that SLPs and audiologists implement interventions that are responsive to the individual's need and desire to participate in their home, school, work, and larger community settings (Wallace et al., 2017). Research suggests that areas important to communication participation include developing relationships; engaging in interaction; and being involved in community, social, and civic life (ter Wal et al., 2023). Intervention approaches for specific disorder types are addressed in later chapters.

Best practices in speech-language pathology and early intervention expect a level of collaboration across professional disciplines to ensure a child, teen, or adult with a communication disorder has a comprehensive plan to address their needs. This requires not only expertise that is discipline-specific but also competency in **interprofessional practice (IPP).** ASHA (2015) and the Council for Exceptional Children, Division for Early Childhood (2020) have policies and requirements that highlight the importance of working across disciplines to facilitate desired communication and learning outcomes (Lieberman-Betz et al., 2023). When supporting individuals with complex communication, physical, and health needs, no one discipline has sufficient expertise to address everything. For this reason, **interprofessional education (IPE)** provides an opportunity for students in training across disciplines (e.g., speech-language pathology, physical therapy, occupational therapy, psychology, special education) to learn with and from one another with the expressed goal of collaborating to improve a patient's or client's quality of care. In fact, research indicates that educating students in IPE facilitates teamwork and collaboration with other disciplines (Cusack & O'Donoghue, 2012; Guraya & Barr, 2018). In fact, Liberman and Betz (2023) found that educating students using case-based instruction, interprofessional faculty, and interaction with families are effective ways to foster understanding and skill in implementing interprofessional practice.

Why Is It Important to Understand Speech and Language Development?

A notable milestone in children's speech development is their ability to connect meaning to the sound productions they made. This connection of sound to meaning and ultimately to words is a gradual process in which children approximate the sounds or sound combination in words (Cassidy et al., 2022; Vihman, 2014). Early word productions also reveal both similar and different sound patterns across languages (de Boysson-Bardies et al., 1992). It is important for us to understand the developmental profiles of sound production in young children if we wish to plan for intervention for children who are not demonstrating the expected acquisition of speech sounds. Recognizing cross-cultural differences in speech sound acquisition and production is also important. For example, Davis and colleagues (2018) considered speech sounds production in words for both French- and English-speaking toddlers and noted that **labial** sounds for which both lips are used (e.g., [b, p, m]) occurred more frequently in the early word production of French toddlers than coronal sounds made using the tip of the tongue hitting the **hard palate** (e.g., [t, d, n]). Although English-speaking toddlers also used the labial sounds frequently, there was no real difference in the use of labial and coronal sounds (Davis et al., 2018). Understanding the use of specific consonants in typical development across languages will likely influence what sounds and words are used in intervention for children who are struggling with their speech-sound production.

Major language milestones evolve between ages 1 and 5 years. During this period, children increase their understanding of what is said and advance their ability to formulate a response to share their thoughts and ideas. They also develop the ability to respond to and initiate joint attention—a critical skill to support their later ability to engage in conversation with a communication partner. The first 5 years of life is a critical period of language development, which is why most young children are screened for language challenges at well child check-ups in pediatric and family health care practices. Following children who are late talkers and recognizing those who demonstrate red flags for developmental language disorders are important roles for SLPs. Collaboration with health care providers is also needed so that referral for early assessment and intervention can occur.

Chapter Summary

There is a population of children identified as late-talking children whose expressive vocabulary at age 2 years is typically 10% below what we would expect for children who are not late talking and are developing language as we would expect (Cheung et al., 2022; Desmarais et al., 2008). This population is also at risk for DLDs, although vocabulary is usually not a good predictor of later language development or delay (Leonard, 2009); however, there are few consistent factors that predict risk for a DLD. Children who are late talkers may also have persistent delays in language through their preschool years and possibly show lags through the teenage years on measures of language (Rescorla, 2009). Furthermore, late-talking children may have difficulty accessing all available mechanisms that support word learning, such as making more differences in encoding and repeating words as well as weaker phonological and lexical development (Cheung et al., 2022; Edwards et al., 2004).

Children with language challenges with no known cause are usually identified as having a DLD, a heterogeneous condition that can affect components of language, including pragmatics, syntax, semantics, phonology, and/or morphology (Spicer-Cain et al., 2023). DLDs can also affect receptive language or the ability to decode and understand what is said, as well as expressive language or the ability to encode a response to share a message. DLDs should not be confused with children identified as late talkers because early language delays do not always predict whether a child will have a language impairment. Children with DLDs, however, have persistent expressive language challenges (Botting et al., 2020; Spicer-Cain et al., 2023) that can impact their academic performance and social communication.

SLPs are important collaborators with other health professionals because they have a critical role in early identification, assessment, and early intervention for children with DLDs. Sharing what they know about the development of speech and language with pediatricians, families, and other health care providers will ensure young children receive the services they require.

Chapter Review Questions

1. What are some signs of late talkers?
2. In what circumstances might an SLP recommend early intervention services for a late talker?
3. What is the difference between speech and language?
4. What are some examples of morphemes that give additional meaning to words?

5. What does speech production look like in the prelinguistic developmental period?
6. When does a child typically say their first word?
7. When do children begin putting words together to form simple phrases and sentences?
8. What is the difference between a criterion-referenced and a norm-referenced assessment tool?
9. Why is interprofessional education important to the delivery of care?
10. What is the difference between response to and initiation of joint attention?

Learning Activities

1. Observe an infant or toddler and document the sounds and words you hear in their interactions with a caregiver or other adult. Identify if they are using any consonants or vowels in their speech, explain what those are, and give examples. Also identify if they are using underextensions or overextensions in their use of words. Finally, determine what words they understand versus what words they use during your observation.

2. Shadow an SLP or audiologist in a clinic, hospital, or school and describe how they collaborate with other professionals in the delivery of their services to infants, children, youth, or adults with communication disorders. How are they demonstrating the principles of interprofessional education and practice in the work they are doing?

3. Complete the following table, indicating the manner of articulation (how a sound is produced), the place of articulation (where the sound is produced and the articulators involved), a list of the consonants in each category, and examples of the sounds in words. One column for each manner of articulation is completed for you.

Manner of Articulation	Description of the Place of Articulation and How the Sound Is Produced	Consonants	Examples in Words
Stop	Closing the lips, placing the tongue behind the teeth or raising the tongue against the palate to stop air from escaping when producing a sound.		
Nasal		[m, n, ng]	
Liquid			lake, red

Manner of Articulation	Description of the Place of Articulation and How the Sound Is Produced	Consonants	Examples in Words
Fricative	Produced by narrowing parts of the vocal tract to let air out to make a hissing sound; fricatives are described by the placement of the articulators in the mouth and vocal tract (i.e., dental, alveolar, alveolo-palatal, and glottal).		
Affricate	_____ _____	[ch, dg]	_____
Glide	_____ _____	_____	yes, wig

Suggested Reading

Haukedal, C. H., Wie, O. B., Schaduber, S. K., & von Koss Torkildsen, J. (2023). Children with developmental language disorder have lower quality of life than children with typical development and children with cochlear implants. *Journal of Speech, Language and Hearing Research, 56,* 3988–4008.

This study investigated the ways in which quality of life (QOL) is related to the language abilities of children with developmental language disorder (DLD) compared to children without DLD and children with cochlear implants. Parents of the DLD group indicated poorer performance on QOL measures for their children than the parents of children without DLD or those with cochlear implants. The study results suggested poorer QOL is related to a child's level of language difficulties.

Paul, D., & Roth, F. R. (2011). Guiding principles and clinical applications for speech-language pathology practice in early intervention. *Language, Speech, and Hearing Services in Schools, 42*(3), 320–330.

Principles for early intervention are described, and the ways in which SLPs apply these principles to address the communication challenges of infants and toddlers are presented. Principles guiding services include family-centered and culturally responsive care, use of natural environments to promote development, collaborative and coordinated care about team members serving the child and family, and implementation of evidence-based practice. Infants and toddlers with or at risk for communication disorders should be receiving early intervention services designed to meet their individual and changing needs. With early intervention, communication is more likely to develop.

Paul, R., & Roth, F. (2011). Characterizing and predicting outcomes of communication delays in infants and toddlers: Implications for clinical practice. *Language, Speech, and Hearing Services in Schools*, *42*(3), 331–340.

The use of data to assist in decision making for early intervention services provided to young children is described. A review of the literature identified the characteristics of young children who typically receive early intervention services. The literature indicates that early intervention makes a difference in communication as well as other developmental domains. Guidance is provided to SLPs who evaluate and determine risk factors for young children where their presentation is less clear.

Wankoff, L. S. (2011). Warning signs in the development of speech, language, and communication: When to refer to a speech-language pathologist. *Journal of Child and Adolescent Psychiatric Nursing*, *24*, 175–184.

A link exists between communication and psychiatric disorders, so it is crucial to understand the red flags indicating a need for a speech and language evaluation, especially during infancy and early childhood. This article summarizes the developmental outcomes for infants and young children through age 5 years in speech, language, and communication, and it highlights red flags suggesting a need for further assessment. Although early signs of communication challenges may be subtle, the potential impact on multiple learning domains is noteworthy. Early detection of difficulties leads to early support, without which ongoing learning and social–emotional problems may be revealed in later childhood and adolescence.

Additional Resources

- ASHA Practice Portal: Clinical Topics
  http://www.asha.org/Practice-Portal/Clinical-Topics
- Identify the Signs
  http://identifythesigns.org

References

American Speech-Language-Hearing Association. (2010). *Guidelines for the roles and responsibilities of the school-based speech-language pathologist*. http://www.asha.org/policy

American Speech-Language-Hearing Association. (2015). *Interprofessional education/interprofessional practice (IPE/IPP)*. https://www.asha.org/practice/interprofessional-education-practice

Bamford, K., Masso, S., Baker, E., & Ballard, K. (2022). Dynamic assessment for children with communication disorders: A systematic scoping review and framework. *American Journal of Speech-Language Pathology*, *31*(4), 1878–1893.

Bauman-Waengler, J. (2009). *Introduction to phonetics and phonology: From concepts to transcription*. Pearson.

Bawayan, R., & Brown, J. A. (2022). Diagnostic decisions of language complexity using informal language assessment measures. *Language, Speech and Hearing Services in Schools, 53*, 466–478.

Baylor, C., & Darling-White, M. (2020). Clinical focus achieving participation-focused intervention through shared decision making: Proposal of an age- and disorder-generic framework. *American Journal of Speech-Language Pathology, 29*(3), 1335–1360.

Bono, M., Daley, T., & Sigman, M. (2004). Relations among joint attention, amount of intervention and language gains in autism. *Journal of Autism and Other Developmental Disabilities, 34*, 495–505.

Bornstein, M., Cote, L., Maital, S., Painter, K., & Park, S. (2004). Crosslinguistic analysis of vocabulary in young children: Spanish, Dutch, French, Hebrew, Italian, Korean, and American English. *Child Development, 75*, 1115–1139.

Botting, N. (2020). Language, literacy and cognitive skills of young adults with developmental language disorder (DLD). *International Journal of Language & Communication Disorders, 55*(2), 255–265.

Botting, N., Durkin, K., Toseeb, U., Pickles, A., & Conti- Ramsden, G. (2016). Emotional health, support, and self- efficacy in young adults with a history of language impairment. *British Journal of Developmental Psychology, 34*(4), 538–554.

Brown, R. (1973). *A first language: The early stages*. Harvard University Press.

Carpenter, M., & Tomasello, M. (2000). Joint attention, cultural learning, and language acquisition. In A. M. Wetherby & B. M. Prizant (Eds.), *Autism spectrum disorders* (pp. 31–54). Brookes.

Cassidy, R., Aoyama, K., & Davis, B. L. (2022). Phonetic characteristics of children's early words in German: Data from typically developing children with clinical implications. *Perspectives of the ASHA Special Interest Groups, 7*, 885–896.

Cheung, R.W., Hartley, C., & Monaghan, P. (2022). Multiple mechanisms of word learning in late-talking children: A longitudinal study. *Journal of Speech, Language, Hearing Research, 65*, 2978–2995.

Clifford, S. M., & Dissanayake, C. (2008). The early development of joint attention to infants with autistic disorder using home video observation and parental interview. *Journal of Autism and Other Developmental Disabilities, 38*, 791–805.

Coplan, J., & Gleason, J. (1988). Unclear speech: Recognition and significance of unintelligible speech in preschool children. *Pediatrics, 82*(3), 447–452.

Council for Exceptional Children, Division for Early Childhood. (2020). *Initial practice-based standards for early interventionists/early childhood special educators*. https://exceptionalchildren.org/standards/initial-practice-based-standards-early-interventionists-early-childhood-special-educators

Cusack, T., & O'Donoghue, G. (2012). The introduction of an interprofessional education module: Students' perceptions. *Quality in Primary Care, 20*(3), 231–238.

Cycyk, L. M., De Anda, S., Moore, H., & Huerta, L. (2021). Cultural and linguistic adaptations of early language interventions: Recommendations for advancing research and practice. *American Journal of Speech-Language Pathology, 30*(3), 1224–1246.

Danahy Ebert, K., & Scott, C. M. (2014). Relationships between narrative language samples and norm-referenced test scores in language assessments of school-age children. *Language, Speech, and Hearing Services in Schools, 45*(4), 337–350.

Davis, B. L., Chenu, F., & Yi, H. (2018). Phonological selection patterns in early words: A preliminary cross-linguistic investigation. *Canadian Journal of Linguistics, 63*(4), 556–579.

de Boysson-Bardies, B., Vihman, M. M., Roug-Hellichius, L., Landberg, I., & Arao, F. (1992). Material evidence of infant selection from the target language: A cross-linguistic phonetic study. In C. A. Ferguson, L. Menn, & C. Stoel-Gammon (Eds.), *Phonological development: Models, research, implications* (pp. 369–393). York Press.

Desmarais, C., Sylvestre, A., Meyer, F., Bairati, I., & Rouleau, N. (2008). Systematic review of the literature on characteristics of late-talking toddlers. *International Journal of Language & Communication Disorders, 43*(4), 361–389.

Edwards, J., Beckman, M. E., & Munson, B. (2004). The interaction between vocabulary size and phonotactic probability effects on children's production accuracy and fluency in nonword repetition. *Journal of Speech, Language, and Hearing Research, 47*(2), 421–436.

Ellis, E., & Thal, D. (2008). Early language delay and risk for language impairment. *Perspectives on Language Learning and Education, 15*(3), 89–126.

Ellis Weismer, S. (2007). Typical talkers, late talkers, and children with specific language impairment: A language endowment spectrum? In R. Paul (Ed.), *The influence of developmental perspectives on research and practice in communication disorders* (pp. 83–102). Erlbaum.

Fenson, L., Marchman, V., Thal, D., Dale, P., Reznick, J. S., & Bates, E. (2007). *MacArthur–Bates Communicative Development Inventories* (2nd ed.). Brookes.

Ganger, J., & Brent, M. (2004). Reexamining the vocabulary spurt. *Developmental Psychology, 40*, 621–632.

Gordon, K. R., Lowry, S., Ohlmann, N. B., & Fitspatrick, D. (2022). Word learning by preschool-age children: Differences in encoding, re-encoding, and consolidation across learners during slow mapping. *Journal of Speech, Language, and Hearing Research, 65*, 1956–1977.

Gordon-Brannan, M., & Hodson, B. W. (2000). Intelligibility/severity measurements of prekindergarten children's speech. *American Journal of Speech Language Pathology, 9*(2), 141–150.

Guraya, S. Y., & Barr, H. (2018). The effectiveness of interprofessional education in healthcare: A systematic review and meta-analysis. *Kaohsiung Journal of Medical Sciences, 34*(3), 160–165.

Hoff, E. (2001). *Language development* (2nd ed.). Wadsworth.

Individuals With Disabilities Education Act, 20 U.S.C. § 1400 (2004).

Kasari, C., Freeman, S. F. N., & Paparella, T. (2001). Early intervention in autism: Joint attention and symbolic play. *International Review of Research in Mental Retardation, 23*, 207–237.

Klee, T., Pearce, K., & Carson, D. (2000). Improving the positive predictive value of screening for developmental language disorder. *Journal of Speech, Language, and Hearing Disorders, 43*, 821–833.

Leonard, L. B. (2009). Is expressive language disorder an accurate diagnostic category? *American Journal of Speech-Language Pathology, 18*(2), 115–123.

Lieberman-Betz, R. G., Brown, J. A., Wiegand, S. D., Vail, C. O., Fiss, A. L., & Carpenter, L. J. (2023). Building collaborative capacity in early intervention preservice providers through interprofessional education. *Language, Speech, and Hearing Services in Schools, 54*, 504–517.

Mundy, P., Block, J., Delgado, C., Pomares, Y., Vaughan van Hecke, A., & Venezia, M. (2007). Individual differences and the development of joint attention in infancy. *Child Development, 78*(3), 938–954.

Mundy, P., Delgado, C., Block, J., Venezia, M., Hogan, A., & Seibert, J. (2003). *A manual for the abridged early social communication scales (ESCS)*. Available through the University of Miami Psychology Department.

Mundy, P., & Stella, J. (2000). Joint attention, social orienting, and nonverbal communication in autism. In A. M. Wetherby & B. M. Prizant (Eds.), *Autism spectrum disorders* (pp. 55–77). Brookes.

Murray, D. S., Creaghead, N. A., Maning-Courtney, P., Shear, P. K., Bean, J., & Prendeville, J. (2008). The relationship between joint attention and language in children with autism spectrum disorders. *Focus on Autism and Other Developmental Disabilities, 23*(1), 5–14.

Nelson, H. D., Nygren, P., Walker, P., & Panoscha, R. (2006). Screening for speech and language delay in preschool children: Systematic evidence review for the US Preventive Services Task Force. *Pediatrics, 117,* 297–315.

O'Fallon, M., Alper, R. M., Beiting, M., & Luo, R. (2022). Assessing shared reading in families at risk: Does quantity predict quality? *American Journal of Speech-Language Pathology, 31,* 2108–2122.

Paul, R. (1991). Maternal linguistic input to toddlers with slow expressive language delay. *Journal of Speech and Hearing Research, 34,* 982–988.

Paul, R., & Norbury, C. (2012). *Language disorders: From infancy through adolescence* (4th ed.). Elsevier.

Peña, E. D., Gillam, R. B., & Bedore, L. M. (2014). Dynamic assessment of narrative ability in English accurately identifies language impairment in English language learners. *Journal of Speech, Language, and Hearing Research, 57*(6), 2208–2220.

Petersen, D. B., Chanthongthip, H., Ukrainetz, T. A., Spencer, T. D., & Steeve, R. W. (2017). Dynamic assessment of narratives: Efficient, accurate identification of language impairment in bilingual students. *Journal of Speech, Language, and Hearing Research, 60*(4), 983–998.

Peterson, P., Carta, J., & Greenwood, C. (2005). Teaching enhanced milieu language teaching skills to parents of multiple risk families. *Journal of Early Intervention, 27,* 94–109.

Prelock, P., Gulbronson, M., Hutchins, T., Green, E., & Glascoe, F. (2013). Psychosocial risk, language development, and bilingual/dual language learners. In F. P. Glascoe, K. P. Marks, J. K. Poon, & M. M. Macias (Eds.), *Identifying & addressing developmental–behavioral problems: A practical guide for medical and non-medical professionals, trainees, researchers and advocates* (pp. 199–234). PEDStest.com.

Prelock, P. A., & Hutchins, T. L. (2018). *Clinical guide to assessment and treatment of communication disorders.* F. R. Volkmar, Editor. NY: Springer.

Reilly, S., McKean, C., Morgan, A., & Wake, M. (2015). Identifying and managing common childhood language and speech impairments. *British Medical Journal, 350,* Article h2318.

Rescorla, L. (2009). Age 17 language and reading outcomes in late-talking toddlers: Support for a dimensional perspective on language delay. *Journal of Speech, Language, and Hearing Research, 52*(1), 16–30.

Rescorla, L. (2011). Late talkers: Do good predictors of outcome exist? *Developmental Disabilities, 17,* 141–150.

Rescorla, L., Bernstein-Ratner, N., Jusczyk, P., & Jusczyk, A. (2005). Concurrent validity of the Language Development Survey: Associated with the MacArthur–Bates Communicative Development Inventories–Words and Sentences. *American Journal of Speech-Language Pathology, 14,* 146–153.

Roos, E., & Weismer, S. (2008). Language outcomes of late talking toddlers at preschool and beyond. *Perspectives on Language Learning in Education, 15*(3), 119–126.

Schietecatte, I., Roeyers, H., & Warreyn, P. (2012). Exploring the nature of joint attention impairments in young children with ASD: Associated social and cognitive skills. *Journal of Autism and Developmental Disorders, 42*(1), 1–12.

Shipley, K. G., & McAfee, J. G. (2009). *Assessment in speech-language pathology* (4th ed.). Delmar Cengage Learning.

Spicer-Cain, H., Camilleri, B., Hasson, N., & Botting, N. (2023). Early identification of children at risk for communication disorders: Introducing a novel battery of dynamic assessments for infants. *American Journal of Speech-Language Pathology, 32*, 523–544.

Stoel-Gammon, C., & Menn, L. (2013). Phonological development: Learning sounds and sound patterns. In J. Berko Gleason & N. Bernstein Ratner (Eds.), *The development of language* (pp. 52–88). Pearson.

Sullivan, M., Finelli, J., Marvin, A., Garrett-Mayer, E., Bauman, M., & Landa, R. (2007). Response to joint attention in toddlers at risk for autism spectrum disorder: A prospective study. *Journal of Autism and Developmental Disorders, 37*, 37–48.

ter Wal, N., van Ewijk, L., Dijkhuis, L., Visser-Meily, J. M. A., Terwee, C. B., & Gerrits, E. (2023). Everyday barriers in communicative participation according to people with communication problems. *Journal of Speech, Language, and Hearing Research, 66*, 1033–1050.

Toth, K., Munson, J., Meltzoff, A. N., & Dawson, G. (2006). Early predictors of communication development in young children with ASD: Joint attention, imitation and toy play. *Journal of Autism and Developmental Disorders, 36*, 993–1005.

Vihman, M. M. (2014). *Phonological development: The first two years*. Wiley.

Wallace, S. J., Worrall, L., Rose, T., le Dorze, G., Cruice, M., Isaksen, J., . . . Gauvreau, C. A. (2017). Which outcomes are most important to people with aphasia and their families? An international nominal group technique study framed within the ICF. *Disability and Rehabilitation, 39*(14), 1364–1379.

Wankoff, L. S. (2011). Warning signs in the development of speech, language, and communication: When to refer to a speech-language pathologist. *Journal of Child and Adolescent Psychiatric Nursing, 24*, 175–184.

Zukowski, A. (2013). Putting words together: Morphology and syntax in the preschool years. In J. Berko Gleason & N. Bernstein Ratner (Eds.), *The development of language* (pp. 120–162). Pearson.

Chapter 4

Anatomy and Physiology of the Speech Mechanism

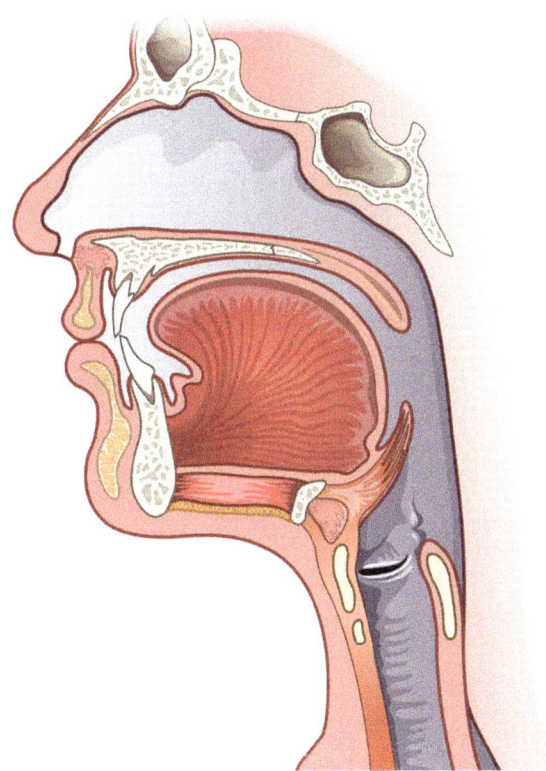

Learning Objectives

After reading this chapter, you will be able to:

- Explain the role of the respiratory system in speech production.
- Describe the phonatory system and associated speech mechanisms.
- Identify the cartilages of the larynx and their role in supporting speech production.
- Explain the role of resonance in speech sound production.
- Identify the parts of the articulatory system.

Key Terms

abduction	maxilla bone
active articulator	medulla oblongata
adduction	myoelastic–aerodynamic theory
alveolar process	nasopharynx
alveolar ridge	orbicularis oris muscle
amplitude	oropharynx
arytenoid cartilage	palatine bone or process
Bernoulli effect	passive articulator
cartilages	pharynx
cricoarytenoid joint	posterior cricoarytenoid muscle
cricoid cartilage	premaxilla
cricothyroid muscle	soft palate
diaphragm	subglottal air pressure
fundamental frequency	temporal bone
glottis	temporomandibular joint
hard palate	thorax
hyoid bone	thyroarytenoid muscle
intensity	thyroid cartilage
interarytenoid muscle	trachea
intercostal muscles	uvula
internal thyroarytenoid muscles	velopharyngeal closure
larynx	velopharyngeal mechanism
lateral cricoarytenoid muscle	velum
levator veli palatini	vertebral column
loudness	vocal folds
mandible	vocalis muscle
maxilla	

Introduction

In this chapter, you will learn about the anatomy and physiology of the speech mechanism. When you speak, your voice is powered by several factors that support your airflow to make sound. Speech production requires coordination of several subsystems (i.e., respiratory, phonatory, articulatory, resonance), as well as the activation of the laryngeal muscles and the engagement of the pharynx, the oral cavity, and nasal cavities.

In the sections that follow, the structures and physiological mechanisms needed for speech production are described. You will learn about the respiratory system, which we need for both breathing and speech, and the phonatory system, which is needed for not only speech but also eating. In addition, you will learn about the articulatory structures involved in various speech productions and the resonance cavities that determine whether sound travels through the nose or mouth.

The central nervous system (CNS), including the brain, is described in Chapter 9. The CNS is responsible for initiating and coordinating with other structures that help an individual produce speech and develop language. In addition, the auditory system, important for sound awareness and regulating speech production, is fully described in Chapter 13.

Respiratory System

The respiratory system is responsible not only for the air we use to breathe but also the air we use to speak. When we speak, we typically do so during exhalation, which is when we breathe out from the lungs. Breathing and speaking together require the coordination of several structures, including the rib cage, the diaphragm, the lungs, and many muscles that are controlled by the nervous system.

The rib cage, also known as the thoracic cage, provides the structural frame for respiration. We have 12 pairs of ribs that form a cylinder-like structure and are attached to the **vertebral column**. There are both upper and lower ribs. Seven upper ribs are attached to the breastbone (or **sternum**) in the front and are typically identified as the true ribs. Three additional ribs are attached to the breastbone; these are known as the false ribs. The two lowest ribs are not attached to the breastbone and are often referred to as the floating ribs. Both the lungs and the heart are housed in the rib cage. The muscles in between the ribs, known as **intercostal muscles**, and muscles in the neck, chest, and stomach are involved in breathing.

At the floor of the chest is the **diaphragm**. This is a thick muscle that is shaped like a dome and separates the stomach from the **thorax**. The lungs rest on the diaphragm, so it has an important role in our breathing. The lungs are also part of the pulmonary system, which includes both lower and upper airways. The lower airway includes the trachea, which is made up of 20 rings of cartilage, whereas the upper airway includes the mouth, nose, and upper portion of the throat.

When we breathe in, oxygen goes into the blood, and when we breathe out, we expel carbon dioxide (Owens & Farinella, 2019). When carbon dioxide accumulates in our bodies, a need for oxygen is created, and the **medulla oblongata** in the brainstem ignites impulses to the respiration muscles. Thus, the process of inhalation and exhalation creates the respiration cycle. On average, we breathe about 12 times per minute, but for younger children that rate is much faster. In fact, infants breathe at rates of 60 times per minute or higher (Hedge, 2010).

Speech is produced when we exhale, and the duration is usually longer than when we inhale or when we are silent. To produce speech, air needs to move through the **vocal folds** to help them vibrate, and respiration provides the needed air flow. To produce a louder sound or longer utterances, breathing is adjusted.

video

Check out the YouTube video **"How Does the Human Body Produce Voice and Speech?"** from the National Institutes of Health.

Phonatory System

The phonatory system involves the **larynx** (also known as the voice box), which is an organ that makes it possible to phonate or produce voice. Where the lungs provide the air supply for speech, the larynx is a valve that opens and closes, allowing air to pass through to facilitate the sound we use for speech. Importantly, the larynx has both a speech function and a biological function. Biologically, it closes the **trachea** (windpipe) so that food and other substances cannot get into the lungs, protecting the lungs from foreign substances. It also helps build up **subglottal air pressure** necessary when lifting heavy objects.

The larynx is in the front of the neck and sits on top of the trachea. It includes cartilages, membranes, and muscles, and it is suspended by the **hyoid bone**. The hyoid bone floats under the jaw, and the muscles of the tongue, skull, larynx, and jaw are attached to it. Several cartilages support the larynx, including the **thyroid**, **cricoid**, and **arytenoid cartilages**. The thyroid cartilage makes up the front and side walls of the larynx. The **cricoid cartilage**, the most important of the three, is at the top of the ring of the trachea and is linked with the thyroid and arytenoid cartilages. There are two small pyramid-like arytenoid cartilages that are connected to the cricoid cartilage via the **cricoarytenoid joint**. This allows for sliding and circular movements, and because the vocal folds are connected to the arytenoid cartilages, this joint is important for facilitating the opening and closing movements of the vocal folds during voicing.

The muscles that comprise the larynx allow us to make the movements needed to phonate. Like other muscles, they can shorten, lengthen, tense, or relax to help the vocal folds come together or move apart. An important pair of internal and external muscles that helps with vibration and sound production are the **thyroarytenoid muscles**, which are attached to the thyroid and arytenoid cartilages. The **internal thyroarytenoid muscles** are most important to the vibration and production of sound and are most often referred to as the **vocalis muscle** or the densest part of the vocal folds. Interestingly, the muscles that bring the vocal folds together and pull them apart usually work in opposition of each other such that the vocal folds can be **adducted** (pulled together) or **abducted** (pulled apart). The two pairs of muscles that bring the vocal folds together are called the **lateral cricoarytenoid** and the **interarytenoid muscles**. The **posterior cricoarytenoid muscle** serves the opposite function, abducting or pulling apart the vocal folds. The **cricothyroid muscle** (attached to the cricoid and thyroid cartilages) is responsible for lengthening (thinning) and tensing (thickening) the vocal folds. The muscles discussed here are known as intrinsic because their attachments are within the larynx. See Figure 4–1 for a visual of the intrinsic laryngeal muscles. There are also extrinsic muscles that are attached to at least one other structure besides the larynx and help keep the laryngeal mechanism in place.

Understanding the muscles and cartilages involved in the phonatory system is important if we think about the timing and coordination that must occur when we engage in conversational speech. Phonation requires that the vocal folds are flexible, can move quickly, to produce speech. At rest, the vocal folds are usually open or abducted, with the opening between them known as the **glottis**, which is usually V-shaped. When the vocal folds are closed or adducted, air pressure builds up beneath them. Because the pressure below the vocal folds is higher than that above the vocal folds, they begin to vibrate and open, starting from the bottom and moving to the top. Once this opening phase reaches the top of the vocal folds, the bottom part of the vocal folds begins to close, with the vocal folds ultimately closing for just a brief period (known as the closed phase) until air pressure builds beneath them and the entire process begins again. See Figure 4–2 for a display of phonation and inspiration and the positioning of the vocal folds when they are adducted versus abducted.

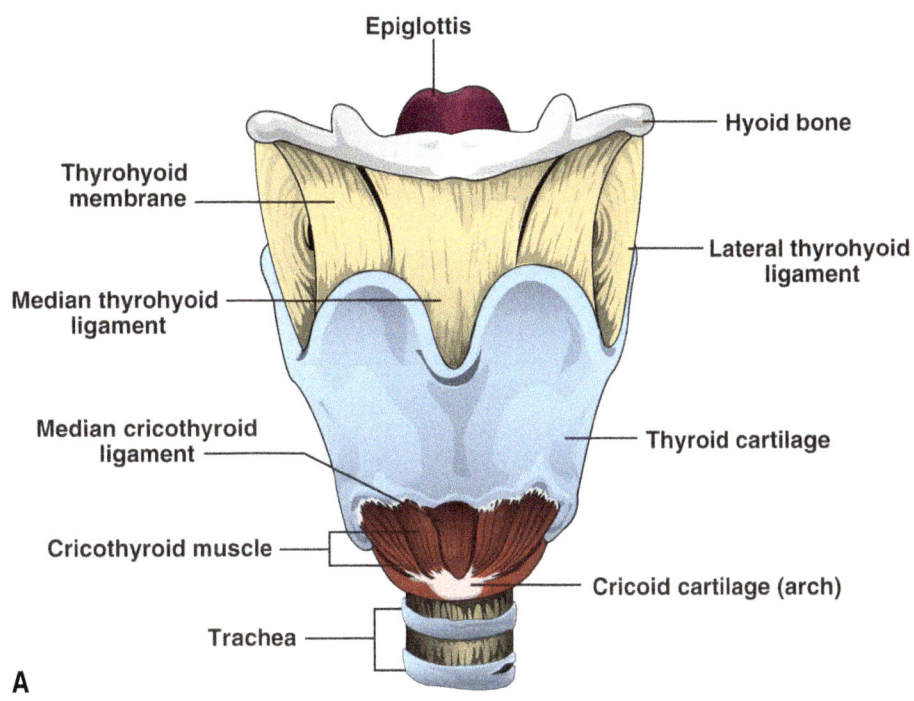

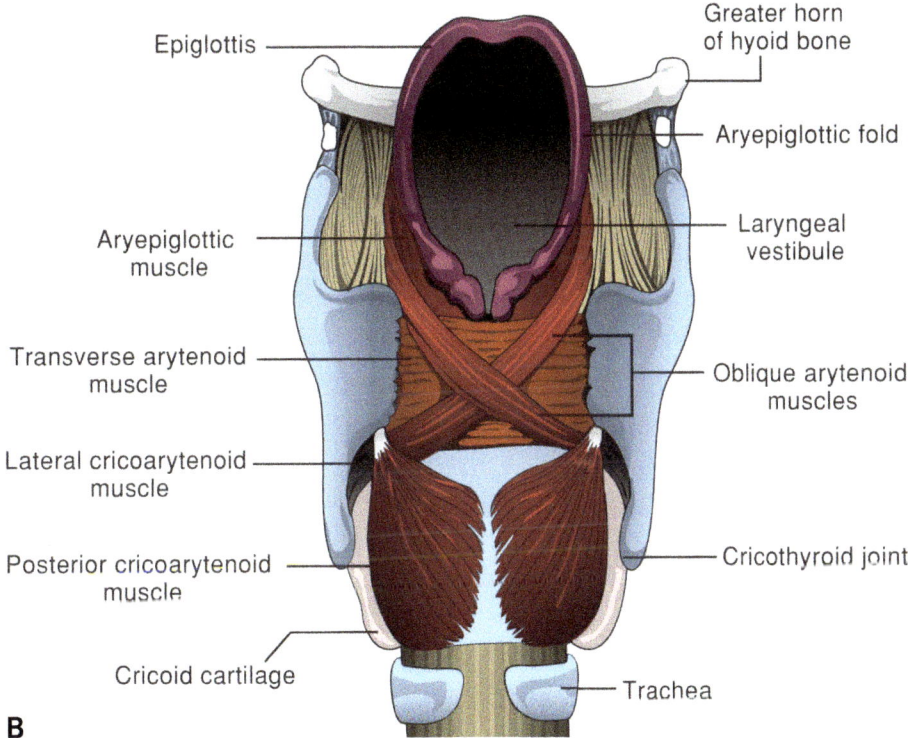

FIGURE 4–1. **A.** Anterior view of the intrinsic laryngeal muscles. *Source:* Modified from *Speech and Voice Science, Fourth Edition* (pp. 1–517) by Behrman, A. Copyright © 2022 Plural Publishing, Inc. All rights reserved. **B.** Posterior view of the intrinsic laryngeal muscles. *Source:* Modified from *Speech and Voice Science, Fourth Edition* (pp. 1–517) by Behrman, A. Copyright © 2022 Plural Publishing, Inc. All rights reserved.

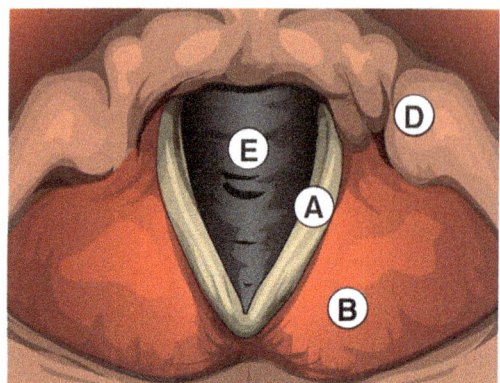

FIGURE 4–2. Phonation and inspiration with vocal folds adducted and abductors. (A) True vocal fold; (B) ventricular fold; (C) aryepiglottic fold; (D) arytenoid complex; (E) glottis. *Source:* Modified from *Speech and Voice Science, Fourth Edition* (pp. 1–517) by Behrman, A. Copyright © 2022 Plural Publishing, Inc. All rights reserved.

Interestingly, the opening of the vocal folds is explained by the buildup of air pressure beneath the vocal folds, where the closing is described by a process known as the **Bernoulli effect**. Bernouilli developed a theory that suggests when gases or liquids move through a constricted passage, the quickness of the motion, or velocity, increases while the force distributed over an area, or pressure, decreases (Hegde, 2010). In phonation, air pressure from the lungs moves through the laryngeal area and passes through the vocal folds, which represent a constricted area. This causes increased velocity and decreased pressure between the folds. Lower air pressure draws the vocal folds together, and increased pressure pushes them apart. The elasticity of the vocal folds helps explain the opening and closing action of the vocal folds, indicating that the folds are strong enough to resist the air pressure beneath them but are sufficiently elastic enough to be blown apart and then closed again. The combination of the air pressure build-up, the pressure differences, and the vocal fold elasticity is known as **myoelastic–aerodynamic theory**.

▶ video

Check out the YouTube video **"How the Larynx Produces Sound,"** which shows the components of the larynx and how they are used to produce sound.

Characteristics of Voice Production: Pitch and Loudness

There are both perceptual and physiological components of the voice we hear in others and in ourselves. **Pitch** and **loudness** are the perceptual or psychological components of the sound we hear. Yet, there are real physical changes and physiological behaviors that explain the differences in the sounds we hear.

Pitch, for example, can be explained by the actual rate of vocal fold vibration (physical characteristic) and the tension, thickening, and elasticity of the vocal folds (physiological characteristics). Vibration frequency is measured in hertz (Hz); for example, 50 Hz is equal to 50 vibrations per second (physical characteristic). The greater the frequency of vocal fold vibration, the higher the pitch we perceive (perceptual characteristic). **Fundamental frequency** describes the rate at which the vocal folds vibrate, and this is different for each person. Male fundamental frequency is approximately 125 Hz, whereas female fundamental frequency is approximately 225 Hz, meaning that males typically have a lower pitch than females. Younger children tend to have an even higher pitch, with a fundamental frequency of approximately 400 Hz (Hegde, 2010). Remember that the elasticity, mass, and tension of the vocal folds also influence the fundamental frequency, as well as the perceived pitch. Thus, longer and thicker vocal folds vibrate at a lower fundamental frequency and have a lower pitch (as you might expect in males), whereas the shorter and thinner vocal folds of females and children vibrate with a higher frequency and have a higher pitch.

Loudness also has physical and physiological features. The loudness you perceive is influenced by the amount of subglottal air pressure below the vocal folds. To increase air pressure, the vocal folds must be adducted (drawn together), and when a person is asked to speak louder, they will likely take in more air and exhale that air more forcibly.

The physiological features of loudness are **intensity** and **amplitude**. For example, greater subglottal air pressure causes higher phonation intensity—or the intensity with which the vocal folds open and close. This high intensity is associated with an increased amplitude or the extent to which the vocal folds move. With greater vocal fold movement, amplitude is higher, such as when the vocal folds abduct farther apart. So, what you hear as loudness is influenced by the increased subglottal air pressure, intensity, and amplitude of the vibrations of the vocal folds.

Articulatory System

The articulatory system is involved with both the movement of the structural elements of articulation and the production of sounds. There are several parts to the vocal tract necessary for speech production, including the pharynx, the oral cavity, and nasal cavities. These cavities serve as the resonance chambers for speech sound production.

You learned earlier in the chapter that breathing is important for producing sounds, but breathing alone is not sufficient for speech production, as several other structures are involved. Cognitively, an individual decides that they want to use exhalation of air and sound energy to produce speech. Ultimately, air is rapidly converted into speech because once you decide to speak, you activate several parts of the systems needed for speech starting from the vocal folds.

Articulators are points or places along the vocal tract involved in the production of speech sounds. They are divided into two parts: **active** and **passive articulators**.

Active articulators are those that move during the production of speech, whereas passive articulators do not move. Both are critical for sound production. For example, when you make the sounds /t/ and /d/, the vocal folds do not vibrate for /t/ (a voiceless sound), but they do vibrate for /d/ (a voiced sound). The production of /t, d/ involves the **alveolar ridge** (the bumpy ridge behind the front teeth), which is considered a passive articulator because it does not move. The tongue, on the other hand, is an active articulator that moves during sound production for /t/ and /d/. Again, both passive and active articulators are critical to sound production.

The tongue, a lingual muscle, is extremely important because it is the most active articulator. It moves throughout the oral cavity to produce various speech sounds, including to the upper part of the mouth, toward the teeth, and even down toward the bottom of the oral cavity. The tongue is the largest articulator and is divided into four parts:

- Tip: Thinnest and most flexible part of the tongue
- Blade: Small area right behind the tip and below the alveolar ridge
- Body or dorsum: Largest part of the tongue; described as having a front (or anterior part), a middle (or medial part), and a back (or posterior part) and is in contact with the hard and soft palate
- Root: Very back of the tongue

Sometimes the same sound may be produced by the blade of the tongue or the tip, depending on the phonological context and the person. The muscles of the tongue move quickly, and they can lengthen, shorten, curl up, flatten, and pull down—all important movements to support articulation. The tongue is also important for eating, including tasting food and moving food throughout the oral cavity in support of chewing and swallowing.

▶ video

Check out the YouTube video **"Active Articulators"** for an explanation of the tongue as an active articulator.

As an active articulator, the tongue works with several passive articulators to produce sounds, including the teeth, alveolar ridge, and hard palate. Although these articulators do not move, they provide an important place for the articulation of specific sounds and are important to accurate speech sound production.

▶ video

Check out the YouTube video **"Passive Articulators"** for an explanation of passive articulators.

The lower jaw, or **mandible**, is the bone on which the lower teeth are located; it is also the floor of the mouth and the frame for the lower lip and tongue. It is a single bone in adults that was the result of the fusion of two bones that connected the midpoint of the chin (Hedge, 2010). Notably, the mandible is hinged to the **temporal bone** of the skull at the **temporomandibular joint**. There are several muscles that help the jaw open and close, not just for sound production but also for chewing food.

The teeth also have an important role in articulation, and the sockets that house them are known as the **alveolar process**. The teeth are primarily used for chewing or mastication, but they also help make some speech sounds. For example, the teeth are an important articulator for the /f/ and /v/ sounds, where the lips and teeth come together.

The lips and cheeks are part of the facial musculature. The lips are made up of the **orbicularis oris muscle** to which several muscles of the chin and cheeks are connected, making lip movements possible. Lips are important to the production of labial sounds, such as /p/ and /b/, where both lips are used. Lip closure helps build intraoral (within the mouth) air pressure, which can be released in a plosive manner to help produce sounds such as /p, b/.

Resonatory System

There are several structures important to normal resonance during speech production, including the facial structures, the soft and hard palates, the articulators, and the pharynx (Fogle, 2019). The **soft palate** or **velum** is a musculature structure that is flexible and is positioned at the juncture of the **oropharynx** and the **nasopharynx**. It is in the back of the mouth beyond the **hard palate** (i.e., the roof of the mouth). There is a small cone-shaped tip of the velum, which is known as the **uvula**. The soft palate is an active articulatory structure, which can be raised or lowered. When the velum is raised, it helps close off the nasal cavity from the oral cavity to produce non-nasal sounds. When the velum is lowered, the nasal cavity is open and allows air to travel through the nose. Figure 4–3 shows the **velopharyngeal mechanism** needed for

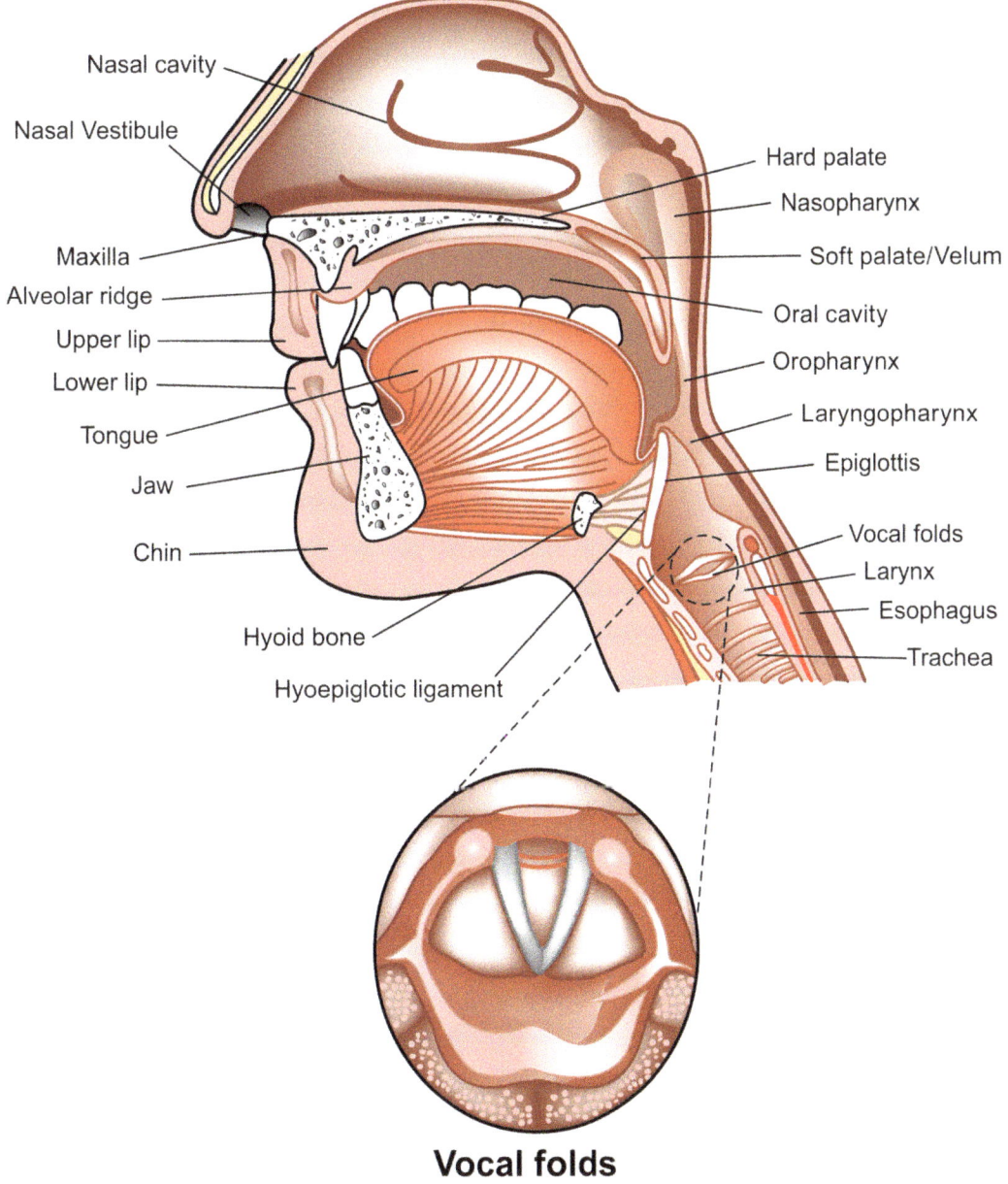

FIGURE 4–3. Velopharyngeal mechanism for speech production.

speech production. "The velopharyngeal (VP) mechanism is a muscular valve that controls the amount of nasal acoustic energy and oral pressure for speech production through opening and closing, respectively" (Kotlarek et al., 2022, p. 3365). It is located behind the hard palate and includes the **velum** as well as the walls of the **pharynx**. The muscle that elevates the velum, known as the **levator veli palatini** muscle, has a critical role in the closure required for speech production (Kotlarek et al., 2022). Figure 4–4 provides an example of how non-nasal versus nasal sounds are produced by the elevation or lowering of the velum. Growth of the velopharyngeal mechanism continues through adolescence. If the muscle is insufficient, however, then **velopharyngeal closure** of the nasal cavity may not occur. An individual will sound more nasal than they should, especially for sounds for which the nasal cavity should be closed off. This often occurs when an individual has a **cleft palate**. Figure 4–5 shows an example of a complete cleft palate.

The hard palate is the bony part of the roof of the mouth and provides the floor of the nose. The hard palate is composed of two bones called the **maxillae** (singular: maxilla). The front part of the maxillae bone is the **premaxilla**, which comprises the incisors or upper front four teeth. During the growth process, the premaxilla grows separately and then fuses with the **maxillary bone**. Most of the hard palate is made up of the **palatine bone** (or palatine process). The palatine process occurs when two pieces of the bone grow and come together at midline; this typically occurs in the fetal stage of development. If the fusion of the bones does not occur, this can result in palatal clefts that impact speech production and resonance.

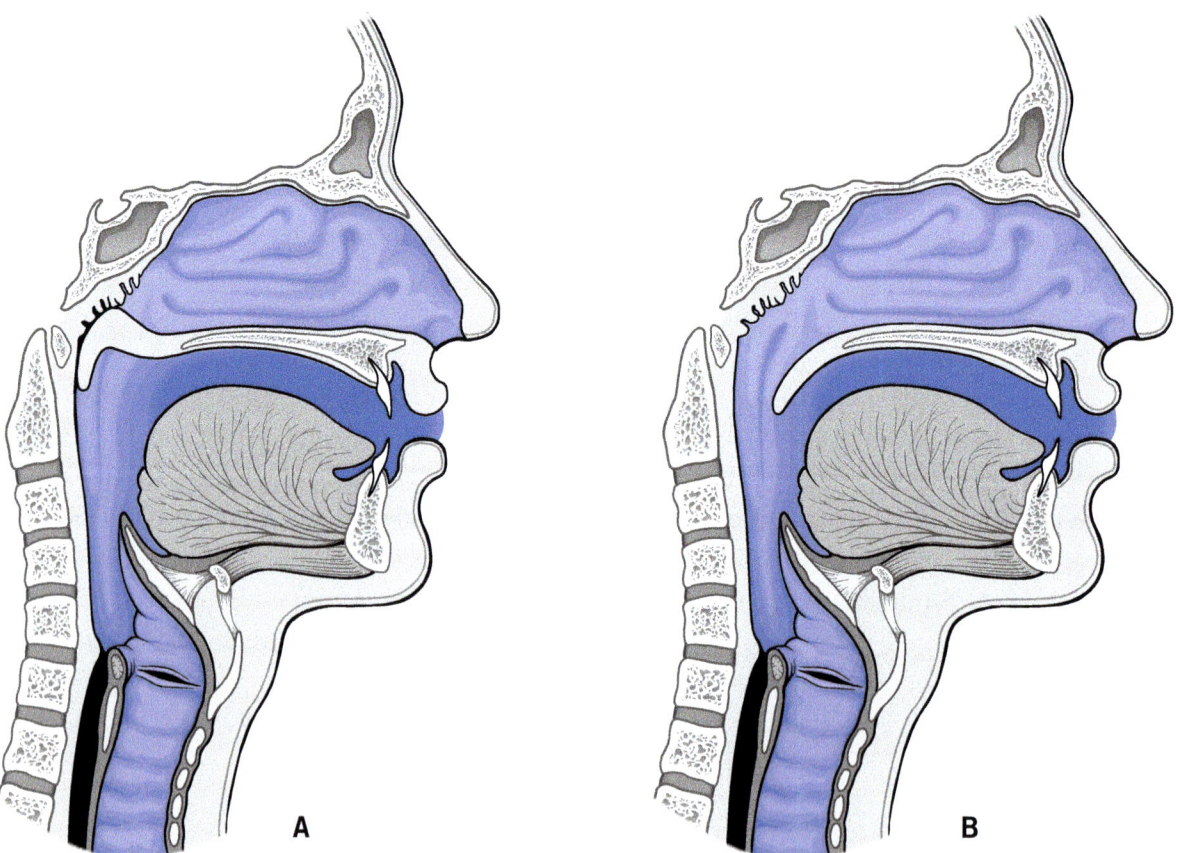

FIGURE 4–4. Elevation of the velum for non-nasal sounds (**A**) and lowering of the velum for nasal sound production (**B**). *Source:* From *Speech and Voice Science, Fourth Edition* (pp. 1–517) by Behrman, A. Copyright © 2022 Plural Publishing, Inc. All rights reserved.

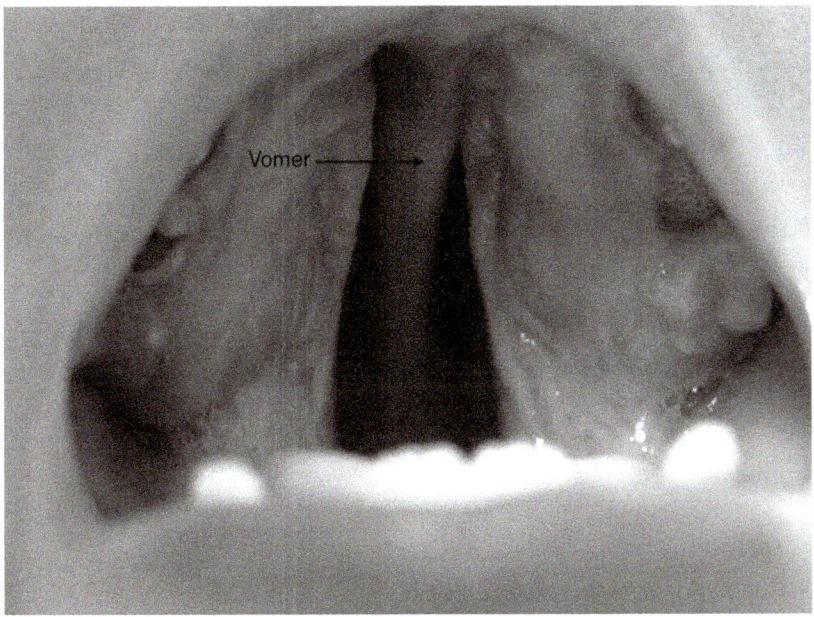

FIGURE 4–5. A view of a complete cleft palate with midline nasal septum visible. *Source:* From *Evaluation and Management of Cleft Lip and Palate: A Developmental Perspective* (pp. 1–418) by Zajac, D. J., & Vallino-Napoli, L. D. Copyright © 2017 Plural Publishing, Inc. All rights reserved.

Chapter Summary

When we speak, several structures are activated, including the abdomen, chest, mouth, and throat. The brain helps regulate these actions. A speaker uses air to vibrate the vocal folds, and the tongue, teeth, and soft and hard palates help shape recognizable speech sounds (Hegde, 2010). The mouth, nose and throat cavities help adjust sound quality.

The respiratory system involves the lungs, ribs, diaphragm, and several muscles that function to expel carbon dioxide from the body through exhalation and take oxygen in through inhalation (Baker, 2018). This breathing process is ultimately needed for speech production. The vocal folds are critical to sound production because vibration of the vocal folds determines if a sound is produced as voiced or voiceless. The tongue is a major articulator for phonation because its movement and ability to change shape facilitate the production of several different sounds. Articulators such as the tongue, lips, teeth, and so on can be active (move) or passive (do not move), both of which are crucial to the kinds of sounds we are able to make. The resonatory system—or how air flows through the oral, nasal, and pharyngeal cavities—also impacts our ability to produce sounds in words that increase the intelligibility of the speech we produce.

Chapter Review Questions

1. What are the roles of the three primary cartilages of the vocal mechanism?
2. Compare and contrast active versus passive articulators, and give an example of each during sound production.

3. What is the Bernoulli effect and why is it important to speech sound production?
4. Describe the four primary parts of the tongue and the importance of the tongue to sound production.
5. What is the importance of the respiratory system to speech production?
6. Describe the biological and speech functions of the larynx.
7. Explain the perceptual and physiological features of the voice we hear.
8. What is the role of the soft palate in determining resonance?
9. What are the components of the oropharynx and nasopharynx, and why are they important to speech production?
10. What is the importance of subglottal air pressure to speech production?

Learning Activities

1. Check out the YouTube video "Larynx Anatomy (Cartilage, Ligaments, Joints, Wall, Cavity)" for a description of the larynx. Draw the larynx and label the primary cartilages and muscles of the vocal mechanism.

▶ video

"Larynx Anatomy (Cartilage, Ligaments, Joints, Wall, Cavity)"

2. Draw an example of the vocal folds as abducted and one that represents adduction. Identify some sounds that are made when the vocal folds are abducted (voiceless) and some sounds that are made when the vocal folds are adducted (voiced).
3. Draw and label the parts of the tongue. Describe what parts of the tongue are involved in the productions of the following sounds: /t, g, l, r, ʃ, dʒ, j/.
4. Create a visual to explain respiration.
5. Look up the cranial nerves that are important to speech production, and describe what structures in the vocal mechanism are affected by which nerves.

References

Baker, L. (2018). Anatomy and physiology of the speech mechanism and features of the human body. *Fishladder: A Student Journal of Art and Writing, 16*(1), Article 32.

Fogle, P. T. (2019). Anatomy and physiology of speech and language. In *Essentials of communication sciences and disorders* (pp. 36–56). Jones & Bartlett.

Hegde, M. N. (2010). Anatomy and physiology of speech and language. In *Introduction to communicative disorders* (pp. 93–132). Pro-Ed.

Kotlarek, K. J., Levene, S., Piccorelli, A. V., Barhaghi, K., & Neuberger, I. (2022). Growth effects on velopharyngeal anatomy within the first 2 years of life. *Journal of Speech, Language and Hearing Research, 65*(9), 3365–3376.

Owens, R. E., & Farinella, K. A. (2019). Overview of the anatomy and physiology of the speech production mechanism. In *Introduction to communication disorders* (6th ed., pp. 45–62). Pearson.

Chapter 5

Developmental Speech Sound Disorders

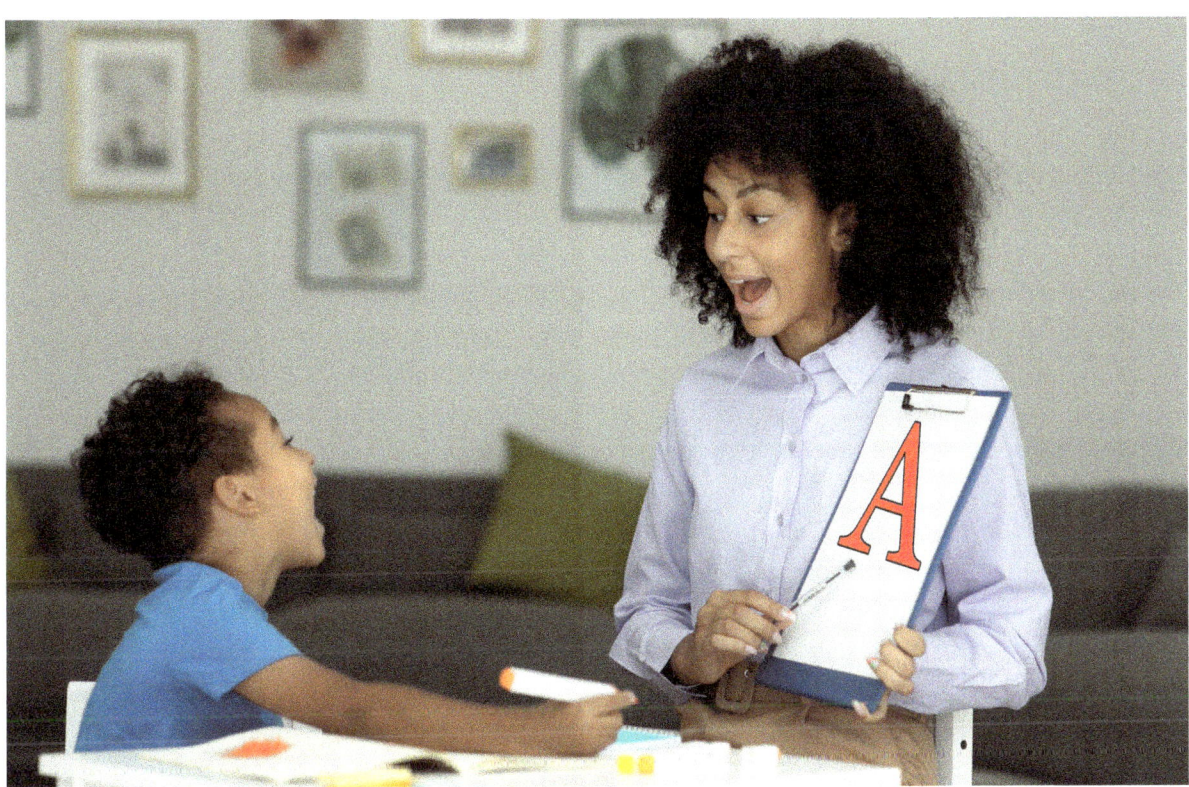

Learning Objectives

After reading this chapter, you will be able to:

- Explain the development of speech sounds.
- Describe and differentiate articulation and phonological disorders.
- Identify the social–cultural differences in speech sound disorders.
- Discuss the disparities in access to assessment and intervention for speech sound disorders in children.

Key Terms

accent	lateral lisp
articulation	manner
articulation disorder	organic speech sound disorders
dialect	phonological awareness
final consonant deletion	phonological disorder
fronting	place
functional speech sound disorders	stimulability
gliding	submucous cleft palate
initial consonant deletion	voicing
interdental (frontal) lisp	

Introduction

Have you ever known someone, perhaps even you as a child, who had difficulty producing sounds (e.g., /r/ or /s/), which resulted in mispronunciation of words (e.g., saying "wed" for "red" or "thit" for "sit")? You may also remember having difficulty producing multisyllabic words such as "banana" or "telephone," leaving out syllables and saying instead "nana" or "tephone." Still others of you may have dropped off the ends of words, saying "ca" for "cat" or "do" for "dog." Speech disorders are characterized by challenges with the speech component of communication, including difficulty saying sounds (speech sound disorders), voice disorders (see Chapter 11), and fluency disorders (see Chapter 10). This chapter focuses on a child's speech sound disorders with unknown causes, typically called articulation and phonological disorders. **Articulation** is the ability to make sounds involving the coordinated movement of the tongue, lips, teeth, hard and soft palates, and the respiratory system that provides the air necessary for speech sound production. **Articulation disorders** occur when an individual produces errors on individual speech sounds (sometimes multiple individual sounds) that are typically mastered by their age. A **phonological disorder** is a type of speech sound disorder in which individuals produce errors on patterns of sounds, and these errors are predictable based on the rules of language. Like articulation disorders, production of these errors is not age appropriate. It can often be tricky to differentiate articulation and phonological disorders, so understanding the two is key!

The *Diagnostic and Statistical Manual of Mental Disorders* (American Psychiatric Association, 2022) describes speech sound disorders as part of the broader category of communication disorders and describes the characteristics of a speech sound disorder as follows:

- Ongoing difficulty producing speech sounds that impacts a child's ability to be understood
- Limits a child's effectiveness as a communicator and their social participation
- Symptoms are seen early on
- Not the result of other acquired (e.g., traumatic brain injury or stroke) or congenital conditions (e.g., cerebral palsy, cleft palate, hearing loss)
- Can co-occur with other conditions such as Down syndrome, 22q deletion, and so on

Articulation and phonological disorders with no known cause occur at a rate of 8% or 9% (Law et al., 2000; Shriberg et al., 1999). In the sections that follow, you will learn more about the risk factors for articulation and phonological disorders, the variance in prevalence, the symptoms that might be observed, what type of assessments are important to identify a speech delay or speech sound disorder, cultural considerations in assessment, and a range of interventions used to treat a speech sound disorder.

What We Know About This Topic

Speech sound disorder refers to any difficulty or combination of difficulties with perception, motor production, or phonological representation of speech sounds, including the rules governing allowable speech sound sequences in a language. A speech sound disorder can be organic, resulting from an underlying neurological, structural, sensory, or motor impairment, or it can be functional (no known cause). Figure 5–1 provides a visual of the speech sound disorder categories you might see in children.

An example of a motor or neurological difference that affects speech production is childhood apraxia of speech, which is discussed in Chapter 6. A structurally involved speech sound disorder is cleft palate, as mentioned and visualized in Chapter 4. Hearing loss is an example of a sensory disorder that affects speech sound production, and it is further described in Chapter 13

Functional speech sound disorders do not have a known cause and are related to the linguistic and the motor aspects of speech sound production. These speech sound disorders include articulation and phonological disorders. Articulation disorders focus on the errors that children make in their individual speech production (e.g., substituting one sound for another), whereas phonological disorders focus on rule-based errors (e.g., deleting the final consonant in the production of words). Because it is sometimes difficult to differentiate between these two disorder types, clinicians and researchers often use the term "speech sound disorders" as a broader category. The focus of this chapter is functional speech sound disorders.

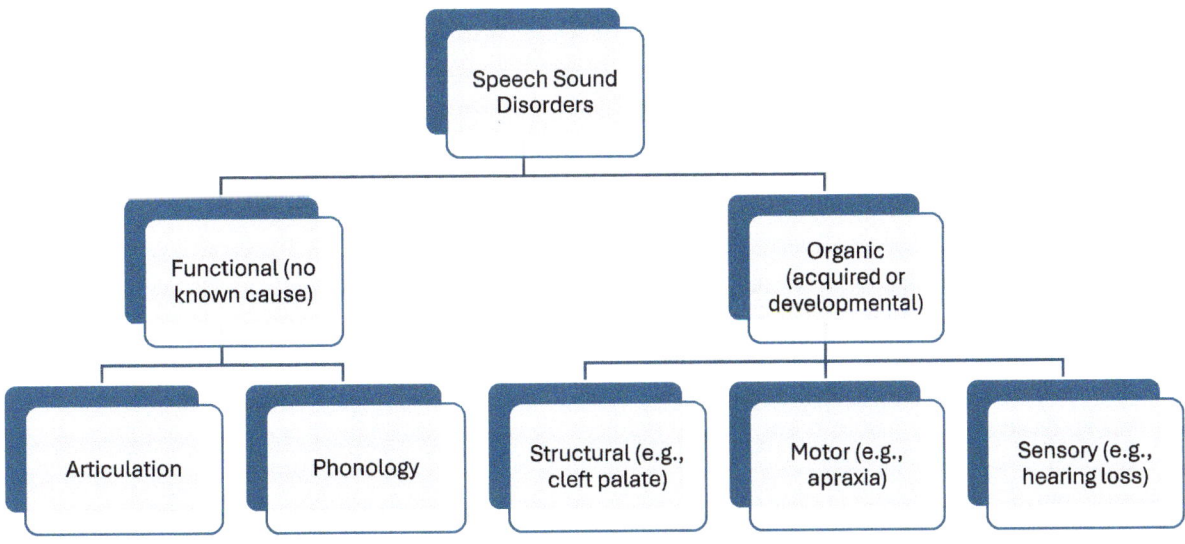

FIGURE 5–1. Speech sound disorders in children.

See the **ASHA Childhood Apraxia of Speech Practice Portal** and the **ASHA Cleft Lip and Palate Practice Portal** to learn more about two common organic speech sound disorders in children.

Importantly, speech sound production difficulties in young children are frequently connected to poor literacy outcomes (Overby et al., 2012) and an increased likelihood of reading disorders (Peterson et al., 2009).

Risk Factors for Functional Speech Sound Disorders

Although the causes of functional speech sound disorders are unknown, several risk factors are relevant. For example, biological sex seems to be an influencing factor, with higher occurrences in males than females (Shriberg et al., 1999). Prenatal and perinatal difficulties such as complications in delivery, infections or stress during pregnancy, low birthweight, and premature birth have been associated with difficulties in acquiring speech sounds along the expected developmental trajectory (Fox et al., 2002). In fact, children born very preterm who show speech sound problems at age 2½ years continue to exhibit persistent speech problems and expressive language disorders at age 4 years (Van Noort-van der Sepk et al., 2022). A family history of speech or language difficulties increases the likelihood of having a speech sound disorder (Campbell et al., 2003; Fox et al., 2002). In addition, as described in Chapter 13, persistent otitis media with effusion (fluid within the middle ear), which is often associated with hearing loss, can impact speech development.

Incidence/Prevalence of Childhood Speech Sound Disorders

Estimated prevalence rates of speech sound disorders—that is, children living with a speech sound disorder at any point in time—vary because of inconsistent classifications and age ranges under investigation. Prevalence rates for speech delay or speech sound disorders vary from 2.3% to 24.6% of school-aged children (Black et al., 2015; Law et al., 2000; Shriberg et al., 1999; Wren et al., 2016). In a 2012 survey from the Center for Health Statistics, nearly half of 3- to 10-year-old children and one-fourth of 11- to 17-year-old children had speech sound problems, with an estimated two-thirds of them receiving intervention support (Black et al., 2015). It appears that speech sound disorders are more common in males than females, and persistent speech errors occur for 1% to 2% of adolescents and adults (Flipsen, 2015; Shriberg et al., 1999; Wren et al., 2016). Notably, research indicates that 11% to 40% of children with speech sound disorders also have a language disorder (see Chapter 7; see also Eadie et al., 2015).

See the **ASHA Speech Sound Disorders Evidence Map** for research summaries on speech sound disorders.

Characteristics of Speech Sound Disorders

There are several signs and symptoms that suggest the presence of a speech sound disorder. A child might omit or delete a particular sound in a word, or they might substitute one sound for another. Sometimes, a child will insert an extra sound in a word, delete a syllable, or distort the production of a sound. These signs and symptoms may occur as independent articulation errors, such as producing a **lateral lisp** or **interdental lisp** to produce the /s/ sound or substituting a /w/ for an /r/ sound (e.g., saying "wed" for "red").

Speech sound errors might also occur because of a rule-based error pattern such as deleting all final consonants from words. It is important to explore in greater detail the rule-based error patterns typically seen in children with phonological disorders. There are times in early speech development when error patterns exist. These error patterns are known as **phonological processes** and are common in the speech development of young children. For example, a child might delete the final consonants of words, such as saying [ca] for "cat," which is known as **final consonant deletion**. A child might also drop a consonant from a cluster of consonants in a word, such as saying "sop" for "stop," which is known as **cluster reduction**. In addition, they might replace a sound that is more difficult to produce in the back of the mouth (e.g., [g]) with an easier sound that is produced in the front of the mouth (e.g., [d]), such as when producing "dot" for "got"—a process known as **fronting**. These are some of the ways that a child might simplify their production of words as they are developing their speech sound system. These phonological processes are not necessarily cause for concern, as children with typically developing speech and language often produce these error patterns as they are developing speech and language skills. These phonological processes tend to be reduced or eliminated on their own as children grow older. Table 5–1 shows the most common phonological processes you might see in young children who are English speakers. Notably, different languages will have different phonological processes as children are learning the sound systems of their language.

There are some processes, however, that are less common in young children as they are learning their speech sound system. These more rare processes would likely be a red flag and might suggest a possible speech sound disorder. For example, deleting the initial consonant of a word (known as **initial consonant deletion**) is an unusual developmental pattern for English but might be a more common pattern in another language (e.g., Japanese). Typically, children learning English will stop using these simplification processes (as seen on the left side of Table 5–1) by age 3 years, but some processes (as seen on the right side of Table 5–1) will persist until age 8 years (Prelock & Hutchins, 2018; Stoel-Gammon & Dunn, 1985). When phonological processes continue to persistent beyond the expected developmental period, the child will likely be identified as having a speech sound disorder.

www

See the **ASHA Selected Phonological Processes (Patterns) Practice Portal** for some examples of these rule-based error patterns.

Cultural Considerations in Speech Production

Speech sound production might also be influenced by an individual's accent or dialect. An **accent** is the unique pronunciation of speech by people who speak the same language. Accents can be regional (e.g., Boston, MA, vs. New Orleans, LA) or can be foreign when the phonetic characteristics of one language

TABLE 5–1. Common Phonological Processes in Typical English Development

Processes Seen Prior to Age 3 Years	Processes Seen After Age 3 Years
Unstressed syllable deletion: Dropping the unstressed syllable within a word Example: "gorilla" → "rilla"	**Consonant cluster reduction:** Dropping a consonant sound when two or more consonants are together Examples: "stop" → "top"; "street" → "teet"
Final consonant deletion: Dropping the consonant at the end of a word Examples: "cat" → "ca"; "bag" → "ba"	**Gliding:** Replacing a vowel-like sound known as a **glide** [w, y] for a liquid sound [l, r] Examples: "red" → "wed"; "pillow" → "piwow"
Reduplication: Repeating a syllable for a word Examples: "bottle" → "bobo"; "water" → "wawa"	**Epenthesis:** Adding an extra vowel sound in a word Examples: "clock" → "calock"; "play" → "palay"
Doubling: Repeating a word Examples: "no" → "no no"; "pop" → "pop pop"	**Stopping:** Replacing a sound where the air is blocked by closing the lips (stops) for a sound where air escapes like a hissing sound (fricatives or affricates) Examples: "sip" → "tip"; "perch" → "pert"
Diminutization: Adding "eee" at the end of a word Examples: "dog" → "doggie"; "bird" → "birdie"	**Vocalization:** Replacing a liquid with vowel at the end of a word or syllable Examples: "butter" → "butto"; "paddle" → "paddo"

Sources: Adapted from Prelock and Hutchins (2018).

are carried over to the new language a person is learning or speaking. Furthermore, for people who speak more than one language, the speech sound productions of their first language may influence the production of speech sounds in subsequent languages. Accents are not speech sound or language disorders and are instead a reflection of speech and language differences seen in different regional or international populations.

www

See the **ASHA Cultural and Linguistic Diversity (CLD) Evidence Map** for research on cultural and linguistic diversity.

Some sound substitutions and omissions may not be speech errors and instead are related to a speaker's **dialect**. Dialects are rule-governed and reflect the regional and social background of a speaker. Variations in language dialects can impact phonology, morphology, syntax, semantics, and pragmatics. For example, a phonological dialectal variation for speakers of African American English (AAE) is the use of the /d/ sound for the "th" sound, such as saying "dis" for "this." This variation would not be considered a speech sound disorder but instead a dialectal variation and phonological feature of AAE.

It is important for speech-language pathologists (SLPs) to recognize the difference between accents, dialects, and speech sound disorders. It is also important to be familiar with assessment procedures that are nondiscriminatory, to evaluate potential sources of bias, and to analyze information considering what is known about accent and particularly dialect use (McLeod et al., 2017).

See ASHA's document **"Speech Characteristics: Selected Populations"** (PDF) for a brief summary of selected populations and characteristic speech problems.

What Can We Do to Address This Communication Challenge?

Delays in speech and language can lead to challenges for children and their families. In fact, research suggests that schoolchildren with such delays may be at increased risk for having a learning disorder that affects their reading and writing. In this section, we describe approaches to screening, assessment and intervention for speech sound disorders in children.

Assessment

When a speech sound disorder is suspected, screening usually occurs first to determine if a child requires further assessment. There are several components to a speech screening, including the following:

- Informally examining individual speech sound productions in single words and connected speech
- An oral motor examination to assess strength and range of motion of the articulators
- A hearing screening
- An orofacial examination to assess symmetry of the face and possible structural reasons for a speech sound problem, such as a **submucous cleft palate**
- An informal screening of the child's language comprehension and production

Several potential outcomes could be determined from a screening, such as a recommendation to monitor the child's speech and rescreen later, refer the child for a comprehensive speech sound assessment, and/or refer the child to other health professionals (e.g., an audiologist if hearing screening suggests a potential hearing loss or an otolaryngologist if a submucous cleft is suspected). Importantly, the U.S. Preventive Services Task Force (2024) conducted a systematic review to determine the likely benefits and potential harms of screening children younger than age 5 years with no symptoms or reported concerns for speech and language delays. They found insufficient evidence to require screening when no symptoms or parental concerns were noted. This is important because it helps the SLP focus their screening efforts on children with observed signs and symptoms or reported concerns.

See the **assessment section** of the **ASHA Speech Sound Disorders Evidence Map** that provides relevant evidence on assessment in speech sound disorders.

When a screening does reveal speech delays or suggests a possible speech sound disorder, a comprehensive speech sound assessment is often the next step. Notably, speech sound acquisition is a developmental process. Recall that children will exhibit typical errors or phonological patterns that would be expected in younger children. This is taken into consideration before a comprehensive assessment is implemented to differentiate between a typical error that is age appropriate and a speech sound disorder.

Assessment will involve the use of a variety of tools, some of which are standardized assessment, as well as informal and formal measures. The selection of measures (and interpretation of results) should consider the child's cultural and linguistical background as well as the presence of a dialect (McLeod et al., 2017). If the assessment measures selected were not normed on the child's linguistic and/or cultural group, standard scores are not used because they are not representative of the child's language.

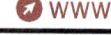

See the **ASHA Assessment Tools, Techniques, and Data Sources Practice Portal** for more information.

The speech sound assessment should also be aligned with the World Health Organization's (WHO) *International Classification of Functioning, Disability, and Health* (ICF) framework, described in Chapter 2 (ASHA, 2016; WHO, 2001). This alignment provides a description of the child's speech sound characteristics in each of the following areas:

- Impairments in body structure and function: Includes the child's speech sound strengths and challenges
- Comorbid deficits or conditions: Identification of any other co-occurring conditions such as a syndrome or medical condition that could explain the speech sound disorder
- Limitations in activity and participation: If/how the speech sound disorder interferes with the child's ability to communicate functionally and engage in interactions with their peers, family members, and others
- Contextual (environmental and personal) factors: Barriers and facilitators of communication in the child's environment

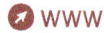

See ASHA's document **"Person-Centered Focus on Function: Speech Sound Disorder"** (PDF) for an example of information collected for a speech sound assessment consistent with the ICF.

There are several specific elements to a speech sound disorder assessment, including taking a case history; performing an oral mechanism examination; completing a hearing screening if one was not already done during screening (see Chapter 13 for a discussion of hearing assessment); and implementing a speech sound assessment including measures of severity, intelligibility, and stimulability. In addition, a language assessment might also be warranted because speech sound disorders and language disorders often co-occur (see Chapter 7 for a discussion of language assessment).

A case history obtains information about the family's concerns; any history of middle ear infections; languages spoken in the home and the child's primary language; and any family history of speech sound disorders or related language, reading, and writing difficulties. During the case history, it is also important to gather information about the parents' and teachers' perceptions of intelligibility and how the child participates in conversations at home and at school.

In an oral mechanism examination, the clinician evaluates the structure and function of the child's speech mechanism to determine adequacy for speech production. The clinician will look for dental occlusion; hard and soft palate structures; and the strength and mobility of the tongue, velum, jaw, and lips.

The assessment of speech sound samples speech production in single words and in sentences. Testing sound production in single words and at the sentence level provides opportunities to assess specific consonants in several phonetic contexts. Note, however, that this may not accurately reflect a child's sound production in connected speech. Therefore, speech sound sampling in connected speech, including at the sentence and conversational levels, is important. Speech sound production in connected speech is best assessed through describing pictures, telling stories, or engaging in conversation. Some connected speech tasks provide more structure than others, such as picture descriptions versus spontaneous, conversational speech. It is important to get a sense of what a child's speech is like in both structured and spontaneous settings.

When completing a speech sound assessment, clinicians examine production of sounds at the beginning, in the middle, and at the end of words. They are also interested in the child's accuracy in producing different vowel sound combinations and consonant clusters. When assessing speech sound errors, clinicians look for consistency in the errors produced, the types of errors (e.g., additions, deletions, distortions, omissions, substitutions), and the position in which the error occurs within a word. They also look for error patterns or phonological simplifications that affect different sound classes (see Table 5–1).

Understanding the severity of a child's speech sound disorder and its impact on intelligibility are important qualitative judgments clinicians make that help them determine priority of intervention needs. Severity is usually assessed with rating scales and some quantitative measures, although there is no agreement on the best way to evaluate speech sound disorder severity. Two common strategies are (a) the use of a numerical scale from mild (few substitutions; omissions uncommon) to profound (Prezas & Hodson, 2010) and (b) the percentage of consonants correct (PCC) within a speech sample. PCC is calculated by counting the correctly produced consonants and dividing this by the total number of consonants, and then multiplying this by 100. A score of 85% or higher is considered to be mild in severity, and a score of lower than 50% is considered to be severe (Shriberg & Kwiatkowski, 1982a, 1982b).

An assessment of intelligibility is a perceptual judgment that indicates the percentage of a child's speech that a communication partner understands. Like severity, intelligibility varies along a continuum from *intelligible* (completely understood) to *unintelligible* (not understood; Bernthal et al., 2017). Several factors influence a child's intelligibility, including the number and type of errors produced, the rate of the child's speech, their utterance complexity, and the listener's familiarity with the child's unique speech pattern. Rating scales have also been used to estimate intelligibility using anchors such as *not at all, seldom, sometimes, most of the time,* or *always* (Ertmer, 2010).

Stimulability is the ability to correctly produce or imitate a sound the child has previously misarticulated when the clinician provides an accurate model for the sound (Glaspey & Stoel-Gammon, 2007). Assessing stimulability is important because it helps determine a child's ability to produce that sound in different contexts (e.g., isolation syllable, word, phrase) and identifies the cueing (e.g., visual, tactile, auditory) needed to achieve the most accurate sound production. Stimulability testing also helps determine if a sound is likely to be learned without intervention and which sounds might be the most appropriate for intervention (Tyler & Tolbert, 2002).

Both stimulability and intelligibility are useful predictors of children who may or may not require intervention. Children with decreased intelligibility and limited stimulability are more likely to be priorities for intervention, whereas children who have speech sound errors but are relatively intelligible and their error sounds are highly stimulable are less likely to be identified as a priority for intervention (To et al., 2022).

There are several possible outcomes of a comprehensive speech sound assessment, including the following:

- A profile of the child's speech sound characteristics is developed.
- A speech sound disorder is identified.
- The severity of the child's speech sound disorder is identified.
- Possible speech sound targets for intervention are identified.
- Co-occurring conditions that may explain the child's speech sound disorder are determined.
- A language disorder is recognized.
- No speech sound disorder is identified.
- Referrals to other professionals are made.

Cultural Considerations for Assessing Bilingual Children

As previously mentioned, assessment of a bilingual (or multilingual) child requires knowledge about both (or all) languages because the sound system of one may influence that of another. In the assessment, the clinician's task is to determine whether sound production differences are the result of a speech sound disorder or are the typical differences that are evident in the speech of children speaking more than one language. It is important to gather a history of the child's language use to determine which language(s) should be assessed. Clinicians also must understand the phonemic inventory as well as the phonological and syllable structures of the child's non-English language. Speech sound assessments should occur at the single word and connected speech levels in both (or all) of the child's languages. The clinician should focus on identifying the child's substitution patterns and the linguistic effects of the child's native language on English (Fabiano-Smith & Goldstein, 2010). Understanding the child's dialect is also crucial to the assessment.

www

See ASHA's resources for **Phonemic Inventories and Cultural and Linguistic Information Across Languages** for more information on determining language differences versus language disorders.

Intervention for Childhood Speech Disorders

Intervention strategies that focus on the motor production of speech sounds are called articulation approaches, whereas interventions that emphasize the linguistic aspects of speech production are called phonological/language-based approaches. Articulation intervention approaches target accurate production of individual sounds. In contrast, phonological or language-based approaches target sound error patterns. The goal is to teach the child the phonological rule so that they can generalize this rule to other sounds in that pattern (e.g., initial consonant deletion, final consonant deletion, syllable reduction). Both approaches can be used in the treatment of speech sound disorders, which ultimately lead to three different levels of skill acquisition:

- Establishment—the ability to consistently and correctly produce a target sound deliberately
- Generalization—the ability to carry over correct production of the target sound to other linguistic contexts (e.g., syllables to words, words to phrases, phrases to sentences, sentences to conversational speech)
- Maintenance—the ability to produce target sounds automatically as well as monitor speech production, recognize when an error is made, and self-correct that error

See the **treatment section** of the **ASHA Speech Sound Disorders Evidence Map** for relevant research evidence on treatment approaches to speech sound disorders.

Choosing a Target

An important component to speech sound intervention is the selection of the target sound(s) for intervention. Typically, sounds are selected based on their developmental appropriateness; that is, sounds that are acquired earlier in development are likely to be the initial targets selected. However, there are other approaches to target sound selection that are less developmental and consider the child's phonological system to encourage generalized sound learning (Storkel, 2018). Another approach focuses on the phonological function of the sound and selecting targets from the child's errors in terms of **place** (i.e., where the articulators are positioned), **manner** (i.e., the way the sound is produced), and **voicing** (i.e., whether the vocal folds vibrate to produce the sound) that are distinct (Williams, 2003). See Table 5–2 for the place, manner, and voicing for English consonants. Targets might also be specific to the child and the relevance of the sound to the child and their family (e.g., sounds in the child's name), whether the sound is stimulable, and whether the production of the sound is visible. In addition, targets might be selected based on errors that most affect intelligibility.

Techniques and Strategies to Support Intervention

There are several techniques and strategies that clinicians use to increase a child's awareness of the placement and articulatory movement for accurate production of the target sound(s), including the following:

- Providing visual cueing for place or manner of production
- Using ultrasound imaging to visualize the configuration and position of the tongue (Lee et al., 2015; Preston et al., 2014)
- Amplifying target sounds to increase sound awareness and discrimination through auditory bombardment (Hodson, 2010)

TABLE 5–2. Place, Manner, and Voicing for English Consonants

Place	Manner	Voicing Voiced	Voiceless
	Stop		
Bilabial		b	p
Alveolar		d	t
Velar		g	k
Glottal			ʔ
	Fricative		
Labiodental		v	f
Linguadental		ð	θ
Alveolar		z	s
Palatal			
Glottal			h
	Affricate		
Palatal		dʒ	tʃ
	Glide		
Bilabial		w	—
Palatal		j	—
	Liquid		
Alveolar		l	—
Palatal		r	—
	Nasal		
Bilabial		m	—
Alveolar		n	—
Velar		ŋ	

- Providing biofeedback through a visual representation of the acoustic signal of speech (McAllister Byun & Hitchcock, 2012)
- Using speech-to-text as a form of biofeedback to improve speech production of targeted phonemes (Findley & Gasaryan, 2022)
- Implementing target "attack strategies" that incorporate different ways to provide sound practice
  - Vertical strategy: Focusing practice on one or two sounds until the child reaches a criterion level (usually connected speech) before moving to another target (Fey, 1986)

- Horizontal strategy: Multiple sounds individually targeted with less intense practice, increasing exposure to the broader sound system (Fey, 1986)
- Cyclical strategy: Using both horizontal and vertical strategies where the child practices given sounds for a set period before moving on to other sounds for a set period and then cycling through all the sounds again (Hodson, 2010)

Intervention Approaches for Supporting Sound Production

Intervention approaches are dependent on several considerations, such as a child age, speech error type, speech sound severity, and the impact on intelligibility (Williams et al., 2010). Table 5–3 provides brief descriptions of a few options that might be selected to support speech sound production in children (ASHA, n.d.).

Intervention approaches

Intervention Considerations for Culturally and Linguistically Diverse Populations

As you learned previously, one linguistic sound system may influence the other, and it is important for the SLP to identify whether differences are the result of a communication difference or disorder. Several strategies might be considered when designing an intervention plan for a culturally and linguistic diverse child. First, it is important to determine if a bilingual approach will be used and what language will be used when providing services. The SLP may need to find alternative ways to provide accurate speech sound models in the child's language protocol. Assessing generalization of accurate sound production across the child's languages will also be important to determining treatment success (Goldstein & Fabiano, 2007).

Service Delivery Options

Once an SLP determines the target for intervention and the type of intervention approach to use for a child with a speech sound disorder, they will need to determine the model for service delivery that will likely achieve the most promising outcomes. First, a determination will need to be made about the frequency, intensity, and duration of service. This could be influenced by the type of speech sound intervention selected. Second, the format for intervention must be identified, particularly whether services will be provided individually or in a small group setting. Third, a decision about who will implement the intervention needs to be made, whether it be the SLP, the SLP assistant, or someone else. Fourth, the setting for intervention must be determined. Will it occur in the child's natural school environment (e.g., classroom, playground, cafeteria), in the SLP's office or resource room, or in the home? Finally, timing is important because once the diagnosis of a speech sound disorder is made, early intervention makes a difference.

TABLE 5–3. Intervention Approaches for Supporting Sound Production

Intervention Approach	Description	References
Complexity approach	The more complex errors in a child's speech are targeted before the less complex errors. When complex errors (determined by manner and stimulability) are targeted, production accuracy can generalize to less complex sounds.	Baker & Williams (2010), Peña-Brooks & Hegde (2015)
Contextual utilization	Speech sound errors are targeted in syllable/word contexts that are facilitative for accurate production of the target sound. Targeting sounds in contexts that are easier for the child can build and be supportive of accurate production in other contexts. For example, producing /d/ may be easier for a child when it is followed by a vowel sound (i.e., "ee") that is produced in the front of the mouth with the tongue raised (e.g., "dee" or "deed").	Bernthal et al. (2017)
Core vocabulary approach	Sound errors are targeted in words that are important to the child's functional communication and those that are used frequently (as determined by observation of the child and collaboration with the child's family and teachers).	Dodd et al. (2006)
Distinctive feature approach	Features of sounds that the child is not producing (e.g., nasality, voicing) are highlighted and compared to sounds without those features. Without targeting each individual *sound* with that specific feature (e.g., all voiced sounds), teaching and targeting the *feature* tends to generalize to accurate production of sounds that share the same features.	Blache & Parsons (1980), Blache et al. (1981)
Metaphon approach	Metaphonological awareness (awareness of the phonological structure of language) is taught specifically for the phonological structures/rules the child is not producing. This includes substitution processes (e.g., fronting, backing, gliding) and syllable structure processes (e.g., final consonant deletion, cluster reduction)—for example, teaching that CVC words have ending sounds for students who engage in the phonological process of final consonant deletion.	Dean et al. (1995), Howell & Dean (1994)
Naturalistic speech intelligibility approach	Production of target sound(s) in natural activities where the sound occurs frequently. This can include when reading books, playing games, ordering food at a restaurant, etc. Using this intervention approach, the clinician recasts the utterances, repeating the error production correctly.	Camarata (2010)
Phonological contrast approach	Emphasizes sound contrasts that are important for differentiating words from one another. Words pairs are the target of intervention instead of individual sounds. The minimal pairs approach may be best for children with fewer errors, whereas the maximal opposition approach may be best for children with multiple speech sound errors.	Storkel (2022), Gierut (1989), Gierut & Neumann (1992)

TABLE 5–3. *continued*

Intervention Approach	Description	References
Phonological contrast approach *continued*	*Minimal pairs approach:* Using word pairs that differ by only one sound and feature that change the meaning of the word (e.g., "go"/"doe," "pay"/"play"). *Maximal opposition approach:* Using word pairs containing a contrastive sound that differs in more than one way (e.g., place, manner, voicing) that changes the meaning of the word (e.g., "fit"/"bit").	
Speech sound perception training	Teaches the child to attend to the phonological structure of words through the acoustic cues of target sounds produced in context. *Auditory bombardment:* The clinician orally presents many words with the target sound while the child listens (and is not asked to produce those sounds). *Identification tasks:* The child identifies correct and incorrect production of target sounds produced by the SLP (e.g., when the clinician says "red" vs. "wed" when talking about the color red).	Brosseau-Lapré et al. (2020), Brosseau-Lapré & Schumaker (2020), Brosseau-Lapré & Roepke (2022)

Source: Adapted from ASHA (n.d.).

Why Is This Topic Important?

Speech sound disorders can have an adverse effect on a child's educational performance in that they may impact the child's ability to fully participate in the classroom (e.g., responding to questions, giving oral presentations). Speech sound disorders may also affect a child's social engagement with their peers, such as during lunch or recess. A speech sound disorder might also indicate difficulties in a child's **phonological awareness** skills that may impact their ability to spell, read, and write. For example, a child's spelling may resemble the sound errors that the child makes in spoken language.

Speech difficulties may persist throughout and beyond the school years to adulthood. Children with persistent speech difficulties will vary in their severity, etiology, and the overall nature of the difficulties they are having with their speech (Shriberg et al., 2010; Wren et al., 2012). Persistent speech difficulties put children at risk for ongoing difficulty communicating with a variety of communication partners, and they may compromise their ability to acquire skills in reading and writing. In addition, reductions in self-esteem, increased risk for bullying, and other psychosocial concerns have been reported for children with speech difficulties (McCormack et al., 2012).

Intervention approaches will vary and are dependent on the child's specific difficulty and related language and literacy concerns. When determining the most appropriate intervention approach, the SLP supports the child to use self-monitoring strategies so they have agency in their communication and can apply the skills they have learned to support their speech production across settings. It will also be important for the SLP to collaborate with school personnel to facilitate the child's access to the academic curriculum and manage any emerging psychosocial challenges (Pascoe et al., 2006).

Application to a Child

 CJ is a 5-year-old boy who will be attending kindergarten in the fall. He was identified at age 4 years with a severe phonological disorder as he exhibited several error patterns, some of which appeared age appropriate when he was 3 years old. These patterns have persisted, resulting in increased frustration with communication. In fact, some of the speech sound error patterns noted were atypical (e.g., initial consonant deletion). A speech sound sample was collected in connected speech using a story retell task. A formal measure of speech sound production was completed and revealed several distortions, omissions, and substitutions of sounds within words. He exhibited several phonological processes that led to an intelligibility rating of less than 50%, with little stimulability for many sounds impacted. He consistently omitted the ending sounds of words (final consonant deletion), as well as inconsistently deleted the initial sounds of words, specifically those with more complex sounds and consonant clusters or blends. In addition, he substituted sounds produced in the front of the mouth (e.g., /t/, /d/) for more complex sounds that were produced in the back of the mouth (e.g., /k/, /g/), a process known as fronting. He also exhibited some difficulty articulating the /r/ and /l/ sounds; that is, he had challenges getting his tongue in the correct position to produce these sounds, especially in the middle of words. Voiceless sounds were easier to produce for CJ than voiced sounds.

Intervention focused on a phonological contrast approach and metaphon therapy to address his speech sound errors. Minimal pairs were used to help CJ learn the rules for speech sound production, specifically addressing "fronting" and "cluster reduction" so that CJ could learn to differentiate one word from another depending on the sound he produced and whether it matched the picture 'seen' (e.g., "tea" for "key"; "pot" for "spot"). He was shown pictures of minimal pairs with the words written under the pictures so that he could see the words and letters that represented the sounds in the words. Increasing his phonological awareness was also a primary goal for addressing his phonological processing errors. For example, CJ often substituted voiceless sounds for voiced sounds or omitted the ends of words. He learned that voiced sounds bring the vocal folds together to make a noisy sound and voiceless sounds are made with the vocal folds apart and that when he substituted a quiet sound for a noisy sound, the words that he produced did not have the meaning he intended (e.g., saying "dock" for "dog"). He also learned that words have ending sounds and that the meanings of words change depending on what the last sounds of the words are (e.g., "see" vs. "seed").

Knowing the challenges that CJ faces with his multiple speech sound errors, consider the following questions:

1. How would you determine the target sound selection for intervention?
2. How might you design an intervention approach that supports both his speech sound production and his letter sound knowledge?
3. How might other aspects of his spoken language be impacted by his tendency to omit the final consonants in words (HINT: think morphology)?
4. What strategies might you suggest to his teacher and parents to support his speech sound production at preschool and in the home?

Chapter Summary

Articulation is the ability to make sounds by coordinating articulatory movements. Articulators important to speech production are the tongue, lips, teeth, and hard and soft palates. A phonological disorder is a type of speech sound disorder in which a child produces errors on patterns of sounds, and these errors are predictable based on the rules of language. Functional speech disorders usually occur without a known cause, although there are several risk factors, including premature birth, chronic ear infections, gender, low birthweight, and delivery complications, that could explain speech difficulties in some children.

A comprehensive speech sound assessment that includes taking a case history, performing an oral mechanism examination, collecting a spontaneous speech sample, testing individual sound productions, and screening hearing could result in several possible outcomes. These include the following:

- No identification of a speech sound disorder
- Identification of a speech sound disorder
- A profile of the child's speech sound characteristics
- Indication of the severity of the child's speech sound disorder
- Considerations for selecting intervention targets
- Existence of other conditions that might explain the child's speech sound disorder

When deciding whether a speech sound disorder exists, it is important to recognize the role of accents and dialects within cultural groups where speech sound differences are expected and appropriate.

Several strategies and techniques are used to support a child in learning about accurate speech sound production, including the following:

- Providing visual cues for the place and manner of sounds
- Using imaging to visual articulator configurations
- Amplifying target sounds to increase sound awareness
- Providing a visual representation of the acoustic signal of speech
- Focusing practice on one or two sounds until the child reaches a criterion level
- Treating multiple sounds with less intense practice but increasing exposure to the broader sound system
- Cycling practice with different sounds for a set period

Several intervention approaches are used to support speech sound production that emphasizes the context and complexity of the child's speech sound difficulties as well as the phonological processes that indicate an underlying language difficulty. The following are some of the approaches highlighted in this chapter:

- Complexity approach
- Contextual utilization
- Core vocabulary
- Cycles intervention
- Distinctive feature therapy
- Metaphon therapy
- Naturalistic speech intelligibility
- Phonological contrast

Chapter Review Questions

1. What is the difference between an articulation disorder and a phonological disorder?
2. What are the risk factors for speech sound disorders in children?
3. What factors are important to consider when selecting a target sound for intervention?
4. What phonological processes are typically seen prior to age 3 years? After age 3 years?
5. Describe the voicing, place, and manner of articulation for the /b, p, k, g, v, f, s, z/ sounds.
6. What are the primary components for screening a possible speech sound disorder?
7. What are three key goals in the treatment of speech sound disorders?
8. What is phonological awareness and how might a child's phonological awareness be impacted by their speech sound disorder?
9. Describe some of the assessment considerations that a clinicians should attend to when evaluating the speech sound abilities in culturally and linguistically diverse children?
10. Select two interventions that could be used to facilitate a child's speech sound production and explain how and when a clinician might use those interventions.

Learning Activities

1. Learn about the occurrence of a partial and a complete cleft palate or cleft lip and palate in different countries. What are the typical causes of this condition in the United States and more globally? Describe the speech sound characteristics of a child with a cleft palate. What manner of speech sound production is most impacted and why?
2. Consider CJ's speech sound challenges (see "Application to a Child" section in this chapter) and outline the aspects of the ICF that would most likely be impacted. Remember to consider the following elements:
   a. Impairments in body structure and function
   b. Limitations in activity and participation
   c. Contextual (environmental and personal) factors
3. Review Table 5–2 and draw a picture that shows the place of articulation for each of the sounds listed and which articulators are active versus passive (as described in Chapter 4).

Suggested Reading

DeVeney, S. L., Cabbage, K., & Mourey, T. (2020). Target selection considerations for speech sound disorder intervention in schools. *Perspectives of the ASHA Special Interest Groups, 5,* 1722–1734.

This is a clinical focus article that describes what SLPs consider when identifying sounds for intervention that are most appropriate for a specific child with a speech sound disorder. There are many considerations, however, in the selection of clinical targets, and SLPs need to be clear about their rationale for target sound selection. This article shares several considerations and offers the reasoning behind what should be a priority consideration for intervention: stimulability, complexity, and intelligibility.

Mues, M., Zuk, J., Norton, E. S., Gabrieli, J. D. E., Hogan, T. P., & Gaab, N. (2023). Preliteracy skills mediate the relation between early speech sound production and subsequent reading outcomes. *Journal of Speech, Language, and Hearing Research, 66*, 2766–2782.

Research suggests that children with speech sound disorders may have different word reading outcomes than children without speech production problems and that this could be indicative of later reading challenges for this population. This article reports on a longitudinal study that examined the relationships between speech sound production and reading outcomes in kindergarteners, with additional focus on potential mediating factors. Researchers found that a child's phonological awareness and letter name knowledge early on can influence the impact of their incorrect speech sound productions and later reading outcomes, including decoding, reading fluency, and reading comprehension.

Roepke, E. (2024). Assessing phonological processes in children with speech sound disorders. *Perspectives of the ASHA Special Interest Groups, 9*, 14–34.

This article is a tutorial on what assessment tasks might be most suited to use with children exhibiting speech sound disorders to identify their phonological processing challenges (i.e., difficulty using phoneme knowledge to process language). The author recommends several phonological processing tasks for this population, including rapid automatized naming (i.e., how quickly a child can name letters) for phonological retrieval, syllable repetition to assess phonological memory, and receptive tasks to assess phonological awareness.

Additional Resources

- University of Arizona, English consonant and vowel charts
  https://www.u.arizona.edu/~ohalad/Phonetics/docs/Cvchart.pdf
- Learning for Justice, "Everyone Has an Accent"
  https://www.learningforjustice.org/magazine/fall-2000/everyone-has-an-accent
- Charles Sturt University, "Multilingual Children's Speech: Intelligibility in Context Scale"
  https://www.csu.edu.au/research/multilingual-speech/ics
- Charles Sturt University, "Multilingual Children's Speech: Speech Participation and Activity Assessment of Children (SPAA-C)"
  https://www.csu.edu.au/research/multilingual-speech/spaa-c
- Reading Rockets, "The Development of Phonological Skills"
  https://www.readingrockets.org/topics/developmental-milestones/articles/development-phonological-skills

References

American Psychiatric Association. (2022). *Diagnostic and statistical manual of mental disorders* (5th ed., text rev.).

American Speech-Language-Hearing Association. (n.d.). *Speech sound disorders: Articulation and phonology*. https://www.asha.org/practice-portal/clinical-topics/articulation-and-phonology

American Speech-Language-Hearing Association. (2016). *Code of ethics* [Ethics]. https://www.asha.org/policy

Baker, E., & Williams, A. L. (2010). Complexity approaches to intervention. In A. L. Williams, S. McLeod, & R. J. McCauley (Eds.), *Intervention for speech sound disorders in children* (pp. 95–115). Brookes.

Bernthal, J., Bankson, N. W., & Flipsen, P., Jr. (2017). *Articulation and phonological disorders: Speech sound disorders in children*. Pearson.

Blache, S. E., & Parsons, C. (1980). A linguistic approach to distinctive feature training. *Language, Speech, and Hearing Services in Schools, 11*, 203–207.

Blache, S. E., Parsons, C. L., & Humphreys, J. M. (1981). A minimal-word-pair model for teaching the linguistic significant difference of distinctive feature properties. *Journal of Speech and Hearing Disorders, 46*, 291–296.

Black, L. I., Vahratian, A., & Hoffman, H. J. (2015). *Communication disorders and use of intervention services among children aged 3–17 years: United States, 2012* (NHS Data Brief No. 205). National Center for Health Statistics.

Brosseau-Lapré, F., & Roepke, E. (2022). Implementing speech perception and phonological awareness intervention for children with speech sound disorders. *Language, Speech and Hearing Services in Schools, 53*, 646–658.

Brosseau-Lapré, F., & Schumaker, J. (2020). Perception of correctly and incorrectly produced words in children with and without phonological speech sound disorders. *Journal of Speech, Language, and Hearing Research, 63*(12), 3961–3973.

Brosseau-Lapré, F., Schumaker, J., & Kluender, K. R. (2020). Perception of medial consonants by preschoolers with and without speech sound disorders. *Journal of Speech, Language, and Hearing Research, 63*(11), 3600–3610.

Camarata, S. (2010). Naturalistic intervention for speech intelligibility and speech accuracy. In A. L. Williams, S. McLeod, & R. J. McCauley (Eds.), *Interventions for speech sound disorders in children* (pp. 381–406). Brookes.

Campbell, T. F., Dollaghan, C. A., Rockette, H. E., Paradise, J. L., Feldman, H. M., Shriberg, L. D., . . . Kurs-Lasky, M. (2003). Risk factors for speech delay of unknown origin in 3-year-old children. *Child Development, 74*, 346–357.

Dean, E., Howell, J., Waters, D., & Reid, J. (1995). Metaphon: A metalinguistic approach to the treatment of phonological disorder in children. *Clinical Linguistics & Phonetics, 9*, 1–19.

Dodd, B., Holm, A., Crosbie, S., & McIntosh, B. (2006). A core vocabulary approach for management of inconsistent speech disorder. *International Journal of Speech-Language Pathology, 8*, 220–230.

Eadie, P., Morgan, A., Ukoumunne, O. C., Eecen, K. T., Wake, M., & Reilly, S. (2015). Speech sound disorder at 4 years: Prevalence, comorbidities, and predictors in a community cohort of children. *Developmental Medicine & Child Neurology, 57*, 578–584.

Ertmer, D. J. (2010). Relationship between speech intelligibility and word articulation scores in children with hearing loss. *Journal of Speech, Language, and Hearing Research, 53*, 1075–1086.

Fabiano-Smith, L., & Goldstein, B. A. (2010). Phonological acquisition in bilingual Spanish–English speaking children. *Journal of Speech, Language, and Hearing Research, 53*, 160–178.

Fey, M. (1986). *Language intervention with young children*. Allyn & Bacon.

Findley, B. R., & Gasparyan, D. (2022). Use of speech-to-text biofeedback in intervention for children with articulation disorders. *Perspectives of the ASHA Special Interest Groups, 7*, 926–937.

Flipsen, P. (2015). Emergence and prevalence of persistent and residual speech errors. *Seminars in Speech Language, 36*, 217–223.

Fox, A. V., Dodd, B., & Howard, D. (2002). Risk factors for speech disorders in children. *International Journal of Language and Communication Disorders, 37*, 117–132.

Gierut, J. A. (1989). Maximal opposition approach to phonological treatment. *Journal of Speech and Hearing Research, 54*, 9–19.

Gierut, J. A., & Neumann, H. J. (1992). Teaching and learning /θ/: A non-confound. *Clinical Linguistics & Phonetics, 6*(3), 191–200.

Glaspey, A. M., & Stoel-Gammon, C. (2007). A dynamic approach to phonological assessment. *Advances in Speech-Language Pathology, 9*, 286–296.

Goldstein, B. A., & Fabiano, L. (2007, February 13). Assessment and intervention for bilingual children with phonological disorders. *The ASHA Leader, 12*, 6–7, 26–27, 31.

Hodson, B. (2010). *Evaluating and enhancing children's phonological systems: Research and theory to practice.* PhonoComp.

Howell, J., & Dean, E. (1994). *Treating phonological disorders in children: Metaphon—Theory to practice* (2nd ed.). Whurr.

Law, J., Boyle, J., Harris, F., Harkness, A., & Nye, C. (2000). Prevalence and natural history of primary speech and language delay: Findings from a systematic review of the literature. *International Journal of Language and Communication Disorders, 35*, 165–188.

Lee, S. A. S., Wrench, A., & Sancibrian, S. (2015). How to get started with ultrasound technology for treatment of speech sound disorders. *Perspectives on Speech Science and Orofacial Disorders, 25*, 66–80.

McAllister Byun, T., & Hitchcock, E. R. (2012). Investigating the use of traditional and spectral biofeedback approaches to intervention for /r/ misarticulation. *American Journal of Speech-Language Pathology, 21*, 207–221.

McCormack, J., McAllister, L., McLeod, S., & Harrison, L. (2012). Knowing, having, doing: The battles of childhood speech impairment. *Child Language Teaching and Therapy, 28*, 141–157.

McLeod, S., Verdon, S., & The International Expert Panel on Multilingual Children's Speech. (2017). Tutorial: Speech assessment for multilingual children who do not speak the same language(s) as the speech-language pathologist. *American Journal of Speech-Language Pathology, 26*, 691–708.

Overby, M.S., Trainin, G., Smit, A. B., Bernthal, J. E., & Nelson, R. (2012). Preliteracy speech sound production skill and later literacy outcomes: A study using the Templin Archive. *Language, Speech, and Hearing Services in Schools, 43*, 97–115.

Pascoe, M., Stackhouse, J., & Wells, B. (2006). *Persisting speech difficulties in children: Children's speech and literacy difficulties, Book 3.* Whurr.

Peña-Brooks, A., & Hegde, M. N. (2015). *Assessment and treatment of articulation and phonological disorders in children.* Pro-Ed.

Peterson, R. L., Pennington, B. F., Shriberg, L. D., & Boada, R. (2009). What influences literacy outcome in children with speech sound disorder? *Journal of Speech, Language, and Hearing Research, 52*, 1175–1188.

Prelock, P. A., & Hutchins, T. L. (2018). *Clinical guide to assessment and treatment of communication disorders.* F. R. Volkmar, Editor. NY: Springer.

Preston, J. L., McCabe, P., Rivera-Campos, A., Whittle, J. L., Landry, E., & Maas, E. (2014). Ultrasound visual feedback treatment and practice variability for residual speech sound errors. *Journal of Speech, Language, and Hearing Research, 57*, 2102–2115.

Prezas, R. F., & Hodson, B. W. (2010). The cycles phonological remediation approach. In A. L. Williams, S. McLeod, & R. J. McCauley (Eds.), *Interventions for speech sound disorders in children* (pp. 137–158). Brookes.

Shriberg, L. D., & Kwiatkowski, J. (1982a). Phonological disorders II: A conceptual framework for management. *Journal of Speech and Hearing Disorders, 47,* 242–256.

Shriberg, L. D., & Kwiatkowski, J. (1982b). Phonological disorders III: A procedure for assessing severity of involvement. *Journal of Speech and Hearing Disorders, 47,* 256–270.

Shriberg, L. D., Tomblin, J. B., & McSweeny, J. L. (1999). Prevalence of speech delay in 6-year-old children and comorbidity with language impairment. *Journal of Speech, Language, and Hearing Research, 42,* 1461–1481.

Storkel, H. L. (2018). The complexity approach to phonological treatment: How to select treatment targets. *Language, Speech, and Hearing Sciences in Schools, 49,* 463–481.

Storkel, H. L. (2022). Minimal, maximal, or multiple: Which contrastive intervention approach to use with children with speech sound disorders? *Language, Speech and Hearing Services in Schools, 53,* 632–645.

To, C. K. S., McLeod, S., Sam, K. L., & Law, T. (2022). Predicting which children will not normalize without intervention for speech sound disorders. *Journal of Speech, Language, and Hearing Research, 65,* 1724–1741.

Tyler, A. A., & Tolbert, L. C. (2002). Speech-language assessment in the clinical setting. *American Journal of Speech-Language Pathology, 11,* 215–220.

U.S. Preventive Services Task Force. (2024). Screening for speech and language delay and disorders in children: US Preventive Services Task Force recommendation statement. *Journal of the American Medical Association, 331*(4), 329–334.

Van Noort-van der Spek, I. L., Dudink, J., Reiss, I. K., & Franken, M.-C. J. P. (2022). Early speech sound production and its trajectories in very preterm children from 2 to 4 years of age. *Journal of Speech, Language, and Hearing Research, 65,* 1294–1310.

Williams, A. L. (2003). Target selection and treatment outcomes. *Perspectives on Language Learning and Education, 10,* 12–16.

Williams, A. L., McLeod, S., & McCauley, R. J. (2010). Direct speech production intervention. In A. L. Williams, S. McLeod, & R. J. McCauley (Eds.), *Interventions for speech sound disorders in children* (pp. 27–39). Brookes.

World Health Organization. (2001). *International classification of functioning, disability and health.*

Wren, Y., Miller, L. L., Peters, T. J., Emond, A., & Roulstone, S. (2016). Prevalence and predictors of persistent speech sound disorder at eight years old: Findings from a population cohort study. *Journal of Speech, Language, and Hearing Research, 59,* 647–673.

Wren, Y. E., Roulstone, S. E., & Miller, L. L. (2012). Distinguishing groups of children with persistent speech disorder: Findings from a prospective population study. *Logopedics Phoniatrics Vocology, 37,* 1–10.

Chapter 6

Motor Speech Disorders

With Dorothy Yang

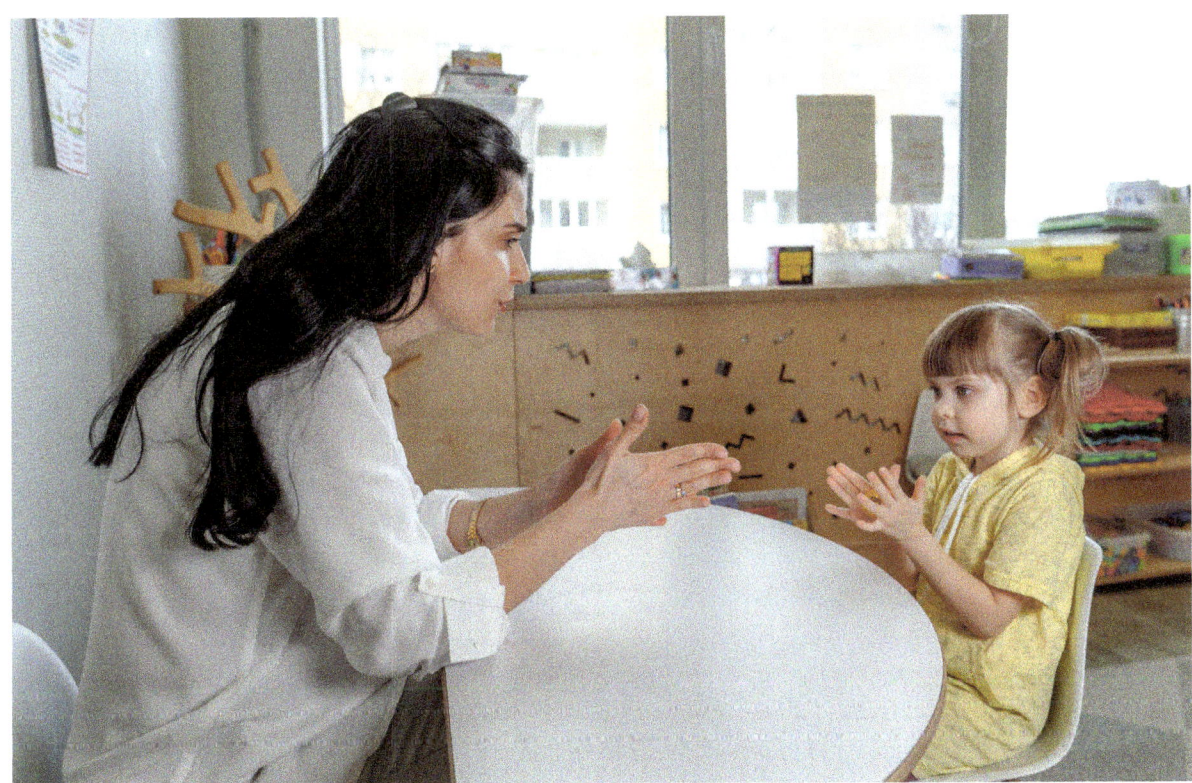

Learning Objectives

After reading this chapter, you will be able to:

- Describe the different motor speech disorders in pediatric and adult populations.
- Identify the importance of differential diagnosis for individuals with motor speech disorders.
- Explain why differential diagnosis is important to intervention.
- Reflect on the value of principles of motor learning to support speech production in children and adults with motor speech disorders.

Key Terms

apraxia of speech
ataxic dysarthria
Bell's palsy
blocked practice
central nervous system
cerebral palsy
childhood apraxia of speech
chorea
communicative efficiency
comprehensibility
cranial nerves
Creutzfeldt–Jakob disease
direct activation pathway
distributed practice
dynamic temporal and tactile cueing (DTTC)
dysarthria
dystonia
electromagnetic articulography (EMA)
electromyography (EMG)
extrapyramidal tract
flaccid dysarthria
Friedreich's ataxia
functional magnetic resonance imaging (fMRI)
Guillain–Barré
hyperadduction
hyperkinetic dysarthria
hypernasality
hypokinetic dysarthria
indirect activation pathway

laryngoscopy
lower motor neuron system
massed practice
melodic intonation therapy
motor speech disorder
myasthenia gravis
nasoendoscopy
nasometry
naturalness (of speech)
palatal lift
peripheral nervous system
positron emission tomography (PET)
progressive bulbar palsy
Prompts for Restructuring Oral Muscular Phonetic Targets (PROMPT) system
pyramidal tract
random practice
rapid syllable transition (ReST)
spastic dysarthria
speech intelligibility
spinal nerves
spirometry
tics
training specificity
tremors
unilateral upper motor neuron dysarthria
upper motor neuron system
videofluoroscopy
videostroboscopy

Introduction

Speech is often the primary modality through which we express our thoughts, ideas, wants, and needs to others. However, communicating is much more than producing the words and sentences that you want to say; it also encompasses *how* you say those words and sentences (e.g., to convey sarcasm or specific emotions). When speech production is impaired, this can impact our ability to communicate our needs and thoughts, to be understood, and to engage socially. In this chapter, we describe several motor speech disorders in pediatric and adult populations, including various dysarthrias and apraxia of speech. We explain how speech-language pathologists (SLPs) are integral to the assessment of motor speech disorders and discuss the importance of (and challenges associated with) differential diagnosis of motor speech disorders in children and adults. Finally, we discuss some common intervention strategies that can be used to treat the different types of motor speech disorders.

The Brain

In Chapter 9, we describe the various structures of the brain that contribute to the complexities associated with language production. The same is true for speech motor control important for speech production. The frontal lobe plays a key part in the movements associated with speech production because it is home to the primary motor cortex. Because the primary motor cortex spans both the left and the right hemisphere of the brain, and the sensory and motor regions of the brain operate contralaterally, damage to the primary motor cortex in one hemisphere of the brain impacts muscle movements on the opposite side of the body. Descending from the primary motor cortex is the **direct activation pathway** (also known as the **pyramidal tract**). It is via this pathway that messages get sent from the cortex to the muscles initiating complex and voluntary muscle movements (of both the limbs and the muscles necessary for speech production). But it is not just voluntary muscle movements that are necessary for speech production. Various involuntary muscle movements and reflexes support movement and motor control, and these messages get sent from the brainstem to the spinal cord via the **indirect activation pathway** (also known as the **extrapyramidal tract**). The direct and indirect activation pathways work in tandem, forming the **upper motor neuron system**, to support the motor control necessary for speech production. Once the motor plan is determined, messages get sent from the motor cortex via the pyramidal and extrapyramidal tracts to the muscles that are used for speech production. At the same time, the cerebellum (also important for motor learning) coordinates the timing of the complex muscle movements, as well as appropriate posture/muscle tone that is necessary for movement.

Whereas the upper motor neuron system consists of the extrapyramidal and pyramidal tracts, the **lower motor neuron system** is composed of cranial nerves and spinal nerves (located in the **peripheral nervous system**). This is how information from the brain and spinal cord (the **central nervous system**) communicates with the rest of the body (Figure 6–1). Primarily originating in the brainstem are 12 pairs of **cranial nerves**, many of which are important to the muscle movements associated with various aspects of speech production (Table 6–1; Figure 6–2). The **spinal nerves**, on the other hand, are important for supporting the respiration functions that are specifically associated with speech production. When all these systems are working properly, the result is smooth and effortless speech production. But what happens when these neurological systems are damaged?

Motor Speech Disorders

When any of the systems or structures that are important for speech production are damaged, the result is often a **motor speech disorder** (MSD). MSDs are a group of disorders associated with neurological conditions that impact a person's muscle movements and/or motor planning necessary for speech production. As such, an MSD is not a disorder of language or cognition but, rather, a disorder of speech. The primary MSDs are dysarthria and apraxia of speech.

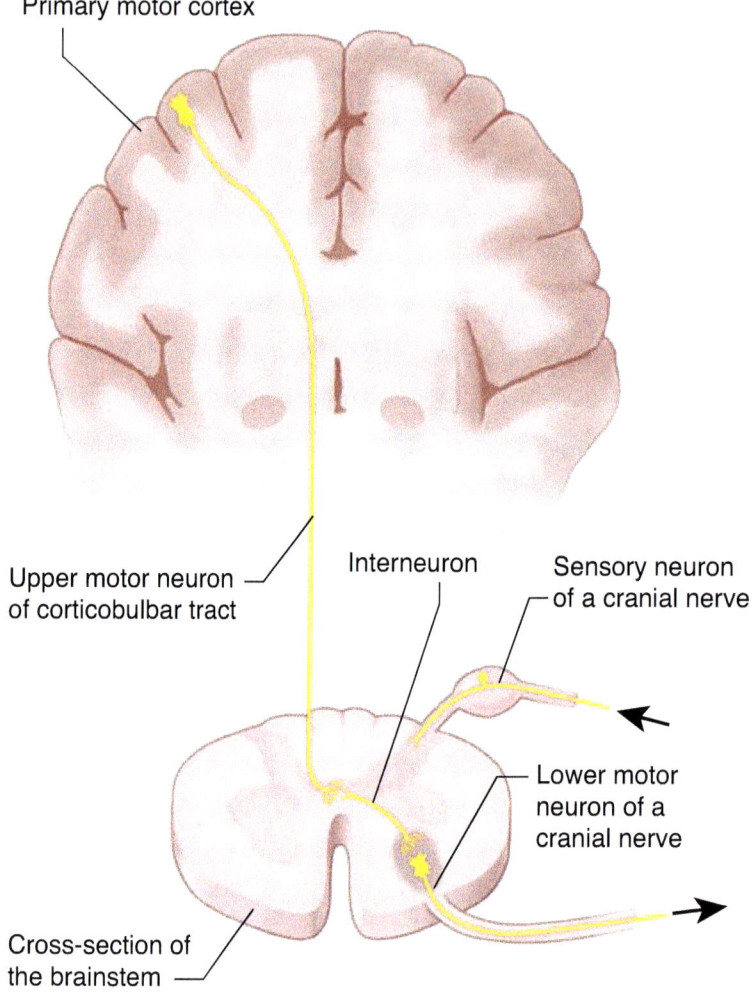

FIGURE 6–1. Upper motor neurons transmit motor impulses within the central nervous system and ultimately send these impulses to the lower motor neurons in the cranial or spinal nerves. *Source:* From *Motor Speech Disorders: Diagnosis and Treatment, Fourth Edition* (pp. 1–381) by Freed, D. B. Copyright © 2025 Plural Publishing, Inc. All rights reserved.

Dysarthria

Dysarthria is an MSD that is concerned with the actual production of speech. That is, the muscles and movements (in terms of speed, strength, range of motion, tone, and accuracy) that are required for the processes associated with speech production (i.e., respiration, phonation, resonance, articulation, and prosody) are impacted. Moreover, dysarthrias are considered in terms of their accompanying physical and perceptual speech characteristics. Physical speech characteristics include muscle weakness, reduced tone, increased rigidity, and so on. Perceptual speech characteristics include reduced rate, decreased loudness, abnormal pitch, reduced vocal quality, and so on. It is important to note that perceptual speech characteristics can be a result of a disturbance in any or all the speech processes: respiration, phonation, articulation,

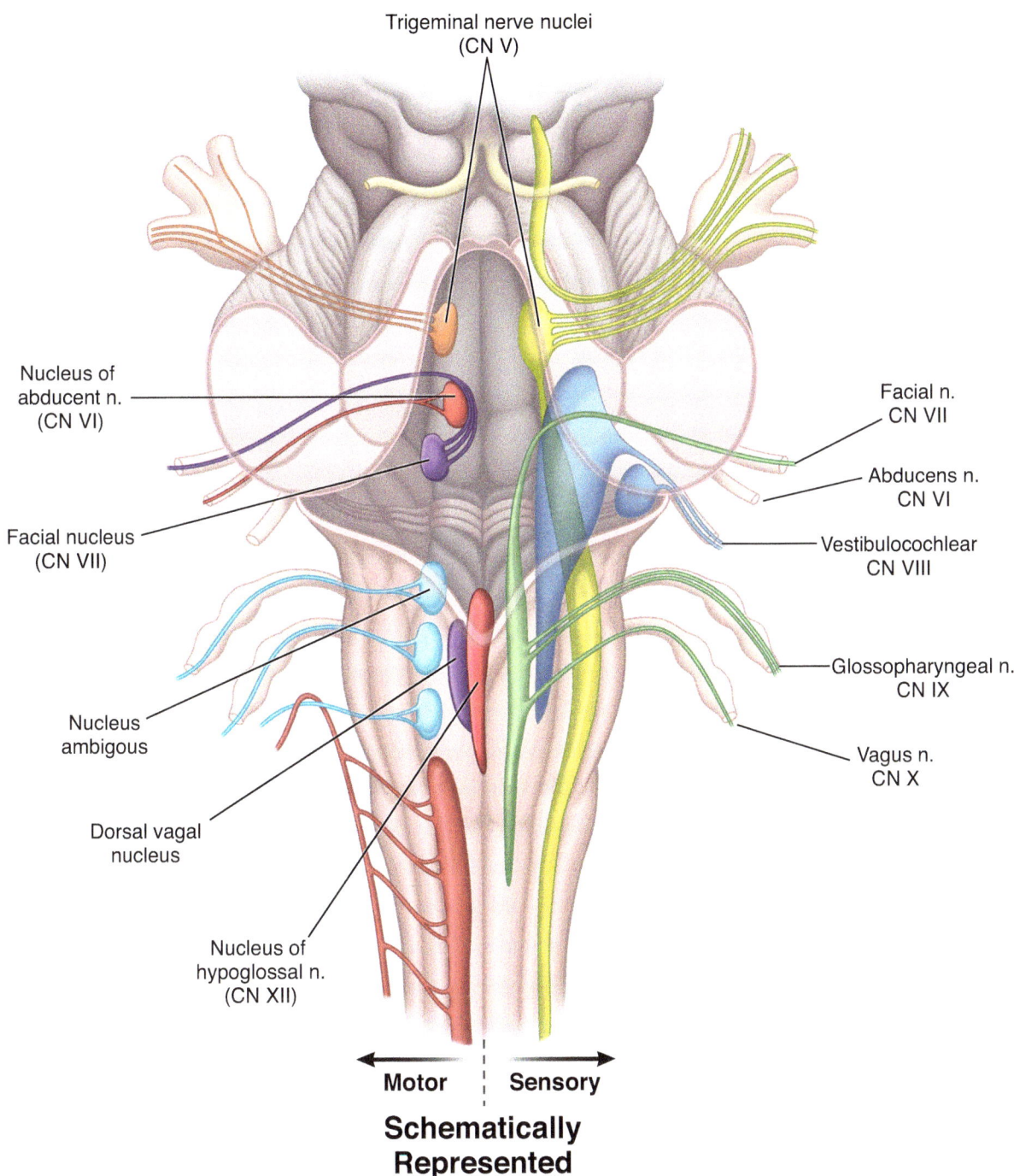

FIGURE 6–2. Cranial nerves, posterior view. On the left side showing the motor nuclei; on the right side showing the sensory nuclei. *Source:* From *Clinical Management of Swallowing Disorders, Sixth Edition* (in press) by Murry, T., Chan, K., & Walsh. E. H. Copyright © 2026 Plural Publishing, Inc. All rights reserved.

TABLE 6–1. Cranial Nerves

	Cranial Nerve	Function
I	Olfactory	Smell
II	Optic	Vision
III	Oculomotor	Eye movement; pupil restriction
IV	Trochlear	Eye movement
V	Trigeminal[a]	Jaw movement; face, mouth, jaw sensation
VI	Abducens	Eye movement
VII	Facial[a]	Facial movement; hyoid elevation; salivation; taste
VIII	Cochleovestibular	Hearing; balance
IX	Glossopharyngeal[a]	Pharyngeal movement; pharynx and tongue sensation; taste
X	Vagus[a]	Pharyngeal, palatal, and laryngeal movement; pharyngeal sensation; control of visceral organs
XI	Accessory[a]	Shoulder and neck movement
XII	Hypoglossal[a]	Tongue movement

Note: [a]Cranial nerves associated with speech production.
Source: Adapted from Duffy (2013).

resonance, and prosody. As you may have guessed, because there are myriad neurons, pathways, brain structures, and cranial nerves that are responsible for different components of speech production, there are various dysarthrias. Although all of the dysarthria types share some common features, each is unique in its clinical presentation (discussed in the following sections).

Dysarthria types include flaccid, spastic, ataxic, hypokinetic, hyperkinetic, and unilateral upper motor neuron. Of course, it is possible that a person experiences damage to various motor systems, which results in a mixed dysarthria.

Flaccid Dysarthria

A **flaccid dysarthria** typically results from damage to the lower motor neuron system (which is made up of cranial and spinal nerves) and is characterized by muscle weakness and flaccidity (i.e., softness). The speech characteristics associated with a flaccid dysarthria include hypernasality, breathiness, abnormalities with speech–breath coordination, and reduced vocal quality with vocal use. Some of the common causes of flaccid dysarthrias include **Bell's palsy, progressive bulbar palsy**, and **myasthenia gravis**.

Spastic Dysarthria

Whereas a flaccid dysarthria is a result of damage to the lower motor neuron system, **spastic dysarthria** occurs because of damage to the upper motor neuron system (remember this encompasses the direct and indirect activation pathways). Spastic dysarthria is characterized by spasticity, which can be described as resistance to passive stretch. The speech characteristics that are associated with a spastic dysarthria include slowed rate of speech, strained vocal quality, and abnormal pitch.

Ataxic Dysarthria

Ataxic dysarthria is localized in the cerebellum (as opposed to the upper or lower motor neuron system) and is primarily concerned with incoordination of muscles. The perceptual speech characteristics that are often present in those with ataxic dysarthria include articulatory breakdowns, slurring of speech, excessive variation in loudness, as well as excess and equal stress.

Hypokinetic Dysarthria

Hypokinetic dysarthria is an MSD that occurs because of damage to the basal ganglia control circuit in the extrapyramidal tract. Whereas spastic dysarthria is associated with resistance to passive stretch, a person with hypokinetic dysarthria experiences rigidity of movement or a reduced range of motion. Because of this, someone with a hypokinetic dysarthria will likely present with monotonous speech, reduced loudness, a rapid speech rate, word repetition, and inappropriate silences. Most individuals diagnosed with Parkinson's disease eventually present with speech characteristics that are associated with a hypokinetic dysarthria. Parkinson's disease is a neurodegenerative disease associated with genetic and environmental causes (although the exact etiology is unknown; National Institute on Aging, 2022). Not surprisingly, disease progression is associated with worsening dysarthria and overall communication and social interaction in general (Pinto et al., 2017).

Hyperkinetic Dysarthria

Like hypokinetic dysarthria, **hyperkinetic dysarthria** occurs due to damage to the basal ganglia circuit. The difference, however, is that hyperkinetic dysarthria is associated with involuntary and abnormal muscular movements necessary for respiration, phonation, articulation, resonance, and prosody. This can result in vocal tremors, breathiness, vocal strain/harshness, variation in loudness, deterioration of vocal quality, and inappropriate vocal noises. Moreover, dysarthria may result from several hyperkinetic disorders, including **tremors** (i.e., involuntary movements associated with rhythmic movements; includes musculature and vocal tremors), **tics** (i.e., rapid patterned movements that are not necessarily involuntary; includes motor and vocal tics), **dystonia** (i.e., slow, involuntary movements that are abnormal in their posture), or **chorea** (i.e., rapid and unpredictable movements). Individuals who are diagnosed with Huntington's disease often present with speech characteristics resembling hyperkinetic dysarthria. Huntington's disease is a hereditary, neurodegenerative condition associated with the basal ganglia region of the brain. It is associated with progressive decline in voluntary movements, cognition, and personality.

Unilateral Upper Motor Neuron Dysarthria

A **unilateral upper motor neuron dysarthria** occurs because there is damage to one side of the upper motor neuron system, resulting in weakness to one side of the lower face and tongue. This translates into a slow rate of speech, as well as imprecise articulation, reduced loudness, and a strained vocal quality.

Mixed Dysarthria

A mixed dysarthria occurs when an individual presents with symptoms of more than one dysarthria. One of the most common examples of this is a person who has **amyotrophic lateral sclerosis (ALS)**, which is commonly known as Lou Gehrig's disease. ALS is a neurodegenerative motor neuron disease in which degeneration occurs in both the upper and motor neurons. As such, a person with ALS exhibits symptoms of both spastic and flaccid dysarthria, and speech function steadily declines with disease progression from normal speech to no verbal speech. A description of the loss of speech function is provided in Table 6–2. ALS tends to occur in individuals aged 40 to 70 years and is more common in men than women (Hanson et al., 2011). Another condition that can be associated with a mixed dysarthria is traumatic brain injury (see Chapter 9).

TABLE 6–2. Loss of Speech Function in Amyotrophic Lateral Sclerosis

Normal Speech Processes	
Normal speech	Speech is normal.
Minimal speech changes	Patient may notice slight changes in speech production; patient maintains normal speaking rate and volume.
Detectable Speech Differences	
Perceivable speech changes	Others notice speech changes, particularly when the individual is tired or stressed; patient maintains normal speaking rate.
Obvious speech changes	Although the patient is generally understood, speech is consistently impaired, including rate, articulation, and resonance.
Behavioral Changes	
Repetition of messages	Patient repeats some words. Rate of speech is slow, but complexity of messages is not impacted.
Repetition or translator required	Patient must repeat messages frequently or require a known communication partner to translate message. Rate of speech is slow, and complexity of messages is reduced.
Use of AAC	
Verbal speech + AAC	Patient uses speech to answer questions; however, intelligibility is impacted to the point where writing and/or a translator are used to help with communication breakdowns.
One-word utterances	Patient uses one-word responses to answer questions. Writing or a spokesperson is used when longer messages are required.
Loss of Verbal Speech	
Vocalizations	Patient uses vocalizations for affirmations and negations, as well as to express emotions.
No vocalizations	Vocalizations are rarely used except for when in pain or crying.
Tracheostomy	Patient receives a tracheostomy.

Note: AAC, augmentative and alternative communication.
Source: Adapted from Hanson et al. (2011).

Causes

As briefly indicated, dysarthria can be caused by several neurologic conditions, including congenital conditions (e.g., cerebral palsy), degenerative conditions (e.g., ALS, Parkinson's disease, Huntington's disease, Friedreich's ataxia), demyelinating and inflammatory diseases (e.g., multiple sclerosis, Guillain–Barré), infectious diseases (e.g., Creutzfeldt–Jakob disease), brain tumors, seizure disorders, toxic diseases, trauma associated with the head/neck/brain, and vascular diseases (e.g., stroke). Dysarthria is common in these conditions, such that it is estimated that 78% to 93% of individuals with Huntington's disease, 40% to 51% of those with multiple sclerosis, 44% to 88% of those with Parkinson's disease, 30% to 86% of those with traumatic brain injury, and 26% to 62% of those with neuromuscular diseases are diagnosed with a dysarthria (American Speech-Language-Hearing Association, n.d.).

Apraxia of Speech

Whereas dysarthria is a disorder of speech production, apraxia of speech (AoS; also called verbal apraxia) is a disorder of the motor planning or programming of speech that usually results from damage in motor areas in the left hemisphere. Individuals with an AoS do not have muscle weakness or otherwise impaired musculature; rather, they have deficits in retrieval of the motor plan required for speech production. The speech characteristics associated with AoS include articulation (vowel and consonant) and prosody errors, a reduced speech rate, as well as groping for sounds. Production of multisyllabic words and words that are complex and unfamiliar pose a particular challenge. A hallmark feature of AoS that can distinguish it from other MSDs is the inconsistent articulatory errors that are produced by an individual even on repeated attempts. A person with an AoS is aware of their speech production errors and will make attempts to correct these errors, often unsuccessfully. Although this is true for volitional speech production, persons with AoS tend to have intact automatic speech (e.g., naming the months of the year, counting). Note that AoS is a motor *speech* disorder, meaning that persons with this condition will have intact language functioning (unless of course they have a co-occurring language disorder such as aphasia).

Childhood Apraxia of Speech

Whereas adults can acquire AoS from damage to the left hemisphere, children can be diagnosed with childhood apraxia of speech (CAS) without neurological insult. Despite being a neurological speech sound disorder, in fact, most of the time the cause of CAS is unknown, although recent evidence shows that CAS may be linked to genetics (Morgan & Webster, 2018). The speech characteristics of CAS are like those of adults with AoS and include inconsistent articulation errors (particularly on multisyllabic and complex words), difficulty with co-articulatory transitions (e.g., groping during speech, sequencing challenges, vowel errors), and inappropriate prosody (Morgan & Webster, 2018). Moreover, children with CAS often have co-occurring language disorders (Lewis et al., 2004).

Cerebral Palsy

The MSDs that we have discussed so far in this book are primarily disorders that happen in adulthood (aside from CAS), although of course children and adolescents can have neurological injury resulting in dysarthria or AoS. A common condition that is associated with dysarthria in childhood is cerebral palsy. Cerebral palsy (CP) is a group of neurological congenital conditions that occur as the fetus is developing in the womb, during birth, or after birth (up to age 5 years) due to disruptions in brain development. These include oxygen deprivation, brain hemorrhages, infections of the brain, exposure to toxins, and malnutrition, although data suggest that roughly half of the children who are born with CP do not have any risk factors (Patel et al., 2020). Prevalence data suggest that roughly 1 million people (children and adults) are living with CP in the United States and that CP affects 1 in every 345 children. CP has been found to be more common in males compared to females, as well as Black children compared to White children (Cerebral Palsy Guide, 2024).

Cerebral palsy affects a person's muscle tone and strength, motor control, posture, and balance. Like dysarthria in adults, there are various types of CP based on how an individual's movement is impacted: spastic, dyskinetic, ataxic, and mixed CP. The most common subtype of CP is spastic CP (comprising approximately 85% of CP cases; Sanger, 2015), which is associated with muscle stiffness and jerky movements. Spasticity can affect various parts of the body, including primarily the lower body (i.e., spastic diplegia), the limbs on one side of the body (i.e., spastic hemiplegia), or the arms and legs on both sides of the body (i.e., spastic quadriplegia). Individuals with spastic hemiplegia and diplegia tend to have intact cognitive and language skills, although those with spastic hemiplegia may have language delays. Those with spastic quadriplegia often have associated language deficits and intellectual disabilities (Patel et al., 2020). Dyskinetic CP (7% of cases; Sanger, 2015) is associated with slow and jerky movements of the extremities (i.e., arms, hands, legs, feet) that are uncontrollable, as well as hyperactive movements of the face that may cause an individual to drool unexpectedly. Those with dyskinetic CP often have challenges with walking and coordinating the muscles for speech production, but they do not have associated intellectual impairments. Unlike spastic and dyskinetic CP, ataxic CP (4% of CP cases; Sanger, 2015) is not associated with jerky musculature movements but instead impacts a person's balance and depth perception. This results in challenges with muscle coordination for walking as well as completing tasks that require fine motor coordination, such as tying a shoelace and doing and undoing buttons. Individuals who have mixed CP present with symptoms of multiple types of CP described above. Table 6–3 lists the different types of CP and their characteristics.

Children with CP often have co-occurring conditions, including musculoskeletal problems that result from the involuntary muscle movements associated with CP, epilepsy, intellectual disability, dysphagia, and speech/language deficits. Complications with respiratory function and challenges with coordinating breathing with speech production are common problems in children with CP, as are laryngeal and velopharyngeal functioning. Proper laryngeal functioning is important for pitch modulation and vocal quality, and intact velopharyngeal functioning impacts resonance. As such, those with CP may present with hypernasality due to velopharyngeal dysfunction (Hustad, 2010). Because of the motor challenges that are present, challenges associated with speech production are not uncommon, including disorders of articulation or phonology, CAS, or dysarthria. Mild-to-moderate dysarthria is the most common speech disorder associated with CP in children (78%), followed by articulation delay/disorder (54%), phonological delay/disorder (43%), and CAS (17%). Of these, dysarthria has been found to be associated with the poorest intelligibility ratings (Mei et al., 2020).

Impact of Motor Speech Disorders Across the Lifespan

Children who are born preterm are at an increased risk for being diagnosed with CP (O'Shea, 2002). This is particularly important because parents who give birth to preterm infants are faced with challenges as they must navigate the emotional experience of their infant receiving intensive care at the hospital, as

TABLE 6–3. Types of Cerebral Palsy

Type	Characteristics	Subtypes (If Applicable)
Spastic	• Muscle stiffness • Jerky movements	*Spastic diplegia:* Lower body primarily affected; intact cognitive and language skills *Spastic hemiplegia:* Limbs on one side of the body affected; intact cognitive and language skills *Spastic quadriplegia:* Limbs on both side of the body affected; associated with cognitive and language deficits
Dyskinetic	• Uncontrollable slow and jerky movements of arms, legs, hands, feet • Hyperactive movements of the face • Challenges walking • Challenges coordinating muscles for speech production • Intact cognitive functioning	
Ataxic	• Balance and depth perception impacted • Challenges with gross motor coordination for walking • Challenges with fine motor coordination	
Mixed	• Combination of dysarthria symptoms	

well as the atypical behaviors that the infant may be displaying (e.g., irritability, regulation challenges, muscle stiffness). For these reasons, it is particularly important that parents receive support from health care professionals to help facilitate parent–infant bonding and attachment (Hadders-Algra et al., 2016).

As children with CP age, they may experience academic and behavioral challenges that accompany their motor deficits, all of which have an impact on their ability to participate in various activities. Moreover, many of these children require assistance from adults in school due to their motor challenges and any accompanying language or cognitive deficits. As is the case with many children who require intensive adult support at school, children and adolescents with CP may have a more difficult time connecting with their peers, particularly peers without disabilities, and may be less socially involved than their nondisabled peers (Chang et al., 2014; Voorman et al., 2009). In addition, evidence suggests that children with CP who have greater cognitive and linguistic challenges exhibit fewer self-determined behaviors (defined in the literature as identifying and pursuing wants and needs, making choices, and engaging in problem-solving techniques; Chang et al., 2014). These self-determined behaviors, which can be facilitated through play and peer interactions, are associated with self-advocacy skills, which are critical components to an individual's ability to build and maintain relationships, as well as their overall quality of life. As children with CP become adults, they may develop other conditions associated with aging, and it has been found that adults with CP receive fewer supports after they age out of the school system. Moreover, adults with CP report engaging in few social activities, which impacts their overall well-being (Furukawa et al., 2001).

Just as CP can have lifelong impacts, so too can CAS, albeit in different ways. Whereas motor functioning is associated with individuals with CP, speech and language impacts are associated with CAS. Because of the high co-occurrence of language disorders with CAS, these children may be at risk for reduced academic achievement compared to their peers without a co-occurring language disorder. At the same time, children with CAS may present with deficits in literacy due to the motor programming challenges that are associated with speech production (Lewis et al., 2004).

Individuals who acquire MSDs in adulthood are likely to experience a host of unexpected challenges like those experienced by adults with acquired language disorders (see Chapter 9). This is because these individuals had normal speech and motor functioning until the onset of their disorder. In addition to the physical changes that a person with an MSD undergoes, there are also social and emotional consequences of an MSD. The person may feel embarrassed by their speech mannerisms as well as frustrated at being unable to communicate in the same way that they had prior to the disorder. In fact, adults with acquired MSDs may limit their social interactions to avoid communicating with others and feeling any associated negative emotions. Because those with strictly MSDs do not have deficits in language and know what they want to say (albeit have difficulty executing speech production), it can be frustrating to be unable to articulate words and have others attempt to speak for them.

In addition, adults with dysarthria resulting from degenerative diseases may progress in their disease to the point where they are unable to care for themselves and perform acts of daily living. For those individuals, quality of life is severely impacted. In fact, Leite and Constantini (2017) found that greater dysarthria severity was correlated with lower ratings of quality of life in adults with ALS and that these individuals reported a low self-image.

Limited research has examined caregiver burden for family caregivers of adults with MSDs. Evidence does suggest, however, that caregivers of individuals with dysarthria resulting from stroke experience higher levels of stress, anxiety, and depression, as well as lower quality of life. Caregiver depression is associated with the severity and duration of the disability and co-occurring conditions, as well as the caregiver's education level (Maratab et al., 2024). As such, it is important that clinicians working with patients with MSDs provide intervention and training for caregivers to support overall health and well-being outcomes for both the patient and the caregivers (Chen et al., 2021).

Cross-Cultural Information

Many of the conditions that are associated with MSDs have neurological underpinnings and impact an individual's neurophysiology regardless of their cultural or linguistic background. Moreover, voice concerns, such as ease of being understood by others, loudness, misarticulations, and vowel centralization, have been acknowledged in individuals with dysarthria (compared to individuals without dysarthria) across several languages, including but not limited to, Spanish, Mandarin, Italian, and Korean (Moya-Galé et al., 2023). Despite this, the impact that the speech characteristics associated with MSDs has on an individual's interaction abilities will differ across languages. For example, not all features that are associated with intelligibility in English are associated with intelligibility in Spanish speakers. Because English has a larger vowel repertoire than Spanish, vowel centralization may not impact intelligibility and ease of understanding in Spanish speakers to the same extent that it does in English speakers (Moya-Galé et al., 2023). Intelligibility may also differ among individuals who speak tonal versus non-tonal languages because tonal languages require more precise control over syllable productions (Whitehall & Wong, 2007).

Assessment

Assessment for Adult Populations

Assessment of MSDs begins with a thorough chart review and case history collected from the patient and/or their caregiver. Some important factors to consider include medical etiology (if known) and its prognosis, problem onset and progression over time, the presence of any associated deficits such as dysphagia (i.e., a swallowing disorder), the patient's perception of their speech problem and its impact on their ability to participate in meaningful activities, and goals that the patient hopes to accomplish in therapy.

After reviewing the patient's medical chart and collecting a thorough case history, the next step is to conduct an oral mechanism examination (OME) to assess the anatomy and physiology (i.e., the sensory and motor functions) of the structures involved in producing speech, such as the face, lips, tongue, jaw, palate, and larynx. If deviations in any of the structures are identified, the SLP must determine whether these deviations are purely anatomical in nature or if they reflect an underlying neurological problem.

Following an OME, the SLP assesses the patient's speech as they perform a variety of speech tasks. These speech tasks highlight patterns of aberrant speech characteristics unique to specific MSDs. There are four speech tasks essential to any motor speech evaluation: (a) discourse, such as speaking in conversation and reading aloud; (b) vowel prolongation (or maximum phonation time), in which the patient is instructed to take a deep breath and hold out an "ah" for as long as they can; (c) alternating motion rates, also known as diadochokinetic rates, in which the patient repeats the syllables "puh," "tuh," and "kuh" as fast and as steadily as possible; and (d) sequential motion rates, in which the patient repeats the sequence "puh–tuh–kuh" or the word "buttercup" as fast and as steadily as possible. If the SLP suspects that the patient has a neurological disorder that results in rapid deterioration or fatigue in speech (e.g., myasthenia gravis), stress testing can be used in which the patient continuously counts or reads a passage for approximately 2 to 4 minutes without rest. If the SLP suspects that the patient has a motor planning and/or programming disorder, the SLP may administer additional tasks that assess these underlying motor planning and/or programming processes, such as producing sounds in isolation, single-syllable words, single and repeated productions of multisyllabic words, sentences, and automatic speech. There are also a few published assessments designed to evaluate MSDs, such as the Frenchay Dysarthria Assessment (FDA-2; Enderby & Palmer, 2008) and the Apraxia Battery for Adults – 2nd Edition (ABA-2; Dabul, 2000); however, administering the four aforementioned speech tasks, along with stress testing and tasks that assess motor planning/programming if indicated, is sufficient to determine diagnosis.

It is important to know that auditory perceptual analysis is the clinical gold standard for differentially diagnosing MSDs. All motor speech evaluations begin with the SLP's ear, meaning that MSDs are diagnosed based on the unique groupings of speech characteristics that the SLP hears which reflect damage to specific areas of the motor system. Furthermore, listening to the patient's speech is the foundation for clinical practice. It allows the SLP to make judgments about the severity of the MSD at any point in time, informs treatment planning, and helps determine whether treatment has been successful.

Although auditory perceptual analysis is the clinical gold standard for differentially diagnosing MSDs, this method of assessment can be highly unreliable if the clinician is not well trained in sharpening their ability to distinguish the perceptual speech characteristics that highlight a specific dysarthria or an AoS. Even if a clinician is well trained in this method, there will still be some degree of subjectivity, making it difficult to quantify certain aspects of speech by ear alone. If quantification is desired, then other assessment techniques, such as acoustic analyses, physiological methods, and visual imaging, may be useful. Acoustic methods yield a visual display of the speech signal (e.g., as a waveform, spectrogram, etc.) and allow the SLP to obtain quantifiable measurements of variables such as frequency, intensity, and duration. Physiologic methods aim to evaluate the sources of activity involved in speech and include aerodynamic approaches, kinematic tracking systems, and neuroimaging. Aerodynamic approaches (e.g., **spirometry**, **nasometry**) measure how air passes through the oral and nasal cavities during speech, kinematic tracking systems (e.g., **electromagnetic articulography [EMA]**, **electromyography [EMG]**) allow for examination of speech structure movement, and neuroimaging techniques (e.g., **functional magnetic resonance imaging [fMRI]**, **positron emission tomography [PET]**) provide visualization of the underlying physiologic activity that occurs in the central nervous system during speech. Finally, if direct visualization of the speech structures and their function is needed, then imaging techniques such as **videofluoroscopy**, **nasoendoscopy**, **laryngoscopy**, and **videostroboscopy** can be considered (note that these tools are also frequently utilized to assess voice and swallowing).

In addition to auditory perceptual analysis and the completion of other supporting objective measures (i.e., acoustic analyses, aerodynamic approaches, kinematic analyses, neuroimaging, direct visual imaging), the SLP should make judgments of the patient's speech intelligibility, comprehensibility, and communicative efficiency. **Speech intelligibility** refers to the degree to which a listener can understand the auditory speech signal produced by the speaker. To assist with calculating intelligibility, several published tests are available, including the Speech Intelligibility Test (SIT) of the Assessment of Intelligibility in Dysarthric Speech (AIDS; Yorkston et al., 1984) and the Frenchay Dysarthria Assessment (FDA-2; Enderby & Palmer, 2008). In contrast to speech intelligibility, **comprehensibility** refers to the extent to which a listener can understand the message a speaker is trying to communicate using the auditory speech signal generated by the speaker as well as all other information relevant to the communicative exchange (setting, nonverbal cues, context, listener familiarity, etc.). Finally, **communicative efficiency** refers to the rate at which a speaker conveys intelligible and/or comprehensible information to their listener. Communicative efficiency is directly determined by a speaker's level of intelligibility and comprehensibility; that is, poor speech intelligibility and comprehensibility will increase the amount of time it takes for a speaker to successfully communicate their message to their listener, thus reducing overall communicative efficiency, whereas a speaker who can convey their message quickly to their listener would be considered highly efficient in their communication. Clinicians will often use information about speech intelligibility, comprehensibility, and communicative efficiency to judge the severity of a patient's MSD (see, for example, the Motor Speech Disorders Severity Rating Scale; Duffy, 2020).

The final component of a motor speech evaluation is to assess the patient's functional communication skills, the effectiveness of their communication, and the psychosocial impact of their MSD on their self-image and daily life. Acquiring this information not only assists with treatment planning but also provides a baseline for comparison after treatment when determining whether therapy was successful (recall that a desired outcome of treatment is to lessen adverse effects of the disorder on the patient's day-to-day living, thereby increasing their ability to engage and participate in meaningful activities). To examine functional communication, communicative effectiveness, and psychosocial impact, SLPs can administer surveys and questionnaires to patients and/or their caregivers to better understand their feelings about the patient's communication, specifically speech, as it occurs in various situations and conditions. Examples of such surveys and questionnaires include the Communicative Effectiveness Survey (CES; Donovan et al., 2007), the Dysarthria Impact Profile (Walshe et al., 2009), Living With Dysarthria (Hartelius et al., 2008), and the Communicative Participation Item Bank (CPIB; Baylor et al., 2013).

Assessment Considerations for Pediatric Populations

As we have seen for the various communication disorders described throughout this book, SLPs are part of an interprofessional team when it comes to diagnosing MSDs in children. The goal of the assessment is to make an accurate diagnosis, which often means using critical thinking clinical skills to differentially diagnose an MSD. The first step in this process is to collect a complete case history that provides information about the child's medical, family, and speech-language therapy histories, as well as current strengths and challenges associated with communication and learning. It is also important to collaborate with the client and family around their goals for assessment and any subsequent intervention.

Considering the importance of differential diagnosis for adults with MSDs, and the difficulty often associated with distinguishing between the various dysarthrias, do you think that differential diagnosis is important for the pediatric populations? The answer is yes!

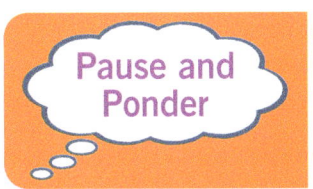

Why do you think that differential diagnosis is important for children with MSDs? What value does this component of assessment bring to intervention?

Diagnosis of MSDs in children can be challenging, particularly because many of the speech characteristics of dysarthria and CAS overlap with one another and with other disorders of articulation (and can even co-occur with one another). Having the textbook knowledge of the characteristics of each condition is one thing; disentangling these diagnoses from one another in practice is another thing (especially when a child has multiple disorders). As is the case with adults, SLPs are in the prime position to differentially diagnose MSDs in children. The first step in this process is to complete an OME to observe the structures and function of the child's oral structures required for speech production. In addition, the SLP must gather data on respiration, phonation, prosody, and loudness in various speaking contexts (e.g., single words, connected speech, repetition, spontaneous speech, reading). Conducting a dynamic assessment, in which the SLP provides cues to help determine if the child has emerging skills in any area, can further support accurate diagnosis. Dynamic assessment also provides information about the severity of the child's impairment, which will be informative for intervention. When working with children, it may also be important to assess language skills because MSDs can co-occur with language disorders. With this information, SLPs will have a complete picture of the client's communication abilities, which will help support differential diagnosis. Here, we describe common differential diagnosis considerations for children with dysarthria as well as those with CAS.

Differential Diagnosis: Dysarthria and Childhood Apraxia of Speech

Assessment of both dysarthria and CAS is often considered a daunting task to clinicians, particularly because of the limited validated assessment measures that are available. An SLP must use clinical judgment in making these diagnoses, which is complicated by the overlap in speech characteristics of each condition. In general, the three primary speech characteristics that are associated with a diagnosis of CAS (and thus examined during an assessment) are inconsistency in consonant and vowel production, coarticulation errors, and inappropriate prosody (Chenausky et al., 2020). Clinical judgment of the presence of these features has been considered the gold standard for assessment of CAS. However, evidence suggests that features of CAS can change over time, with improvements seen in articulation, and that this may be due to the intervention that the children receive (Lewis et al., 2004).

Several studies have been conducted to disentangle CAS from non-motor-based speech sound disorders (SSDs), and it is suggested that CAS and SSDs differ on the following speech characteristics during the production of multisyllabic words: voicing, structurally correct words, correct lexical stress, and syllable deletions. That is, children with CAS present with more voicing changes, fewer structurally correct words, inaccurate lexical stress, and greater number of syllable deletions on multisyllabic words compared to children with SSDs (Benway & Preston, 2020). Table 6–4 highlights the differences between CAS, dysarthria, and SSDs.

Iuzzini-Seigel and colleagues (2022) created a tool for SLPs to help with differential diagnosis of dysarthria and CAS. They identified several speech characteristics that are associated with dysarthria, CAS, or both in the areas of respiration, phonation, resonance, rate, prosody, and articulation. They also created a flowchart to help clinicians determine a child's likely diagnosis based on the speech features that are present (or absent). Furthermore, recent evidence has suggested that in addition to these features, clinicians should consider the **naturalness** of the child's speech, as children who present with dysarthria are perceived to have less natural-sounding speech compared to typically developing same-aged peers (Schölderle et al., 2023). In addition, one standardized test that uses dynamic assessment to facilitate differential diagnosis of CAS in children aged 3 years or older is the Dynamic Evaluation of Motor Speech Skill (DEMSS; Strand & McCauley, 2019). The DEMSS is designed to examine articulatory accuracy, vowel accuracy, prosodic accuracy, and consistency in various utterance types and lengths from CV and VC structures to multisyllabic words to utterances of greater length while providing the child with cueing as necessary (Strand et al., 2013). Finally, it is important to gather information about the child's intelligibility across people and contexts. For this reason, McLeod and colleagues (2012) developed the Intelligibility in Context Scale (ICS), a rating scale that asks about how well caregivers and others (e.g., extended family, peers, strangers) understand the child's speech.

Explore and Find Out!

Iuzzini-Seigel, J., Alison, K., & Stoekel, R. (2022). A tool for differential diagnosis of childhood apraxia of speech and dysarthria in children: A tutorial. *Language, Speech, and Hearing Services in Schools, 53*, 926–946.

▶ video

Check out the YouTube video series **"Childhood Apraxia of Speech"** by Dr. Edythe Strand for more information about CAS and differential diagnosis.

Cross-Cultural Considerations in Assessment

Given that MSDs are linked to damage to specific areas of the motor system, there are likely more similarities than differences in the ways that AoS or the various types of dysarthria affect speech across languages. In fact, preliminary evidence appears to support this (see, for example, Chakraborty et al.,

TABLE 6–4. Primary Characteristics of Childhood Apraxia of Speech, Dysarthria, and Speech Sound Disorders in Children

Speech Subsystem	Childhood Apraxia of Speech	Dysarthria	Speech Sound Disorders

Respiration/ phonation	• Volume not affected
	• Speech breathing not affected
	• Vocal quality not affected
		• Volume affected, including
		  ○ Low volume
		  ○ Volume decay with fatigue
		  ○ Excessive loudness
		  ○ Loudness variation
		• Effortful inspiration for speech breathing
		• Short breaths used when speaking
		  ○ Sounds like the speaker has run out of air when speaking
		• Atypical vocal quality depending on the type of dysarthria
		  ○ Strained
		  ○ Hoarse
		  ○ Rough
		  ○ Breathy
		  ○ Effortful
			• Volume not affected
			• Speech breathing not affected
			• Vocal quality not affected

Resonance	• Resonance affected
	  ○ Speech may sound intermittently hypernasal or hyponasal.
		• Resonance affected
		  ○ Speech may sound intermittently hypernasal or hyponasal.
		  ○ Consistent hypernasality
			• Resonance not affected

Rate/ prosody	• Slow rate of speech
	  ○ Slow articulatory movements
	  ○ Increased pausing
	• Atypical stress, including
	  ○ Monotone
	  ○ Monopitch
	  ○ Excess–equal stress across syllables
	• Stress errors at the word level
	• Atypical pausing between sounds, syllables, and words resulting in reduced flow of speech
		• Slow rate of speech
		  ○ Slow articulatory movements
		  ○ Increased pausing
		• Atypical stress, including
		  ○ Monotone
		  ○ Monopitch
		  ○ Excess–equal stress across syllables
			• Rate/prosody not affected

continues

TABLE 6–4. *continued*

Speech Subsystem	Childhood Apraxia of Speech	Dysarthria	Speech Sound Disorders

Articulation	• Consonant errors
	• Vowel errors
	• Voicing errors
	• Inappropriate use of schwa
	  ○ Schwa added at the beginning, middle, or end of words
	  ○ Vowels may be produced as schwa
	• Coarticulation errors
	  ○ Oral groping during speech production
	  ○ Challenges sequencing sounds
	• Inconsistent articulation errors
	• Articulation errors increase as length of word increases
	• Automatic speech easier to produce than spontaneous speech
		• Imprecise articulation
		• Consonant errors
		• Vowel errors
		• Voicing errors
		• Articulation errors consistent
			• Consonant errors
			• Articulation errors consistent
			• Articulation errors consistent as length of word increases

Sources: Adapted from Iuzzini-Seigel et al. (2022) and Stoeckel and Hammer (2001).

2008; Whitehill, 2010; Wong et al., 2024). Although additional research in this area is warranted, good assessment principles can still be applied when working with multicultural and linguistically diverse populations. When assessing for MSDs in individuals who speak languages other than English, clinicians should carefully consider the tasks that they are administering and evaluate whether the tasks are sensitive to detecting changes in speech that deviate from the normal speech patterns of the patient's native language. This is because languages vary widely in terms of their phonetic inventory and prosodic structure (e.g., stress, tone, rate of speech). For example, assessment of alternating and sequential motion rates in English involves the rapid production of the syllables "puh," "tuh," and "kuh"; however, not all languages have /p/, /t/, and /k/ in their phonetic inventory. As such, the clinician may need to select anterior and posterior sounds that are in the patient's phonetic inventory to allow for examination of the rapid production of these sounds in isolation and when sequenced together. Clinicians should also be sensitive to possible influences of speech in the primary language on speech in the secondary language because this may impact how articulation and prosody are realized in the second language. Furthermore, stimuli should be graded in complexity appropriate to the speech of the patient's native language and presented systematically so that areas of breakdown can be better identified. Thoughtful consideration of all tasks and stimuli will require considerable preparation from the clinician in advance.

Treatment

Treatment for Adult Populations

A strong understanding of the principles of motor learning is foundational to treating MSDs. There are six principles that one must consider: (a) drill, (b) instruction and self-learning, (c) feedback, (d) training specificity, (e) consistent and variable practice, and (f) speed–accuracy trade-offs. To rehabilitate impaired speech movements, intensive drill or training via repetition of target stimuli is essential. The clinician should aim to elicit as many accurate productions of the target as possible from the patient during their treatment sessions. Throughout treatment, particularly during the initial stages, the clinician will likely need to provide some degree of articulatory instruction to the patient regarding how they should produce speech movements. It is also important for the clinician to encourage self-learning in therapy and to provide the patient with opportunities to monitor their own speech and self-correct their errors when they occur. In addition to articulatory instruction, the clinician will need to consider the timing, frequency, and form of feedback that they will offer to the patient. Types of feedback can include clinician feedback, where the clinician informs the patient about the accuracy of their production, or instrumental feedback, where the patient receives information about the movement of their articulators for speech in real time or the outcome of their production (e.g., electromagnetic articulography, acoustic analyses, ultrasound). As a rule of thumb regarding the timing and frequency at which feedback should be provided, feedback should not exceed 60% of trials in a given treatment session, and there should be at least a 3- or 4-second delay following an elicited response before feedback is given. Ensuring that feedback is not provided too often and too quickly promotes better generalization of learned skills and encourages self-reflection and self-monitoring. The principle of **training specificity** states that training should be specific to the targeted skills required for the activity being practiced (in this case, speech). In other words, to improve speech, one must practice speech. As such, clinicians should prioritize practicing words and phrases (vs. individual speech sounds or nonspeech oral movements such as blowing, tongue pushing, and smiling) because these are more functional and lead to better generalization for speech. The clinician must also determine and set the patient's practice schedule in therapy. There are two options for practice: consistent practice (i.e., blocked practice) and variable practice (i.e., random practice). In consistent practice, multiple repetitions of the target (e.g., a word, a phrase) are elicited from the patient in the absence of any intervening stimuli. In variable practice, many different targets are practiced but in random order, requiring the patient to remain flexible in their responses; because this form of practice is more complex and more challenging compared to consistent practice, it may lead to greater acquisition, retention, and generalization of learned skills. Finally, the clinician must recognize that there is a trade-off between speed and accuracy of movement when learning any new motor skill. Generally, when treating individuals with MSDs, the clinician must reduce the rate at which the patient is speaking, even if the patient's rate of speech is already slower than normal at baseline, to increase articulatory accuracy. Once the patient has achieved greater articulatory accuracy, the clinician can proceed to work on improving the naturalness of the patient's speech by increasing their rate.

Recall that AoS is a disorder of motor planning and/or programming; therefore, the goal of intervention is to reestablish the motor plans and/or programs required for speech. Research supports the use of articulatory kinematic and rate and/or rhythm approaches to treat AoS. Examples of articulatory kinematic approaches include integral stimulation, sound production treatment (SPT), and motor learning guided

(MLG) intervention. In integral stimulation, the protocol begins with the clinician instructing the patient to watch, listen, and say the target with them (Rosenbek et al., 1973). The treatment then proceeds to follow a hierarchy of cues that move from most supportive (e.g., mouthing the target) to least supportive (e.g., providing a written cue) to elicit multiple and accurate productions of the target from the patient. SPT incorporates the "watch, listen, and say it with me" component of integral stimulation as well as other forms of explicit feedback (e.g., articulatory placement) to help patients accurately produce the target, specifically minimal pairs/contrasts, such as "sun"/"fun" (Bailey et al., 2015; Wambaugh, 2010; Wambaugh et al., 1999; Wambaugh & Mauszycki, 2010). Finally, MLG can be used to help patients increase their ability to independently monitor their own speech and develop strategies to self-correct their errors (Hageman et al., 2002; Johnson, 2018; Johnson et al., 2018). In this treatment, the patient produces the target stimulus three times; each iteration is separated by a 2- or 3-second delay. During each delay, the patient is instructed to analyze their most recent production and make modifications if necessary for their next production. After the patient is done with their three productions of the target stimulus, the clinician invites the patient to share their perceptions of their performance (e.g., "How do you think you did?"). The clinician also provides the patient with feedback; however, feedback in MLG primarily focuses on the outcome of the patient's productions (e.g., "You were more accurate on your second production. I heard you making changes with each try") versus instruction on articulatory placement.

In contrast to AoS, dysarthria is a disorder of motor execution or motor control. Because dysarthria can affect a single subsystem or multiple subsystems of speech (i.e., respiration, phonation, resonance, articulation, prosody), treatment will largely depend on which subsystem(s) is involved. Some techniques that can be used to address impairments in respiration, phonation, resonance, articulation, and prosody are outlined in this section.

Because good breath support is fundamental to speech production, clinicians should consider initiating therapy with an introduction to diaphragmatic (i.e., abdominal) breathing. Diaphragmatic breathing involves contracting the diaphragm, a dome-shaped muscle separating the thorax from the abdomen, to fill the lungs more efficiently with air and encourage full oxygen exchange. Patients can perform this breathing technique with or without phonation (i.e., a prolonged vowel) to build adequate breath support for speech. If other physiologic respiratory impairments are identified, the clinician may work to increase the patient's respiratory drive for speech by altering the patient's posture (i.e., individuals with inspiratory weakness benefit more from speaking in an upright position, whereas individuals with expiratory weakness benefit more in a supine position); prescribing an expiratory muscle strength training program (see Chapter 12); or instructing the patient to push, pull, or bear down during speech. Also, the clinician can work on phrasing to help the patient expand the number of words they can produce in a single breath.

If a patient is not initiating phonation at the beginning of exhalation, the clinician must address and correct this behavior in therapy to eliminate air wastage so that there is adequate breath support to support phonation. If a patient has vocal fold weakness preventing them from achieving complete vocal fold adduction or closure, closure techniques (e.g., exercises that involve pushing, pulling, or bearing down), postural adjustments (e.g., a head turn to the weak side), and physical manipulation of the larynx may be helpful. Individuals with **hyperadduction** who present with too much tension in the vocal folds may benefit from producing a breathy onset or sigh at the start of voicing to promote easy, more relaxed phonation. Vocal exercise programs such as Lee Silverman Voice Treatment (LSVT; Ramig et al., 1995), Phonation Resistance Training Exercises (PhoRTE; Ziegler et al., 2014; Ziegler & Hapner, 2013), and vocal function exercises (Angadi et al., 2019; Bane et al., 2017; Gorman et al., 2008; Stemple et al., 1994) can also help strengthen the voice and improve vocal flexibility. Examples of some voice exercises that are incorporated into these programs include holding out a prolonged vowel (e.g., /i/, /a/, /o/), producing pitch glides from a high to low pitch and vice versa, and using the voice that is practiced in speech (e.g., words, phrases, sentences); some of these programs also include components in which the patient produces voice at various loudness levels. See Chapter 11 for more information about treating voice disorders.

Medical management is usually required to address physiologic impairments in resonance. If an individual has difficulties elevating their velum during speech and therefore suffers from **hypernasality** (i.e., too much resonance in the nasal cavity due to sound being channeled through the nose), then surgery or a prosthetic device may be indicated. Surgically, a physician may perform a velar injection; for this procedure, material is inserted into the velum to increase its size so that better approximation between the velum and the posterior pharyngeal wall can be achieved during activities that require velar elevation. If surgery is not indicated or is undesirable, a prosthetic device such as a **palatal lift** (i.e., a retainer-like device with a posterior projection to help keep the velum in a raised position) may be appropriate. In terms of behavioral management, SLPs can introduce clear speech to their patients. Clear speech, a speaking technique in which patients are taught to over-articulate their words, may help reduce the amount of air flowing through the nasal cavity; decrease the length of time at which an individual needs to sustain pressure in the oral cavity for pressure consonants; and increase loudness, thereby improving overall speech intelligibility.

Patients with articulatory impairments can benefit from clear speech as well. Not only does over-articulating sounds in words improve articulatory clarity and precision but it also helps decrease the patient's rate of speech, which is often necessary to improve intelligibility, as stated previously in this section, given the speed–accuracy trade-off. LSVT has also been shown to improve articulation; when the patient focuses solely on speaking in a loud voice, the effects of loudness transcend the entire speech system, resulting in improvements across all subsystems of speech (Sapir et al., 2011). If individual sounds are being targeted in treatment, then a patient with dysarthria may respond well to articulatory kinematic approaches such as integral stimulation or articulatory instruction. Similarly to treatment for AoS, treatment for dysarthria should yield generalization of skills practiced in the therapy room to real-world situations. Intelligibility drills in which a speaker (i.e., the individual with dysarthria) must communicate a target word, phrase, or sentence that is unknown to their listener are particularly helpful in increasing overall speech intelligibility, enhancing self-awareness, and promoting discovery learning. Furthermore, these drills provide the patient with opportunities to apply speaker–listener strategies in a communicative context (i.e., recognizing communication breakdowns and working to repair them). Finally, it is important to note that evidence from the literature supporting the use of nonspeech oral motor exercises to strengthen weakened articulatory structures is lacking. In fact, clinicians must exercise extreme caution when considering using any nonspeech oral movement or gesture to facilitate speech (e.g., performing blowing exercises for a /u/ sound). Recall the motor learning principle of training specificity: The best way to improve speech is to practice speaking!

Some of the treatment techniques already discussed in this section can be used to target speaking rate and prosody. For example, clear speech gives a patient more time to produce the full range of motion required to reach their articulatory targets and to coordinate their movements for speech. As another example, working on various aspects of phrasing (e.g., increasing the pause length between words and phrases, chunking utterances into their natural syntactic units, producing the prosodic pattern that is consistent with a given phrase) can help modify rate and increase the naturalness of speech. Furthermore, patients with reduced prosody may benefit from tasks that focus on the production of stress, such as converting a statement into a question, conveying different emotions through stress, and varying the word that is stressed in a phrase (e.g., "I *have* a book" vs. "I have a *book*"). External cues such as hand or finger tapping, a metronome, or pacing boards can also be incorporated into therapy to support speech rate and prosody.

In some cases (consider, for example, patients with severe dysarthria), augmentative and alternative communication (AAC) may be warranted to facilitate more efficient and effective communication; these tools may be speech-generating devices, or they may be low-tech in nature (e.g., an alphabet board that a patient simultaneously uses during speech to point to the initial letter of the word that they are saying to provide additional context for their listener).

Treatment Considerations for Pediatric Populations

There is currently minimal research on the effectiveness of intervention for children with MSDs. Although the presentation of MSDs often looks similar across pediatric and adult populations, it is important to remember that adults usually *acquire* their disorder, whereas children develop *with* the disorder. That is, adults likely had fully functioning speech and language functioning prior to their condition, and therapy will focus on rehabilitation or management of skill. Children, however, often have co-occurring language deficits, cognitive deficits, and/or a developmental disorder, making intervention techniques more about developing skills in various areas. As such, intervention considerations for pediatric populations must fundamentally differ from those used with adults (Levy, 2014). However, as with adults who have MSDs, intervention for pediatric populations should incorporate the principles of motor learning for optimal outcomes. Although more research is needed on the effectiveness of interventions that adhere to the principles of motor learning, interventions that occur with many practice trials are more likely to result in changes in the neuroplasticity of the brain. (For a systematic review of motor speech interventions that have been used with children with dysarthria resulting from CP, see Korkalainen et al., 2023.)

Two primary approaches have been studied for use with children with dysarthria: Speech Systems Intelligibility Treatment (SSIT) and LSVT LOUD. Both are intensive interventions that have shown promising results for improving speech function in children with dysarthria, although they differ in their approach. SSIT targets the subsystems that are important for speech function: respiration, phonation, resonance, and articulation. Because the focus is on the specific subsystems, this technique is tailored to the individual needs of the child and their unique presentation of dysarthria. Targeting respiration, phonation, and speech rate using SSIT has been found to be associated with loudness control and increased utterance length, both of which indicate that children developed better breath control and were better able to coordinate breathing with speaking (Pennington et al., 2018). Whereas SSIT focuses on multiple subsystems of speech, LSVT LOUD focuses on one mechanism of speech: intensity (i.e., loudness). Children are taught to "think loud," initiating positive effects throughout the speech production system. Evidence suggests that for children with CP, LSVT LOUD results in increased loudness, as well as increased intelligibility of speech (Langlois et al., 2020). Moreover, parents indicate a preference for the quality of their child's speech production after having completed LSVT LOUD compared to prior to the intervention (Fox & Boliek, 2012).

As much as it is important to address speech functioning in children with MSD, it is also critical to support families and caregivers through the process, including very early on in the child's development. Early intervention for children who are at risk for CP suggests that providing parents with education and support is associated with decreases in anxiety and depression (Hadders-Algra et al., 2016).

A variety of treatment approaches for CAS have been proposed, with each approach unique in how it attempts to support communication. Although nonspeech oral motor exercises (nonspeech-related activities that target the structures used in speech, such as the tongue, lips, and jaw) can be used initially to bring attention to the child's articulators and movement of these muscles, they should not be used as a treatment technique because evidence suggests that they do not support speech production (Lee & Gibbon, 2015; Strand, 2021). Moreover, the child should understand *why* they are being asked to participate in therapy (*so that they can communicate with others*). The following intervention types are used in CAS: motor-based approaches, linguistic approaches, and multimodal communication approaches (for a review, see Morgan et al., 2018).

Motor-based approaches are grounded in the principles of motor learning and involve several repetitions of successful productions (i.e., *practice, practice, practice*). Clinicians must decide between four practice schedules, with the best choice depending on the severity of the child's disorder. These include **massed practice** (i.e., the child practices a skill [e.g., production of CVC words] repeatedly and all at once in a single session), **distributed practice** (i.e., the child practices various skills [e.g., several syllable shapes] in a single session), **random practice** (i.e., mixed stimuli are practiced throughout a session), and **blocked practice** (i.e., one stimulus is practiced repeatedly before moving on to the next stimulus). According to Strand and colleagues (Strand, 2017; Yorkston et al., 2010), massed practice leads to skill development more quickly with poorer generalization, whereas skill development is more time-consuming with distributed practice, although it leads to better motor learning. Similarly, these authors suggest that blocked practice leads to better motor performance in a short period of time (and less effective motor learning over time), whereas random practice is more time-consuming for skill development but leads to better motor learning. As children demonstrate improvements in speech production through therapy, clinicians often move from mass and blocked practices to distributed and random practices.

Feedback is integral to motor-based approaches as well, and this includes intrinsic and extrinsic feedback. **Intrinsic feedback** involves the child being aware of the sensory information associated with speech production (e.g., what they hear, how their articulators feel), whereas **extrinsic feedback** is feedback provided by others. Two types of extrinsic feedback are related to (a) accuracy of the actual production and (b) information about the movement of articulators as it relates to the production. As you might have guessed, extrinsic feedback is particularly important to provide if a child is unable to access sensory information required for intrinsic feedback, as well as for children with more severe impairments who are early in the treatment process. Naturally, extrinsic cues and feedback become faded over time as the client becomes more independent and successful with the intervention. Examples of motor-based approaches are the **Prompts for Restructuring Oral Muscular Phonetic Targets (PROMPT) system**, **melodic intonation therapy**, **dynamic temporal and tactile cueing (DTTC)**, and **rapid syllable transition (ReST)**. Several interventions that adhere to the principles of motor learning have been found to support speech production in CAS (see Morgan et al., 2018; Murray et al., 2014; Strand, 2017, 2019).

Linguistic approaches are particularly useful for children who have co-occurring language disorders, where the focus is less on motor speech production and more on targeting semantics, phonology, and/or syntax (see Chapter 7). One intervention that has been shown to be effective for children with CAS and a co-occurring language disorder is integrated phonological awareness intervention (Murray et al., 2014).

Multimodal communication approaches aim to support verbal communication through other means, such as AAC (see Chapter 14). These methods are often used with children who have minimal or no verbal speech or whose speech intelligibility is quite low. AAC can include high-tech devices, such as computers or tablets, or low-tech systems such as communication boards. In addition, a child might use gestures or signs to communicate. Evidence suggests that AAC supports communication in children with CAS. This may be due to children having access to communication during times when verbal speech is not adequate (Murray et al., 2014).

Explore and Find Out!

Levy, E., & Moya-Galé, G. (2023). Revisiting dysarthria treatment across languages: The hybrid approach. *Journal of Speech, Language, and Hearing Research*, 1–10. https://doi.org/10.1044/2023_JSLHR-23-00629

Why Is This Topic Important?

As stated at the beginning of this chapter, speech is the primary modality through which many of us express our thoughts, ideas, wants, and needs to others. Although this observation alone illustrates the importance of speech to our everyday lives, communicating through speech is much more than producing the words and sentences that you want to say; it also encompasses *how* you say those words and sentences (e.g., to convey sarcasm or specific emotions). Furthermore, speech can be a fundamental aspect of our identity; consider, for example, the defining characteristics of our voice that make up our unique vocal fingerprint or an accent, which may suggest ties to a specific region and/or culture. Given that speech serves a variety of purposes and functions, it is not difficult to recognize how an adverse change in one's ability to speak could negatively impact their quality of life.

As discussed in this chapter, MSDs result from neurologic damage to the structures and processes involved in speech motor planning, programming, execution, and/or control (Duffy, 2020). These include AoS, flaccid dysarthrias, spastic dysarthria, ataxic dysarthria, hypokinetic dysarthria, hyperkinetic dysarthrias, unilateral upper motor neuron dysarthria, and mixed dysarthrias. Each disorder is associated with clusters of deviant speech characteristics, which make accurate differentiation and diagnosis possible if the clinician can identify their auditory–perceptual features. Differential diagnosis serves several important purposes. As stated previously, injury to different parts of the central and peripheral nervous systems results in distinct perceptual speech patterns, and although an MSD cannot suggest a specific neurological diagnosis in isolation (e.g., ALS, multiple sclerosis, traumatic brain injury), it can assist with localization of the disease. An SLP's skills and expertise in this area can therefore be extremely valuable to the medical team, especially if the patient does not yet have an official medical diagnosis, because it helps the team make decisions that will result in more focused and expedited care to determine the root cause of the patient's complaints. In fact, subtle but adverse speech changes are sometimes the first sign of an underlying neurological disease, and SLPs are the ones on the interprofessional health care team who are trained to recognize those changes. In contrast, if a patient has a known medical condition, the MSD diagnosis should be consistent with what is known about the underlying medical etiology and provide further confirmation and support for the medical diagnosis. If there is any misalignment, then this may indicate a misdiagnosis or the presence of some other co-occurring disease.

Accurate differentiation also influences treatment planning and helps the SLP select the most appropriate treatment approach for their patient with an MSD. Not all treatment approaches are appropriate for every MSD, and it is important for the SLP to recognize when an approach is contraindicated for a given

MSD diagnosis. Finally, being able to recognize the speech patterns associated with neurologic damage can assist with the identification of functional speech disorders (i.e., speech disorders that cannot be attributable to an organic cause, specifically a neurological lesion or disease). Functional speech disorders are becoming increasingly common and are often misdiagnosed due to a poor understanding of these disorders and an inability to differentiate them from MSDs. For SLPs, correct diagnosis of functional speech disorders is critical because they cannot be managed with traditional motor speech approaches.

Finally, recall the *International Classification of Functioning, Disability and Health* (ICF) model (World Health Organization, 2001) from Chapter 2. Let's apply the ICF framework to an adolescent (Landon) with CP (Figure 6–3). To get a better sense of how Landon's disability interacts with various environmental and personal factors to support or hinder his participation in activities throughout his day, let's look at a completed ICF diagram. Here, we want to know about Landon's ability to participate in one of his favorite activities: playing video games with his friends. We consider the factors that are both supportive of and barriers to his participation in this activity. Several factors contribute to Landon's ability to play video games with his friends. Because Landon presents with dyskinetic CP, the movements of his arms and legs are often slow and jerky, and he has trouble coordinating the muscles for speech production (body function and structure). This impacts his ability to walk as well as to efficiently and effectively use verbal speech. He uses a motorized wheelchair that is connected to an eye-gaze AAC system which allows him to communicate with his friends and play video games using his eyes. Environmental factors that may impact his participation in this activity include his eye gaze system being calibrated properly to ensure accuracy of use, as well as whether the eye gaze device and his wheelchair are charged. If Landon's Bluetooth-to-AAC system is working properly, he will not have to worry about any wires for his AAC

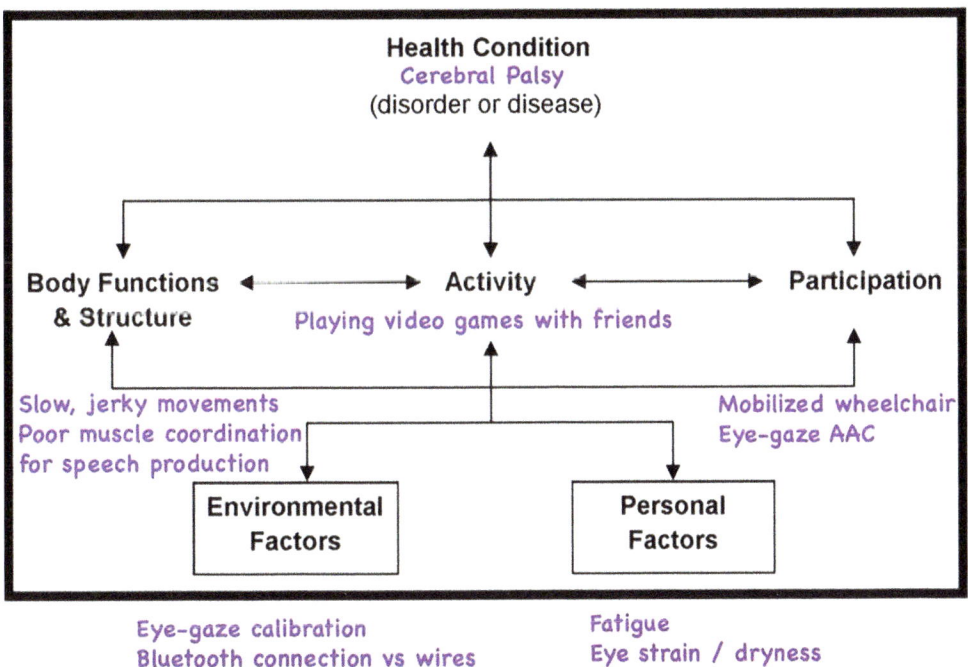

FIGURE 6–3. ICF model example. AAC, augmentative and alternative communication. *Source:* Adapted from the World Health Organization (2002).

device/eye gaze system getting caught in his wheelchair while he plays video games with his friends. Personal factors may also impact Landon's ability to play video games with his friends, including his level of overall fatigue, eye strain, and eye pain or dryness. If Landon is experiencing eye strain, for example, continuing to use his eye gaze system to communicate and control the video game may result in further pain (e.g., a headache) and reduce his ability or desire to continue the activity.

Application to a Child

Boeden is a 5-year-old boy who was recently diagnosed with CAS. Boeden lives with his mother in a one-bedroom apartment and visits his grandparents regularly. He is fascinated by dinosaurs, and each week when he goes to the library, he checks out a new book on the prehistoric creatures. Boeden loves playing dinosaurs with friends at school, although he has difficulty connecting with his peers during this play. Dinosaur names are often multisyllabic, and Boeden struggles producing any word that is more than one syllable. Even so, Boeden is highly motivated to communicate with others and is persistent in his communication attempts.

During his most recent assessment, it was found that he demonstrates average receptive and expressive language skills and cognitive functioning. He shows challenges in early literacy skills, including letter–sound correspondence. The assessment process revealed that Boeden has good, focused attention to tasks, even those that are somewhat challenging. Boeden is receptive to adult feedback and guidance, and he seeks help from others on complicated tasks. Teacher report during the assessment also revealed that Boeden is having difficulty connecting with his peers, despite his best efforts. His peers often do not understand what he is saying and have begun to ignore his messages or interjections into the conversation. Despite being persistent in attempting to be understood, his teacher worries that Boeden will soon become discouraged from initiating play with his peers and prefer to engage in isolated activities.

Based on Boeden's speech patterns prior to the assessment, the SLP at his school suspected that he may present with CAS. The SLP noticed that Boeden had a limited consonant inventory and was only able to produce some vowels. In addition, Boeden primarily produced one-syllable words, and occasionally he produced two-syllable words, although these were usually segmented and said in a monotonous voice. The SLP noted that Boeden did not attempt to produce anything more complex than two-syllable words.

To assess Boeden's speech, the SLP first completed an OME to view the structures of his oral cavity. She found nothing remarkable that indicated muscle weakness or reduced range of motion. The SLP then completed a checklist of diagnostic features across several speaking tasks to gather information about each of Boeden's speech subsystems (i.e., respiration, phonation, resonance, rate, prosody, and articulation). For a standardized assessment, the SLP decided to use DEMSS to help determine if Boeden presented with CAS. She found that he was able to say one-syllable words, and his ability to produce two-syllable words was significantly aided by her cueing. Cueing also helped Boeden say two-syllable words with appropriate stress and prosody, instead of in a monotonous tone. Furthermore, she noted that with several forms of cueing, he demonstrated some ability to say multisyllabic words, although these were always said in a monotonous voice.

In addition to DEMSS, the SLP completed a spontaneous speech sample on which she conducted a speech/language analysis, as well as assessed the intelligibility of his oral communication across people and contexts using the ICS.

After a comprehensive assessment that resulted in a diagnosis of CAS, the SLP concluded that the best treatment approach would be a motor learning approach to support communication. Based on the evidence of the program, the SLP chose to implement DTTC, where the clinician first modeled the target and then Boeden imitated the target. Following DTTC guidelines, first the SLP and Boeden produced the target words simultaneously, and the SLP provided visual, tactile, and gestural feedback. The SLP also targeted producing the words with varying prosody, including using loud and soft voices as well as different emotions. After successful productions at this stage, the SLP moved to having Boeden directly imitate her. This stage was more complicated for Boeden, especially for multisyllabic words with varying prosody. As such, the SLP planned to stay at this stage until Boeden was ready to move on to delayed imitation and then spontaneous speech.

How do you think targeting Boeden's speech production will impact him in other areas of his life? How might it support his social engagement and connection with his peers? What about his literacy skills might be impacted and how should those be addresses?

Application to an Adult

Gary is a 70-year-old male who was brought to the hospital by his daughter for an unwitnessed fall. Gary's daughter told the physician in the emergency department that she found him on the floor when she went to pick him up for their weekly lunch outing. She further added that he had been having multiple falls during the past 3 or 4 months. In addition to the falls, she expressed some concerns about his speech, endorsing that she has noticed some recent and significant changes during the past several months. She commented that he often mumbles, making it difficult for her and others to hear what he is saying. She often tells him to speak louder, but he insists that his speech is just fine. Gary was admitted to the hospital for further workup regarding these concerns. Because Gary fell, a computed tomography head scan was ordered; results of the head scan were unremarkable and yielded negative findings of brain swelling, hemorrhages, or skull fractures. In addition, a consult was placed to speech-language pathology for further evaluation of Gary's communication skills.

The SLP stopped by Gary's room the next day to conduct the evaluation. While conversing with Gary, the SLP noted that Gary's speech was monopitch and monoloud, and his overall stress during speech was reduced. He also spoke in short phrases and would produce prolonged pauses at inappropriate times when speaking. Some dysfluencies such as sound prolongations and sound, syllable, and word repetitions were observed. His vocal quality was harsh, his vocal loudness attenuated, and his articulation imprecise as it appeared that he was not achieving full range of motion of his articulators during speech. In addition, his speech rate was slow. These features of Gary's speech continued to be highlighted across the motor speech evaluation, particularly during a short reading task, production of alternating motion rates, and prolongation of the vowel /a/. Together, these groupings of deviant speech characteristics strongly suggested the presence of a hypokinetic dysarthria, pointing to a lesion somewhere in the basal ganglia and/or basal ganglia control circuit.

The SLP relayed their findings back to the medical team, which in turn consulted neurology for further examination to determine whether a possible medical condition could explain the symptoms that Gary was experiencing during the past few months. With the information provided by the SLP, the neurologist was able to perform focused testing that confirmed a medical diagnosis of Parkinson's disease.

In terms of Gary's speech, the SLP, who was certified in LSVT, determined that Gary would be a good candidate for this therapy program. After 16 sessions following the LSVT protocol, Gary made significant gains in his speech. He demonstrated improvements in vocal loudness, articulatory precision, prosody, and overall speech intelligibility. He also reported less frustration around communication; other people seemed to better understand what he was saying, and he was no longer receiving requests to repeat himself (this was also confirmed by his daughter). Furthermore, Gary could independently implement the skills practiced in therapy in his day-to-day communication with others.

What role did the SLP play in Gary's diagnosis? Why was working together as an interdisciplinary team important for Gary's quality of life? What might be some of the ongoing implications for supporting Gary and his family as his Parkinson's progresses.

Chapter Summary

Motor speech disorders arise from neurological damage to structures vital for speech production, resulting in difficulties with muscle movements or motor planning and/or programming. Dysarthria is an MSD that may present in many forms—flaccid, spastic, ataxic, hypokinetic, hyperkinetic, unilateral upper motor neuron, and mixed dysarthria—each with distinct characteristics and causes. AoS is another MSD characterized by deficits in motor planning and/or programming rather than muscle weakness due to damage to motor planning/programming areas of the left hemisphere of the brain. CAS, which appears in the pediatric population, can occur without neurological insult, and it shares similar characteristics with AoS. CP is a common condition associated with dysarthria in childhood, and it includes spastic, dyskinetic, ataxic, and mixed CP. CP affects muscle tone, strength, and motor control, and it can be accompanied by speech, language, and/or cognitive deficits.

Assessment of MSDs begins with a comprehensive chart review and case history, considering factors such as medical etiology, problem onset, associated deficits, and patient goals. This is followed by an OME to assess speech-related anatomy and physiology. Speech tasks, including discourse, vowel prolongation, and alternating and sequential motion rates, can help identify patterns indicative of specific MSDs. Auditory perceptual analysis serves as the gold standard for diagnosis; however, other objective measures, such as acoustic analyses and physiological methods, can be used to further characterize the patient's speech. Speech intelligibility, comprehensibility, and communicative efficiency are assessed to judge disorder severity. Finally, evaluating functional communication skills and the psychosocial impact of the

MSD on the patient's life through surveys and questionnaires completes the assessment process, aiding in treatment planning and outcome evaluation.

When assessing MSDs in children, it is crucial to conduct a thorough evaluation to differentiate between dysarthria and CAS. This process involves collecting a comprehensive case history, conducting an OME, and evaluating the patient's speech through various tasks. Differential diagnosis is important due to the overlapping characteristics of dysarthria and CAS, along with the potential co-occurrence of other speech disorders. Clinicians rely on clinical judgment and validated assessment tools to differentiate between the two conditions, considering features such as inconsistency in speech production, coarticulation errors, and inappropriate prosody for CAS, while also assessing features associated with dysarthria. Dynamic assessment and standardized tests such as DEMSS aid in this process, along with gathering information about the child's intelligibility across different contexts.

Understanding the principles of motor learning is crucial for treating MSDs, with six key principles to consider: drill, instruction and self-learning, feedback, training specificity, consistent and variable practice, and speed–accuracy trade-offs. Rehabilitation involves intensive drill of target stimuli, providing articulatory instruction, encouraging self-learning, and offering appropriate feedback. For AoS, articulatory kinematic approaches such as integral stimulation, sound production treatment, and motor learning guided methods are effective. Dysarthria treatment varies based on the affected subsystems, including techniques for respiration, phonation, resonance, articulation, and prosody. These may involve exercises to strengthen breath support and vocal fold musculature and interventions to improve articulation, speech rate, and prosody (e.g., LSVT, clear speech). In severe cases, AAC methods may be necessary for effective communication.

Research on intervention effectiveness for children with MSDs is limited, but it is essential to distinguish between interventions for adults who acquire MSDs and children who develop with them. Whereas adult therapy typically focuses on rehabilitation, pediatric interventions often address co-occurring deficits, requiring a developmental approach. Despite the need for more research, interventions following motor learning principles show promise in altering brain neuroplasticity. Two primary approaches for children with dysarthria are SSIT and LSVT LOUD; both emphasize intensive interventions with promising outcomes. Early intervention also supports families, reducing caregiver anxiety and depression. Treatment approaches for CAS include motor-based, linguistic, and multimodal communication approaches, with interventions such as the PROMPT system and integrated phonological awareness showing positive gains in speech and overall communication skills. In addition, AAC methods are valuable for children with minimal verbal speech or low speech intelligibility.

Chapter Review Questions

1. What is the difference between the indirect activation pathway and the direct activation pathway?
2. What is the difference between the upper motor neuron system and the lower motor system?
3. What are the speech characteristics that are commonly associated with spastic dysarthria? Flaccid dysarthria? Ataxic dysarthria? Hyperkinetic dysarthria? Hypokinetic dysarthria? Unilateral upper motor neuron dysarthria?
4. What condition is commonly associated with flaccid dysarthria? Hypokinetic dysarthria? Hyperkinetic dysarthria? Mixed dysarthria?

5. In what ways does dysarthria differ from apraxia of speech?
6. What is a common speech characteristic of children with cerebral palsy?
7. Why is it important to differentially diagnose motor speech disorders in children, such as dysarthria and childhood apraxia of speech? What value does this component of assessment bring to intervention?
8. What is the difference between speech intelligibility, comprehensibility, and communicative efficiency?
9. What are the six principles of motor learning crucial for treating motor speech disorders?
10. How do intervention considerations for children with motor speech disorders differ from those for adults?
11. What are the primary differences between LSVT LOUD and SSIT for children with motor speech disorders?

Learning Activities

1. Watch and listen to the YouTube video "Adult Apraxia of Speech." What speech characteristics do you hear that are consistent with an apraxia of speech diagnosis? Where is the neurological site(s) of lesion?

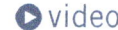

"Adult Apraxia of Speech"

2. Watch and listen to the YouTube video "Flaccid Dysarthria." What speech characteristics do you hear that are consistent with a flaccid dysarthria diagnosis? Where is the neurological site(s) of lesion? Which cranial nerve(s) do you think is involved?

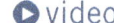

"Flaccid Dysarthria"

3. Watch and listen to the YouTube video "Spastic Dysarthria." What speech characteristics do you hear that are consistent with a spastic dysarthria diagnosis? Where is the neurological site(s) of lesion?

"Spastic Dysarthria"

4. Watch and listen to the YouTube video "Ataxic Dysarthria." What speech characteristics do you hear that are consistent with an ataxic dysarthria diagnosis? Where is the neurological site(s) of lesion?

"Ataxic Dysarthria"

5. Watch and listen to the YouTube video "LSVT LOUD Speech Therapy for Parkinson Disease" of a person with hypokinetic dysarthria prior to LSVT (up to 1:00 minute). What speech characteristics do you hear that are consistent with a hypokinetic dysarthria diagnosis? Where is the neurological site(s) of lesion? Now watch and listen to the remainder of the video (after 1:00 minute). How does this individual's speech change after LSVT?

"LSVT LOUD Speech Therapy for Parkinson Disease"

6. Watch and listen to the YouTube video "Huntington's Disease Clinic—Nebraska Medicine" of a person with hyperkinetic dysarthria. Then watch and listen to the YouTube video "Confessions of a Girl With Spasmodic Dysphonia" of a person with spasmodic dysphonia, another form of hyperkinetic dysarthria. How are the two individuals' speech similar? How are they different? What speech characteristics do you hear in both video clips that are consistent with a hyperkinetic dysarthria diagnosis? Where is the neurological site(s) of lesion?

"Huntington's Disease Clinic—Nebraska Medicine"
"Confessions of a Girl With Spasmodic Dysphonia"

Suggested Reading

Duffy, J. R., Utianski, R. L., & Josephs, K. A. (2021). Primary progressive apraxia of speech: From recognition to diagnosis and care. *Aphasiology, 35*(4), 560–591.

Apraxia of speech resulting from neurodegenerative disease is called primary progressive apraxia of speech (PPAOS). In this article, clinical guidance regarding the diagnosis and management of PPAOS is provided. The authors describe the clinical features of PPAOS, including speech characteristics and subtypes. In addition, they discuss other problems that may emerge as the disease progresses, such as dysarthria, aphasia, and/or other cognitive–linguistic impairments. Finally, the article concludes with some suggestions for managing PPAOS. Because PPAOS is degenerative in nature, the purpose of intervention is less about restoring function and more about helping the patient and their caregiver adopt compensatory strategies that will enhance the speaker–listener interaction (e.g., clear speech, rate reduction techniques, intelligibility drills, AAC). Management of PPAOS will also likely require ongoing education, counseling, and support because the disorder is often poorly understood by the medical community.

Gomez, M., McCabe, P., & Purcell, A. (2022). A survey of the clinical management of childhood apraxia of speech in the United States and Canada. *Journal of Communication Disorders, 96*, Article 106193.

This was a survey design study that examined SLPs' perspectives of CAS treatment in the United States and Canada. The researchers developed a survey to examine what CAS treatment approaches SLPs use, in what frequency and duration are these treatments implemented, what are SLPs' attitudes and perspectives of evidence-based practice in CAS, and what are the barriers to using evidence-based intervention strategies when working with children with CAS. The researchers identified that SLPs use a variety of interventions when working with children with CAS, often combining strategies from different approaches, and that they tend to use interventions that have worked for them in the past (compared to what has been evaluated through research). Clinicians noted that they do not always have a strong understanding of what the evidence is for CAS treatments. This finding is important because it suggests one of two things: Clinicians must be more mindful about engaging in the research on best practices for CAS intervention or researchers must conduct more rigorous studies on what it is that clinicians are doing in practice. Moreover, clinicians noted that time is a barrier to determining and using evidence-based practice strategies, as well as reduced access to research articles. This article provides important information about how CAS intervention is being conducted by SLPs. To ensure that children with CAS receive the most appropriate intervention, it is necessary for researchers and clinicians to come together to support best practice implementation.

Utianski, R. L., & Duffy, J. R. (2022). Understanding, recognizing, and managing functional speech disorders: Current thinking illustrated with a case series. *American Journal of Speech-Language Pathology, 31*(3), 1205–1220.

In this article, an overview of functional speech disorders (i.e., speech disorders that cannot be attributable to a neurological lesion or known neurological disease) is provided. The information presented in this article underscores the importance of understanding the clinical features associated with various neurogenic MSDs so that a correct diagnosis of a functional speech disorder is not overlooked. To illustrate the various ways in which functional speech disorders can manifest, four clinical case studies are described. For each case study, the authors detail how the patient presented at the start of the evaluation and the results of the patient's speech examination that led to a diagnosis of a functional speech disorder. The authors also document how each patient's functional speech disorder was addressed and the outcomes of intervention. Finally, the article concludes with the authors offering some guiding principles regarding the assessment, diagnosis, and treatment of functional speech disorders. This article also highlights how successful management of functional speech disorders requires a different approach from the traditional methods that are frequently used to treat neurogenic MSDs.

Voorman, J., Dallmeijer, A., van Eck, M., Schuengel, C., & Becher, J. (2009). Social functioning and communication in children with cerebral palsy: Association with disease characteristics and personal and environmental factors. *Developmental Medicine & Child Neurology, 52*, 441–447.

This was a longitudinal study that examined social functioning and communication in children with CP. Researchers followed 110 children aged 9 to 16 years (with an average age of 11;3) over a period of 3 years and gathered information about the children's CP diagnosis and severity, social functioning and communication, behavioral challenges, as well as parental stress. The researchers found that social functioning was associated with several factors, including the severity of the child's CP as well as age, behavioral challenges, and parental level of education. That is, children who were older, had a more severe diagnosis of CP, had more behavioral challenges, and whose parents had a lower education level tended to have worse social functioning. Similarly, children's communication skills were associated with several factors, including severity of CP, co-occurring diagnoses, behavioral challenges, number of siblings, and parental stress. To elaborate, less good communication abilities were observed in children with more severe CP as well as those who had co-occurring epilepsy and speech challenges, those who had more behavioral challenges, and those who did not have any siblings. In addition, communication skills were lower in children whose parents experienced higher levels of stress. This study offers important findings about children with CP. Although supporting speech and language abilities in this population is of utmost importance, clinicians must also consider how the child's social functioning impacts their ability to participate in daily activities. Moreover, it is widely recognized that social functioning is strongly related to overall quality of life. As clinicians, it is necessary to provide support in the areas of social functioning and overall communication to help ensure optimal outcomes for clients with CP.

References

American Speech-Language-Hearing Association. (n.d.). *Dysarthria in adults.* https://www.asha.org/practice-portal/clinical-topics/dysarthria-in-adults/#collapse_1

Angadi, V., Croake, D., & Stemple, J. (2019). Effects of vocal function exercises: A systematic review. *Journal of Voice, 33*(1), 124.e13–124.e34.

Bailey, D. J., Eatchel, K., & Wambaugh, J. (2015). Sound production treatment: Synthesis and quantification of outcomes. *American Journal of Speech-Language Pathology, 24*(4), S798–S814.

Bane, M., Angadi, V., Dressler, E., Andreatta, R., & Stemple, J. (2017). Vocal function exercises for normal voice: The effects of varying dosage. *International Journal of Speech-Language Pathology, 21*(1), 37–45.

Baylor, C., Yorkston, K., Eadie, T., Kim, J., Chung, H., & Amtmann, D. (2013). The Communicative Participation Item Bank (CPIB): Item bank calibration and development of a disorder—generic short form. *Journal of Speech, Language, & Hearing Research, 56*(4), 1190–1208.

Benway, N., & Preston, J. (2020). Differences between school-age children with apraxia of speech and other speech sound disorders on multisyllable repetition. *Perspectives of the ASHA Special Interest Group, 5*(4), 794–808.

Cerebral Palsy Guide. (2024). *Cerebral palsy incidence.*

Chakraborty, N., Roy, T., Hazra, A., Biswas, A., & Bhattacharya, K. (2008). Dysarthric Bengali speech: A neurolinguistic study. *Journal of Postgraduate Medicine, 54*(4), 268–272.

Chang, H.-J., Chiarello, L., Palisano, R., Orlin, M., Bundy, A., & Gracely, E. (2104). The determinants of self-determined behaviors of young children with cerebral palsy. *Research in Developmental Disabilities, 35*(1), 99–109.

Chen, C., Shune, S., & Namasivayam-MacDonanld, A. (2021). Understanding clinician perspectives and actions to address caregiver burden in caregivers of adults. *Perspectives of the ASHA Special Interest Groups, 6*, 1452–1469.

Chenausky, K., Brignell, A., Morgan, A., Gangé, D., Norton, A., Tager-Flusberg, H., . . . Green, J. (2020). Factor analysis of signs of childhood apraxia of speech. *Journal of Communication Disorders, 87*, Article 106033.

Dabul, B. (2000). *Apraxia Battery for Adults–2nd Edition (ABA-2)*. Pro-Ed.

Donovan, N. J., Velozo, C. A., & Rosenbek, J. C. (2007). The Communicative Effectiveness Survey: Investigating its item-level psychometric properties. *Journal of Medical Speech Language Pathology, 15*, 433–447.

Duffy, J. (2013). *Motor speech disorders: Substrates, differential diagnosis, and management* (3rd ed.). Elsevier.

Duffy, J. (2020). *Motor speech disorders: Substrates, differential diagnosis, and management* (4th ed.). Elsevier.

Enderby, P. M., & Palmer, R. (2008). *Frenchay Dysarthria Assessment–2nd Edition (FDA-2)*. Pro-Ed.

Fox, C., & Boliek, C. (2012). Intensive voice treatment (LSVT LOUD) for children with spastic cerebral palsy and dysarthria. *Journal of Speech, Language, and Hearing Research, 55*(3), 930–945.

Furukawa, A., Iwatsuki, H., Nishiyama, M., Nii, E., & Uchida, A. (2001). A study on the subjective well-being of adult patients with cerebral palsy. *Journal of Physical Therapy Science, 13*, 31–35.

Gomez, M., McCabe, P., & Purcell, A. (2022). A survey of the clinical management of childhood apraxia of speech in the United States and Canada. *Journal of Communication Disorders, 96*, Article 106193.

Gorman, S., Weinrich, B., Lee, L., & Stemple, J. C. (2008). Aerodynamic changes as a result of vocal function exercises in elderly men. *The Laryngoscope, 118*(10), 1900–1903.

Hadders-Algra, M., Boxum, A., Hielkema, T., & Hamer, E. (2016). Effect of early intervention in infants at very high risk of cerebral palsy: A systematic review. *Developmental Medicine & Child Neurology, 59*(3), 246–258.

Hageman, C. F., Simon, P., Backer, B., & Burda, A. N. (2002, November). *Comparing MIT and motor learning therapy in a nonfluent aphasic speaker* [Paper presentation]. Annual meeting of the American Speech-Language-Hearing Association, Atlanta, GA.

Hanson, E., Yorkston, K., & Britton, D. (2011). Dysarthria in amyotrophic lateral sclerosis: A systematic review of characteristics, speech treatment, and augmentative communication options. *Journal of Medical Speech-Language Pathology, 19*(3), 12–30.

Hartelius, L., Elmberg, M., Holm, R., Lövberg, A. S., & Nikolaidis, S. (2008). Living with dysarthria: Evaluation of a self-report questionnaire. *Folia Phoniatrica et Logopaedica, 60*(1), 11–19.

Hustad, K. (2010). Childhood dysarthria: Cerebral palsy. In K. Yorkston, D. Beukelman, E. Strand, & M. Hakel (Eds.), *Management of motor speech disorders in children and adults* (pp. 359–384). Pro-Ed.

Iuzzini-Seigel, J., Alison, K., & Stoekel, R. (2022). A tool for differential diagnosis of childhood apraxia of speech and dysarthria in children: A tutorial. *Language, Speech, and Hearing Services in Schools, 53*, 926–946.

Johnson, R. K. (2018). Motor learning guided treatment for acquired apraxia of speech. *Speech, Language and Hearing, 21*(4), 202–212.

Johnson, R. K., Lasker, J. P., Stierwalt, J. A., MacPherson, M. K., & LaPointe, L. L. (2018). Motor learning guided treatment for acquired apraxia of speech: A case study investigating factors that influence treatment outcomes. *Speech, Language and Hearing, 21*(4), 213–223.

Korkalainen, J., McCabe, P., Smidt, A., & Morgan, C. (2023). Motor speech interventions for children with cerebral palsy: A systematic review. *Journal of Speech, Language, and Hearing Research, 66,* 110–125.

Langlois, C., Tucker, B., Sawatzky, A., Reed, A., & Boliek, C. (2020). Effects of an intensive voice treatment on articulatory function and speech intelligibility in children with motor speech disorders: A phase one study. *Journal of Communication Disorders, 86,* Article 106003.

Lee, A., & Gibbon, F. (2015). Non-speech oral motor treatment for children with developmental speech sound disorders. *Cochrane Database of Systematic Review,* 2015(3), Article CD009383.

Leite, L., & Constantini, A. (2017). Dysarthria and quality of life in patients with amyotrophic lateral sclerosis. *Revista CEFAC, 19*(5).

Levy, E. (2014). Implementing two treatment approaches to childhood dysarthria. *International Journal of Speech-Language Pathology, 16*(4), 344–354.

Lewis, B., Freebairn, L., Hansen, A., Iyengar, S., & Taylor, H. (2004). School-age follow-up of children with childhood apraxia of speech. *Language, Speech, and Hearing Services in Schools, 35*(2), 122–140.

Maratab, S., Naz, S., Asghar, E., Kausar Yousuf, K., Badar, F., & Ahmed, A. (2024). The influence of training on alleviating stress and enhancing quality of life among caregivers of individuals with dysarthria following stroke. *Journal of Population Therapeutics & Clinical Pharmacology, 31*(1), 766–775.

McLeod, S., Harrison, L., & McCormack, J. (2012). The Intelligibility in Context Scale: Validity and reliability of a subjective rating measure. *Journal of Speech, Language, and Hearing Research, 55*(2), 648–656.

Mei, C., Reilly, S., Bickerton, M., Mensha, F., Turner, S., Kumaranayagam, D., . . . Morgan, A. (2020). Speech in children with cerebral palsy. *Developmental Medicine & Child Neurology, 62*(12), 1374–1382.

Morgan, A., Murray, E., & Liégeois, F. (2018). Interventions for childhood apraxia of speech. *Cochrane Database of Systematic Reviews, 5*(5), Article CD006278.

Morgan, A., & Webster, R. (2018). Aetiology of childhood apraxia of speech: A clinical practice update for paediatricians. *Journal of Paediatrics and Child Health, 54,* 1090–1095.

Moya-Gale, G., Kim, Y., & Fabiano, L. (2023). Raising awareness about language- and culture-specific considerations in the management of dysarthria associated with Parkinson's disease within the United States. *Journal of Speech, Language, and Hearing Research.* https://doi.org/10.1044/2023 _JSLHR-23-00365

Moya-Galé, G., Wisler, A., Walsh, S., McAuliffe, M., & Levy, E. (2023). Acoustic predictors of ease of understanding in Spanish speakers with dysarthria associated with Parkinson's disease. *Journal of Speech, Language, and Hearing Research, 66*(8S), 2999–3012.

Murray, E., McCabe, P., & Ballard, K. (2014). A systematic review of treatment outcomes for children with childhood apraxia of speech. *American Journal of Speech-Language Pathology, 23,* 486–504.

National Institute on Aging. (2022). *Parkinson's disease: Causes, symptoms, and treatments.* https://www.nia.nih.gov/health/parkinsons-disease/parkinsons-disease-causes-symptoms-and-treatments#:~:text=While%20genetics%20is%20thought%20to,such%20as%20exposure%20to%20toxins

O'Shea, T. (2002). Cerebral palsy in very preterm infants: New epidemiological insights. *Mental Retardation and Developmental Disabilities, 8*, 135–145.

Patel, D., Neelakantan, M., Pandher, K., & Merrick, J. (2020). Cerebral palsy in children: A clinical overview. *Translational Pediatrics, 9*(Suppl. 1), S125–S135.

Pennington, L., Lombardo, E., Steen, N., & Miller, N. (2018). Acoustic changes in the speech of children with cerebral palsy following an intensive program of dysarthria therapy. *International Journal of Language & Communication Disorders, 53*(1), 182–195.

Pinto, S., Chan, A., Guimarães, I., Rothe-Neves, R., & Sadat, J. (2017). A cross-linguistic perspective to the study of dysarthria in Parkinson's disease. *Journal of Phonetics, 64*, 156–167.

Ramig, L., Pawlas, A., & Countryman, S. (1995). *The Lee Silverman Voice Treatment (LSVT): A practical guide to treating the voice and speech disorders in Parkinson disease.* National Center for Voice and Speech.

Rosenbek, J. C., Lemme, M. L., Ahern, M. B., Harris, E. H., & Wertz, R. T. (1973). A treatment for apraxia of speech in adults. *Journal of Speech and Hearing Disorders, 38*(4), 462–472.

Sanger, T. (2015). Movement disorders in cerebral palsy. *Journal of Pediatric Neurology, 13*(4), 198–207.

Sapir, S., Ramig, L. O., & Fox, C. M. (2011). Intensive voice treatment in Parkinson's disease: Lee Silverman Voice Treatment. *Expert Review of Neurotherapeutics, 11*(6), 815–830.

Schölderle, T., Haas, E., & Ziegler, W. (2023). Speech naturalness in the assessment of childhood dysarthria. *American Journal of Speech-Language Pathology, 32*(4), 1633–1643.

Stemple, J. C., Lee, L., D'Amico, B., & Pickup, B. (1994). Efficacy of vocal function exercises as a method of improving voice production. *Journal of Voice, 8*(3), 271–278.

Strand, E. (2017). *Diagnosis and management of childhood apraxia of speech (CAS) using dynamic tactile and temporal cueing (DTTC).* https://childapraxiatreatment.org/wp-content/uploads/2021/06/Handout-for-Diagnosis-and-Treatment-of-CAS-Using-DTTC.pdf

Strand, E. (2019). Dynamic temporal and tactile cueing: A treatment strategy for childhood apraxia of speech. *American Journal of Speech-Language Pathology, 29*(1), 30–48.

Strand, E., & McCauley, R. (2019). *Dynamic Evaluation of Motor Speech Skill (DEMSS).* Brookes.

Strand, E., McCauley, R., Weigand, S., Stoeckel, R., & Baas, B. (2013). A motor speech assessment for children with severe speech disorders: Reliability and validity evidence. *Journal of Speech, Language, and Hearing Research, 56*, 505–520.

Voorman, J., Dallmeijer, A., van Eck, M., Schuengel, C., & Becher, J. (2009). Social functioning and communication in children with cerebral palsy: Association with disease characteristics and personal and environmental factors. *Developmental Medicine & Child Neurology, 52*, 441–447.

Walshe, M., Peach, R. K., & Miller, N. (2009). Dysarthria Impact Profile: Development of a scale to measure psychosocial effects. *International Journal of Language & Communication Disorders, 44*(5), 693–715.

Wambaugh, J. (2010). Sound production treatment for acquired apraxia of speech. *Perspectives on Neurophysiology and Neurogenic Speech and Language Disorders, 20*(3), 67–72.

Wambaugh, J. L., Martinez, A. L., McNeil, M. R., & Rogers, M. A. (1999). Sound production treatment for apraxia of speech: Overgeneralization and maintenance effects. *Aphasiology, 13*(9–11), 821–837.

Wambaugh, J. L., & Mauszycki, S. C. (2010). Sound production treatment: Application with severe apraxia of speech. *Aphasiology, 24*(6–8), 814–825.

Whitehall, T., & Wong, L. (2007). Effect of intensive voice treatment on tone-language speakers with Parkinson's disease. *Clinical Linguistics & Phonetics, 21*(11–12), 919–925.

Whitehill, T. L. (2010). Studies of Chinese speakers with dysarthria: Informing theoretical models. *Folia Phoniatrica et Logopaedica, 62*(3), 92–96.

Wong, E. C., Wong, M. N., Chen, S., & Lin, J. Y. (2024). Pitch variation skills in Cantonese speakers with apraxia of speech after stroke: Preliminary findings of acoustic analyses. *Journal of Speech, Language, and Hearing Research, 67*(1), 1–33.

World Health Organization. (2001). *International classification of functioning, disability and health.*

Yorkston, K. M., Beukelman, D. R., & Traynor, C. (1984). *Assessment of intelligibility of dysarthric speech.* Pro-Ed.

Ziegler, A., & Hapner, E. (2013). Phonation Resistance Training Exercise (PhoRTE) therapy. In A. Behrman & J. Haskell (Eds.), *Exercises for voice therapy* (2nd ed.). Plural Publishing.

Ziegler, A., Verdolini Abbott, K., Johns, M., Klein, A., & Hapner, E. R. (2014). Preliminary data on two voice therapy interventions in the treatment of presbyphonia. *The Laryngoscope, 124*(8), 1869–1876.

Chapter 7

Childhood Language Disorders

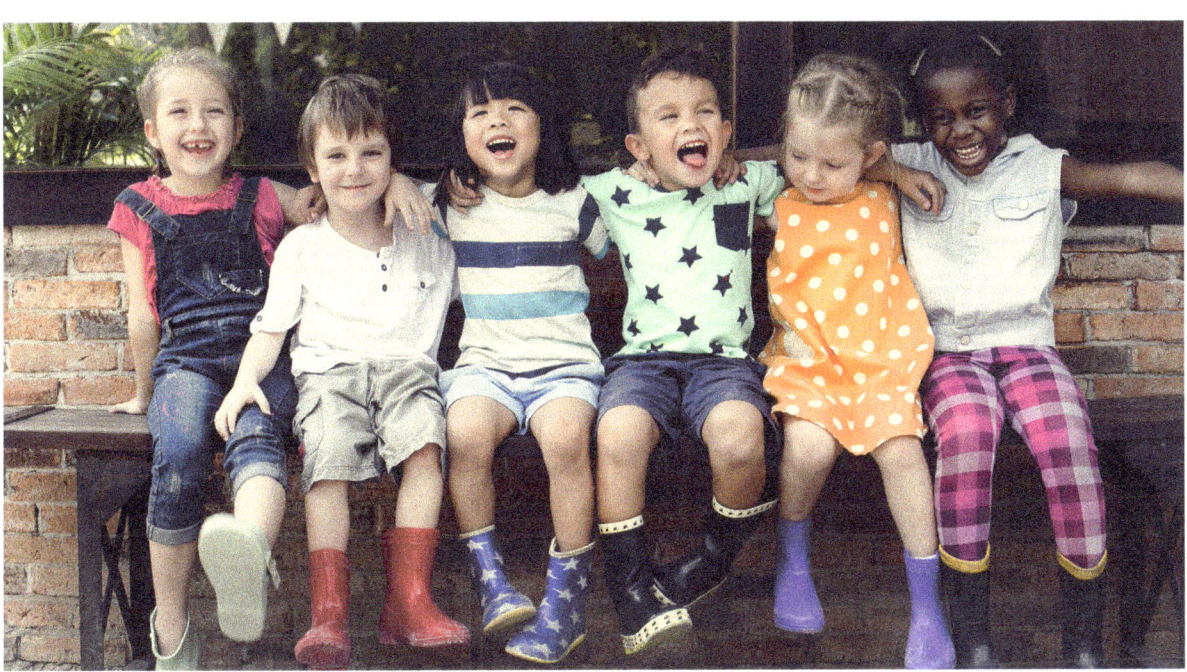

Learning Objectives

After reading this chapter, you will be able to:

- Describe the impairments in language form, content, and use associated with developmental language disorders.
- Explain the language characteristics seen in common genetic syndromes.
- Identify the cultural and linguistic considerations in the assessment of diverse populations.
- Compare and contrast the language intervention targets for preschool and school-age children and adolescents.
- Describe at least three interventions that are appropriate to support language in preschool children.

Key Terms

enhanced milieu teaching
features of an alternative response
focused stimulation
functional equivalence
language scaffolding
natural communities of reinforcement
neurodevelopmental disorder
parallel talk

prelinguistic milieu teaching
recasting
reliability
sensitivity
sequential bilingualism
simultaneous bilingualism
specificity
validity

Introduction

Typically, children develop their language skills with little effort, but there are those who demonstrate delays or differences in their development (Crespo & Kaushanskaya, 2022). When children have trouble understanding what people say or difficulty expressing their thoughts or ideas, they may have a language disorder, which may also be referred to as a language impairment, language delay, or specific language impairment (Gillam et al., 2021). Most recently, the term used to describe childhood language disorders is developmental language disorder (DLD). DLD tends to be diagnosed in children who have language challenges with no known cause, which affects approximately 8% of school-age children (Bishop et al., 2017). Importantly, children with DLD do not have other conditions that would explain their language challenges (e.g., impaired hearing or neurological functioning).

DLD is characterized by difficulties in the social use of language (pragmatics), grammar (syntax), vocabulary or the use of words (semantics), speech sound development and the rules or processes that govern that development (phonology), and/or difficulty understanding and using the smallest units of meaningful language (morphology; Spicer-Cain et al., 2023). Children with language disorders may have difficulties understanding language (comprehension) and/or expressing their ideas (production), and their symptoms can shift over time but usually persist into adulthood.

DLD should not be confused with children who are late talking as described in Chapter 3. Early language delays do not always predict whether a specific child will have a later impairment in their language, yet we know many children with DLD have persistent expressive language challenges that affect their overall health and well-being as well as opportunities for post-secondary education and employment (Botting, 2020; Botting et al., 2016; Dubois et al., 2020; Spicer-Cain et al., 2023). In this chapter, you will learn about the breakdown that can occur in children's spoken language as well as their language understanding. Furthermore, you will learn about other disorders that share the characteristics of a language disorder, including social communication disorder, autism, intellectual developmental disorders, and disorders associated with specific genetic syndromes.

What We Know About This Topic

The development of language is one of the most important milestones in early development. Helping children communicate their thoughts, ideas, and beliefs is crucial to the development of their ability to interact and learn in school. In this section, you will learn about the prevalence and incidence of DLD, signs and symptoms that characterize the disorder, and the likely causes. In addition, you will learn about other disorders that share the characteristics of a language disorder.

DLD is one of the most common disorders of childhood (Botting et al., 2016; Dubois et al., 2020). It is categorized under the larger umbrella term of **neurodevelopmental disorder**. Like other neurodevelopmental disorders, language disorders are observed early in development, usually before a child begins school, and are characterized by differences in the way that linguistic information is processed in the brain (American Psychiatric Association [APA], 2022).

Children who have difficulty with language, either receptive or expressive, may also have challenges in reading and writing, both of which are language-based skills. In fact, 65% of fourth graders with DLD read below what is expected for their age, and those reading below expected levels are likely to experience limited communication progress compared to children who perform at or above grade level in reading (National Center for Education Statistics, 2019; O'Fallon et al., 2022). Early reading difficulties also lead to greater developmental challenges and negatively impact language development and academic performance (Duff et al., 2015; Mol & Bus, 2011).

DLD is most often characterized by difficulties learning and using language to speak, write, or engage in other forms of expressive communication such as sign language, as well as understanding and using words, formulating sentences, and engaging in conversations. It occurs early in development without associated hearing, motor, or other neurological impairments. Risks for DLD can be environmental, genetic, and/or physiological, and language impairments similar to those in DLD often co-occur with other disorders, such as autism, intellectual disorders, and learning disorders.

Notably, both executive function (EF) difficulties and reading challenges are often seen in children with DLD. EF skills help us attend to relevant information, manage competing thoughts, plan and organize our behavior, and keep information in our working memory (Senter et al., 2023). Challenges in EF are a frequent characteristic of DLD (American Speech-Language-Hearing Association [ASHA], 2020), requiring both assessment and intervention in the areas of attention, organization, and regulation to help ensure that children are available to learn (Meltzer et al., 2021). It remains unclear if the challenges in EF are verbal, nonverbal, or both and how this impacts a child's language function. Everaert and colleagues (2023) compared the nonverbal performance of preschoolers with DLD with typically developing (TD) peers to examine the relationship between DLD and EF. The authors tested nonverbal EF using three different visual tasks tapping attention, memory, and broad EF abilities. Using standardized language tasks, they also measured vocabulary and morphosyntax. They found that TD peers outperformed the children with DLD on all nonverbal EF tasks.

Reading requires two important skills relevant to language development: word recognition and comprehension. When children learn to read, they begin to recognize letters and manipulate sounds in the words they are trying to read. They learn about sound–letter correspondence and when there are exceptions to how words are written versus how they sound. Children learn to make sense of the printed words that they read and how words are produced—an ability that is related to vocabulary growth. Typically, children with DLD have an increased incidence of reading disorders (25–90%) and overall poorer reading achievement compared to children without DLD (Duff & Tomblin, 2018). Also well-established is the relationship between spoken and written language because children with language problems frequently have difficulty learning to write (Hulme & Snowling, 2013). Furthermore, school-age children with poorer language often have difficulty managing classroom expectations because language competence is necessary for social and academic success. Thus, assessment and intervention are key to creating a learning environment that supports a child's literacy development.

See the **ASHA Language in Brief Practice Portal** and the **ASHA Written Language Disorders Practice Portal** for more information.

In addition, children with language disorders may experience social–emotional difficulties that impact their relationships with their peers, such as a tendency to withdraw, difficulty judging the emotion of others, or difficulty regulating their own emotions, and this could result in misperceptions of their behavior (Brinton et al., 2007; Fujiki et al., 2002, 2004). As adolescents, they may be less emotionally engaged in relationships and may be at risk for being bullied (Blood, 2014; Brownlie et al., 2007; Wadman et al., 2011). Behavioral difficulties such as attentional problems are also likely (Dockrell et al., 2007).

Signs and Symptoms of Language Disorders

Language abilities vary across children and are dependent on age, the language domains affected, the stage of language development, and the severity of disruption to communication (ASHA, n.d.). The signs and symptoms associated with language disorders discussed below fall into skills that emphasize language form (phonology, syntax, morphology), language function (semantics), and language use (pragmatics), as discussed in Chapter 3 (Figure 7–1). Although they are described as separate skills, it is important to note that there is a synergistic relationship among them, and together they form a dynamic whole to ensure effective communication (Berko Gleason, 2005).

See the **ASHA Spoken Language Disorders Practice Portal**.

Language Form: Phonology, Morphology, and Syntax

As described in Chapter 3, deficits in phonology are represented by the patterning of speech sounds in the language a child is acquiring. For example, if a child is unaware of how to use a speech sound in their language, this could impact their awareness of how words are formed. Children with language disorders tend to use less mature syllable structures and have greater inconsistency of their phonological skills. Challenges with speech sound development may impact intelligibility and could co-occur with poor **phonological awareness**, which facilitates a child's ability to rhyme words, segment words into sounds, and blend sounds into words. Phonological awareness is a **metalinguistic skill** (awareness of language and of one's own thinking about language) important to the development of more advanced spoken and written language skills. As a type of metalinguistic skill, phonological awareness is important to the development of later reading and writing skills (Al Otaiba et al., 2009).

Difficulties in morphology and syntax are demonstrated in the later acquisition of word combinations; limited mean length of utterance; as well as errors in verb endings (e.g., past tense), function words (e.g., prepositions), and pronouns (e.g., he, she, they). Errors are often characterized by the omission of words

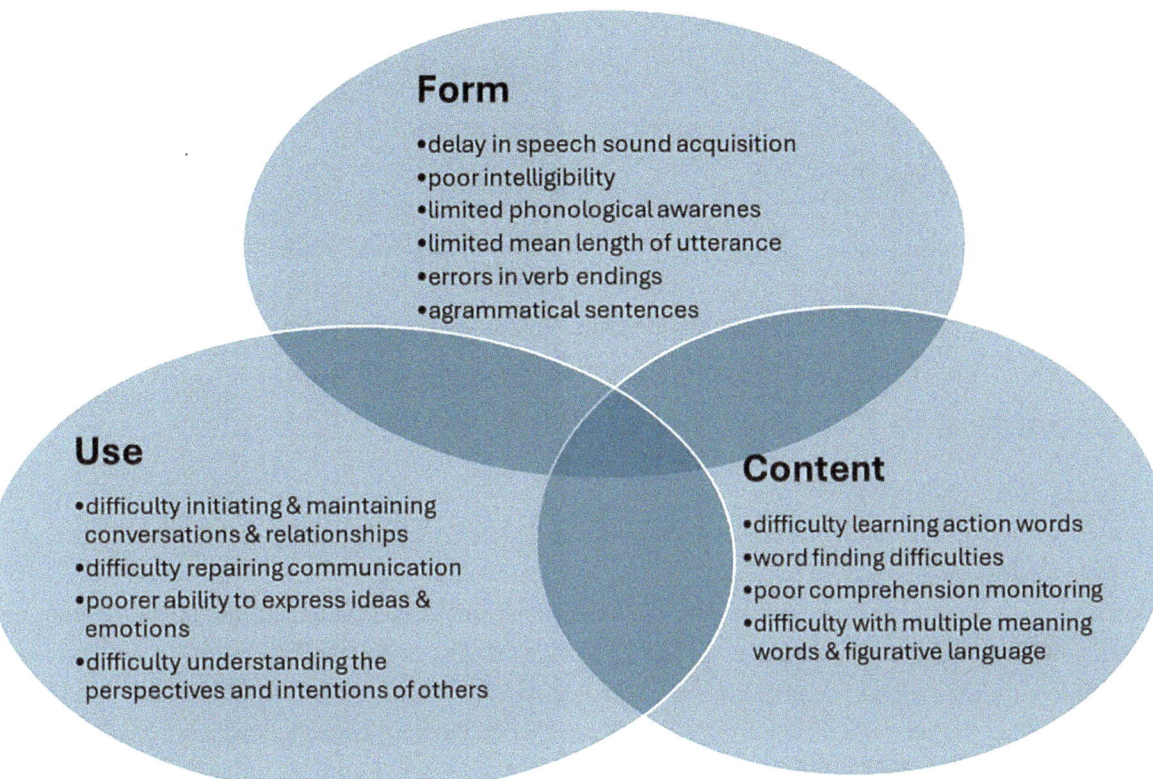

FIGURE 7–1. Selected examples of breakdowns in language form, function, and use in children with DLD.

or word endings that impact meaning. Less mature word forms are used, and prefixes and suffixes, as well as tense markers, may be omitted or used incorrectly. A child might have difficulty judging the grammatical accuracy of a sentence and correcting grammatical errors. Understanding different parts of speech, such as nouns, verbs, adjectives, and adverbs, is challenging, as is comprehending and using complex syntactic structures. Both narrative and expository language are less well developed, and the language of the curriculum often poses difficulties with learning in the classroom.

Language Content: Semantics

Vocabulary development, particularly verbs, may also be slower than expected for the child's developmental age. **Fast mapping**, the ability to learn new words or concepts after minimal exposure, is also impacted in these children because they often require several exposures to learn new vocabulary. Some children with language disorders will have word finding difficulties and may have less elaborate memory networks for words. Monitoring their own comprehension, following along with what is being said in a conversation, understanding questions that are being asked, and understanding what they read are often challenging, and these children may seldom request clarification. In addition, these children may have difficulty using multiple-meaning words and figurative language (e.g., metaphors, proverbs, idioms), as well as understanding synonyms and antonyms. Comprehending narrative and expository text presents a challenge, especially if the child is asked to draw inferences (ASHA, n.d.).

Language Use: Pragmatics

Difficulties in using language in social situations range from initiating play and maintaining conversations with peers to understanding the perspectives and intentions of others. Children with pragmatic challenges struggle to express their ideas, emotions, and personal experiences, and they are less effective at participating in reciprocal conversations and taking turns. They seem to have difficulty repairing breakdowns in communication and demonstrate more limited discourse skills in the classroom. Often, they have difficulty knowing what to say, when to say something, and when not to say something. When telling stories, they often omit key story components, which impacts story cohesion.

Incidence and Prevalence of Language Disorders

Remember that incidence refers to the number of new cases identified in a specified period, whereas prevalence refers to the number of individuals living with the disorder at a point in time. No reliable data on incidence for child language disorders are available, and much of this information is dated. Available prevalence data are likely the result of how language impairment is defined and the actual populations examined (Pinborough-Zimmerman et al., 2007). With that said, approximately 3.3% of children aged 3 to 17 years in the United States were identified as having a language disorder that lasted for 1 week or longer during the previous 12 months (Black et al., 2015). Earlier research examining kindergartners in the United States indicated that 7.4% of children overall presented with a language disorder (with a higher prevalence in boys compared to girls), with the highest prevalence of language disorders occurring in Native Americans, followed by African Americans, Hispanics, Whites, and Asians (Gray, 2003; Lahey & Edwards, 1999; Tomblin et al., 1997).

In the United Kingdom, the median prevalence of receptive language disorder ranged from 2.63% to 3.59%, with expressive language disorder ranging from 2.81% to 16% and combined receptive and expressive language disorder ranging from 2.02% to 3.01% for children aged 7 years or younger (Law et al., 2000). For Canadian kindergarten children, the prevalence was closer to that reported for children in the United States, with language disorders at 8.04% overall, 8.37% for girls, and 8.17% for boys (Beitchman et al., 1986).

Causes of Language Disorders

A DLD is described as a primary disorder, but a language disorder can co-occur (often as a secondary condition) with other disabilities such as autism, traumatic brain injury (TBI), intellectual disability, and genetic conditions such as Down syndrome. Co-occurring language disorders are typically associated with, and linked to, the primary condition. There might be an environmental cause such as a TBI as the result of a car accident, a single gene variation (e.g., Down syndrome), or multiple gene variations (e.g., autism). When a language disorder is not the result of another condition, the cause is more difficult to identify. Some have suggested it is the result of a cognitive processing problem (Leonard et al., 2007), a biological difference (Ellis Weismer et al., 2005), or a genetic variation (Rice, 2013), although these factors are not necessarily independent of each other (Reed, 2012).

We also offer a causal modeling approach to explain the foundational elements of language development so that you can see where breakdowns might occur in DLD. Figure 7–2 provides a graphic representation of a causal modeling approach that has three components: biological, behavioral, and cognitive (Hutchins & Prelock, 2015). The role of the environment is also represented and viewed as having contributions across all three levels. At the biological level, genes, brain structures, and the cranial

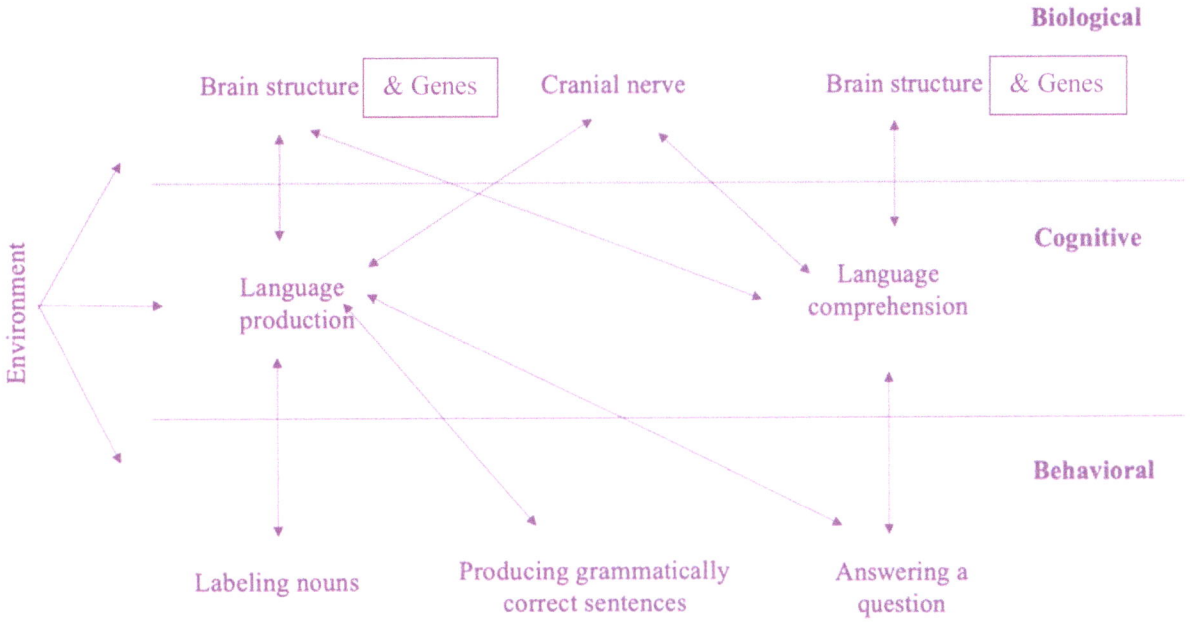

FIGURE 7–2. Causal model for language.

nerves related to speech, language, and hearing are represented. At the behavioral level in this example, you see some of the skills involved in language production and comprehension. It is at the cognitive level where we will do most of our intervention to improve both language production and language comprehension—recognizing there is a synergistic relationship between a child's capacity for language learning (biological level) and what they produce (behavioral level). Working at the cognitive level allows us to capitalize on a child's current skill level and expand upon it across several behavioral domains and contexts. Thinking about DLD from a causal modeling framework has two specific advantages. First, it allows us to describe several interacting components associated with, in this case, a language disorder, while providing a framework for advancing our clinical practice. Second, it allows us to represent the cause and outcome of a disorder with a level of detail and complexity that is not often considered (Hutchins & Prelock, 2015).

Other Disorders That Share Characteristics of a Language Disorder

In the following sections, several disorders that share characteristics of a language disorder are briefly described. These include social communication disorder, learning disorder, autism, intellectual developmental disorder, and several genetic syndromes with accompanying language disorders (i.e., Angelman syndrome, Down syndrome, fetal alcohol syndrome, fragile X syndrome, William syndrome, and velocardiofacial syndrome).

Social Communication Disorders

A social communication disorder is characterized by challenges in the use of both verbal and nonverbal communication during social situations. This might include difficulties greeting a potential communication partner, sharing information, and adapting communication based on the listener (e.g., teacher, peer, child, adult). It might also involve difficulties following the rules of conversation, such as taking turns, initiating and ending conversations, and observing the interest level of others. Telling stories that are cohesive and coherent is often challenging, as is understanding more complex and abstract language (e.g., idioms, sarcasm, humor). These differences ultimately lead to problems developing and maintaining social relationships (e.g., friendships, romantic relationships, collegial relationships)—an expectation that increases as individuals get older. Importantly, although some symptoms of social communication disorder are similar to those of other neurodevelopmental conditions such as autism and intellectual disability, a social communication disorder is its own diagnostic entity and is not attributed to other conditions (APA, 2022). Notably, some children with language disorders may have a social communication difficulty because there are several components that make up social communication, including social interaction, social cognition, pragmatics, and language processing.

See the **ASHA Social Communication Disorder Practice Portal** for more information.

Learning Disorders

Learning disorders or learning disabilities are also linked to language disorders, although there is little agreement on the exact relationship. Typically, a language disorder is diagnosed prior to a learning disorder, and both impact a child's academic performance. When a child is identified as having a learning disability, a language disorder usually underpins the child's academic difficulties, particularly those related to reading and writing. See Chapter 8 for more information on learning disorders and literacy impairment.

Autism

Autism is a neurodevelopmental condition and one of the most common childhood disorders, with approximately 2% of the child population affected worldwide (Roman-Urrestarazu et al., 2021). In 2020, 1 in 36 children in the United States, aged 8 years, was estimated to have autism, with approximately 4% of boys and 1% of girls affected (Maenner et al., 2023). The prevalence estimate for autism continues to increase, and this was the first time that the prevalence for autism was lower among White children (24.3%) compared to Black (29.3%), Hispanic (31.6%), and Asian/Pacific Islander (33.4%) children. In addition, Black, Asian, and Hispanic children are more likely than White children to be diagnosed with both autism and a co-occurring intellectual disability and autism (Maenner et al., 2023).

The diagnostic criteria used to determine the presence of autism include two primary deficit areas: (a) social communication and social interaction; and (b) restricted, repetitive, and stereotyped patterns of behavior (APA, 2022). Children with autism have difficulty with social–emotional reciprocity or back-and-forth conversation; poor integration of their nonverbal (e.g., eye contact, gestures) and verbal behaviors; and challenges with developing and maintaining relationships with peers, particularly in complex social contexts (APA, 2022). Symptoms are usually seen in early development, although some individuals may be diagnosed later in life. Children with autism may have co-occurring conditions such as attention-deficit/hyperactivity disorder, speech sound disorder, and language disorder. The criteria that differentiate children with social communication disorder and autism is that in the latter there is the presence of restricted, repetitive, and stereotyped patterns of behavior. These include motor movements (e.g., hand flapping, repetitive jumping, rocking back and forth), speech (e.g., echolalia), and interests (e.g., a focused interest on trains) that interfere with daily life. An autistic child will likely experience ongoing challenges throughout their lifetime, including employment and mental health issues (Harmuth et al., 2018; Hollocks et al., 2019), and may also experience a co-occurring language disorder (Botting et al., 2016; Dubois et al., 2020).

See the **ASHA Autism Spectrum Disorder Practice Portal** and resources from the **Centers for Disease Control and Prevention** and **National Institute of Mental Health** for more information.

Intellectual Developmental Disorder

An intellectual disability, more recently named an intellectual developmental disorder (IDD), is characterized by impairments in general mental abilities that affect an individual's adaptive functioning and ability to manage daily tasks in three primary areas: conceptual, social, and practical (APA, 2022). The conceptual area characterizes challenges in language, reading, writing, math, reasoning, memory, and general knowledge. In the social area, difficulties are seen in the development of social judgment, interpersonal skills, and developing friendships. The practical area involves challenges with self-management, including personal care, money management, organizing required school or job tasks, implementing job responsibilities, and so on. Usually, symptoms begin in the early developmental period and are assessed based on the severity of adaptive functioning. IDD often co-occurs with other conditions, such as autism, Down syndrome, fetal alcohol syndrome, and brain injury.

See the **ASHA Intellectual Disability Evidence Map** for the most recent research on IDD.

Genetic Syndromes

There are many genetic syndromes that have accompanying language disorders. In the following sections, we briefly describe some of the most common genetic syndromes that have notable language disorders. Each of these syndromes (i.e., Angelman syndrome, Down syndrome, fetal alcohol syndrome, fragile X syndrome, Williams syndrome, and velocardiofacial syndrome) are described briefly below, and a summary of their characteristics is provided in Table 7–1.

TABLE 7–1. Language Disorders in Genetic Syndromes

Type of Disorder/ Characteristics	Williams Syndrome	Fragile X Syndrome	Down Syndrome	Velocardiofacial Syndrome	Angelman Syndrome	Fetal Alcohol Syndrome
Cause	Deletions of genetic material from adjacent genes located on the long arm of chromosome 7	Mutations in the *FMR1* gene	*Trisomy*: Full or partial extra copy of chromosome 21 *Mosaicism*: Some cells have an extra chromosome and some do not *Translocation*: Extra copy of chromosome 21 is attached to another chromosome	Unknown, but appears individuals are missing a piece of chromosome 22	Deficiency of the *UBE3A* gene	Alcohol exposure in utero
Physical/health	Long philtrum Wide mouth Full lips Small upturned nose Heart disease Failure to thrive Hearing loss Motor control and planning differences	Prominent jaw Large ears Long and narrow face Flat feet	Large tongue Narrow, high arched palate Small oral cavity Flattened nasal bridge Upward eye slant Deep crease in palm of hand Small stature Poor muscle tone	Cleft palate Thin upper lip Prominent nose with narrow nasal passages Low-set ears Scoliosis Calcium deficiency Hypo-/hyperthyroidism Recurrent seizures Strabismus Cardiovascular malformations	Abnormally wide mouth Widely spaced teeth Prominent chin Deep-set eyes Walking and balance difficulties Gastrointestinal issues Seizures	Thin upper lip Smooth skin between nose and upper lip Upturned nose Small eyes Vision and hearing problems

154

Cognitive/ psychological profile	Intellectual or learning disability Discrepancies between verbal and nonverbal reasoning Gregarious Non-social anxiety	Delayed developmental milestones Moderate to severe intellectual disability that worsens with age Afraid or anxious in new situations Trouble making eye contact ADHD or ADD symptoms Problems with certain sensations	Mild to moderately severe intellectual disability	65% have a nonverbal learning disability Higher verbal than performance scores on measures of intelligence	Delayed development Severe to profound intellectual disability Outgoing personality	Low to average IQ, learning disabilities Difficulty with self-regulation, working memory, response inhibition, attention and hyperactivity, reasoning and judgment
Speech and language	Delay in canonical babbling, gestures, and joint attention Challenges with relational and pragmatic language Relative strengths in concrete vocabulary and phonological skills	Unintelligible conversational speech with consonant substitutions, omissions, and distortions Repeats multisyllabic sequences Problems with tone and atypical pragmatic and abstract language Boys frequently stutter, leaving out parts of words Problems for girls are not as severe	Delayed speech with phonological errors and poor speech intelligibility Delay syntax comprehension Boys less skilled at speech motor functions and coordinated speech movements	Hypernasal speech Severe articulation disorder Higher frequency of glottal stop use Lower receptive than expressive language skills	Receptive language more developed than expressive language Verbal speech limited, with 71% to 90% never or rarely producing speech	Expressive language delays Difficulty with speech discrimination, comprehension, syntax, prosody, conversational rules, sentence combinations, and semantic elaboration Some speech delays, with errors in certain consonants; others have more involved speech difficulties leading to poor intelligibility

Note: ADD, attention deficit disorder; ADHD, attention-deficit/hyperactivity disorder.

Angelman Syndrome. Angelman syndrome is caused by loss of function of the *UBE3A* gene. Typically, children inherit one copy of the gene from both parents, and both copies are active in the body's tissues. In the case of Angelman syndrome, only the maternal copy of the gene is active, but because of a mutation in which the *UBE3A* gene is lost, the individual has no active copies of the gene in most parts of the brain (Mayo Foundation for Medical Education and Research, 2022; National Organization for Rare Disorders, 2018). The physical manifestation of Angelman syndrome is characterized by an abnormally wide mouth, widely spaced teeth, a prominent chin, and deep-set eyes. Children with Angelman syndrome might also exhibit walking and balance problems, gastrointestinal difficulties, as well as seizures. From a cognitive perspective, they usually have delayed language, severe to profound intellectual disability, and an outgoing personality. Evidence suggests that receptive language is more well-developed than expressive language and that verbal speech is impacted, with 71% to 90% of children affected never or rarely producing verbal speech (Angelman Syndrome Foundation, 2022; Pearson et al., 2019).

See the **National Organization for Rare Disorders** and **Mayo Foundation for Medical Education and Research** for more information on Angelman syndrome.

Down Syndrome. Approximately 1 in 700 live births in the United States and 1 in 1,000 throughout the world result in a child born with Down syndrome, a common genetic condition in which the child has 47 compared to the expected 46 chromosomes—an extra chromosome on the 21st pair (Mai et al., 2019). Children with Down syndrome are often born with several physical, communication, and cognitive differences, from hearing and swallowing problems to muscle weakness, communication delays, and cognitive challenges (Boliek et al., 2022; Kaczorowska et al., 2019). Generally, receptive language tends to be stronger than expressive language, with difficulties often noted in the areas of syntax and phonology (Martin et al., 2009).

See the **Centers for Disease Control and Prevention** and **National Down Syndrome Society** for more information on Down syndrome.

Fetal Alcohol Syndrome. Fetal alcohol syndrome (FAS) encompasses a range of disorders caused by prenatal alcohol exposure leading to congenital anomalies and an array of cognitive, behavioral, emotional, and adaptive functioning impairments with mild to severe effects (APA, 2022; Lange et al., 2017). Physical features usually include a thin upper lip, upturned nose, and small eyes with the potential for hearing and vision problems. Children with FAS usually have low to average intelligence and associated learning disabilities, with difficulties in self-regulation, response inhibition, attention, and hyperactivity (Kodituwakku, 2009). Working memory, reasoning, and social judgment are also areas of challenge. Children with FAS are likely to have expressive language delays and difficulty with speech discrimination and comprehension (Vega-Rodríguez et al., 2020). There are also reported challenges in syntax, semantics, prosody, and following conversational rules (Hendricks et al., 2018). Intelligibility may also be impacted in some cases.

See the **Centers for Disease Control and Prevention** and **Mayo Foundation for Medical Education and Research** for more information on FAS.

Fragile X Syndrome. Fragile X syndrome is caused by a mutation in the *FMR1* gene. The physical features often seen in children with fragile X include large ears, a prominent jaw, and a long and narrow face. Cognitively, children exhibit delayed developmental milestones and moderate to severe intellectual abilities that usually worsen over time. Children with fragile X often have a co-occurring diagnosis of autism and/or attention-deficit/hyperactivity disorder and portray fear and anxiousness in new situations. They also have difficulty making eye contact. Speech and language are impacted in several ways. Research suggests that children with fragile X syndrome tend to have impairments in several domains of receptive and expressive language, including vocabulary, morphology, and syntax, as well as in the social use of language (pragmatics) and narrative discourse (Finestack et al., 2009). Research on speech sound production and intelligibility is less well-established, but evidence suggests that children with fragile X syndrome do not present with similar phonological skills as younger neurotypical children; however, their intelligibility in conversational speech may be reduced (Barnes et al., 2009).

See the **Cleveland Clinic** and **U.S. National Library of Medicine** for more information on fragile X syndrome.

Williams Syndrome. Approximately 1 in 7,500 to 10,000 people worldwide (approximately 20,000–30,000 in the United States) have a diagnosis of Williams syndrome, which occurs equally in males and females across cultures. Children with Williams syndrome have a deletion of genetic material (genes 26–28) on chromosome 7 that leads to differences in physical features (e.g., hearing loss, small, upturned nose, wide mouth, full lips, etc.) and often is associated with intellectual disabilities or learning disorders. Children with Williams syndrome are usually friendly and highly social, and their relatively good verbal skills may mask or hide their cognitive challenges. Speech and language are characterized by delays in early gestural development and joint attention, as well as difficulties in pragmatic language (Mervis & Velleman, 2011). Speech sound production and vocabulary appear to be relative strengths in this population.

See the **Williams Syndrome Association** for more information on Williams syndrome.

Velocardiofacial Syndrome. The cause of velocardiofacial syndrome remains unclear, but it appears that children with this condition are missing a piece of chromosome 22. Several physical features characterize velocardiofacial syndrome, including a cleft palate, a prominent nose with narrow nasal passages, and low-set ears. Children usually have scoliosis, a calcium deficiency, and either an over- or underactive thyroid. Seizures are also prominent, as are cardiovascular malformations and strabismus. Approximately 65% of children with velocardiofacial syndrome have a nonverbal learning disability (see description in Chapter 8), exhibiting higher verbal than nonverbal performance scores on intelligence measures. Speech is described as hypernasal, and articulation is poor, with frequent use of glottal stops (D'Antonio et al., 2001). Interestingly, children with velocardiofacial syndrome tend to have better receptive language skills than expressive language skills (Glaser et al., 2002).

See the **National Human Genome Research Institute** for more information on velocardiofacial syndrome.

What Do We Do to Address This Communication Challenge?

In this section, you will learn about approaches to screening, assessment, and intervention. You will also learn about cultural considerations when assessing a child for a DLD. Screening is a first step to determine if there is a need for further assessment of a language disorder. Assessment is an important part of our discovery of how individuals understand and communicate their needs, wants, and ideas. Understanding the impact of cultural and linguistic differences is a critical consideration in the ultimate determination of a language disorder. If, through a comprehensive assessment, a language disorder is identified, intervention is the step taken to support the facilitation of a child's language across communication contexts.

Assessment of Childhood Language Disorders

Speech-language pathologists (SLPs) have a crucial role in the diagnosis and assessment of children with language disorders. Some of these roles include the following:

- Screening children for language difficulties
- Identifying the need for further assessment
- Determining whether referrals are needed for services beyond speech and language
- Recognizing that students with language disorders are at greater risk for literacy difficulties
- Conducting culturally and linguistically appropriate assessments
- Understanding language differences based on dialect and when English is not the child's first language
- Diagnosing a language disorder
- Making referrals to other service providers to rule out medical and other conditions that might impact language development

See the **ASHA Scope of Practice in Speech-Language Pathology** for more information.

Screening

If a child is suspected of having a language disorder, the first step is to screen the child's language. Although this does not result in a diagnosis, it does guide the SLP in determining whether additional testing is indicated. To conduct a language screening, the SLP often gathers information about any language concerns from a variety of sources, including teachers and parents, and conducts a hearing screening to rule out any possible hearing loss that might be influencing the child's language skills. In addition to seeking information about the child's language skills from others, the SLP also uses age-appropriate screening tools that are normed or have cut-off scores to determine whether a child should undergo a full language evaluation.

Screening results may indicate a need for a more comprehensive assessment of language, hearing, and/or speech sound development. Language assessment should be culturally relevant and consider the child's functional needs. It should also involve the child's family, teachers, and other professionals as appropriate. Considering the child's age and their current stage of language development, an assessment would include several components, such as the following:

- Birth and medical history as well as any family history of language disorders or learning challenges
- Clarity on the family's concerns about their child's language, as well as child strengths and the family's goals and desires for the assessment, intervention, and child outcomes
- Description of teacher's concerns, if any, regarding the child's language and learning
- Hearing assessment if not previously obtained
- An examination of the child's oral mechanism
- Language testing examining phonology, semantics, morphology, syntax, and pragmatics

Assessment should also include all languages and/or dialects used in the home, in what situations they are used, and the frequency/mastery of other languages used by the child and caregivers.

In addition, SLPs will often include a literacy assessment as part of their comprehensive language assessment because this falls under their scope of practice due to the strong association between language and literacy skills. A speech sound assessment might also be included (see Chapter 5) because speech sound difficulties can be the result of a language disorder in phonology. Also, children may present with a language disorder and a co-occurring speech sound disorder.

See ASHA's documents and references for the **"Assessment and Evaluation of Speech-Language Disorders in Schools"** for more information.

Assessment Approaches

Several types of assessment procedures can be used to conduct a comprehensive language assessment, as shown in Table 7–2. Standardized assessments are formal measures that have been empirically tested to identify specific elements of language functioning. Standard measures usually have standard scores and percentile ranks, as well as report on their **reliability, validity, sensitivity**, and **specificity**. Although standardized tools provide general information on language functioning, they are insufficient to be used on their own to create language profiles for children. Standardized assessments should be paired with other measures of language to help ensure that the assessment captures the child's true language abilities. One such technique is language sampling, which is an approach that allows the SLP to observe a child's language in a variety of communication contexts. This can include during structured conversations, a story retell, telling of a personal narrative, or during spontaneous conversations with various communication partners (e.g., peers, teachers, parents). Language sampling across contexts allows the SLP to examine several components of the child's language content, function, and use, including length of utterances, number of different words produced, types of words produced, and complexity of the sentences they use.

Another approach to assessment is called **dynamic assessment**. During this approach, language is tested, challenge areas are treated, and the child is then retested to determine the effects of the intervention. Dynamic assessment focuses on the learning process and an individual child's capacity for learning with scaffolded support (e.g., modeling, cueing, prompting). Evolving from Vygotsky's (1978) sociocultural theory, dynamic assessment aligns with the **zone of proximal development** (ZPD), which is the area between what a child can do completely unaided and what they cannot do even with adult support. Supporting a child's skills within the ZPD means identifying a child's skills in specific learning areas and their capacity for learning when supported by an adult. Typically, dynamic assessment uses a test–teach–retest framework in which children complete a static assessment, receive a brief intervention, and then complete the assessment again to reveal the amount of change that occurred. With dynamic assessment, the "teach" phase typically includes a metacognitive component that facilitates the child's ability to learn a strategy for completing a specific task (Peña et al., 2014; Petersen et al., 2017). Dynamic assessment is often used in combination with language sampling and standard assessments, and it is a helpful tool for differentiating between a language disorder and a language difference, particularly when no standardized assessments are available in the child's language(s). For this reason, dynamic assessment is important for all individuals, especially bi- and multilingual speakers.

See ASHA's micro courses on **dynamic assessment** for more information.

Another technique that is often used in the assessment of bi- and multilingual speakers is **ethnographic interviewing**. This type of interview gathers in-depth and descriptive information from the child, their family, and their teachers to better understand what language looks like in different contexts with different people. It is characterized by using open-ended questions, listening and restating what an individual describes, and getting clarification on what a student and their family or teacher reported. When possible, ethnographic interviewing can include observations of the child across contexts.

TABLE 7–2. Type, Description, and Examples of Language Assessments

Type of Assessment	Description	Examples/Resources
Standardized assessment	Empirically developed with established reliability and validity. Designed to assess an individual's skills in a structured and standardized way	*Clinical Evaluation of Language Fundamentals–5th Edition: CELF-5* (Wiig et al., 2013) *Clinical Evaluation of Language Fundamentals–Preschool–3rd Edition: CELF-3* (Wiig et al., 2020) *Comprehensive Assessment of Spoken Language–2nd edition: CASL-2* (Carrow-Woolfolk, 2017) *Test of Language Development–Primary (5th Edition) TLD-P-5* (Newcomer & Hammill, 2019) *Test of Language Development–Intermediate (5th Edition) TLD-I-5* (Hammill & Newcomer, 2020)
Language sampling	Gather spontaneous language during a variety of communication exchanges (e.g., storytelling, conversation, picture description tasks). Can provide information about an individual's utterance length, complexity of sentences, number of different words used, etc.	Developmental sentence score (Lee & Canter, 1971) Systematic Analysis of Language Transcripts (SALT), https://www.saltsoftware.com Heilmann & Miller (2023) Nippold (2021)
Dynamic assessment	Language is assessed, specific language skills are taught, language is retested to determine influence of intervention on outcome (test–teach–retest); often used with linguistically and culturally diverse populations	Bamford et al. (2022) Orellana et al. (2019) Peña et al. (2014) Petersen et al. (2020) Spicer-Cain et al. (2023) Bilinguistics' Dynamic Assessment Protocol, https://bilinguistics.com/evaluation-resources Pearson's YouTube tutorial on "Dynamic Assessment With English Language Learners," https://www.youtube.com/watch?v=Z_GU0dgEv_A
Systematic observation	Observation of language in the classroom	CELF-5 Observational Rating Scale (Wiig et al., 2013)
Ethnographic interviewing	Interviews designed to gather the perspective of the parent, teacher, or child in different contexts; often used with linguistically and culturally diverse populations	Westby et al. (2003)

continues

TABLE 7–2. *continued*

Type of Assessment	Description	Examples/Resources
Parent report measures	Checklists or questionnaires completed by the parent	Children's Communication Checklist–2 (Bishop, 2006) Girolametto (1997) Hutchins, & Prelock (2016) IMPACT Language Rating Scale, https://videoassessmenttools.com/impact-language-rating-scale Language Development Survey (LDS; (Rescorla, 1989) Rescorla & Alley (2001) MacArthur–Bates Communication Development Inventories (MB-CDIs-Third edition; Marchman et al., 2023) Social Skills Improvement System (SSIS) Rating Scales–Parent form (Gresham & Elliott, 2008) Speech and Language Assessment Scale (SLAS), https://www.phenxtoolkit.org/protocols/view/200302
Teacher Report Measures	Checklists or questionnaires completed by the teacher	Social Skills Improvement System (SSIS) Rating Scales–Teacher form (Gresham & Elliott, 2008)
Child report measures	Self-report measures completed by the child	Social Skills Improvement System (SSIS) Rating Scales–Child form (Gresham & Elliott, 2008)
Curriculum-based assessment	An assessment of the language demands of the classroom	Prelock et al. (1993)

This technique is effective in gathering different perspectives about the child and others who know the child well to affirm or contradict what was observed or reported in other assessments, ultimately leading to a more holistic picture of the child's language profile.

Classroom observation is also used to assess communication in natural contexts. This information can be used to create an individual profile for a student who may have language challenges that look different in the classroom than on a standard measure or in a spontaneous language sample. Informant measures, such as parent, teacher, and/or child questionnaires or rating scales, are often used to gain a more comprehensive understanding of the child's language strengths and challenges from many who know the child. This is especially important when the child is learning English as a second language so that information can be gathered about what language is spoken in the home and if there are difficulties with the child's native language as well as English.

A final technique that is often used for the school-age child is a curriculum-based assessment. This approach incorporates probes to assess the child's understanding of the language demands of the curriculum and how effectively a child can navigate those curricular demands.

Ultimately, a comprehensive assessment should include many of the elements listed in Table 7–2 and will lead to one of several outcomes that can help a clinician answer the following questions:

- Does the child have a language disorder?
- Does the language disorder impact the child's receptive language, expressive language, or both?
- Is there a language delay as opposed to a language disorder due to environmental influences?
- What are the characteristics and severity of the child's language difficulties?
- How does the child's language performance change in different contexts?
- Is the child also showing challenges with literacy?
- Does the child also have a speech sound disorder?
- Is the child's hearing within normal range?
- Should the child be referred to other specialists?
- What are the support needs for the child and what type of intervention will best meet the child's needs?

See the **assessment section** of the **ASHA Spoken Language Disorders Evidence Map** for available evidence.

Cultural Considerations

Language systems and rules, as well as how language is used socially, differ across cultures. These variations reflect the communication differences (including dialect) shared by a group of individuals who share regional, social, cultural, and/or ethnic factors. These communication variations are not considered to be language disorders. Furthermore, children who are dual language learners and exhibit patterns that are expected when learning English as a second language should also not be identified as having a developmental language disorder unless they are exhibiting difficulty in developing their first language as well as English. There are some unique challenges for SLPs when tasked with identifying a language disorder for children who speak a specific dialect in English, are bilingual, or are learning English as a second language because this requires both familiarity with and understanding of specific dialectal rules as well as how dual language learning develops and the process for learning a second language. Interestingly, some of the linguistic characteristics of children learning two languages simultaneously (**simultaneous bilingualism**) and those acquiring a second language (**sequential bilingualism**) are similar to the linguistic features sometimes seen in children with language impairments who are monolingual, including similar morphosyntactic profiles (Paradis & Crago, 2000, 2004) and impairment in vocabulary development (Paradis et al., 2011). It is important to remember, however, that bilingualism does not indicate a language impairment, and some language processes observed in bilingualism (e.g., code mixing) also occur in bilingual children who have a language disorder (Gutiérrez-Clellen et al., 2009).

Some standardized language assessment tools have been adapted and translated into other languages, with Spanish being the most frequent. Although this is an important step for assessment of a child's skills in their native language, a bilingual SLP and/or the presence of an interpreter is required. Interestingly, many countries do not recommend early diagnosis of developmental language disorders because of unreliable early assessments for children younger than age 3 years across cultures (Jullien, 2021; Reilly et al., 2015; I. Wallace et al., 2015).

See the **ASHA Cultural Responsiveness Practice Portal**, the **ASHA Multilingual Service Delivery Practice Portal**, and ASHA's resources for **"Phonemic Inventories and Cultural and Linguistic Information Across Languages"** for more information on determining language differences versus language disorders.

Intervention for Childhood Language Disorders

In addition to the critical role of SLPs in assessment, they have an equally important role in the intervention process for children with language disorders. Their role includes, but is not limited to, the following:

- Making decisions about how to address a language disorder
- Developing plans for intervention, implementing those plans, and documenting the child's performance
- Providing counseling regarding the impact of a language disorder
- Educating, consulting, and collaborating with families, teachers, and other professionals on the needs of children with language disorders
- Keeping informed about available research and evidence-based practices in childhood language disorders
- Determining when it is appropriate to dismiss a child from intervention
- Advocating for children with language disorders at a local, state, and national level

The goal of language intervention is to stimulate language development and support the child's ability to participate in daily life, including (but not limited to) their ability to express themselves in complex and meaningful ways, access academic content, and develop and maintain relationships with others. Intervention goals should be specific to each individual child's specific needs and developmental level to support their communication effectiveness and social success. There are several principles that should be considered when selecting and developing an intervention plan for children, including the following (Roth & Worthington, 2015):

- Using strategies that facilitate communication rather than teach isolated skills
- Ensuring ongoing assessment and monitoring of a child's progress, making adjustment to the intervention as needed
- Individualizing the intervention in consideration of the child's unique communication profile

- Establishing goals that scaffold the child's knowledge a step beyond their current performance level

In the following sections, we provide several strategies to support language development across age levels with the intent of helping children build as much independence and autonomy in functional language use as possible in daily settings.

Language Intervention for Preschoolers

Language usually develops at a rapid rate in preschool children when their vocabularies grow, and they begin to master basic sentence structures. For children with language difficulties, however, this process is often delayed. Therefore, SLPs use targeted areas for intervention across phonology, morphology and syntax, semantics, and pragmatics.

Intervention at the phonological level focuses on improving the child's awareness of patterns in language, particularly as it relates to how sounds combine to form words and reducing their use of phonological processes. When a child has a phonological disorder, reducing phonological processes leads to an increase in intelligibility, which ultimately serves to decrease a child's frustration in communicating their message. Support at the phonological level may also involve expanding a child's phonological awareness skills (e.g., rhyming, segmenting words).

At the semantic level, intervention focuses on increasing the child's vocabulary, including, but not limited to, basic concepts, action words, and pronouns, as well as increasing their understanding and use of semantic relationships (e.g., agent + action, action + object). Morphology instruction with preschool children focuses on awareness of morphemes in words, as well as how morphemes (e.g., prefixes, suffixes, base words) can be combined to form new words. When working on syntax, SLPs may focus on increasing sentence length and complexity.

When supporting preschool-aged children in pragmatics, SLPs may teach different levels of play, including pretend play, and the language that is associated with imaginative play. SLPs may also work on turn-taking, maintaining topics in conversation, initiating conversation, requesting information, and developing skills in storytelling and narrative language.

Table 7–3 outlines four commonly used evidence-based strategies for supporting early language development in preschool children with DLD: **focused stimulation**, **language scaffolding**, **parallel talk**, and **recasting**. Focused stimulation incorporates predetermined vocabulary in a highly concentrated way to support a child's vocabulary development. For example, if a child is talking about going to the beach, the clinician identifies relevant concepts that can be the focus of the conversation (e.g., water, ocean, lake, waves, swimming, fish, sand, umbrella, bathing suit, shovel, bucket). A language scaffolding approach would incorporate parts of a child's utterance into the clinician's response, who would then add new vocabulary or more complex grammar. For example, if a child says "water" while pointing to a picture of an ocean wave, the clinician might say, "The ocean water has big waves." In parallel talk, the clinician comments on what a child is doing while they are doing it, including naming their actions and identifying new words. While the child is coloring a picture of a beach, the clinician might say, "You are coloring the ocean blue and the sun yellow." Finally, recasting is a strategy in which the clinician repeats back what a child says while expanding their utterance to include accurate and new semantic and syntactic information. For example, if a child says, "Put sand bucket," the clinician would say, "You are putting sand in the red bucket. The bucket is almost full."

TABLE 7–3. Evidence-Based Interventions to Support the Language of Young Children With Developmental Language Disorder

Intervention Strategy	Description	Example
Focused stimulation	Using predetermined vocabulary in a highly concentrated way to support vocabulary development	When discussing making an ice cream sundae, the clinician identifies particular toppings (e.g., sprinkles, whipped cream, nuts, cherry, chocolate sauce, caramel) and types of ice cream that can be used.
Language scaffolding	Incorporating segments of a child's utterance into an adult response that adds new information such as new vocabulary or more complex grammar	When a child says "ice cream," the clinician can say "put in two scoops of ice cream."
Parallel talk	Commenting on what a child is doing while they are doing it; naming the actions and identifying new words	When making the ice cream sundae, the clinician talks about everything the child is doing: "Nice job scooping the ice cream out of the bucket and putting it in the bowl."
Recasting	Repeating what a child says but expanding their utterance to include accurate and new semantic and syntactic information	When the child is making the sundae and says, "Put ice cream," the clinician says, "You want to put two scoops of ice cream in the bowl."

Source: Adapted from Freeman (2023).

There are other strategies that may also be useful to young children with DLD, such as facilitating word learning and group language intervention with typical peers. Implicit word learning is a challenge for children with DLD, leading to poorer vocabulary development, which impacts listening comprehension, reading, and writing as well as educational achievement (Haebig et al., 2015; Lervåg et al., 2018; Spencer et al., 2017). Levlin and colleagues (2022) examined the outcomes of two different learning methods to support vocabulary development in children with DLD: retrieval practice (RP) and rich vocabulary instruction (RVI). RP is a learning approach that helps us remember information on later tasks by recalling newly learned information from memory rather than repeatedly studying, relearning, or encoding the information (Levlin et al., 2022). Research suggests that RP improves vocabulary learning and retention to a greater extent than other learning strategies (Dunlosky et al., 2013). Repeating words in context also increases exposure to new words, and better word learning was found for children in seventh through ninth grade using retrieval practice (Levlin et al., 2022). RVI is an instructional strategy that provides the child with tools to become an active and independent word learner. It involves teaching the child the phonological and morphological information about the word (Beck et al., 2013) and using context to establish word meaning variations.

Schmitt and colleagues (2022) measured the effects of including children with typical language development in an 8-week group language intervention with peers who had DLD. Children with DLD were randomly assigned to language intervention with a TD peer or to intervention with a peer who also had DLD. All children showed gains in their language on measures of semantics, syntax, morphology, and narratives.

Effect sizes from pre to post intervention, however, indicated that children with DLD who were assigned to groups with peers without DLD performed better in the areas of syntax, morphology, and narratives.

Language Intervention for School-Age Children

Language intervention for elementary school-age children with DLD is designed to provide them with the skills they need to learn and succeed in the classroom environment. Usually, interventions are curriculum-based with goals addressing the concepts and language used and taught in the classroom. Literacy skills might also be a focus of the intervention, including support for reading comprehension, as well as narrative and expository writing. An emphasis on metacognitive and metalinguistic skills might also be a priority to increase the student's awareness of language rules for using various language forms as well as the ability to self-monitor the accuracy of their language understanding and use. An effective language intervention program requires the SLP to collaborate with the classroom teacher, special education teacher (where appropriate), paraprofessionals (as appropriate), and related service providers (e.g., psychologist, physical therapist, occupational therapist) who are also supporting the child with a DLD.

Intervention goals may target a variety of language components. Children may continue to require instruction in phonological awareness as well as reducing any residual phonological processes. From a semantics perspective, vocabulary knowledge would continue to be a focus, with special attention to the vocabulary used in the curriculum. Intervention might also require increased depth in the understanding and use of figurative language, abstract vocabulary, multiple meaning words, and word meaning differences influenced by context. Morphologically, the student will now be expected to use and understand morphemes for more complex vocabulary words (e.g., support/supportive, ideal/idealistic). Complex sentence use, such as compound sentences and sentences with dependent and relative clauses, may be an intervention focus, as will recognizing and correcting grammatical errors. Pragmatic intervention may focus on using language for various purposes, including to persuade, clarify, engage in discourse, and contribute to classroom discussions.

Notably, the classroom environment is a primary place where children listen, comprehend, and learn. In fact, children spend 45% to 65% of their time "listening" in school (Rosenberg et al., 1999). Therefore, it is important to create an environment in which children can hear the teacher and noise is minimized. Several characteristics of the environment (e.g., shape, furnishings, surrounding noises) can influence a child's ability to hear and understand what is being presented (Murgia et al., 2023). Often, however, classroom acoustics fall short, which impacts a child's ability to discriminate what is being said and attending to relevant information being presented (Shield et al., 2015). When the level of classroom noise is greater than the level of speech information, this speech-to-noise ratio (SNR) can affect the intelligibility of the speech signal being delivered to the student and ultimately impact their academic achievement (Caviola et al., 2021; Connolly et al., 2019; Prodi et al., 2019; Rudner et al., 2018). Typically, it is expected that classroom SNR varies, but optimal benefit occurs when speech is +15 dB greater than the classroom noise (ASHA, 2005). Ultimately, appropriate acoustics in the classroom helps ensure that a child can hear what the teacher says, which can increase their likely success in the classroom.

Language Intervention for Adolescents

Curriculum demands only increase as students enter middle school and high school. If by this time a student has still not acquired the basic language skills needed to close the gap between their ability and grade-level expectations, language intervention may focus on explicitly teaching language skills as well as ways to compensate for the language challenges the adolescent continues to exhibit. At this stage, the role of the adolescent in their intervention is critical to empower a sense of responsibility and self-advocacy to achieve the best possible outcomes.

The focus of intervention at this level includes teaching the rules, principles, and strategies that will help facilitate knowledge acquisition across settings, with a focus on *how* to learn versus *what* specific content to learn. Strategies might include any of the following:

- How to infer meaning from text
- Identifying main ideas
- Deconstructing morphologically complex words in the curriculum to make sense of their meaning
- Using checklists and graphic organizers to plan presentations and research papers
- Using electronic tools (e.g., spell check, grammar check, speech-to-text) to help with written work
- Implementing technology to access, share, and evaluate information in collaboration with peers for shared projects

Intervention Applications in Cultural Groups

Bilingual children with DLD have difficulty with complex syntax as well as morphology and vocabulary (Castilla-Earls et al., 2021; Peña et al., 2020). Complex syntax is often untreated in bilingual children, yet it is critical to academic success (Curran, 2020). Castilla-Earls and Van Home (2023) examined the feasibility of delivering recast therapy to support complex syntax to bilingual children speaking Spanish and English using telepractice. They included 15 bilingual children with DLD who were assigned to one of three conditions: Spanish only, English only, and Spanish + English. Children completed a 16-hour treatment and completed pre- and post-intervention testing of the ability to produce conditional adverbs (therapy target) and subject relative clauses (not targeted in therapy). The use of recast therapy improved syntactic structures that were part of therapy more than structures that were not directly targeted. For those receiving intervention in only one language, gains were similar in both the treated and untreated languages.

Additional Intervention Approaches

There are several different intervention approaches and strategies for use with individuals with language disorders that vary along a continuum of naturalness ranging from drill-based activities in a therapy room (clinician directed) to modeling play in more natural settings (child centered) to those that combine both approaches. Some language intervention approaches target specific language skills (e.g., semantics, syntax), whereas others are more holistic and target a range of language skills. When making any decision about an intervention, it is important to consider the child's language profile, severity of the language disorder, and any other co-occurring conditions, as well as their cultural background and overall communication needs. Included in this section are brief descriptions of several general and specific treatments for addressing language disorders, many with a behavioral basis and others with a more naturalistic framework. Many of these approaches are used with children with autism or social communication disorders, although many are appropriate for children with any DLD.

Functional Communication Training

Functional communication training (FCT) is a common intervention technique that is designed to replace challenging behaviors (which often serve a communicative purpose) with alternative communicative behaviors. FCT is a multistep process that assesses the function of a challenging behavior, selects an appropriate alternative communicative behavior (e.g., using gestures or words), and teaches that form of communication. It is guided by three basic principles: functional equivalence, natural communities of reinforcement, and features of the alternative response (Durand, 2021). **Functional equivalence** is the idea that one behavior can be replaced by another behavior if the new behavior serves the same function and is more efficient at gaining the desired reinforcers. For example, if child learns to say "want" to indicate that they want their toys, this should serve the same function and be more efficient at obtaining their toys than banging on the box of toys that they are unable to open. **Natural communities of reinforcement** use communication as a replacement behavior and help recruit desired reinforcers. **Features of an alternative response** include how the alternative response matches the intention of the original response or what is known as the response match and also whether the alternative response is successful, efficient, acceptable, and recognizable to the communicator.

Milieu Communication Therapy

Milieu communication theory (MCT) is an intervention designed to facilitate early communication and language development. It includes both **prelinguistic milieu teaching** for children who have not yet developed language and **enhanced milieu teaching** for children with early language development. MCT incorporates behavioral strategies (e.g., task analysis, predictable structure, attention to antecedent, consequent events) to help shape functional language. It incorporates several strategies that foster communication acts such as requesting and commenting. Strategies include the following (Kaiser et al., 2021):

- Placing items in sight but out of reach
- Using expectant waiting
- Briefly withholding materials of interest
- Giving small portions of objects/materials
- Minorly sabotaging familiar routines
- Slightly protesting a child's actions
- Creating silly or unexpected situations
- Imitating contingent actions
- Modeling language forms and vocabulary
- Reinforcing natural language attempts

Narrative Interventions

These interventions support a child's ability to engage in storytelling using story grammars to organize events. Narrative interventions teach children to utilize microstructures (e.g., syntactic complexity, conjunctions, elaborated phrases) to enhance narrative clarity. Narratives can provide a natural way to target specific language difficulties.

Parent-Mediated Intervention

Parent-mediated interventions are used to increase parent–child interaction and support children's early language and communication. Parents are important to supporting a child's language success. Parents learn to use direct and individualized strategies that increase their child's skill acquisition.

Pivotal Response Treatment

The pivotal response treatment (PRT) intervention emphasizes functional language use and incorporates teaching techniques that motivate children to use language to communicate. Core motivational variables are used, including giving the child choices, reinforcing attempts at communication, varying tasks in which language is expected, providing natural reinforcers, and interspersing learned tasks with new tasks. PRT is a play-based intervention with six primary targets—motivation, responsivity to multiple cues, self-initiation, empathy, self-regulation, and social interaction—all of which are skills central to social language development and a wide range of other communication skills (Koegel & Koegel, 2006).

Video Modeling

In this intervention, the target child watches a scripted video of adults or children performing a particular task that is a target area for the child (e.g., engaging in conversation, playing, completing an activity) and modeling targeted behaviors such as conversational scripts, self-help skills, greetings, labeling, and so on. Video modeling helps the target child focus their attention on the relevant information in the task that they are learning. With practice, the child begins to use the targeted language and behaviors that are modeled in the video; repeated viewings support the child's ability to learn specific vocabulary associated with targeted situations (Buggey, 2012). Video modeling also fosters children's ability to take what they have learned in a video modeling session and generalize that information into other areas of their daily life (Shipley-Benamou et al., 2002).

Service Delivery Options

In addition to determining the type of intervention that is appropriate for a child with a language disorder, the SLP should also consider other variables, including the following:

- Dosage: Intervention frequency, intensity, and duration
- Format: Individual or group therapy
- Provider: Who provides the intervention (e.g., SLP, SLP assistant, paraprofessional, parent)
- Setting: Where the intervention occurs (e.g., at home, in the community, at school)
- Timing: When the intervention occurs following a diagnosis

These are important to consider in designing a therapy program for children with DLD.

Why Is This Topic Important?

Understanding the impact of language disorders on a child's ability to fully engage within their environment and to share their experiences, thoughts, and ideas is critical to their long-term success at home, in school, and in their community. Although many approaches have been developed to diagnose children with DLD early on to facilitate early intervention, there remain challenges in our assessment process. Valid assessments for infants and toddlers are lacking in the literature, and those that are available may be impacted by linguistic and cultural biases (Cycyk et al., 2021). Therefore, clinical research must continue to evaluate assessment models and tools to ensure reliable approaches exist so that we do not delay diagnosis and intervention, which can have a long-term impact (Hus & Segal, 2021).

It is also true that more formal or traditional approaches to assessment are generally static, in which a child is tested in a standard testing environment without receiving feedback or support. Scores on these norm-referenced assessments compare a child's performance to the performance of others at a particular point in time (Spicer-Cain et al., 2023). One of the flaws in this approach to assessment is the lack of information on how a child responds in a more natural context and engages with an examiner to show their best response. For the youngest children with or at risk for DLD, it is important to gather information from direct observations as well as parental report. SLPs may also consider a dynamic assessment approach in which clinicians measure children's emerging developmental skills as well as their potential for learning (Bamford et al., 2022). A dynamic assessment approach is key to developing a more individualized approach to assessment across cultures.

Difficulty communicating impacts a child's ability to fully participate in daily activities, often resulting in negative outcomes. The ability to participate in daily life activities certainly varies depending on the etiology and severity of the communication challenge, as well as the personal factors that characterize the individual and the environmental context in which they live (Baylor & Darling-White, 2020). It is important, therefore, that SLPs and audiologists implement intervention that is responsive to the child's need and desire to participate in their home, school, and larger community (S. Wallace et al., 2017). Research suggests that areas important to communication participation, as defined by the *International Classification of Functioning, Disability and Health* (World Health Organization, 2001), include developing relationships and engaging in interaction (66%) and being involved in community, social, and civic life (10%) (ter Wal et al., 2023).

Supporting children with language disorders can and should happen throughout the day. Adult conversations with young children are important to language development, and the early childhood classroom provides a key opportunity to support back-and-forth conversations among children and teachers outside of direct intervention (Hindman et al., 2022). SLPs can teach other adults to informally support children's language development through the common task of book reading. Adults can be guided to both initiate and sustain conversations during interactive book reading by frequently soliciting and responding to children's talk, which then facilitates children's vocabulary development (Hindman et al., 2022).

Best practices in speech-language pathology require a level of collaboration across professional disciplines to ensure a child, teen, or adult with a communication disorder has a comprehensive plan to address their needs. This requires not only expertise that is discipline specific but also competency in interprofessional practice. ASHA (2015) and the Council for Exceptional Children, Division for Early Childhood (2020) have expectations in their accreditation guidelines, policies, and requirements that highlight the importance of professionals working together to facilitate desired communication and learning outcomes (Lieberman-Betz et al., 2023). When supporting children with complex communication, physical, and health needs, no one discipline has sufficient expertise to address all areas. For this reason, students training to be health care professionals are encouraged to engage in **interprofessional education** (IPE), which provides opportunities for students in training across disciplines to learn with and from one another with the expressed goal of collaborating to improve a patient's or client's quality of care. In fact, the research indicates that training students in IPE facilitates teamwork and collaboration with other disciplines. Research suggests that preservice IPE promotes skills in interdisciplinary collaboration and teamwork (Cusack & O'Donoghue, 2012; Guraya & Barr, 2018). For example, Lieberman-Betz and colleagues (2023) found that educating students in training using a combination of case-based instruction, interprofessional faculty, and families is an effective way to foster understanding and skill in implementing interprofessional practice.

Application to a Child

Ethan is a 3-year-old boy with an intellectual disability and a language impairment. As an infant, he was described by his parents as delayed in reaching many of his milestones. He was less responsive than they remember his older sister to be. Even smiling seemed to be delayed. He was diagnosed at 6 months as having a severe developmental delay affecting all major motor and communication milestones. At 16 months, his behaviors approximated that of a much younger child, and the milestones he had achieved were more like those of a 7-month-old. Ethan often communicated through nonverbal behaviors, such as facial expressions and gestures.

An SLP determined that Ethan's goals should include using intentional communication (long-term goal) and promoting intentional behaviors such as behavior regulation, responding to joint attention, reaching and pointing, and following routines (short-term goals). She initiated an intervention, during which she worked with Ethan and his parents to replace less effective behaviors, such as escaping and protesting through hitting, with more effective communicative behaviors, such as requesting and rejecting. The SLP began teaching Ethan requesting and rejecting language (e.g., "want," "not," "stop") by using augmentative and alternative communication (AAC). The SLP employed comprehension checks to ensure that Ethan understood the symbols and language being used, errorless learning to ensure that he responded accurately with support, and a high-tech AAC device with robust vocabulary. After 8 months of intervention, Ethan was successfully showing intentional behaviors. He learned to identify different objects and began vocalizing sounds. At 36 months, he began school with an Individualized Education Plan and was able to attend an inclusive preschool where he continued to develop language with AAC. Eventually, he began forming two- or three-word phrases and started to initiate interactions.

As you think about Ethan and consider what you have read in this chapter and learned in class thus far, reflect on the following questions:

- What other interventions might work to support Ethan's developing language?
- Why was it important for the SLP to use comprehension checks in her intervention with Ethan?
- What is the role of the family in supporting Ethan's communication development?
- How might AAC be used to support Ethan's ability to communicate his wants and needs with his family?

Chapter Summary

Developmental language disorder is characterized by difficulties in grammar (syntax), vocabulary (semantics), the rules or processes that govern speech sound development (phonology), understanding the principles by which words are formed (morphology), and the social use of language (pragmatics). Children with DLD exhibit notable challenges in a variety of communicative situations, and those with receptive–expressive disorder are affected more than those with an expressive disorder only. In fact, compared to parents of children with expressive disorder only, parents of children with receptive–expressive disorder indicate that their children are more limited in their language. Similarly, teachers indicate that the communication abilities and social competencies of children with receptive–expressive language difficulties are poorer than those with expressive language challenges only (Bruinsma et al., 2024).

There are many formal and informal approaches to gathering information about children's comprehension and spoken language. Assessment procedures might include the following:

- Curriculum-based assessment
- Dynamic assessment
- Ethnographic interviewing
- Language sampling
- Parent, teacher, and child report measures
- Standardized testing
- Systematic observation

Intervention is an important step in addressing the language challenges of children with DLD. Intervention strategies should focus on difficulties in morphology, phonology, pragmatics, semantics, and syntax that change over time in preschool and school-age children and adolescents. Interventions commonly used to support language in preschool children include the following:

- Focused stimulation
- Language scaffolding
- Parallel talk
- Recasting

Other interventions that are frequently used to support social communication and children and adolescents include the following:

- AAC
- Functional communication training
- Milieu communication teaching
- Narrative intervention
- Parent intervention
- Pivotal response training
- Video modeling

Chapter Review Questions

1. Compare and contrast the language challenges of children with social communication disorder and those with autism.
2. Describe some of the challenges children with DLD have in language form.
3. Explain the dynamic assessment process and why this process might be more effective for children with cultural and linguistic differences.
4. Identify at least three interventions that are appropriate for supporting a preschool child's expressive language abilities.
5. What components of language are usually impacted for a child with Down syndrome?
6. Describe some of the targets that may be appropriate in supporting the language development of school-age children.
7. What are some of the strategies used to enhance early language development in milieu communication training?
8. What are the central features of pivotal response treatment?
9. Explain the difference between retrieval practice and rich vocabulary instruction to support language content in children with DLD?
10. What are some considerations for supporting adolescents with language disorders?

Learning Activities

1. Spend time with a preschool child and listen to their language. Practice using parallel talk and focused stimulation when interacting with the child. What did you learn about their language?
2. Create a video model for a child who has difficulty taking turns in conversation.
3. Develop an activity for a child with a DLD using the principles of pivotal response treatment.
4. Search the internet for videos that demonstrate the use of at least three of the interventions you learned about in this chapter.
5. Consider the language that is used in a current course you are taking. Write down any multiple-meaning words or figurative speech that the professor used and/or you read in your text for a particular day. How might the complexity of the curriculum you are learning be difficult for a student with DLD?

Suggested Reading

Manwaring, S. S., Mead, D. L., Swineford, L., & Thurm, A. (2017). Modelling gesture use and early language development in autism spectrum disorder. *International Journal of Language & Communication Disorders, 52*(5), 637–651.

This study compared gesture use, language, and fine motor skills between autistic children and neurotypical children or children with other developmental delays. Children were between ages 1 and 4 years at the initial testing. Post-evaluation tests were done on autistic children 8 to 16 months after the initial evaluation. Evaluations included the Developmental Profile Caregiver Questionnaire (CQ); Autism Diagnostic Observation Schedule (ADOS); Mullen Scales of Early Learning (MSEL); Vineland Adaptive Behavior Scales–II (VABS-II); and MacArthur–Bates Communicative Development Inventories, Second Edition (CDI). CQ is a questionnaire for parents regarding their child's prelinguistic communication. ADOS is the gold-standard autism diagnostic tool that examines a child's verbal and nonverbal behavior using semistructured modules in response to social probes. MSEL examines verbal and nonverbal development, including gross and fine motor skills, receptive and expressive language, and visual reception (Manwaring et al., 2017). VABS-II measures adaptive behavior using caregivers reports about communication, motor skills, socialization, and daily living skills. CDI is another parent report on language and communication development.

The authors found that ADOS and CQ scores were highly correlated and that autistic children tend to have fewer early gestures than neurotypical children and children with other developmental delays. Gesture use was also correlated with the severity of autism spectrum disorder. Deficits in fine motor skills were seen in autistic children across these measures as well. Findings suggest that because fine motor and language skills are correlated, intervention should consider both skill areas to facilitate growth.

All the measures used in this study are limited in the way that data are recorded, and future studies should aim to find a measure that incorporates key aspects of the five measures. The use of gestures in language development also requires further investigation. Importantly, both parent report and direct observation measures are accurate in identifying gesture use.

Solot, C. B., Sell, D., Mayne, A., Baylis, A. L., Persson, C., Jackson, O., & McDonald-McGinn, D. M. (2019). Speech-language disorders in 22q11.2 deletion syndrome: Best practices for diagnosis and management. *American Journal of Speech-Language Pathology, 28*(3), 984–999.

This article discusses key features of 22q11.2 deletion syndrome (22qDS) and gives information for clinical management based on these features. Most people diagnosed with DiGeorge syndrome, velocardiofacial syndrome, conotruncal anomaly face syndrome, and/or Cayler cardiofacial syndrome have also been identified to have 22qDS. Some distinct facial features include hooded eyelids, auricular anomalies, nasal crease or dimple, and small mouth.

Feeding and swallowing disorders are also commonly seen in children with 22qDS. Nasal regurgitation, gastroesophageal reflux disease, and recurrent vomiting are the most common. Some children require tube feeding, depending on the severity of their disorder. Other children may develop behavioral feeding problems that require therapy to manage.

Many children with 22qDS have hearing loss. Malformations of the cochlea and vestibule, middle ear fluid, and ossicular chain abnormalities are major contributing factors to hearing loss. Children with 22qDS also have voice and airway disorders. These disorders may require children to have tracheostomies performed on them. Problems with speech may include breathiness, hoarseness, and soft volume.

Significant developmental delays are often seen in preschool-aged children with 22qDS. Some studies have shown that IQ scores can change throughout the life of someone with 22qDS. Strengths in cognition are reading decoding, spelling, verbal memory, and rote processing. However, some language delays are seen, including the emergence of words and phrases, expressive vocabulary, and language use. Even if children do not show delays in language early on, later difficulties may be present. Parents typically seek interventions during the preschool years to facilitate growth in language and communication skills. These interventions are meant to help with speech sound disorders related to cleft palate or velopharyngeal dysfunction (VPD). Notably, children with 22qDS have more difficulties than children who only have cleft palate/VPD, and there may be something intrinsic to 22qDS that makes speech sound production difficult. In fact, most children with 22qDS have VPD and/or palate abnormalities, and surgery is a common intervention for VPD. Strategies to help with speech sounds include whispering, nares compression, and auditory pressure cues. It is important to note that every child is different and therefore should have an individualized treatment plan.

Autism spectrum disorder is also a common comorbidity. Anxiety, later onset psychosis, and attention-deficit/hyperactivity disorder may also be seen in children with 22qDS. Interventions should start early and be ongoing. SLPs can be liaisons and recommend appropriate support to those who may need them. New information is always being produced, and keeping up to date on complex syndromes such as 22qDS is imperative for ensuring quality health care.

Additional Resource

- American Speech-Language-Hearing Association, "Assessment and Evaluation of Speech-Language Disorders in Schools"
https://www.asha.org/slp/assessment-and-evaluation-of-speech-language-disorders-in-schools

References

Al Otaiba, S., Puranik, C. S., Ziolkowski, R. A., & Montgomery, T. M. (2009). Effectiveness of early phonological awareness interventions for students with speech or language impairments. *Journal of Special Education, 43*(2), 107–128.

American Psychiatric Association. (2022). *Diagnostic and statistical manual of mental disorders* (5th ed., text rev.).

American Speech-Language-Hearing Association. (n.d.). *Spoken language disorders* [Practice portal]. Retrieved June, 8, 2024, from https://www.asha.org/Practice-Portal/Clinical-Topics/Spoken-Language-Disorders/

American Speech-Language-Hearing Association. (2005). *Acoustics in educational settings: Technical report*. https://specialedlaw.blogs.com/home/files/AcousticsTR.pdf

American Speech-Language-Hearing Association. (2015). *Interprofessional Education/Interprofessional Practice (IPE/IPP)*. https://www.asha.org/practice/interprofessional-education-practice

American Speech-Language-Hearing Association. (2020). *2020 Schools Survey report: SLP caseload and workload characteristics*. http://www.asha.org/Research/memberdata/Schools-Survey

Bamford, K., Masso, S., Baker, E., & Ballard, K. (2022). Dynamic assessment for children with communication disorders: A systematic scoping review and framework. *American Journal of Speech-Language Pathology, 31*(4), 1878–1893.

Barnes, E., Roberts, J., Long, S., Martin, G., Berni, M., Mandulak, K., & Sideris, J. (2009). Phonological accuracy and intelligibility in connected speech of boys with fragile X syndrome or Down syndrome. *Journal of Speech, Language, and Hearing Research, 52*(4), 1048–1061.

Baylor, C., & Darling-White, M. (2020). Clinical focus achieving participation-focused intervention through shared decision making: Proposal of an age- and disorder-generic framework. *American Journal of Speech-Language Pathology, 29*(3), 1335–1360.

Beck, I. L., McKeown, M. G., & Kucan, L. (2013). *Bringing words to life: Robust vocabulary instruction* (2nd ed.). Guilford.

Beitchman, J. H., Nair, R., Clegg, M., & Patel, P. G. (1986). Prevalence of speech and language disorders in 5-year-old kindergarten children in the Ottawa–Carleton region. *Journal of Speech and Hearing Disorders, 51,* 98–110.

Berko Gleason, J. (2005). *The development of language* (6th ed.). Pearson.

Bishop, C. (2006). *Children's Communication Checklist–2*. Pearson. https://www.pearsonassessments.com/store/usassessments/en/Store/Professional-Assessments/Speech-%26-Language/Children%27s-Communication-Checklist-2-%7C-U-S-Edition/p/100000193.html

Black, L. I., Vahratian, A., & Hoffman, H. J. (2015). *Communication disorders and use of intervention services among children aged 3–17 years: United States, 2012* (NCHS data brief No. 205). National Center for Health Statistics.

Blood, G. (2014). Bullying be gone. *The ASHA Leader, 19,* 36–42.

Boliek, C. A., Halpern, A., Hernandez, K., Fox, C. M., & Ramig, L. (2022). Intensive voice treatment (Lee Silverman Voice Treatment [LSVT LOUD]) for children with Down syndrome: Phase I outcomes. *Journal of Speech-Language-Hearing Research, 65,* 1228–1262.

Botting, N. (2020). Language, literacy and cognitive skills of young adults with developmental language disorder (DLD). *International Journal of Language & Communication Disorders, 55*(2), 255–265.

Botting, N., Durkin, K., Toseeb, U., Pickles, A., & Conti-Ramsden, G. (2016). Emotional health, support, and self-efficacy in young adults with a history of language impairment. *British Journal of Developmental Psychology, 34*(4), 538–554.

Brinton, B., Spackman, M. P., Fujiki, M., & Ricks, J. (2007). What should Chris say? The ability of children with specific language impairment to recognize the need to dissemble emotions in social situations. *Journal of Speech, Language, and Hearing Research, 50*(3), 798–811.

Brownlie, E. B., Jabbar, A., Beitchman, J., Vida, R., & Atkinson, L. (2007). Language impairment and sexual assault of girls and women: Findings from a community sample. *Journal of Abnormal Psychology, 35,* 618–626.

Bruinsma, G. I., Wijnen, F., & Gerrits, E. (2024). Communication in daily life of children with developmental language disorder: Parents' and teachers' perspectives. *Language, Speech, and Hearing Services in Schools, 55,* 105–129.

Buggey, T. (2012). Video modeling applications for persons with autism. In P. A. Prelock & R. J. McCauley (Eds.), *Treatment of autism spectrum disorders: Evidence-based intervention strategies for communication and social interaction* (pp. 345–369). Brookes.

Carrow-Woolfolk, E. (2017). *Comprehensive Assessment of Spoken Language–Second Edition*. Pro-Ed.

Castilla-Earls, A. P., Pérez-Leroux, A. T., Fulcher-Rood, K., & Barr, C. (2021). Morphological errors in Spanish-speaking bilingual children with and without developmental language disorders. *Language, Speech, and Hearing Services in Schools, 52*(2), 497–511.

Castilla-Earls, A., & Van Home, A. O. (2023). Children with developmental language disorder: A feasibility and early efficacy study examining the role of language of intervention on outcomes. *Journal of Speech, Language, and Hearing Research, 66*, 2783–2801.

Caviola, S., Visentin, C., Borella, E., Mammarella, I., & Prodi, N. (2021). Out of the noise: Effects of sound environment on math performance in middle-school students. *Journal of Environmental Psychology, 73*, Article 101552.

Connolly, D., Dockrell, J., Shield, B., Conetta, R., Mydlarz, C., & Cox, T. (2019). The effects of classroom noise on the reading comprehension of adolescents. *Journal of the Acoustical Society of America, 145*(1), 372–381.

Council for Exceptional Children, Division for Early Childhood. (2020). *Initial practice-based standards for early interventionists/early childhood special educators.* https://exceptionalchildren.org/standards/initial-practice-based-standards-early-interventionists-early-childhood-special-educators

Crespo, K., & Kaushanskaya, M. (2022). The role of attention, language, language ability and language experience in children's artificial learning grammar. *Journal of Speech, Language, and Hearing Research, 65*, 1574–1591.

Curran, M. (2020). Complex sentences in an elementary science curriculum: A research note. *Language, Speech, and Hearing Services in Schools, 51*(2), 329–335.

Cusack, T., & O'Donoghue, G. (2012). The introduction of an interprofessional education module: Students' perceptions. *Quality in Primary Care, 20*(3), 231–238.

Cycyk, L. M., De Anda, S., Moore, H., & Huerta, L. (2021). Cultural and linguistic adaptations of early language interventions: Recommendations for advancing research and practice. *American Journal of Speech-Language Pathology, 30*(3), 1224–1246.

Dockrell, J., Lindsay, G., Palikara, O., & Cullen, M. A. (2007). *Raising the achievements of children and young people with specific speech and language difficulties and other special educational needs through school to work and college.* Department for Education and Skills/Institute of Education, University of London.

Dubois, P., St.-Pierre, M. C., Desmarais, C., & Guay, F. (2020). Young adults with developmental language disorder: A systematic review of education, employment, and independent living outcomes. *Journal of Speech, Language, and Hearing Research, 63*(11), 3786–3800.

Duff, F. J., Reen, G., Plunkett, K., & Nation, K. (2015). Do infant vocabulary skills predict school-age language and literacy outcomes? *The Journal of Child Psychology and Psychiatry, 56*(8), 848–856.

Duff, D., & Tomblin, J. B. (2018, October). Literacy as an outcome of language development and its impact on children's psychosocial and emotional development. *Language Development & Literacy*, 1–8.

Dunlosky, J., Rawson, K. A., Marsh, E. J., Nathan, M. J., & Willingham, D. T. (2013). Improving students' learning with effective learning techniques. *Psychological Science in the Public Interest, 14*(1), 4–58.

Durand, M. (2021). Functional communication training: Treating challenging behavior. In P. A. Prelock & R. J. McCauley (Eds.), *Treatment of autism spectrum disorders: Evidence-based intervention strategies for communication and social interaction* (pp. 107–138). Brookes.

Ellis Weismer, S., Plante, E., Jones, M., & Tomblin, J. B. (2005). A functional magnetic resonance imaging investigation of verbal working memory in adolescents with specific language impairment. *Journal of Speech, Language, and Hearing Research, 48*(2), 405–425.

Everaert, E., Boerma, T., Selten, I., Gerrits, E., Houben, M., Vorstman, J., & Wijnen, F. (2023). Nonverbal executive functioning in relation to vocabulary and morphosyntax in preschool children with and without developmental language disorder. *Journal of Speech, Language, and Hearing Research, 66*, 3954–3973.

Finestack, L., Richmond, E., & Abbeduto, L. (2009). Language development in individuals with fragile X syndrome. *Topics in Language Disorders, 29*(2), 133–148.

Freeman, M. (2023). Linking language to action: Enhancing preschoolers' communicative abilities within language stimulation. *Language, Speech, and Hearing Services in Schools, 54*(4), 1308–1322.

Fujiki, M., Brinton, B., & Clarke, D. (2002). Emotion regulation in children with specific language impairment. *Language, Speech, and Hearing Services in Schools, 33*(2), 102–111.

Fujiki, M., Spackman, M. P., Brinton, B., & Hall, A. (2004). The relationship of language and emotion regulation skills to reticence in children with specific language impairment. *Journal of Speech, Language, and Hearing Research, 47*(3), 637–646.

Gillam, S. L., Holbrook, S., & Kamhi, A. G. (2021). Developmental language disorder. In J. S. Damico, N. Muller, & M. J. Ball (Eds.), *The handbook of language and speech disorders* (pp. 171–191). Wiley.

Girolametto, L. (1997). Development of a parent report measure for profiling the conversational skills of preschool children. *American Journal of Speech-Language Pathology, 6*(4), 25–33. https://doi.org/10.1044/1058-0360.0604.25

Glaser, B., Mumme, D., Blasey, C., Morris, M., Dahoun, S., Antonarakis, S., . . . Eliez, S. (2002). Language skills in children with velocardiofacial syndrome (deletion 22q11.2). *Journal of Pediatrics, 140*(6), 753–758.

Gray, S. (2003). Word-learning by preschoolers with specific language impairment: What predicts success? *Journal of Speech, Language, and Hearing Research, 46*, 56–67.

Gresham, F., & Elliott, S. N. (2008). *Social Skills Improvement System (SSIS) Rating Scales*. Pearson. https://www.pearsonassessments.com/store/usassessments/en/Store/Professional-Assessments/Behavior/Social-Skills-Improvement-System-SSIS-Rating-Scales/p/100000322.html

Guraya, S. Y., & Barr, H. (2018). The effectiveness of interprofessional education in healthcare: A systematic review and meta-analysis. *Kaohsiung Journal of Medical Sciences, 34*(3), 160–165.

Haebig, E., Kaushanskaya, M., & Ellis Weismer, S. (2015). Lexical processing in school-age children with autism spectrum disorder and children with specific language impairment: The role of semantics. *Journal of Autism and Developmental Disorders, 45*(12), 4109–4123.

Hammill, D. D., & Newcomer, P. L. (2020). *Test of Language Development-Intermediate-Fifth Edition*. Pro-Ed.

Harmuth, E., Silletta, E., Bailey, A., Adams, T., Beck, C., & Barbic, S. P. (2018). Barriers and facilitators to employment for adults with autism: A scoping review. *Annals of International Occupational Therapy, 1*(1), 31–40.

Heilmann, J., & Miller, J. F. (2023). Systematic analysis of language transcripts solutions: A tutorial. *Perspectives of the ASHA Special Interest Groups, 8*(1), 1–18. https://pubs.asha.org/doi/10.1044/2022_PERSP-22-00148

Hendricks, G., Malcolm-Smith, S., Adams, C., Stein, D. J., & Donald, K. A. (2018). Effects of prenatal alcohol exposure on language, speech and communication outcomes: A review of longitudinal studies. *Acta Neuropsychiatrica, 31*(2), 74–83.

Hindman, A. H., Farrow, J. M., & Wasik, B. A. (2022). Teacher–child conversations in preschool: Insights into how teacher feedback supports language development. *Topics in Language Disorders, 42*(4), 336–359.

Hollocks, M. J., Lerh, J. W., Magiati, I., Meiser-Stedman, R., & Brugha, T. S. (2019). Anxiety and depression in adults with autism spectrum disorder: A systematic review and meta-analysis. *Psychological Medicine, 49*(4), 559–572.

Hulme, C., & Snowling, M. J. (2013). *Developmental disorders of language learning and cognition.* Wiley-Blackwell.

Hutchins, T. L., & Prelock, P. A. (2015). Beyond the theory of mind hypothesis: Using a causal model to understand the nature and treatment of multiple deficits in autism spectrum disorder. In R. Huntley-Bahr & E. R. Silliman (Eds.), *Routledge handbook of communication disorders* (pp. 247–257). Routledge.

Hutchins, T. L., & Prelock, P. A. (2016). *Technical manual for the Theory of Mind Inventory–2.* The Theory of Mind Inventory. http://www.Theoryofmindinventory.com

Jullien, S. (2021). Screening for language and speech delay in children under five years. *BMC Pediatrics, 21*(Suppl. 1), Article 362.

Kaczorowska, N., Kaczorowski, K., Laskowska, J., & Mikulewicz, M. (2019). Down syndrome as a cause of abnormalities in the craniofacial region: A systematic literature review. *Advances in Clinical and Experimental Medicine, 28*(11), 1587–1592.

Kaiser, A. P., Fuller, E. A., & Heidlage, J. K. (2021). Enhanced milieu teaching. In P. A. Prelock (Ed.), *Autism spectrum disorders: Issues in assessment and intervention* (pp. 255–286). Pro-Ed.

Kodituwakku, P. W. (2009). Neurocognitive profile in children with fetal alcohol spectrum disorders. *Developmental Disabilities Research Reviews, 15*(3), 218–224.

Koegel, R. L., & Koegel, L. K. (2006). *Pivotal response treatments for autism: Communication, social, and academic development.* Brookes.

Lahey, M., & Edwards, J. (1999). Naming errors of children with specific language impairment. *Journal of Speech, Language, and Hearing Research, 42,* 195–205.

Lange, S., Rovet, J., Rehm, J., & Popva, S. (2017). Neurodevelopmental profile of fetal alcohol spectrum disorder: A systematic review. *BMC Psychology, 5*(22), 1–12.

Law, J., Boyle, J., Harris, F., Harkness, A., & Nye, C. (2000). Prevalence and natural history of primary speech and language delay: Findings from a systematic review of the literature. *International Journal of Language and Communication Disorders, 35*(2), 165–188.

Lee, L. L., & Canter, S. M. (1971). Developmental sentence scoring: A clinical procedure for estimating syntactic development in children's spontaneous speech. *Journal of Speech and Hearing Disorders, 36*(3), 315–340. https://doi.org/10.1044/jshd.3603.315

Leonard, L. B., Ellis Weismer, S., Miller, C. A., Francis, D. J., Tomblin, J. B., & Kail, R. V. (2007). Speed of processing, working memory, and language impairment in children. *Journal of Speech, Language, and Hearing Research, 50*(2), 408–428.

Lervåg, A., Hulme, C., & Melby-Lervåg, M. (2018). Unpicking the developmental relationship between oral language skills and reading comprehension: It's simple, but complex. *Child Development, 89*(5), 1821–1838.

Levlin, M., Wiklund-Hornqvist, C., Sandgren, O., Karlsson, S., & Jonsson, B. (2022). Evaluating the effect of rich vocabulary instruction and retrieval practice on the classroom vocabulary skills of children with (developmental) language disorders. *Journal of Speech, Language, and Hearing Research, 53,* 542–560.

Lieberman-Betz, R. G., Brown, J. A., Wiegand, S. D., Vail, C. O., Fiss, A. L., & Carpenter, L. J. (2023). Building collaborative capacity in early intervention preservice providers through interprofessional education. *Language, Speech, and Hearing Services in Schools, 54*, 504–517.

Maenner, M. J., Warren, Z., Williams, A. R., Amoakohene, E., Bakian, A. V., Bilder, D. A., . . . Shaw, K. A. (2023). Prevalence and characteristics of autism spectrum disorder among children aged 8 years—Autism and Developmental Disabilities Monitoring Network, 11 sites, United States, 2020. *MMWR Surveillance Summary, 72*(SS-2), 1–14.

Mai, C. T., Isenburg, J. L., Canfield, M. A., Meyer, R. E., Correa, A., Alverson, C. J., . . . National Birth Defects Prevention Network. (2019). National population-based estimates for major birth defects, 2010–2014. *Birth Defects Research, 111*(18), 1420–1435.

Marchman, V.A., Dale, P. S., & Fenson, L. (2023). *MacArthur-Bates Communicative Development Inventories-Third Edition*. Brookes.

Martin, G. E., Klusek, J., Estigarribia, B., & Roberts, J. E. (2009). Language characteristics of individuals with Down syndrome. *Topics in Language Disorders, 29*(2), 112–132.

Mayo Foundation for Medical Education and Research. (2022, March 1). *Angelman syndrome*. Mayo Clinic. Retrieved June 10, 2022, from https://www.mayoclinic.org/diseases-conditions/angelman-syndrome/symptoms-causes/syc-20355621#:~:text=Angelman%20syndrome%20is%20a%20genetic,and%20have%20happy%2C%20excitable%20personalities

Meltzer, L., Greschler, M. A., Davis, K., & Vanderberg, C. (2021). Executive function, metacognition, and language: Promoting student success with explicit strategy instruction. *Perspectives of the ASHA Special Interest Groups, 6*(6), 1343–1356.

Mervis, C. B., & Velleman, S. L. (2011). Children with Williams syndrome: Language, cognitive, and behavioral characteristics and their implications for intervention. *Perspectives on Language Learning and Education, 18*(3), 98–107.

Mol, S.E., & Bus, A.G. (2011). To read or not to read: A meta-analysis of print exposure from infancy to early adulthood. *Psychological Bulletin, 137*(2), 267–296.

Murgia, S., Webster, J., Cutiva, L. C. C., & Bottalico, P. (2023). Systematic review of literature on speech intelligibility and classroom acoustics in elementary schools. *Language, Speech, and Hearing Services in Schools, 54*, 322–335.

National Organization for Rare Disorders. (2018, February 14). *Angelman syndrome*. Retrieved June 10, 2022, from https://rarediseases.org/rare-diseases/angelman-syndrome

Nippold, M. A. (2021). *Language sampling with children and adolescents: Implications for intervention* (3rd ed.). Plural Publishing.

Orellana, C. I., Wada, R., & Gillam, R. B. (2019). The use of dynamic assessment for the diagnosis of language disorders in bilingual children: A meta-analysis. *American Journal of Speech-Language Pathology, 28*(3) 1298-1317.

Paradis, J., & Crago, M. (2000). Tense and temporality: Similarities and differences between language-impaired and second-language children. *Journal of Speech, Language, and Hearing Research, 43*(4), 834–848.

Paradis, J., & Crago, M. (2004). Comparing L2 and SLI grammars in child French. In P. Prevost & J. Paradis (Eds.), *The acquisition of French in different contexts: Focus on functional categories* (pp. 89–107). Benjamins.

Paradis, J., Genesee, F., & Crago, M. (2011). *Dual language development and disorders: A handbook on bilingualism & second language learning* (2nd ed.). Brookes.

Pearson, E., Wilde, L., Heald, M., Royston, R., & Oliver, C. (2019). Communication in Angelman syndrome: A scoping review. *Developmental Medicine & Child Neurology, 61*(11), 1266–1274.

Peña, E. D., Bedore, L. M., Lugo-Neris, M. J., & Albudoor, N. (2020). Identifying developmental language disorder in school-age bilinguals: Semantics, grammar, and narratives. *Language Assessment Quarterly, 17*(5), 541–558.

Peña, E. D., Gillam, R. B., & Bedore, L. M. (2014). Dynamic assessment of narrative ability in English accurately identifies language impairment in English language learners. *Journal of Speech, Language, and Hearing Research, 57*(6), 2208–2220.

Petersen, D. B., Chanthongthip, H., Ukrainetz, T. A., Spencer, T. D., & Steeve, R. W. (2017). Dynamic assessment of narratives: Efficient, accurate identification of language impairment in bilingual students. *Journal of Speech, Language, and Hearing Research, 60*(4), 983–998.

Petersen, D.B., Tonn, P., Spencer, T.D., & Foster, M.E. (2020). The classification accuracy of a dynamic assessment of inferential word learning for bilingual English/Spanish-speaking school-age children. *Language, Speech and Hearing Services in Schools, 51*(1), 144-164.

Pinborough-Zimmerman, J., Satterfield, R., Miller, J., Bilder, D., Hossain, S., & McMahon, W. (2007). Communication disorders: Prevalence and comorbid intellectual disability, autism, and emotional/behavioral disorders. *American Journal of Speech-Language Pathology, 16*, 359–367.

Prelock, P. A., Miller, B. L., & Reed, N. L. (1993). *Working with the classroom curriculum: A guide for analysis & use in speech therapy.* Communication Skill Builders.

Prodi, N., Visentin, C., Peretti, A., Griguolo, J., & Bartolucci, G. B. (2019). Investigating listening effort in classrooms for 5- to 7-year-old children. *Language, Speech, and Hearing Services in Schools, 50*(2), 196–210.

Reed, V. A. (2012). *An introduction to children with language disorders* (4th ed.). Allyn & Bacon.

Reilly, S., McKean, C., Morgan, A., & Wake, M. (2015). Identifying and managing common childhood language and speech impairments. *British Medical Journal, 350*, Article h2318.

Rescorla, L. (1989). The Language Development Survey: A screening tool for delayed language in toddlers. *Journal of Speech and Hearing Disorders, 54*(4), 587–599.

Rescorla, L., & Alley, A. (2001). Validation of the Language Development Survey (LDS): A parent report tool for identifying language delay in toddlers. *Journal of Speech, Language, and Hearing Research, 44*(2), 434–445. https://doi.org/10.1044/1092-4388(2001/035)

Rice, M. L. (2013). Language growth and genetics of specific language impairment. *International Journal of Speech-Language Pathology, 15*(3), 223–233.

Roman-Urrestarazu, A., van Kessel, R., Allison, C., Matthews, F. E., Brayne, C., & Baron-Cohen, S. (2021). Association of race/ethnicity and social disadvantage with autism prevalence in 7 million school children in England. *JAMA Pediatrics, 175*(6), Article e210054.

Rosenberg, G. G., Blake-Rahter, P., Heavner, J., Allen, L., Redmond, B. M., Phillips, J., & Stigers, K. (1999). Improving classroom acoustics (ICA): A three-year FM sound field classroom amplification study. *Journal of Educational Audiology, 7*, 8–28.

Roth, F., & Worthington, C. K. (2015). *Treatment resource manual for speech-language pathology.* Delmar Cengage.

Rudner, M., Lyberg-Åhlander, V., Brännström, J., Nirme, J., Pichora-Fuller, M. K., & Sahlén, B. (2018). Listening comprehension and listening effort in the primary school classroom. *Frontiers in Psychology, 9*, Article 1193.

Schmitt, M. B., Tambyraja, S., & Siddiqui, S. (2022). Peer effects in language therapy for preschoolers with developmental language disorder: A pilot study. *American Journal of Speech-Language Pathology, 31,* 1854–1867.

Senter, R., Chow, J. C., & Willis, E. C. (2023). Speech-language pathology interventions for children with executive function deficits: A systematic literature review. *Language, Speech, and Hearing Services in Schools, 54,* 336–354.

Shield, B., Conetta, R., Dockrell, J., Connolly, D., Cox, T., & Mydlarz, C. (2015). A survey of acoustic conditions and noise levels in secondary school classrooms in England. *Journal of the Acoustical Society of America, 137*(1), 177–188.

Shipley-Benamou, R., Lutzker, J. R., & Taubman, M. (2002). Teaching daily living skills to children with autism through instructional video modeling. *Journal of Positive Behavioral Interventions, 4*(3), 166–177.

Spencer, S., Clegg, J., Stackhouse, J., & Rush, R. (2017). Contribution of spoken language and socioeconomic background to adolescents' educational achievement at age 16 years. *International Journal of Language & Communication Disorders, 52*(2), 184–196.

Spicer-Cain, H., Camilleri, B., Hasson, N., & Botting, N. (2023). Early identification of children at risk for communication disorders: Introducing a novel battery of dynamic assessments for infants. *American Journal of Speech-Language Pathology, 32,* 523–544.

ter Wal, N., van Ewijk, L., Dijkhuis, L., Visser-Meily, J. M. A., Terwee, C. B., & Gerrits, E. (2023). Everyday barriers in communicative participation according to people with communication problems. *Journal of Speech, Language, and Hearing Research, 66,* 1033–1050.

Tomblin, J. B., Records, N. L., Buckwalter, P., Zhang, X., Smith, E., & O'Brien, M. (1997). Prevalence of specific language impairment in kindergarten children. *Journal of Speech, Language, and Hearing Research, 40*(6), 1245–1260.

Vega-Rodríguez, Y. E., Garayzabal-Heinze, E., & Moraleda-Sepúlveda, E. (2020). Language development disorder in fetal alcohol spectrum disorders (FASD): A case study. *Languages, 5*(4), Article 37.

Wadman, R., Durkin, K., & Conti-Ramsden, G. (2011). Close relationships in adolescents with and without a history of specific language impairment. *Language, Speech, and Hearing Services in Schools, 42*(1), 41–51.

Wallace, I., Berkman, N., Watson, L., Coyne-Beasley, T., Wood, C., Cullen, K., & Lohr, K. (2015). Screening for speech and language delay in children 5 years old and younger: A systematic review. *Pediatrics, 136*(2), e448–e462.

Wallace, S. J., Worrall, L., Rose, T., le Dorze, G., Cruice, M., Isaksen, J., . . . Gauvreau, C. A. (2017). Which outcomes are most important to people with aphasia and their families? An international nominal group technique study framed within the ICF. *Disability and Rehabilitation, 39*(14), 1364–1379.

Westby, C., Burda, A., & Mehta, Z. (2003). Asking the right questions the right way. *The ASHA Leader, 8*(8). https://doi.org/10.1044/leader.FTR3.08082003.4

Wiig, E. H., Secord, W. A., & Semel, E. (2020). *Clinical Evaluation of Language Fundamentals–Preschool–Third Edition.* Pearson.

Wiig, E. H., Semel, E., & Secord, W. A. (2013). *Clinical Evaluation of Language Fundamentals–Fifth Edition.* Pearson.

World Health Organization. (2001). *International classification of functioning, disability and health.*

Chapter 8

Specific Learning Disorders and Literacy Impairments

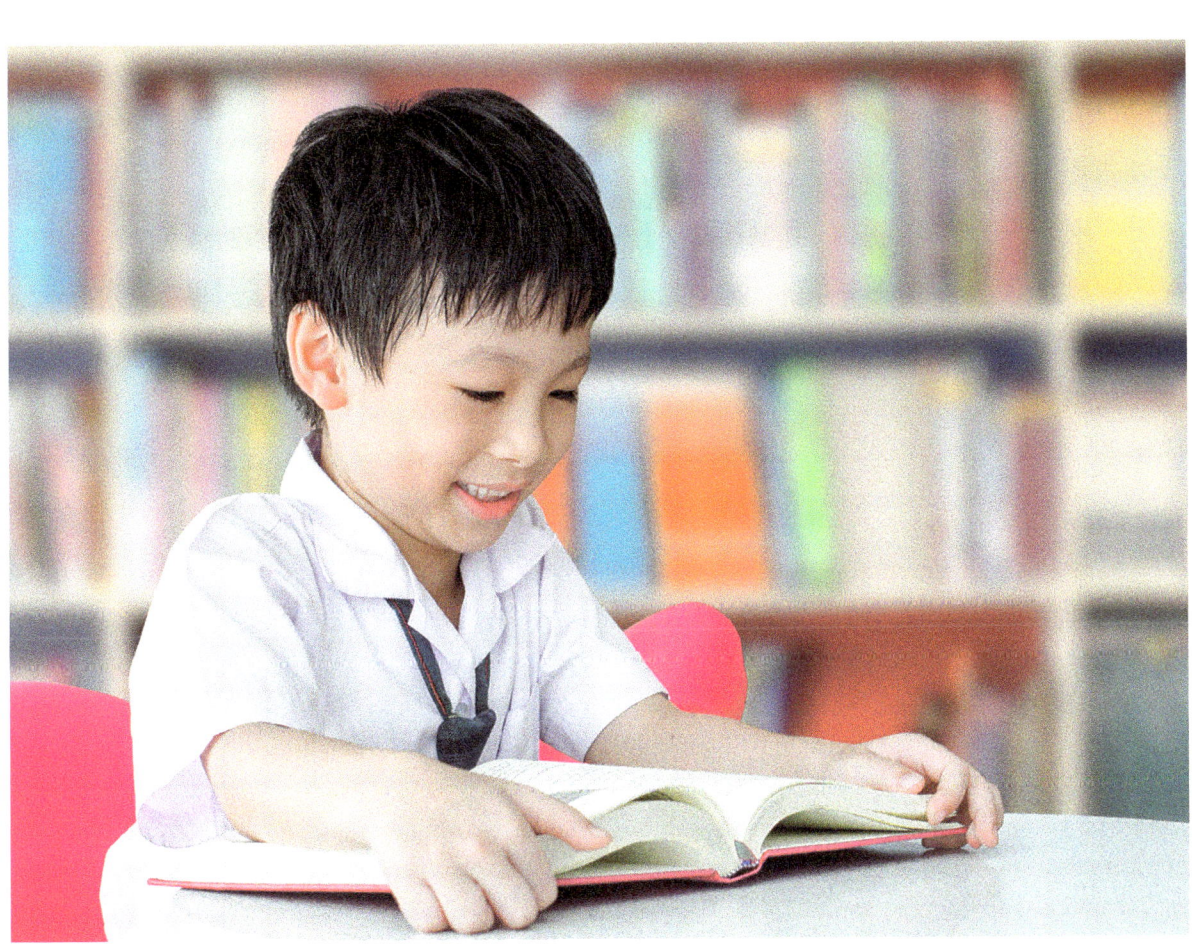

Learning Objectives

After reading this chapter, you will be able to:

- Describe the language associated with challenges in reading, reading comprehension, and writing.
- Explain the social–cultural differences in identification of learning disorders in academic areas.
- Define some of the assessment and intervention approaches that are used to support those with learning disorders.
- Identify the disparities in access to assessment and intervention for language-based literacy impairments.

Key Terms

dyscalculia	parietal–temporal
dysgraphia	phonemic awareness
dyslexia	phonics
executive functions	phonological awareness
gestalt	pragmatic difficulties
gestalt imagery	print awareness
graphic organizers	reading comprehension
learning disability	reading fluency
letter identification	semantic clustering
metacognitive skills	serial clustering
morphology	thinking maps
occipital–temporal	vocabulary development

Introduction

Do you know what Jennifer Aniston, Tom Cruise, Albert Einstein, Whoopi Goldberg, Magic Johnson, Keira Knightley, Steven Spielberg, and Tim Tebow have in common? They have all been diagnosed with a reading disorder, often described as **dyslexia**, which made school particularly difficult for them. Yet, each of them persisted, built on their strengths, and worked to overcome their learning disorder to accomplish great things.

Have you ever had difficulty sounding out words that you are unfamiliar with, seeing letters or numbers backwards, or having difficulty remembering math facts? These are just some of the difficulties that children with specific learning disorders might experience in the way they learn. These learning differences might also lead to difficulties making social connections and managing behavior as frustrations with learning become more evident. In addition, specific learning disorders are often accompanied by language challenges and can impact the individual's learning experience across the lifespan (Prelock & Hutchins, 2018; Sun & Wallach, 2014).

This chapter will provide you with an understanding of what specific learning disorders are, as described in the fifth edition, text revision, of the *Diagnostic and Statistical Manual of Mental Disorders* (*DSM-5-TR*; American Psychiatric Association [APA], 2022), and the literacy challenges this population often experiences. General approaches to assessment and intervention are presented, and two case studies are offered to help you apply your learning.

What Is a Specific Learning Disorder?

A specific learning disorder (also known as learning disorder) is a neurodevelopmental disorder that has a biological basis. When children work hard academically but still struggle in one or more areas of learning, even when intelligence is intact and motivation is not impacted, they likely have a learning disorder (Centers for Disease Control and Prevention [CDC], 2011a).

An individual with a learning disorder has continuous problems with academic skill development, with performance well below what is expected for their age along with behavior that is often typical of younger children (APA, 2022). Six key symptoms characterize a specific learning disorder, and an individual must have persistent demonstration of at least one of the symptoms for 6 months or more despite intervention. These symptoms include having difficulty with (APA, 2022):

- Reading words (e.g., inaccurate word recognition; difficulty decoding or sounding out words; slow, effortful oral reading)
- Reading comprehension (e.g., difficulty making inferences, misunderstanding of character relationships, missing the deeper meaning of what is read)
- Spelling words (e.g., deletes, adds, or substitutes sounds in words)
- Writing (e.g., syntax and punctuation errors, poor organization, ideas are unclear)
- Numerical understanding and math calculation (e.g., weak number understanding, difficulty retrieving math facts, lacking computational skills)
- Math reasoning (e.g., difficulty with mathematical problem-solving)

Previously, specific learning disorders were associated with the term **learning disability**, indicating an individual exhibited a difference in their learning capacity compared to their actual academic achievement, suggesting some underlying neurological differences (Prelock, 2013). Children with a learning disorder have unique educational needs because of the differences in their approach to learning. Often, their learning disorder has a language basis and may be referred to as a language-based learning disability (Sun & Wallach, 2014).

Diagnosis of a learning disorder can have a significant impact on a child's family because there is an ongoing need to manage the child's difficulties across the lifespan. Many disciplines, including primary care and pediatric practitioners, general and special educators, and speech-language pathologists (SLPs), have a critical role in supporting individuals with learning disorders and their families (Prelock & Hutchins, 2018). Children with learning disorders often feel frustrated if they cannot accomplish a task even though they are trying hard to do so. This may lead to acting out behaviorally or withdrawing (CDC, 2011a). Appropriate diagnosis is critical so that support and individualized intervention can begin.

What We Know About This Topic

Individuals who have a learning disorder demonstrate academic skills much lower than would be expected based on their age and overall cognitive ability. The observed learning differences become most evident for the school-age child as the expectations and demands for reading, writing, and math increase. A specific learning disorder is determined following a comprehensive evaluation that includes standardized assessment tools examining a child's academic skills, intellectual ability, and language performance. To be diagnosed with a specific learning disorder, the condition cannot be better explained by an intellectual disability, uncorrected hearing, visual impairment, another mental or neurobiological disorder, or lack of adequate language and/or academic instruction. Table 8–1 displays the likely areas of academic difficulty and subskills that may be impaired in an individual with a specific learning disorder. Generally, impairments are characterized as reading difficulties in accuracy, fluency, and comprehension; written expression challenges in spelling, grammar, and punctuation; and problems in math related to understanding numbers, knowing math facts, and demonstrating an ability to calculate accurately and engage in numerical reasoning (APA, 2022). The *DSM-5-TR* also describes levels of severity for specific learning disorders. These levels are presented in Table 8–2.

You might also hear the term **dyslexia** to describe the reading challenges of some children. Dyslexia is used to describe difficulty decoding and spelling words, and those with dyslexia are often inaccurate in the recognition of words when reading. Their decoding difficulties impact their fluency when reading aloud. They may also have difficulties with understanding what they are reading or demonstrating an ability to reason when figuring out math word problems.

TABLE 8–1. Areas of Impairment and Subskills Impacted in Individuals With Learning Disorders

Primary Area of Impairment	Subskills That Could Be Impacted
Reading	• Recognizing letters and words • Breaking up words into sounds (i.e., phonemic awareness or phonological awareness) • Comprehending what is being read • Reading at a fluent and expected rate • Developing vocabulary skills
Writing	• Handwriting • Spelling • Organizing ideas • Composing ideas
Mathematics	• Understanding math concepts (e.g., quantity, place value, and time) • Remembering math facts • Organizing numbers to complete math problems

TABLE 8–2. Severity Levels for Specific Learning Disorders

Severity Level	Description
Mild	• Difficulties in one or two academic areas. • With accommodations and supports, the student performs well in school.
Moderate	• More significant difficulties in one or more academic areas. • Intensive teaching is needed in the affected academic areas and accommodations used to ensure work is accurate and complete.
Severe	• Significant difficulties in multiple academic areas. • Student requires ongoing intensive teaching and a range of accommodations to complete work.

Source: Adapted from APA (2022).

Another term you might hear is **dyscalculia**. This term is used to describe difficulties with understanding numbers including math facts, completing math calculations, and processing numerical information. A person with dyscalculia might also have problems with math reasoning. You might also hear the term **dysgraphia**, which describes difficulties with writing.

Interestingly, reading and spelling challenges appear to differ in their association with math difficulties. For example, students exhibiting math difficulties also tend to have more difficulties with spelling than reading (Moll et al., 2014). It seems likely that the processes underlying math and reading are different than those for math and spelling. Notably, boys tend to have more difficulties with spelling, whereas girls have greater challenges in math; there does not appear to be a gender difference for reading problems (Moll et al., 2014).

Incidence and Prevalence of Learning Disorders

Approximately 15% of Americans have some type of learning disability or learning disorder (CDC, 2011a). The APA (2022) suggests a school age prevalence of 5% to 15% in the United States, Brazil, and Northern Ireland. The presence of learning disability in the adult population is unclear. Onset usually occurs in young elementary children when they experience the first expectations for reading, writing, and math. Prevalence varies for different cultural groups, with non-Hispanic White children (16%) and non-Hispanic Black children (13%) being more likely to be diagnosed with a learning disorder than Hispanic children (9%) for families with income less than 100% of poverty level (CDC, 2011a, 2011b). Interestingly, diagnosis of a learning disorder appears to decrease as the income of families increases (Prelock & Hutchins, 2018).

More than 13% of school-age children receive special education services (approximately 6.5 million children), and 35% of those children are diagnosed with learning disorders (National Center for Education Statistics, 2019); reading is often the primary area of academic difficulty (National Center for Education Statistics, n.d.; U.S. Department of Education, 2015). Notably, boys receive proportionally more special education services than girls (Bandian, 1999; Coutinho & Oswald, 2005). Similar prevalence statistics are found for learning disorders in other countries. For example, researchers report a prevalence rate of 13.6% for primary school–age children in Turkey, with a greater prevalence reported for boys (17%)

than girls (10.4%), although the occurrence of specific types of learning disorders varied from the North American population, with writing and math impairments more common than reading impairments (Gorker et al., 2017).

Learning disorders occur across cultures and socioeconomic levels, although characteristics may vary depending on the symbols systems (e.g., signs, drawings) for reading and writing in a particular culture. Importantly, however, speaking a language at home that differs in sound and linguistic structure from what children are hearing and speaking in academic settings does not suggest increased risk for a specific learning disability (APA, 2022).

Signs of Learning Disorders

Several signs and symptoms may indicate that a child has a learning disorder. You might notice the child having difficulty determining right from left or reversing letters or numbers. Recognizing size and shape patterns and understanding time concepts might be problematic early on for some children. Others will have difficulty remembering what was said or read and staying organized to complete tasks. Even doing tasks requiring eye–hand coordination, such as cutting, drawing, and writing, may present as difficult.

Understanding the expected developmental milestones for toddlers and preschoolers and knowing when a child lags in their development are important because early delays may be a sign of a later learning disorder (Prelock, 2013). As a heterogeneous group with deficits in both academic and linguistic domains, several factors influence the diagnosis. There could be neurobiological or genetic factors, environmental conditions such as socioeconomic status and parental educational level, and/or cognitive and psychosocial factors such as level of attention and motivation (Prelock & Hutchins, 2018). Table 8–3 summarizes some signs that may suggest a learning disability in preschool children, early and later school-age children, and adolescents.

TABLE 8–3. Signs That Suggest a Learning Disorder in Preschool and School-Age Children and Adolescents

Preschool Children	Elementary School Children	Later Elementary School Children	Adolescents
Delays in speech and language	Difficulty connecting sounds to letters	Persistent letter sequence reversals	Slow, effortful reading
Little interest in sound games like rhyming	Concept knowledge difficulty	Difficulty understanding prefixes, suffixes, root words	Poor written expression
Problems following directions	Errors in spelling and reading	Handwriting challenges	Inaccurate spelling
Limited vocabulary development	Number and letter reversals	Avoidance of reading aloud	Ongoing comprehension difficulties
Trouble learning letters and numbers	Problems telling time	Limited recall affecting comprehension and following instructions	Continued difficulty with math facts and math problem-solving
Difficulty relating to peers	Challenges learning math facts	Difficulty making friends	Avoidance of reading and writing activities
Fine motor delays	Poor coordination		

Source: Adapted from Prelock and Hutchins (2018).

Causes of Learning Disorders

It is unclear what causes learning disorders, but they do appear to run in families and occur slightly more frequently in males than females (APA, 2022). Other identified causal factors include pregnancy difficulties, problems at birth or following birth, anomalies in brain development, and toxin exposure (Prelock & Hutchins, 2018).

Co-Occurring Disorders

Learning disorders may co-occur with other neurodevelopmental disorders such as attention-deficit/hyperactivity disorder (ADHD), communication disorders, anxiety disorders, and behavioral difficulties. In addition, there are certain disorders that might be confused with learning disorders. Individuals with an intelligence quotient (IQ) below 70 are diagnosed with an intellectual disability and not a learning disorder, although learning would likely be compromised because of the individual's cognitive impairment (Prelock & Hutchins, 2018).

Communication difficulties might be characteristic of students with learning disorders because these children often have receptive and expressive language difficulties that impact their ability to understand what they hear in the classroom and their ability to formulate thoughts and ideas required for oral and written assignments. In addition, the student may experience **pragmatic difficulties** that impact how they use language in social situations. ADHD often co-occurs with learning disorders, adding to students' struggles when required to focus on relevant academic information. In fact, ADHD and learning disorders are the most frequently diagnosed conditions in children (Mayes et al., 2000; Zablotsky et al., 2019), although the prevalence of their co-existence differs by race and ethnicity (Morgan et al., 2013, 2015). Between 2016 and 2018, almost 14% of 3- to 17-year-olds were reported to have ADHD or a learning disorder; diagnosis differed for all races and ethnicities by poverty level (Zablotsky, 2019). Notably, learning disorders, communication disorders, and ADHD often share difficulties in working memory, planning, and attention shifting (known as **executive functions**), making differential diagnosis particularly challenging, although not all communication disorders have impaired executive function.

Importantly, many students with learning disorders have underlying challenges in language (Wallach, 2005), such that they have trouble finding the right words to express their ideas, comprehending spoken and written language, selecting appropriate vocabulary, organizing and planning their ideas, and using appropriate grammar (Prelock & Hutchins, 2018). Because language is a critical component of academic tasks, a comprehensive language assessment should be completed for all students with a diagnosed learning disorder.

Reading Disorders

As interest and awareness of literacy emerge, children begin to understand that the world is made up of print. They then develop **phonological awareness** and alphabetic understanding or **letter identification**. Reading, on the other hand, is described as the way in which an individual creates meaning from printed symbols, and it includes the ability to decode words and comprehend the written word.

Children are exposed through auditory or written means to more than 1,000 words each hour within the school day. Many of those words are commonly occurring words in the English language. Interestingly, however, most of those are not academic or curriculum vocabulary, although instances of these words are variable (Wanzek et al., 2023). In addition, the frequency of academic words that teachers use predicts children's vocabulary at the end of the school year (Wanzek et al., 2023). Research also suggests that fifth-grade students who complete 10 minutes of independent reading a day read 622,000 more words each year than students who do not do independent reading (Blachowicz & Fisher, 2004).

Experienced readers exhibit integration of several brain areas in the left hemisphere. The **parietal–temporal** area facilitates word analysis and the sounding out of words, whereas the **occipital–temporal** area stores the recognition and meaning of words that support reading fluency (N. Hudson et al., 2016; R. Hudson et al., 2007). Figure 8–1 displays the areas of the brain that are important for reading. There appears to be a glitch, however, in the neural circuitry of individuals who struggle with reading (S. Shaywitz & Shaywitz, 2004). The parietal–temporal and occipital–temporal areas are underactivated in children with dyslexia, affecting their word analysis and reading fluency (B. Shaywitz et al., 2002). Reading skill was noted with greater activation in the left occipital–temporal area.

Children with a history of language impairment are at high risk for reading difficulties because reading is a language-based skill (Catts et al., 2001). Phonological awareness predicts reading achievement in first and second graders who have a language or articulation impairment in kindergarten. Fifty-six percent of poor readers in second grade had deficits in phonological awareness in kindergarten and 45% had difficulty on a rapid naming task; 57% also had receptive language challenges and 50% had expressive language challenges in kindergarten (Catts et al., 2001). Reading outcomes for children with language impairment are concerning because they perform more poorly on word recognition and reading comprehension tasks in second and fourth grade (Catts et al., 2002).

Sixty-five percent of fourth graders read below what is expected for their age, and those reading below expected levels are likely to experience limited progress in reading compared to children who perform at or above grade level (National Center for Education Statistics, 2019; O'Fallon et al., 2022).

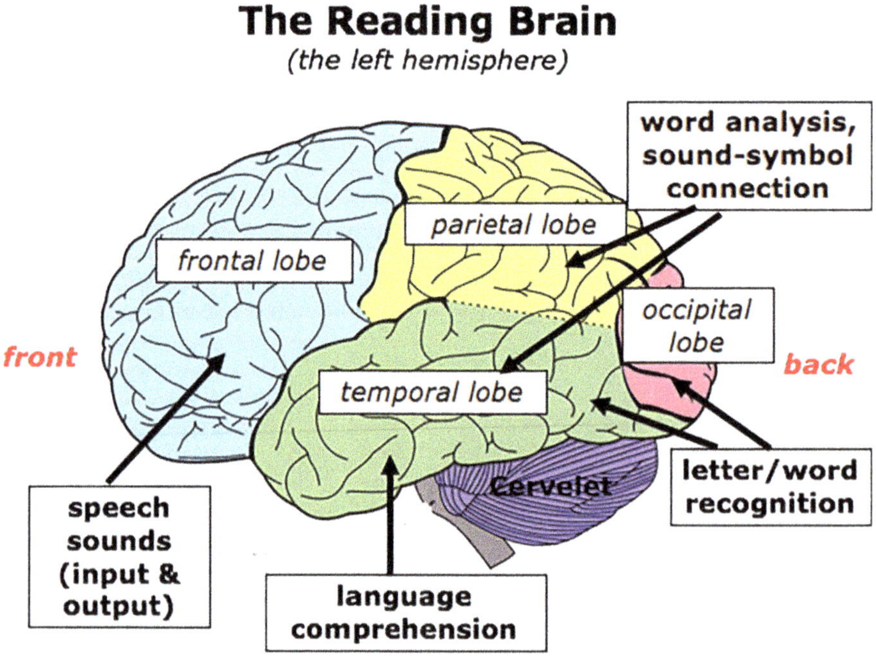

FIGURE 8–1. Areas of the brain affecting reading. *Source:* Keys to Literacy.

Early reading difficulties also lead to greater developmental challenges and impact language development and academic performance (Duff et al., 2015; Mol & Bus, 2011). It is also known that children's early literacy development is influenced by literacy opportunities in the home and how parents perceive the importance of reading interactions with their children (Bingham, 2007). Overall, research suggests that the more understanding a parent has about the value of reading, the greater the chance they will engage in quality literacy interactions with their child. The child's attitude toward reading is also an influencing factor for reading success. Furthermore, the literature indicates that parents spending time reading to their children is related to children's literacy outcomes (Logan et al., 2020).

Cultural Considerations in Reading Disorders

Considering the cultural and linguistic aspects of reading, reading failure appears to be the greatest for children in disadvantaged environments (Lyon & Chhabra, 2004). Preschool children from low-income families have greater difficulty manipulating sound structure along with limited growth in their phoneme knowledge and vocabulary than preschoolers from middle- and high-income families. It has also been suggested that children from families of lower socioeconomic status have significantly fewer experiences of listening and speaking to their parents than those with families from higher socioeconomic statuses (Lyon & Chhabra, 2004). Children who are culturally and linguistically diverse also demonstrate vocabulary skills below what is expected for their age (Crowley & Valenti, 2002). This might occur for several reasons. Students may live in families that provide many quality words with varied meanings, but those words may not be like terms used to assess a child or support their access to their educational curriculum (Crowley & Valenti, 2002). Other children may lose some words in their first language as they are trying to incorporate new vocabulary relevant to their academic curriculum in English, and still others may have a language disorder.

Written Language Disorders

Written language involves the ability to plan, write, and review content at the word, sentence, and discourse level (Koutsoftas, 2023). Children must learn handwriting and spelling skills as well as ways to translate their thoughts and ideas into sentences. A review of the literature on writing and spelling difficulties suggests a delay in transcription and translation abilities for children with language learning disorders compared to their age-matched peers (Williams & Larkin, 2023) and overall deficits in writing and spelling (Koutsoftas & Srivastava, 2020; Williams et al., 2021). Writing errors in children with language disorders are characterized by regular and irregular past tense errors, as well as errors in syntax for simple or complex sentences (Brimo et al., 2023). Compared to typically developing children, children with language learning disorders use fewer words and sentences and produce more errors in their written language samples (Scott & Windsor, 2000). Furthermore, students who have difficulty writing longer texts usually have weaker sentence-level skills (Arfe et al., 2016), although there is not a clear developmental pattern for writing various sentence types (Ritchey et al., 2023). Challenges in sentence-level writing occur across cultures for students with learning disorders (Arfe & Pizzocara, 2016).

The literature suggests that the complexity of syntax or grammar is an important consideration in students' ability to be proficient writers and that proficient writers usually produce more complex sentences than less proficient writers (Jagaiah et al., 2020). Writing also places significant cognitive demands on the learner because they must understand the genre in which they are writing and the structure used to communicate their thoughts while also considering word selection and sentence-level grammatical development (Hall-Mills & Wood, 2023).

Specific problem areas will affect a student's writing competency, from weak concept knowledge and limited vocabulary to significant errors in sentence structure and morphological endings. Writing competency is also impacted by a failure to monitor performance, which leads to reduced editing skills. Students who present with difficulty organizing their ideas to fit a particular writing structure or schema will have problems with appropriate word selection to express their ideas. In addition, challenges with pragmatic skills could lead to written language deficits, such as writing that incorporates irrelevant and off-topic ideas as well as writing that fails to consider the point of view or perspective of the reader. Struggling writers spend less time planning, make fewer revisions to their writing samples, and appear to be less aware of effective strategies for writing compared to their peers who do not struggle with writing (Graham & Harris, 2005).

Writing skills in more culturally and linguistically diverse populations are less well studied. We do know that English language learners with language difficulties are more likely to struggle in their narrative writing samples as well as expository samples, producing simpler syntactic structures (Silverman et al., 2015).

Math Disorders

Some researchers estimate that approximately 25% to 35% of school-age students have difficulties in math knowledge and application, making classroom performance challenging (Mazzocco, 2007). In fact, approximately 5% to 8% of all students have significant difficulties that require special education services to help them with both computational math and application in math word problems (Geary, 2004). Considering brain–behavior connections related to math, the parietal, occipital, and temporal lobes and the cerebellum are all involved in different math functions, including number recognition, calculation, and understanding word problems. Without intensive instruction, students with learning disorders in math will fall behind their peers (Jitendra et al., 2013; Sayeski & Paulsen, 2010). The language of math (e.g., quantitative concepts, word problems) is an important area for SLPs to understand and support.

Nonverbal Learning Disability

You may hear the term nonverbal learning disability (NVLD) to describe children who have challenges academically as well as managing social expectations in an educational setting. Although not part of the learning disorders described in the *DSM-5-TR*, children with an NVLD have difficulty processing nonverbal information and particularly social information, with additional problems in reasoning, visual discrimination and visual–spatial organization, math calculation, and reading comprehension (Prelock & Hutchins, 2018; Rourke et al., 2002; Rourke & Tsatsanis, 1996). They have relative strengths in processing information auditorily as well as in verbal memory, understanding language, and decoding and spelling words. Often, children exhibiting an NVLD will struggle initiating and maintaining peer connections because of their social interaction difficulties and their difficulty recognizing emotions and demonstrating appropriate social judgment (Volden, 2004).

Three primary areas have been identified in the literature to describe an NVLD that could serve as criteria for making a diagnosis. The first area is a deficit in visual–spatial abilities in which performance is at or below the 16th percentile or a significant difference exists in verbal versus spatial abilities with basic reading abilities above the 16th percentile (Margolis et al., 2020). The second area represents performance at or below the 16th percentile in at least two of the following four areas: social skills, math calculation, motor skills, and visual executive functioning (Margolis et al., 2020). The final area is the lack of features representing autism (e.g., restricted, repetitive patterns of behavior).

It is important to identify students who meet the criteria for NVLD so that intervention can be initiated, because such a diagnosis may have a crucial impact on the individual's mental health (Margolis et al., 2020). Frequently, those meeting the criteria for NVLD often have co-occurring diagnoses of ADHD and anxiety disorder (Davis & Broitman, 2011). A differentiating factor for NVLD is the spatial deficits that characterize the disorder (Banker et al., 2020). The prevalence of NVLD was reported to be 3% or 4% in a cross-sectional study of nearly 2,600 children and adolescents, suggesting that between 2 and 3 million children and adolescents have NVLD in North America (Margolis et al., 2020).

Table 8–4 highlights the neuropsychological assets and challenges frequently observed in individuals with NVLD. Their academic patterns align with these neuropsychological strengths and challenges in that they exhibit relative strengths in reading decoding, spelling, and graphomotor output and challenges in reading comprehension, mechanical math, and integration of information and problem-solving. Individuals with NVLD also have some unique social–emotion patterns, including difficulty adapting to new situations, managing transitions, and using good social judgment in their interactions (Volden, 2004). Notably, this population is at risk for emotional difficulties and especially internalizing problems such

TABLE 8–4. Neuropsychological Assets and Challenges Frequently Observed in Individuals With Nonverbal Learning Disabilities

Neuropsychological Assets	Neuropsychological Challenges
• Intact repetitive motor skills	• Bilateral tactile–perceptual and psychomotor deficits
• Responsive to learning through repetition and the auditory modality	• Impaired visual discrimination
• Well-developed auditory perceptual skills	• Impaired visual–spatial organization (e.g., drawing patterns from memory)
• Well-developed rote verbal and verbal memory skills	• Difficulty with novel and complex situations
• Ability to sustain attention to simple, repetitive verbal information	• Difficulties in nonverbal problem-solving concept formation, hypothesis testing, and use of feedback
• Strong receptive language skills, including rote verbal memory and verbal associations	• Difficulty with cause–effect and recognizing incongruities
• Advanced phonemic awareness, including blending and segmentation	• Verbose with poor pragmatics (i.e., miss social cues), including inefficient prosody and overreliance on language for relating socially and decreasing anxiety
• Average single-word reading and spelling skills	• Challenges in math (i.e., functions, decimals, percentages, ratios, estimation; geometry, and any visual–spatial math function)
	• Impairments in social perception, judgment, and interaction skills, including tendency to withdraw
	• Increased risk for suicide

Source: Adapted from Rourke et al. (2002).

as depression, withdrawal, and suicide ideation (Volden, 2004). Interestingly, there are also problems with immediate memory for faces; that is, individuals with NVLD take longer to encode a face, but once the encoding is successful, there is less difficulty with facial recognition (Liddell & Rasmussen, 2005). Furthermore, some research suggests that mothers of children with NVLD display higher levels of difficult interactions (e.g., engaging with their child, managing their social behaviors), and the more severe a child's NVLD is, the greater the parental stress; therefore, social skills training is often recommended to increase positive peer interactions and decrease maternal stress (Antshel & Joseph, 2006). Of interest as well is that children with NVLD rely more on **serial clustering** (recalling items in the order in which they are presented) rather than **semantic clustering** (grouping items into semantic categories such as food, clothing, etc.), leading to stronger rote memory skills than active processing and categorization skills (Volden, 2004).

What Do We Do to Address This Communication Challenge?

Assessment

Early identification of learning disorders is important so that modification of instruction and intervention can be initiated (Padhy et al., 2016). Diagnosis, however, is challenging because it requires not only accurate testing but also comprehensive data collection through a variety of sources, including history-taking, standardized testing, and observation of performance inside the classroom and with peers. Several professionals are involved in the evaluation process, and they must coordinate their efforts to obtain an accurate diagnosis with input from teachers, parents, and the students. Primary care providers often make referrals for a comprehensive learning assessment, which typically includes language, cognitive, neuropsychological, and educational batteries. SLPs complete a comprehensive speech and language assessment as well as a written language assessment to determine the level of language impairment that may be involved in a child with a suspected learning disorder. Psychologists complete a comprehensive cognitive battery and may also perform neuropsychological testing. Special educators complete a comprehensive educational battery in collaboration with the SLP and the psychologist.

Historically, two approaches have been used to identify learning disorder: the IQ-achievement discrepancy approach and the response to intervention approach. Originally, the IQ-achievement discrepancy approach was used to make a diagnosis in which a student would receive intelligence and academic achievement testing. The assessment team would also consider the student's classroom performance and interaction with peers. Speech and language testing and an assessment of attention may or may not have occurred. The results of the assessment determined if the student's academic performance was aligned with their cognitive ability. If a student's cognitive ability (IQ) was above their academic achievement (how they were performing at school), a diagnosis of a learning disorder was made. This approach is called **cognitive referencing**. Cognitive referencing suggests the presence of a learning disorder primarily through a discrepancy between general aptitude as measured by an IQ test and academic achievement (Troia, 2005).

There were problems with this approach, however, in that there is limited evidence that an IQ-achievement discrepancy truly indicates a learning disorder (Barnes et al., 2007; Harrison & Flanagan, 2005).

Furthermore, children should receive services if they need them, and this need can be determined by whether their language skills help them thrive personally, socially, academically, and vocationally (Ehren & Nelson, 2005). Thus, a discrepancy between intelligence and achievement is no longer required to make a diagnosis of a learning disorder (Individuals With Disabilities Education Improvement Act of 2004).

In the response to intervention (RTI) approach, the assessment process is more intervention focused. Students are screened, and those having difficulty receive evidence-based instruction before a diagnosis is made (Prelock & Hutchins, 2018). Progress monitoring is initiated to determine if providing intensive intervention facilitates a student's achievement gains. Students who respond to this intensive evidence-based instruction will not require further intervention or diagnosis, whereas those who do not respond are referred to special education (Prelock & Hutchins, 2018). The advantage of this approach is access to immediate intervention when a student shows they are struggling. The 2004 reauthorization of the Individuals With Disabilities Education Act allows this approach to be used to identify students with learning disorders. Although this is the preferred method for early support, there are some limitations in that a student's individual neuropsychological profile is not considered when designing the intervention, it takes longer to implement, and it requires a strong educational environment delivered by general educators (Fletcher et al., 2007; Prelock & Hutchins, 2018).

If a referral for a comprehensive assessment to diagnose a potential learning disorder is made, several standardized measures are used to assess the student's reading fluency, decoding, and comprehension; math calculation skills and problem-solving; and written language abilities, including organization, narrative development, and spelling. Notably, a comprehensive assessment is a requirement for intervention and should also include an assessment of receptive and expressive language because language impairment often co-occurs with learning disorders.

An additional consideration for assessing written language is identifying the match or mismatch between curricular expectations for written language and the students' communication impairments. It is valuable to establish a process for data collection or ongoing evaluation such as administering periodic probes for the level of written language expected. It is also crucial to create a process for assessing and supporting note-taking. In the assessment, it is important to gather information on the student's use of words and sentence structure and determine if the student understands the underlying scripts or schemas for writing narratives, letters, biographies, book reports, poetry, and so on.

Furthermore, when evaluating written language, it is appropriate to use rubrics to assess levels of writing competencies identified for specific grade levels. You want to analyze adequacy of the length of the written sample, the lexical diversity, and grammatical complexity, as well as any grammatical errors (Scott & Windsor, 2000). Teachers often consider multiple ways to gather a portfolio of written language samples so there is evidence of opportunities for developing, revising, and editing. The data collected during the written language assessment then help guide goal development and an intervention plan for the student.

There are also some specific considerations for the assessment of children with NVLD. These students should have a comprehensive neuropsychological and social–emotional evaluation as well as an academic evaluation. For this reason, assessment is best completed by an interdisciplinary team, including an occupational therapist, SLP, psychologist, developmental pediatrician or child psychiatrist, and general and special educators. Language assessments should examine semantic knowledge and include measures of multiple meaning words, figurative language, explaining inferences, narrative understanding, as well as pragmatic language (Volden, 2004).

Intervention

Often, children with learning disorders require additional help and specialized instruction that is offered as special education services in their school setting. Typically, school systems complete their own assessment to determine a student's intervention needs. If additional concerns exist for the child, such as emotional or behavioral problems, other health care providers may need to be part of the team to determine the most appropriate approach to a comprehensive intervention plan, including additional referrals as needed.

Early intervention leads to fewer children eventually diagnosed with a learning disorder. In fact, National Institutes of Health (NIH) research suggests that 67% of students exhibiting risk for reading disorders who receive intervention early on will achieve average or above average reading. Importantly, however, although some classroom adjustments can improve the learning environment, many of these instructional approaches may not be sufficiently responsive to students' different learning styles (Sternberg & Grigorenko, 1999, 2001).

Therefore, an integrated intervention approach is needed to identify both the strengths and challenges of children with learning disorders (Bradley et al., 2002; Fletcher et al., 2007). An integrated approach considers the RTI model to not only identify children at greater risk for learning challenges but also allow for an evaluation of instructional effectiveness and progress monitoring over time (Prelock & Hutchins, 2018). In addition, an integrated intervention approach helps determine when formal assessment across learning domains is needed (Bradley et al., 2002).

Intervention for learning disorders requires collaboration with multiple team members with specific expertise to address the complexity of needs that a student with a learning disorder might exhibit. Most students are assigned a special education case manager who is responsible for coordinating each student's overall assessment and intervention plan. A special educator is a crucial part of the team because they have specific expertise to address the learning needs of the student with a learning disorder. For some students, a neurologist may be involved if there are questions about the neurological basis of the learning disorder. An SLP is a critical member of the team because they provide language and social communication support for the student with a learning disorder as typically there is an underlying language component to the learning disorder. A psychologist plays an important role in the student's intellectual assessment, and they might also provide guidance regarding any co-occurring behavioral or emotional difficulties.

Strategy instruction is a frequently used approach to support students with language learning disorders. This approach is composed of a series of sequenced steps and cognitive processes that foster a student's ability to complete a task (Reid & Lienemann, 2006a, 2006b). It involves a process of self-regulation in which learners manage their ability to plan a task, monitor or check comprehension, and work to detect a problem in understanding and correct it. There are six stages to a self-regulated strategy development (SRSD) model, which are explained as follows (Reid & Lienemann, 2006a, 2006b):

- Step 1: Develop and activate background knowledge—In this step, the clinician defines the skills that the student needs to perform for a learning task and assess their knowledge of or ability to perform the expected skills.
- Step 2: Discuss the strategy—In this step, the clinician helps the student believe that the strategy they are learning will improve their performance.
- Step 3: Model the strategy—In this step, the clinician models the strategy for the student. For example, if it is a "think-aloud" strategy, the clinician would model "thinking aloud" by stating why they are taking a particular action, how they know to perform that action, and what additional information they might need to complete the task.

- Step 4: Memorize the strategy—The student memorizes the steps in the strategy.
- Step 5: Support the strategy—In this step, the clinician and student practice using the strategy until the student performs the strategy independently and effectively.
- Step 6: Perform independently—In this final step, the student's performance is monitored for appropriate and consistent use.

General interventions typically used to support students with learning disorders are highlighted in Table 8–5. Effective interventions have a scientific basis, are usually intensive, and are always individualized to meet the specific needs of the student (Prelock & Hutchins, 2018). In the sections that follow, interventions that would be appropriate to support children with reading, writing, or math disorders are highlighted, as well as strategies to address the needs of children with nonverbal learning disabilities.

Boosting Language and Literacy

There are several approaches to teach reading, and certainly some methods are more effective than others. Not surprisingly, reading aloud is one of the best ways that families can prepare their child to become a successful reader (Handler & Fierson, 2011). The National Reading Panel (2000) explored the most effective approaches to teach reading and found that effective interventions require the following components: **phonemic awareness** instruction, systematic instruction in **phonics**, strategies to increase **reading fluency**, and methods to support **reading comprehension**. Types of instruction most often used to support students' reading include the following (Camilli & Wolfe, 2004):

TABLE 8–5. Descriptions of Selected Interventions for Specific Learning Disorders

Intervention	Explanation and Examples
Direct instruction	One-on-one instruction that is individually designed and presented in a structured manner and typically offered daily. Academic content is developed prior to the instruction with an effort to have children experience initial success and provide models for correct responses.
Arrangement of classroom context	The academic environment is adjusted to accommodate the needs of the students, from providing quiet study spaces to preferential seating, extended time for test-taking, or completing assignments.
Technology for learning	Increased use of audio books, voice output devices, spell-checkers, calculators, speech-to-print programs, iPads, etc.
Classroom support	Access to proofreaders, notetakers, para-educators, etc. to ensure students remain focused on their academic tasks and engage in the classroom content.
Special education support	Access to resource room supports, instruction, and case management from a special educator; the development of an Individualized Educational Plan; and access to related interventions.
Speech-language pathology support	Support for language learning in the classroom, breaking down the language of the curriculum, support for reading comprehension, facilitation of the use of language in social situations, and the development of written language.

Source: Adapted from Prelock and Hutchins (2018).

- Systematic phonics: Introduces letter–sound correspondences in a predetermined manner (compared to phonics as decoding, which involves looking at words to figure out what they mean in context).
- Differentiated instruction: Students' needs are assessed to determine the best ways to address those needs; both individual and group instructional experiences are designed to address the identified needs.
- Direct instruction: Embedding print-rich literacy experiences in short individual sessions.

Research also suggests that individual tutoring (approximately 30 minutes daily for 70–80 sessions) leads to on-level reading for approximately 50% of students who struggle (Allington, 2004). In addition, peer-mediated tutoring approaches have been used to support reading comprehension in middle school students (Calhoun, 2005).

Teaching vocabulary is an important part of facilitating reading in children. Children with reading comprehension difficulties often confuse similar-sounding words when they are learning new vocabulary (Juel & Deffres, 2004). Word knowledge means knowing how a word sounds, how it is written, how it is used, and whether it has multiple meanings. There are several approaches to vocabulary instruction; two are highlighted here (Juel & Deffres, 2004):

- Anchored word instruction: This approach links the meaning, spelling, and sounds in the word. The teacher might introduce a new word, read aloud a book that uses the new word, talk about the meaning of the word, point out pictures that illustrate the word, have the student point to the word in a book, and then have the child sound out the word.
- Analytic vocabulary instruction: This approach highlights words in the literature being read. The teacher gives clear explanations of the words and provides examples of the words' meanings in various contexts, including relating the words to the student's own experiences and discussing and comparing the words in new contexts.

Teachers can develop word awareness and a student's love of words through word play (e.g., having a word wall in the classroom on which students put new words they have read or heard in conversation or on television). It is important to deliver explicit instruction to facilitate word knowledge, and some teachers use a STAR model (Vlasákova & Manuhutu, 2018).

Select: Draw a story map and have students summarize text related to four to six target words.

Teach: Make sure students understand key words by sharing a few sentences from the text to support their understanding.

Activate: Connect new words to things the students already know or have experienced or demonstrate knowledge of words through art or role play.

Revisit: Use games, writing tasks, and word books to facilitate the review of the new words learned.

Typically, students learn to read words in four ways. First, they might engage in contextual guessing or reading most words in a text as sight words and then use the rest of the text to guess the words they do not know (Gaskins, 2004). They might also engage in letter–sound decoding, making letter–sound matches to read the word. A third way that students learn to read is by making an analogy to another known site word (Gaskins, 2004). Finally, students might engage in sight reading or reading words from memory.

Instruction focused on **morphology** or learning word parts can help students learn new words while reading and will also teach them how to use the dictionary to learn word meanings and pronunciations. Exposure to a variety of literature forms and rereading stories can also enhance and stabilize word meanings for a student. The more students know about how words are systematically structured to represent speech, the more fluent readers they become.

Check out **"NICHD Looks Back on 50 Years of Learning Disabilities Research"** on the National Institute of Child Health and Human Development website to learn more about how NIH researchers have built on the National Reading Panel's findings as well as new discoveries on how certain instruction can lead to brain changes that support reading.

There are several strategies that families can use to support their child's language and literacy awareness. Children can review menus at restaurants to increase their print knowledge, play "I spy" to find different letters in their environment, or think about words that begin with the same letter or sound of their name. Mealtime, whether at home or at a restaurant, is also an excellent time to practice back-and-forth conversation and focus on increasing word knowledge and understanding. Families can think about favorite topics for their child and start a conversation by asking questions and making comments, modeling conversational language for their child. Families can also practice naming foods in similar categories—meats, vegetables, fruits, and so on—and use descriptive words to talk about how the food smells and tastes.

See **"Successful Strategies for Teaching Students With Learning Disabilities"** on the Learning Disabilities Association of America website for additional teaching strategies.

Facilitating Written Language

To improve written language, initial instruction facilitates the student's development of simple sentences and then elaborating on those sentences by adding descriptive words (Ritchey et al., 2023). Strategy instruction based on the SRSD model (Harris & Graham, 1999; Sun et al., 2022) is also used to help create sentences, edit sentences, and construct paragraphs. Most often, explicit instruction is used with the teacher modeling expectations and creating practice opportunities, with explicit feedback provided to the student (Ritchey et al., 2023).

Several strategies are used to help students with written language disorders plan what they are going to write and how they are going to organize their thinking. You may have learned some of these strategies in school as well. **Graphic organizers** are common organizational tools that allow students to visually arrange key words or concepts as they prepare to write. The following are common graphic organizers:

- Semantic webs: A key concept is placed in a center circle, and lines are drawn from the circle to categories of related concepts. Generally, it is a brainstorming tool to get ideas out, but it may not be as useful to help a student begin writing. See Figure 8–2 for an example of a semantic web.
- Flowcharts: These have greater complexity than semantic webs and are similar to outlining. Flowcharts follow a visual hierarchy moving from the most superordinate concept at the top of the flowchart to subcategories placed underneath with lines connecting to the main concept. See Figure 8–3 for an example of a flowchart.
- Semantic feature analysis: This approach is based on a topic a student will read, and words are listed in a column that are related to the topic. This strategy helps increase a student's awareness of story concepts they will be reading and helps facilitate a more accurate reflection of these concepts in their writing. See Figure 8–4 for an example of a semantic feature analysis.
- Venn diagrams: These are used for making comparisons and contrasting concepts. See Figure 8–5 for an example of a Venn diagram.

It is important that students learn to ask themselves the question, What graphic organizers or visual supports do I know, and which one will help me complete the assignment? SLPs can help students understand how and when each graphic organizer might be beneficial to support their learning. There are also eight basic thinking maps that teachers and SLPs have found helpful in supporting students' thought process during written language tasks from learning to categorize, describe, and sequence ideas to analyzing cause–effect and making comparisons (Hyerle, 2000).

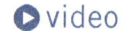 video

 See the Vimeo video "**David Hyerle—Thinking Maps**" for an explanation of how the thinking map process can support students' written language.

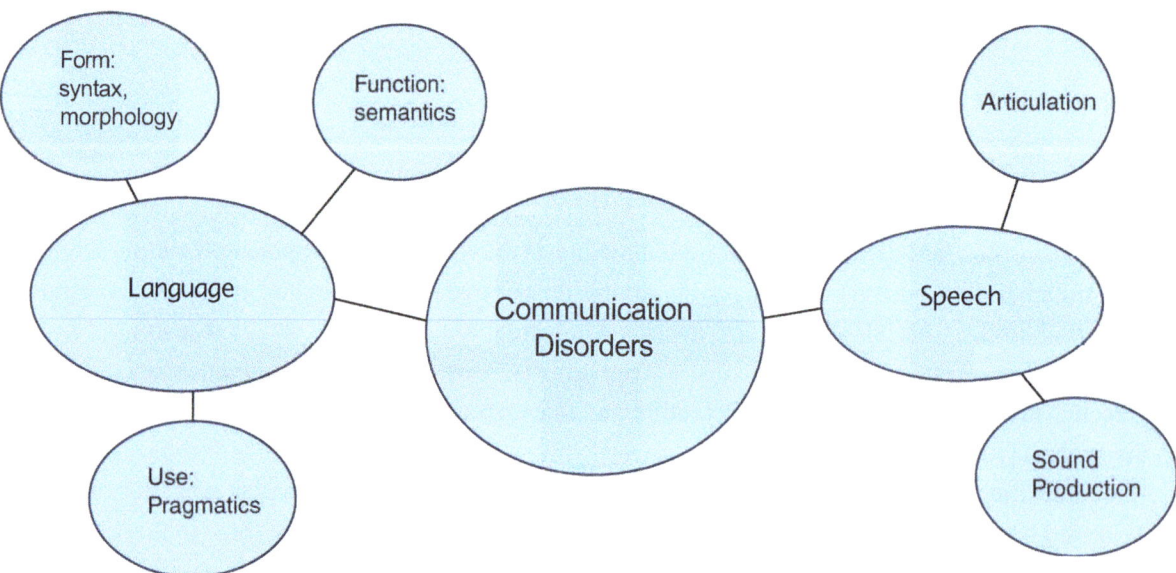

FIGURE 8–2. Example of a semantic web for brainstorming information about communication disorders.

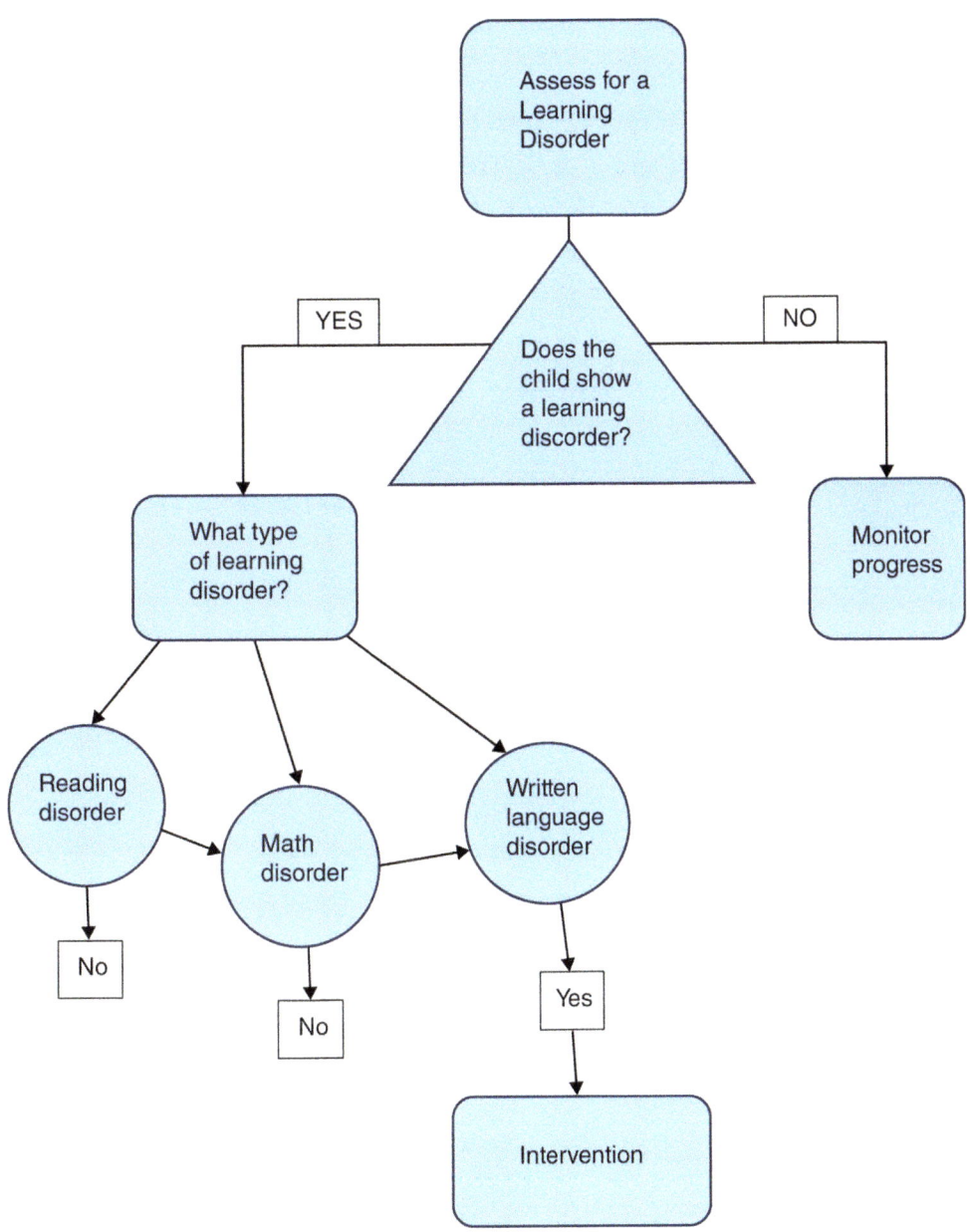

FIGURE 8–3. Example of a flowchart for explaining the process of diagnosis for a learning disorder.

	Apple	Pear	Peach	Plum
Seasonal	+	+	+	+
Taste				
• Sweet	+	+	+	+
• Tart	+	-	-	-
Texture				
• Crispy/Crunchy	+	+	-	-
• Soft & juicy	-	+	+	+
Color				
• Yellow	+	+	+	-
• Red	+	+	-	+
• Orange	-	-	+	-
• Green	+	+	-	-
• Purple	-	-	-	+
Shape				
• Round	+	-	+	+
• Oval	+	-	-	+
• Varies	-	+	-	-

FIGURE 8–4. Example of a semantic feature analysis for fruits.

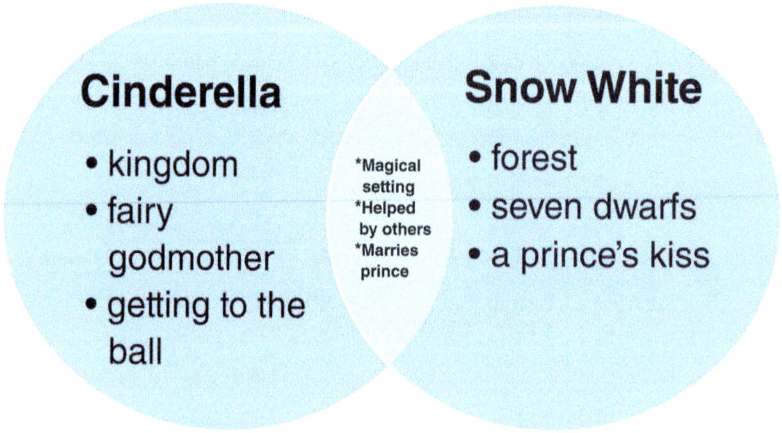

Cinderella
- kingdom
- fairy godmother
- getting to the ball

*Magical setting
*Helped by others
*Marries prince

Snow White
- forest
- seven dwarfs
- a prince's kiss

FIGURE 8–5. Example of a Venn diagram for comparison and contrasting concepts.

The EmPOWER writing strategy (Bashir & Singer, 2006; Singer & Bashir, 2003, 2004b) is a popular approach to supporting written language that balances the writing process with the skill of writing. See Table 8–6 for an outline of the overall approach. The EmPOWER writing strategy considers a hierarchy of instructional targets from text structure to mechanics, and it is the clinician's job to figure out where students are stuck and begin intervention there. When students EmPOWER their writing, they learn to evaluate their assignment, create a plan to complete the assignment, organize their ideas, engage in doing the work of writing, evaluate what they write, and make changes or revisions.

The writing lab approach (Nelson et al., 2004; Nelson & Van Meter, 2006a, 2006b) is another strategy to support written language. This involves SLPs collaborating with teachers to plan and implement curriculum-based writing opportunities. There are three major components: instruction in a curriculum-based writing process with team-taught mini-lessons and peer conferences; computer software support for all stages of the writing process; and inclusive, individualized intervention for students with special needs. Continuous monitoring of student performance is provided during the writing process using interim drafts and story probes with analysis at the word, sentence, and discourse levels.

The approaches described here are just some of the many strategies used to support written language for those with learning disorders or language-based learning disabilities. There are undoubtedly several other strategies that you have found useful in your own efforts to write text across different genres.

Supporting Mathematical Understanding

The 2015 National Assessment of Educational Progress reported that nearly 90% of eighth graders with disabilities were just at or below the basic levels of math proficiency, highlighting the crucial need for effective teaching practices for students with learning disorders.

2015 National Assessment of Educational Progress

TABLE 8–6. Outline of the EmPOWER Writing Strategy Steps and Considerations for Each Step

Step		Considerations	Evaluate & Revise
Understand the assignment/writing goal	Choose strategies to organize	Consider audience	Assess outcomes
Understand the thinking required	Develop a text focus	Translate thesis, main idea, supporting details into sentences and/or paragraphs	Make changes
Brainstorm the needed information	Write initial thesis and map main idea and supporting details	Transcribe ideas to create a draft	Create a final draft

Source: Adapted from Singer and Bashir (2003, 2004b).

Effective math teaching practices are characterized by systematic and explicit instruction; use of visuals, graphs, and manipulatives to teach math concepts; and formative assessment—giving students multiple opportunities and ways to practices their math understanding and application.

An example of a mathematics program that includes current beliefs about the most effective instruction for students with math difficulties is the Early Learning in Mathematics program (Davis & Jungjohann, 2009; Doabler et al., 2012). This program includes several critical elements of systematic and explicit instruction, such as the following:

- Teacher provides clear and specific models.
- Material is sequenced according to difficulty.
- Teacher scaffolds responses to help build understanding.
- Teacher provides feedback on a consistent basis.

Many specific strategies have been identified that support students who are struggling with math. Students must first learn to develop a number sense so that they understand what quantities and numbers mean. For example, a child learns that the number 3 represents three objects and that 3 is greater than 2 but less than 4. Another area that students must develop a level of fluency in is *math facts* so that they can easily add, subtract, multiply, and divide numbers, which will then help them understand fractions and decimals. The use of visuals and manipulatives helps students understand differences in length and area. Problem-solving strategies are used to help students read a problem, organize the information they have been given, and follow a systematic process to answer the question. Technology can be used to support practice in many math concepts, and the use of explicit instruction helps students understand new math concepts being taught. There are also specific steps to tackling a math problem that teachers encourage students to use. First, students are instructed to look for what is being asked in the problem—looking for a question mark is a good indicator of what they are being asked. Students then need to ask what the components of the problem are and write down all the numbers that were specified in the word problem, making sure they place the numbers in the correct order. Students then ask themselves if the problem requires them to add, subtract, multiply, divide, or some combination of operators. Students might also draw the problem out to provide a visualization of what is being asked of them as they read through the problem. This is known as the fast-draw approach and is often used to teach math word problems (Mercer & Miller, 1992). A similar approach to solving word problems is the RIDE approach (Mercer et al., 2011):

- R: Remember the problem.
- I: Identify relevant information.
- D: Determine what mathematical operations are needed.
- E: Enter the answer but recalculate to check for accuracy.

Several strategies are used to teach math vocabulary. Teachers often do some pre-teaching of the vocabulary concepts (Sliva, 2004) and review vocabulary that is introduced in the math textbook to make sure students have an accurate understanding of the terms used. Some teachers will use mnemonic devices to facilitate word meaning, whereas others will use a key word approach. Focusing on developing **metacognitive skills** (the ability to think about and plan activities) is also a frequently used strategy. Metacognitive skills help students focus on what they are doing and create a plan for strategies they will likely employ, as well as adjust when their plan is not following the expected path (Mevarech & Amrany,

2008). Some of these strategies include using "think-alouds" as the student talks through a learning activity, creating graphic organizers or visual images to help complete the various steps of a task, and engaging in self-monitoring to talk through the activity and check for accuracy in their thinking.

Strategies Supporting Students With Nonverbal Learning Disability

Ideally, instruction would be systematic, and material discussed in the classroom would be presented in a slow, step-by-step, and repetitive manner for students with NVLDs. Teachers might teach strategies for problem-solving difficult situations and foster the student's ability to stop–look–listen–examine before talking and take the time to process and store visual information. Presenting explicit verbal instructions is key because many students with NVLDs have difficulty with inner speech (Tuller et al., 2007). Structured peer interactions should be facilitated, and verbal strategies are taught to improve organizational skills. In terms of social skill development, the team should work to increase the student's self-awareness in social interactions. This includes becoming aware of one's own display of emotions, understanding that how one talks and behaves influences other's perceptions, being aware of physical boundaries in social interactions and the reciprocal nature of conversational exchanges, as well as understanding that interactions with peers are different from interactions actions with adults.

A specific intervention strategy that is often recommended for students with NVLDs is **gestalt imagery**. Children with NVLDs have difficulty creating a **gestalt** to support their comprehension; that is, they have difficulty organizing and synthesizing the whole of what they are learning or reading (and instead pay more attention to the smaller details/parts; Berg, 2000). Gestalt imagery involves creating mental models of what is being described by a speaker or writer. It connects incoming language (both oral and written) to prior knowledge and experience. Ultimately, it is the use of language to help us think about what we see, hear, and feel. To stimulate gestalt imagery, the clinician has the student begin by describing a picture or an image of a concept they are thinking about. In this description, the student includes its color, size, shape, where it is, any movement seen, when one might see it, and ideas or perspectives about the concept. The student then moves to imagining a simple sentence and then a short paragraph. The clinician helps the student add interpretation and critical thinking to the imagery they are creating so eventually multiple sentences can be represented. Gestalt imagery can support reading comprehension in that it helps organize information for storing meaning and facilitates the ability to make comparisons.

Academic interventions for students with NVLDs capitalize on their verbal capacity. For example, with handwriting, verbal mediation is used to talk through writing movements. In addition, because of the visual–spatial challenges that are prominent in those with NVLDs, writing on every other line can be helpful. For spelling, imagery can be used in which the student sees the word, says the word, traces the word with their finger, and writes the word in the air. They might also look at the word, create a visual image, spell it with their eyes closed, and then check for accuracy. **Thinking maps** or visual patterns used to map out content to define, classify, describe, sequence, compare, and so on can be used to support writing, which allows the student to create a cohesive story connected to a specific purpose and structure. To support reading comprehension, because students with NVLDs have difficulty identifying the main idea of a story, gestalt imagery can be used to identify major and minor details that lead to an increased understanding of the main idea. For math calculation, each step should be presented in detail, and the student should use their words to describe the different parts of the operation and write out the rules for the operation.

www

Thinking maps

Why Is This Topic Important?

Understanding learning disorders and literacy impairments should give you a better sense of the complexities involved in learning and the thought processes that are critical to being a competent reader, writer, and speller, as well as the role of conceptual thinking required in mathematical success. Learning disorders impact an individual's ability to learn in academic settings and often lead to frustration and decreased motivation because the instruction provided is not explicit, individualized, or sufficiently intensive. Students have different ways of learning, but we often expect all students to learn in the same way. For a student with a learning disorder, it is important to recognize their relative strengths, capitalize on those strengths, and identify where the specific learning breakdown occurs so an adjustment can be made in the teaching approach. Students who do not receive the instruction needed to support their learning success may experience challenges later in adulthood, including securing employment, having fewer opportunities for community engagement, and a reduced number of social relationships. It is also important to recognize that children with learning disorders often have underlying language impairments that complicate their learning success, as well as attention difficulties such as ADHD. It is crucial, therefore, to ensure that a comprehensive assessment is completed for students showing signs of learning disorders to determine if and how other co-occurring conditions are impacting the student's performance, from which an individualized intervention plan can be initiated. SLPs are critical members of the educational team who assess underlying language impairments in children with learning disorders and provide strategies for supporting reading comprehension, understanding math concepts, and developing written language.

Application to a Child

Carlos is in fifth grade. He speaks English and Spanish and knows some Italian. He lives with his mother, who was born in Costa Rica; his father, who was born in Texas; his younger brother; his older sister; and his paternal grandmother, who was born in Italy. Carlos' mother speaks Spanish approximately 50% of the time in the home, and his grandmother speaks primarily Italian in the home, interspersed with limited English. Carlos received speech and language therapy two times a week in kindergarten and first and second grade. Therapy addressed vocabulary development, remediation of a speech sound disorder, and grammar, particularly with the use of questions and embedded sentences. Carlos' speech sound errors were similar in English and Spanish, and his grammatical errors were common in both languages, although English grammatical structure seemed to be more difficult for Carlos to master. Carlos was highly motivated in therapy and made great progress. In third and fourth grade, it was determined that his intervention could move to a collaborative, in-classroom model once a week during which the SLP would collaborate with Carlos' teachers to deliver curriculum-based language intervention.

Fifth grade has begun, and Carlos seems to be struggling more than in the past 2 years. Although Carlos has been a great storyteller, sharing personal stories with expression and focusing on topics of interest to his peers, he continues to have difficulty retelling stories that he has read or creating stories around a specific topic that is less familiar to him. In addition, he is particularly challenged in his written discourse. Spelling, selecting words to represent his intended meanings, and length of written stories are areas of challenge. Furthermore, both his teacher and SLP have noticed that reading comprehension has been more problematic this year than in the past. Carlos' performance is below what is expected for fifth graders, and because the school is following an RTI framework for progress monitoring, the teacher and SLP are reevaluating the type of instruction Carlos is receiving, recognizing the importance of including scientifically based instruction that is both explicit and frequent enough to enhance his language and literacy growth.

Carlos' parents report that although Carlos continues to love school and being with his friends, he seems to be more frustrated during his homework time. They report that he often seems confused by the instructions and seems to miss key points in the content that he is reading. They are worried that Carlos will fall behind but do not want Carlos to be pulled out of class because his peer connections are so important to him.

Currently, Carlos plays football in the fall and baseball in the spring and summer. He is a team player and has shown some real leadership. He is well-liked by his peers and coaches. However, practice and games are taking away from his studies. His parents worry that he may need to give up some of these extracurricular activities to address his academic needs. Carlos is very upset that this may be a possibility, and he is becoming increasingly stressed about his academic performance.

Carlos' mother comes to you with her concerns for her son. Based on this case study and your understanding of the concepts you reviewed in this chapter, do you think Carlos presents with a potential language-based learning disorder? Why or why not? What recommendations will you make to Carlos' mother to address her concerns? What other professionals may need to be involved to facilitate a meaningful assessment and intervention plan for Carlos?

Application to an Adolescent

Michael is a 14-year-old boy who is about to begin his freshman year in high school. He received speech and language therapy from kindergarten through fifth grade, when his annual language assessment indicated that his performance was within 1 standard deviation of the mean expected for his age. He was dismissed from therapy prior to going to middle school.

Michael's past speech and language history was characterized by poor vocabulary development and word-finding difficulties, difficulty identifying and communicating the most relevant information when interacting with adults and peers, poor attention to tasks, a history of chronic ear infections, and poor social relationships. Although he had some early speech sound deficits, these have been resolved and his sentence structure is appropriate. Michael has always been a verbal communicator, yet his expressive language has often masked his difficulties in comprehension. He is a good reader, yet his written language is unorganized, and his spelling is poor. His written language is adequate when adaptations are made for keyboard use and extra time is given to complete the required tasks. However, his expository writing is usually factual with few inferences or integration of ideas. Math performance has been inconsistent, and word problems continue to challenge him. As a middle school student, Michael managed his coursework with some support from teachers who worked with him after school. The summer before high school, he had periodic tutoring for written language, reading comprehension, and math. His middle school teachers were increasingly worried about his transition to high school, as they began to notice increases in social challenges. Michael does not seem to recognize the nonverbal cues of his peers, fails to read their facial expressions, and does not seem to understand idiomatic expressions, all of which are crucial in the high school environment.

Upon beginning high school, Michael is receiving no supports and is participating in a regular academic track in high school. In the first weeks of school, he is showing a real interest in world history and actively participates in class. His English teacher has reported some concerns in his ability to understand select literature, as they are reading *Hamlet* and writing reflection papers on the characters. Michael is challenged in describing the relevant attributes of the characters and making judgments about the story. Because the writing reflections are being completed in class, Michael is doing so without the supports that have been useful for him, including typing his responses with a keyboard and using spell-check. The teacher reports that Michael's writing is often illegible and that his ideas are poorly organized and not fully developed. The algebra teacher is concerned that Michael does not have a logical way in approaching the problems posed in class and those assigned for homework.

Both the English and algebra teachers wonder if Michael should be enrolled in their classes and are concerned about his ability to meet the expectations of the curriculum. When the English teacher talks with Michael after class, Michael expresses his ideas overall, although his word choices are not always accurate, and he often provides as much irrelevant as relevant information. The algebra teacher is concerned that Michael does not get the whole picture when considering the problems he is solving; therefore, he only answers parts of the assigned problems accurately. The world history teacher likes having Michael in class because he is actively engaged in the material. His primary concern is with Michael's expository writing because his written assignments lack cohesiveness, often assume that the reader has background knowledge of the topic, are generally disorganized sequentially, and are replete with inappropriate word choices.

Michael has had difficulty transitioning to high school and currently is having trouble making friends. He struggles to bring the appropriate materials to each of his classes and often forgets assignments. His peers struggle to have conversations with him because he usually talks about his specific interests, which his peers are generally not really interested in. He stands too close to others and does not read their facial expressions or nonverbal behaviors which indicate that they do not understand what he is talking about or wish to leave the conversation.

Michael is interested in movies and has an interest in acting. He wants to join the drama club but is afraid his peers will make fun of him. He is not sure how to approach the club or the faculty advisor.

Knowing Michael's history of language and learning difficulties, what are some of your predictions about why he is struggling in his current classes? What are the specific demands of the curriculum that are likely to be problematic for him? What additional assessment would you do and why? Specifically, what type of services, if any, will be needed to address Michael's current needs and how might these be delivered? Describe the challenges you anticipate in implementing the needed services and how you might manage those barriers. What specific intervention strategies would you initiate to address Michael's difficulties?

Chapter Summary

This chapter focused on the prevalence of learning disorders (i.e., reading, written language, math, and nonverbal learning disabilities) in children, possible causes, and the likelihood that many learning disorders have underlying language impairments. There are six potential areas in which students with learning disorders might fall short. First, they might have difficulty reading words, lacking accurate word recognition and decoding (or sounding out words). Second, they might exhibit problems with reading comprehension and understanding the meaning of what has been read. Third, spelling could be a problem area in which the student omits, adds, or substitutes sounds in words. Writing might also be an area of challenge in which the student demonstrates grammatical errors and exhibits a poor organization structure that makes their ideas unclear. A fifth area of difficulty is numerical understanding and math calculation, in which students have problems retrieving math facts and accurately completing computations. Finally, math reasoning could be impacted, in which a student has difficulty with math problem-solving. Learning disorders suggest continuing problems with academic skill development, with performance well below what is expected for their age.

Diagnosis of a specific learning disorder is made following a comprehensive evaluation with standardized assessment tools examining a child's academic skills, intellectual ability, and language performance. To be diagnosed with a specific learning disorder, a student's observed challenges cannot be better explained by an intellectual disability, uncorrected hearing, visual impairment, another mental or neurobiological disorder, or lack of adequate language and/or academic instruction. Diagnosis of a learning disorder has a significant impact on the family because there will be an ongoing need to navigate the child's difficulties across the lifespan. Many professional disciplines, including pediatric practitioners, general and special educators, psychologists, and SLPs, have a critical role in supporting individuals with learning disorders and their families.

Early intervention is important for students with learning disorders because classroom adjustments and instructional methods can be implemented to address the students' learning differences. An integrated approach to intervention is recommended because this leads to creating profiles of students' areas of strength and challenge and considers an RTI model to not only identify children at greater risk for learning difference but also allow for an evaluation of instructional effectiveness. Intervention for learning disorders also requires collaboration with multiple team members with specific expertise to address a student's complex and individual needs. A case manager usually coordinates the student's intervention plan, with a special educator as a crucial part of the team because of their expertise to address the learning needs of students with learning disorders. An SLP is a critical team member because they provide language and social communication support that students with learning disorders often require. Several strategies were discussed to foster learning across academic areas; strategy instruction seems to be the most frequently used approach because it teaches students a series of ordered steps and cognitive processes that help them complete a variety of academic tasks.

Chapter Review Questions

1. Describe the six areas of potential learning challenges that a student with a learning disorder might exhibit.
2. What are the unique strengths and challenges of a students with a nonverbal learning disability?
3. Explain the language challenges a student with a learning disorder might experience in reading, writing, and math.
4. How is the response to intervention (RTI) model used to support instruction for those at risk for a learning disorder?
5. Which of the following statements is *false* regarding language-based learning disabilities/disorders?
    a. Persistent difficulties in reading, writing, arithmetic, and/or mathematical reasoning during formal schooling must continue for a minimum of 6 months even with intervention.
    b. Several professionals, such as psychologists, occupational therapists, and speech-language pathologists, are involved in the evaluation process and must coordinate to obtain an accurate diagnosis.
    c. Intelligence and academic achievement testing, classroom performance, and social interaction are assessed.
    d. Problems in pregnancy are the only cause of language-based learning disabilities.
6. Describe the steps you might take to assess a student's written language.
7. Identify two strategies you would use to improve a student's word knowledge or vocabulary.
8. Describe the steps of the EmPOWER writing strategy.
9. What is the role of an SLP in the assessment and intervention provided for students with a language-based learning disorder?
10. What strategies are most useful to support students with a learning disorder in math?

Learning Activities

1. Identify an entertainer, athlete, or professional who you admire who has a learning disorder. Read about their learning struggles and the strategies they used to manage their learning difficulties.
2. Review the eight thinking maps described by Hyerle (2000) and explain how you might use any of these maps to facilitate your thinking process when writing a paper. You might even

practice using a few of them as part of your assignments in any of the courses that you are currently taking.

3. You have been assigned to be a tutor for a student with a nonverbal learning disorder. What information do you need about the student and the content areas of difficulty to provide effective tutoring? What strategies might you employ to foster the student's learning success?

Suggested Reading

Hughes, E. M., Powell, S. R., Lembke, E. S., & Riley-Tillman, T. C. (2016). Taking the guesswork out of locating evidence-based practices for diverse learners. *Learning Disabilities Research and Practice, 31,* 130–141.

This article guides educators in their selection of evidence-based practices that will facilitate diverse students' abilities to improve mathematics performance and to give teachers a degree of confidence in the effectiveness of their instruction.

Interventions for Beginning Reading: Review Protocol (retrieved from the U.S. Department of Education, Institute of Education Sciences, What Works Clearinghouse, http://ies.ed.gov/ncee/wwc)

This review from What Works Clearinghouse highlights reading interventions for students in kindergarten through third grade designed to increase skills in alphabetics (**phonemic awareness, phonological awareness, print awareness,** and **phonics**), reading fluency, comprehension (vocabulary and reading comprehension), or general reading achievement. The review examines evidence that answers three key questions: (a) Which interventions improve reading skills among 5- to 8-year-old children? (b) Are some interventions more effective in supporting specific reading skills? (c) What interventions are most effective for particular types of students who have fallen behind in reading?

Serniclaes, W., & Sprenger-Charolles, L. (2015). Reading impairment: From behavior to brain. In R. Huntley Bahr & E. R. Silliman (Eds.), *Routledge handbook of communication disorders* (pp. 34–45). Routledge.

This chapter focused on reading impairments and how reading challenges relate to cognitive differences. The chapter explains the role of speech perception in learning to read. The authors then discuss key competencies needed for acquiring the ability to read and how a challenge in any one of these areas can explain reading impairment. Clinical implications and ideas for intervention are provided.

Stevens, E. A., Walker, M. A., & Vaughn, S. (2017). The effects of reading fluency interventions on the reading fluency and reading comprehension performance of elementary students with learning disabilities: A synthesis of the research from 2001 to 2014. *Journal of Learning Disabilities, 50*(5), 576–590.

The ability to read words fluently is believed to increase a child's reading comprehension because less struggle decoding words allows for increased cognitive capacity to attend to meaning. This article synthesizes research examining reading fluency interventions and outcomes on reading comprehension over a 14-year period. Gains in reading fluency and comprehension were seen following several reading fluency interventions, such as repeated reading and assisted audiobook reading.

Additional Resources

- American Speech-Language-Hearing Association, "Written Language Disorders Practice Portal"
  https://www.asha.org/Practice-Portal/Clinical-Topics/Written-Language-Disorders
- American Speech-Language-Hearing Association, "Written Language Disorders (School-Age) Evidence Map"
  https://apps.asha.org/EvidenceMaps/Maps/LandingPage/29e542a1-d46e-4df9-a361-2293 62674cf4
- Institute of Education Sciences, "Practice Guide: Assisting Students Struggling With Mathematics: Response to Intervention for Elementary and Middle Schools" (2009)
  https://ies.ed.gov/ncee/wwc/PracticeGuide/2
- Center on Instruction, "Mathematics Instruction for Students With Learning Disabilities or Difficulty Learning Mathematics: A Guide for Teachers" (2008)
  https://www.centeroninstruction.org/mathematics-instruction-for-students-with-learning-disabilities-or-difficulty-learning-mathematics-a-guide-for-teachers

References

Allington, R. L. (2004). Setting the record straight. *Educational Leadership*, *61*(6), 22–25.

American Psychiatric Association. (2022). *Diagnostic and statistical manual of mental disorders* (5th ed., text rev.).

Antshel, K. M., & Joseph, G.-R. (2006). Maternal stress in nonverbal learning disorder: A comparison with reading disorder. *Journal of Learning Disabilities*, *39*(3), 194–205.

Arfe, B., Dockrell, J. E., & De Bernardi, B. (2016). The effect of language specific factors on early written composition: The role of spelling, oral language, and text generation skills in a shallow orthography. *Reading and Writing*, *29*, 501–527.

Arfe, B., & Pizzocaro, E. (2016). Sentence generation in children with and without problems of written expression. In J. Perera, M. Aparici, E., Rosado, & N. Salas (Eds.), *Written and spoken language development across the lifespan: Essays in honour of Liliana Tolchinsky* (pp. 327–344). Springer.

Bandian, N. A. (1999). Reading disability defined as a discrepancy between listening and reading comprehension: A longitudinal study of stability, gender differences, and prevalence. *Journal of Learning Disabilities*, *32*(2) 138–148.

Banker, S. M., Ramphal, B., Pagliaccio, D., Thomas, L., Rosen, E., Sigel, A. N., . . . Margolis, A. E. (2020). Spatial network connectivity and spatial reasoning ability in children with nonverbal learning disability. *Scientific Reports*, *10*(1), Article 561.

Barnes, M. A., Fletcher, J., & Fuchs, L. (Eds.). (2007). *Learning disabilities: From identification to intervention*. Guilford.

Bashir, A. S., & Singer, B. D. (2006). Assisting students in becoming self-regulated writers. In T. A. Ukrainetz (Ed.), *Contextualized language intervention: Scaffolding PreK–12 literacy achievement*. Thinking Publications.

Berg, M. (2000, April). *Nonverbal learning disabilities* [Paper presentation]. First annual Pine Ridge School Conference on Learning Disabilities, Burlington, VT.

Bingham, G. E. (2007). Maternal literacy beliefs and the quality of mother–child book-reading interactions: Associations with children's early literacy development. *Early Education and Development, 18*(1), 23–49.

Blachowicz, C. L. Z., & Fisher, P. (2004). Vocabulary lessons. *Educational leadership, 61,* 66–69.

Bradley, R., Danielson, L., & Hallahan, D. P. (2002). *Identification of learning disabilities: Research to practice.* Erlbaum.

Brimo, D., Nallamala, K., & Werfel, K. L. (2023). Writing errors of children with developmental language disorder. *Topics in Language Disorders, 43*(4), 302–316.

Calhoun, M. B. (2005). Effects of a peer mediated phonological skill and reading comprehension program on reading skill acquisition for middle school students with reading disabilities. *Journal of Learning Disabilities, 38*(5), 424–433.

Camilli, G., & Wolfe, P. (2004). Research on reading: A cautionary tale. *Educational Leadership, 61*(6), 26–29.

Catts, H. W., Fey, M. E., Tomblin, J. B., & Zhang, X. (2002). A longitudinal investigation of reading outcomes in children with language impairments. *Journal of Speech, Language, and Hearing Research, 45*(6), 1142–1157.

Catts, H. W., Fey, M. E., Zhang, X., & Tomblin, J. B. (2001). Estimating the risk of future reading difficulties in kindergarten children: A research-based model and its clinical implementation. *Language, Speech, and Hearing Services in Schools, 32,* 38–50.

Centers for Disease Control and Prevention. (2011a). *National Health Interview Survey 2007–2009 data.* http://www.cdc.gov/nchs/nhis.htm

Centers for Disease Control and Prevention. (2011b, July). QuickStats: Percentage of children aged 5–17 years ever receiving a diagnosis of learning disability, by race/ethnicity and family income group: National Health Interview Survey, United States, 2007–2009. *MMWR Morbidity and Mortality Weekly Report, 60*(25), 853. https://www.cdc.gov/mmwr/preview/mmwrhtml/mm6025a6.htm

Coutinho, M. J., & Oswald, D. P. (2005). State variation in gender disproportionally in special education: Finding and recommendations. *Remedial and Special Education, 26*(1), 7–15.

Crowley, C. J., & Valenti, D. M. (2002). Vocabulary development with students who are culturally and linguistically diverse. *Perspectives on Language Learning and Education, 9*(3), 25–29.

Davis, J. M., & Broitman, J. (2011). *Nonverbal learning disability in children: Bridging the gap between science and practice.* Springer.

Duff, D., Tomblin, J. B., & Catts, H. (2015). The influence of reading on vocabulary growth: A case for a Matthew effect. *Journal of Speech, Language, and Hearing Research, 58*(3), 853–864.

Ehren, B. J., & Nelson, N. W. (2005). The responsiveness to intervention approach and language impairment. *Topics in Language Disorders, 25*(2), 120–131.

Fletcher, J. M., Lyon, G. R., Fuchs, L. S., & Barnes, M. A. (2007). Classification, definition and identification of learning disabilities. In M. A. Barnes, J. Fletcher, & L. Fuchs (Eds.), *Learning disabilities: From identification to intervention* (pp. 25–63). Guilford.

Gaskins, I. W. (2004). Word detectives. *Educational Leadership, 61,* 70–73.

Geary, D. C. (2004). Mathematics and learning disabilities. *Journal of Learning Disabilities, 37,* 4–15.

Gorker, I, Bozatu, L., Kormazlar, U., Yucel Karadag, M., Ceylan, C., Sogut, C., . . . Turan, N. (2017). The probable prevalence and sociodemographic characteristics of specific learning disorder in primary school children in Edrine. *Archives in Neuropsychiatry, 54,* 343–349.

Graham, S., & Harris, K. R. (2005). *Writing better: Effective strategies for teaching students with learning difficulties.* Brookes.

Hall-Mills, S., & Wood, C. (2023). Complex syntax production in informational writing by students with language impairment from diverse linguistic backgrounds. *Topics in Language Disorders, 43*(4), 333–348.

Handler, S. M., & Fierson, W. M. (2011). Learning disabilities, dyslexia, and vision. *Pediatrics, 127*(3), e818–e856.

Harrison, P. L., & Flanagan, D. P. (2005). *Contemporary intellectual assessment: Theories, tests, and issues.* Guilford.

Hudson, N., Scheff, J., Tarsha, M., & Cutting, L. E. (2016, Spring). Reading comprehension and executive function: Neurobiological findings. *Perspectives on Language and Literacy.* Retrieved December 30, 2023, from https://mydigitalpublication.com/publication/?i=298764&article_id=2460782&view=articleBrowser

Hudson, R. F., High, L., & Al Otaiba, S. (2007). Dyslexia and the brain: What does current research tell us? *The Reading Teacher, 60*(6), 506–515.

Hyerle, D. (2000). *A field guide to visual tools.* Association for Supervision and Curriculum Development.

Jagaiah, T., Olinghouse, N. G., & Kearns, D. M. (2020). Syntactic complexity measures: Variation by genre, grade-level, students' writing abilities, and writing quality. *Reading and Writing, 33*(10), 2577–2638.

Jitendra, A. K., Rodriguez, M., Kanive, R., Huang, J., Church, C., Conroy, K. A., & Zaslofsky, A. (2013). Impact of small-group tutoring interventions on the mathematical problem solving and achievement of third-grade students with mathematics difficulties. *Learning Disability Quarterly, 36*, 21–35.

Juel, C., & Deffres, R. (2004). Making words stick. *Educational Leadership, 61*, 30–34.

Koutsoftas, A. D. (2023). Issue editor foreword: Sentence-level writing skills in children with and without developmental language disorders. *Topics in Language Disorders, 43*(4), 281–282.

Koutsoftas, A. D., & Srivastava, P. (2020). Oral language contributions to reading and writing in students with and without language-learning disabilities. *Exceptionality, 28*(5), 380–392.

Liddell, G. A., & Rasmussen, C. (2005). Memory profile of children with nonverbal learning disability. *Learning Disabilities Research & Practice, 20*(3), 137–141.

Logan, J. A. R., Justice, L. M., Yumus, M., & Chaparro-Moreno, L. J. (2020). When children are not read to at home: The million-word gap. *Journal of Developmental & Behavioral Pediatrics, 40*(5), 383–386.

Lyon, G., & Chhabra, V. (2004, January). The science of reading research. *Educational Leadership, 61*(6).

Margolis, A. E., Broitman J., Davis, J. M., Alexander, L., Hamilton, A. M., Liao, Z., . . .T Milham, M. P. (2020). Estimated prevalence of nonverbal learning disability among North American children and adolescents. *JAMA Network Open, 3*(4), Article e202551.

Mayes, S. D., Calhoun, S. L., & Crowell, E. W. (2000). Learning disabilities and ADHD: Overlapping spectrum disorders. *Journal of Learning Disabilities, 33*(5), 417–424.

Mazzocco, M. (2007). Defining and differentiating mathematical learning disabilities and difficulties. In D. Berch & M. Mazzocco (Eds.), *Why is math so hard for some children? The nature and origins of mathematics learning difficulties and disabilities* (pp. 29–47). Brookes.

Mercer, C. D., & Miller, S. P. (1992). *Multiplication facts 0 to 81*. Edge Enterprises.

Mercer, C. D., Mercer, A. R., & Pullen, P. C. (2011). *Teaching students with learning problems* (8th ed.). Pearson.

Mevarech, Z. R., & Amrany, C. (2008). Immediate and delayed effects of meta-cognitive instruction on regulation of cognition and mathematics achievement. *Metacognition and Learning, 3*(2), 147–157.

Mol, S. E., & Bus, A. G. (2011). To read or not to read: A meta-analysis of print exposure from infancy to early adulthood. *Psychological Bulletin, 137*(2), 267–296.

Moll, K., Kunze, S., Neuhoff, N., Bruder, J., & Schulte-Körne, G. (2014). Specific learning disorder: Prevalence and gender differences. *PLoS ONE, 9*(7), Article e103537.

Morgan, P. L., Farkas, G., Hillemeier, M. M., Mattison, R., Maczuga, S., Li, H., & Cook, M. (2015). Minorities are disproportionately underrepresented in special education: Longitudinal evidence across five disability conditions. *Educational Research, 44*(5), 278–292.

Morgan, P. L., Staff, J., Hillemeier, M. M., Farkas, G., & Maczuga, S. (2013). Racial and ethnic disparities in ADHD diagnosis from kindergarten to eighth grade. *Pediatrics, 132*(1), 85–93.

National Center for Education Statistics. (n.d.). Common Core of Data (CCD), "State Nonfiscal Survey of Public Elementary/Secondary Education," 2013–14. *Digest of Education Statistics 2015*, Table 204.30 and Table 204.50.

National Center for Education Statistics. (2019). *2019 NAEP reading assessment highlights* (Statistical Analysis Report NCES 2020012). https://www.nationsreportcard.gov/highlights/reading/2019

National Reading Panel. (2000). *Teaching children to read: An evidence-based assessment of the scientific research literature on reading and its implications for reading instruction* (NIH Publication No. 00-4769). https://www.nichd.nih.gov/publications/pubs/nrp/smallbook

Nelson, N. W., Bahr, C. M., & Van Meter, A. M. (2004). *The writing lab approach to language instruction and intervention*. Brookes.

Nelson, N. W., & Van Meter, A. M. (2006a). Partnerships for literacy in a writing lab approach. *Topics in Language Disorders, 26*, 55–69.

Nelson, N. W., & Van Meter, A. M. (2006b). The writing lab approach for building language, literacy & communication abilities. In R. J. McCauley & M. E. Fey (Eds.), *Treatment of language disorders in children* (pp. 383–422). Brookes.

O'Fallon, M., Alper, R. M., Beiting, M., & Luo, R. (2022). Assessing shared reading in families at risk: Does quantity predict quality? *American Journal of Speech-Language Pathology, 31*, 2108–2122.

Padhy, S. K., Goel S., Das, S. S., Sarkar, S., Sharma, V., & Panigrahi, M. (2016). Prevalence and patterns of learning disabilities in school children. *Indian Journal of Pediatrics, 83*(4), 300–306.

Prelock, P. A. (2013). What is a learning disability? In F. R. Volkmar (Ed.), *Encyclopedia for autism spectrum disorders*. Springer

Prelock, P. A., & Hutchins, T. (2018). Children with learning disabilities or specific language disorders. In *Clinical guide to assessment and treatment of communication disorders* (pp. 65–74). Springer.

Reid, R., & Lienemann, T. O. (2006a). Building background knowledge. In *Strategy instruction for students with learning disabilities* (pp. 16–31). Guilford.

Reid, R., & Lienemann, T. O. (2006b). Integrating strategies and self-regulation. In *Strategy instruction for students with learning disabilities* (pp. 109–124). Guilford.

Ritchey, K. D., Coker, D. L., Myers, M. C., & Zhang, F. (2023). Teaching students to write sentences. *Topics in Language Disorders, 43*(4), 317–332.

Rourke, B. P., Ahmad, S., Collins, D., Hayman-Abello, B., Sayman-Abello, S., & Warriner, E. (2002). Child clinical/pediatric neuropsychology: Some recent advances. *Annual Reviews of Psychology, 53,* 309–339.

Rourke, B. P., & Tsatsanis, K. D. (1996). Syndrome of nonverbal learning disabilities: Psycholinguistic assets and deficits. *Topics in Language Disorders, 16,* 30–44.

Sayeski, K. L., & Paulsen, K. J. (2010). Mathematics reform curricula and special education: Identifying intersections and implications for practice. *Intervention in School and Clinic, 46,* 13–21.

Scott, C. M., & Windsor, J. (2000). General language performance measures in spoken and written narrative and expository discourse of school-age children with language learning disabilities. *Journal of Speech, Language, and Hearing Research, 43,* 324–339.

Shaywitz, B. A., Shaywitz, S. E., Pugh, K. R., Mencl, W. E., Fulbright, R. K., Skudlarksi, P., . . . Gore, J. C. (2002). Disruption of posterior brain systems for reading in children with developmental dyslexia. *Biological Psychiatry, 52,* 101–110.

Shaywitz, S. E., & Shaywitz, B. A. (2004). Neurobiologic basis for reading and reading disability. In P. McCardle & V. Chhabra (Eds.), *The voice of evidence in reading research* (pp. 417–442). Brookes.

Silverman, R. D., Coker, D., Proctor, C. P., Harring, J., Piantedosi, K. W., & Hartranft, A. M. (2015). The relationship between language skills and writing outcomes for linguistically diverse students in upper elementary school. *Elementary School Journal, 116*(1), 103–125.

Singer, B., & Bashir, A. (2003, November). *EmPOWERing expository writing for students with LLD* [Paper presentation]. National Convention of the American Speech-Language-Hearing Association, Chicago, IL.

Singer, B., & Bashir, A. (2004a). Developmental variations in writing composition skills. In K. Apel, B. Ehren, E. Silliman, & A. Stone (Eds.), *Handbook of language and literacy development and disorders* (pp. 559–582). Guilford.

Singer, B., & Bashir, A. (2004b). EmPOWER: A strategy for teaching students with language learning disabilities to write expository text. In E. Silliman & L. Wilkinson (Eds.), *Language and literacy learning* (pp. 239–272). Guilford.

Sliva, J. A. (2004). *Teaching inclusive mathematics to special learners, K–6.* Corwin.

Sternberg, R. J., & Grigorenko, E. L. (1999). *Our labeled children: What every parent and teacher need to know about learning disabilities.* Perseus.

Sternberg, R. J., & Grigorenko, E. L. (2001, December). Learning disabilities, schooling, and society. *Phi Delta Kappan,* 335–338.

Sun, L., & Wallach, G. P. (2014). Language disorders are learning disabilities: Challenges on the divergent and diverse paths to language learning disability. *Topics in Language Disorders, 34*(1), 25–38.

Troia, G. A. (2005). Responsiveness to intervention: Roles for SLPs in the prevention and identification of learning disabilities. *Topics in Language Disorders, 25*(2), 106–119.

U.S. Department of Education, Office of Special Education Programs. (2015). *Individuals With Disabilities Education Act (IDEA) database.* Retrieved September 25, 2015, from http://www2.ed.gov/programs/osepidea/618-data/state-level-data-files/index.html#bcc

Vlasákova, J., & Manuhutu, N. (2018). Applying STAR strategy to improve students' vocabulary. *ELS Journal on Interdisciplinary Studies in Humanities, 1*(2), 210–217.

Volden, J. (2004). Nonverbal learning disability: A tutorial for speech-language pathologists. *American Journal of Speech-Language Pathology, 13*, 128–141.

Wallach, G. P. (2005). A conceptual framework in language learning disabilities: School-age language disorders. *Topics in Language Disorders, 25*(4), 292–301.

Wanzek, J., Wood, C., & Schatschneider, C. (2023). Teacher vocabulary use and student language and literacy achievement. *Journal of Speech, Language, and Hearing Research, 66*, 3574–3587.

Williams, G. J., & Larkin, R. F. (2023). Translation and transcription processes in the writing skills of children with developmental language disorder. *Topics in Language Disorders, 43*(4), 283–301.

Williams, G. J., Larkin, R. F., Rose, N. V., Whitaker, E., Roeser, J., & Wood, C. (2021). Orthographic knowledge and clue word facilitated spelling in children with developmental language disorder. *Journal of Speech, Language, and Hearing Research, 64*(10), 3909–3927.

Zablotsky, B., Black, L. I., Maenner, M. J., Schieve, L. A., Danielson, M. L., Bitsko, R. H., . . . Boyle, C. A. (2019). Prevalence and trends of developmental disabilities among children in the United States: 2009–2017. *Pediatrics, 144*(4), Article e20190811.

Chapter 9

Adult Language and Cognitive Communication Disorders

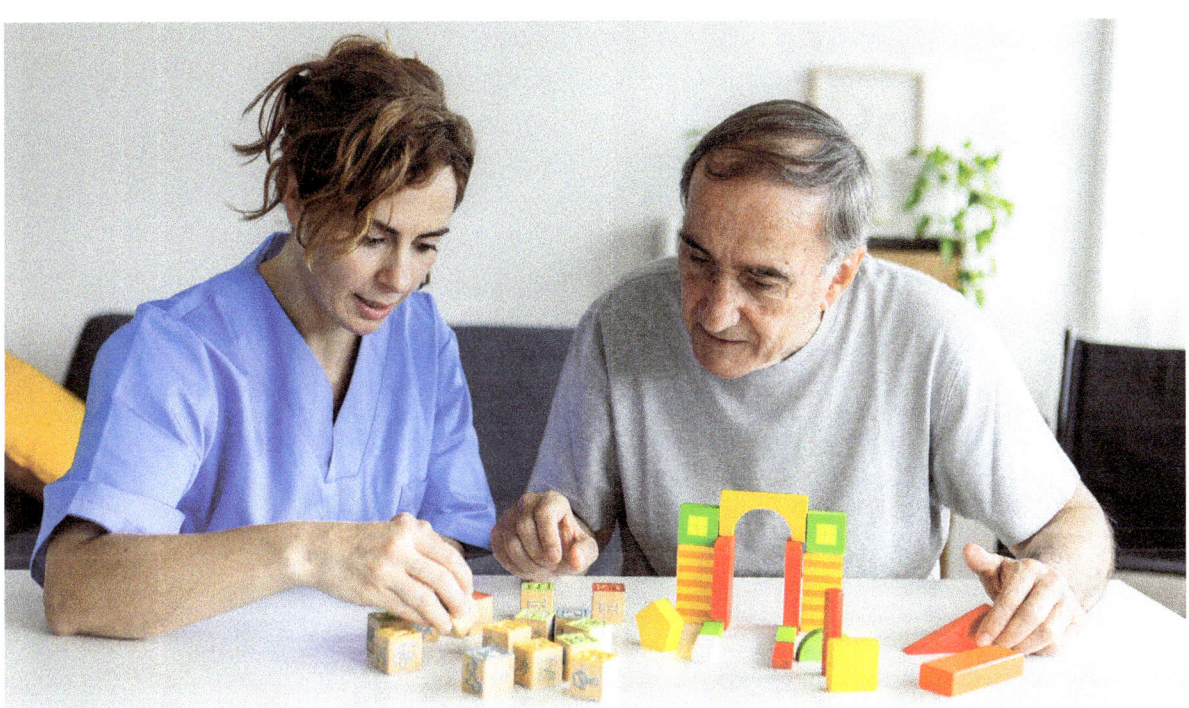

Learning Objectives

After reading this chapter, you will be able to:

- Describe the characteristics associated with aphasia, right hemisphere disorder, traumatic brain injury, and dementia.
- Differentiate between a language disorder and a disorder of cognitive communication.
- Identify ways to assess adult language and cognitive communication disorders.
- Identify intervention approaches and strategies that help support adults with acquired language and communication disorders, including incorporating family members and caregivers in the assessment and intervention processes.

Key Terms

- agrammatical
- Alzheimer's disease
- anomia
- anomic aphasia
- aphasia
- aprosodia
- auditory cortex
- brainstem
- Broca's aphasia
- Broca's area
- cerebellum
- cerebrum
- cognitive communication training
- compensatory strategies
- conduction aphasia
- corpus callosum
- dementia
- discourse
- dysarthria
- dysphagia
- executive functions
- frontal lobe
- frontotemporal dementia
- functional communication training
- global aphasia
- hemorrhagic strokes
- Huntington's disease
- impairment-based approaches
- ischemic stroke
- Lewy body dementia
- neologisms
- occipital lobe
- parietal lobe
- Parkinson's disease
- primary progressive aphasia
- restorative approaches
- right hemisphere disorder
- somatosensory cortex
- temporal lobe
- transcortical motor aphasia
- transcortical sensory aphasia
- traumatic brain injury
- visual cortex
- Wernicke's aphasia
- Wernicke's area

Introduction

The brain is a fascinating organ that we rely on every day, most of the time without even acknowledging or thinking about it. We would not be able to engage in the world around us in the ways that we do—sharing our feelings, asking for help, thinking abstract thoughts, tying our shoes, making a cup of coffee, sending an e-mail, navigating in traffic, and so much more—without the complex interactions that take place in our brains on a biological and neurological level. The importance of our brains for everyday functioning lies not just within the brain structures themselves (e.g., the frontal lobe) but also in the interactions *between* the structures and the pathways through which the brain communicates with the rest of the body. Although it is outside the scope of this book to discuss all of the structures of the brain and why they are important, we review structures that are particularly important for language and communication. Perhaps you are wondering why learning about anatomy is necessary for you as a potential future speech-language pathologist (SLP) or audiologist because you will likely be working with clients on language as a behavior and not language from a biological perspective. Well, remember our causal model (Figure 9–1)?

Through the lens of a causal model for language, we can consider the brain and its structures as part of *biology*. These biological mechanisms interact with language at the *cognitive* level (e.g., comprehension

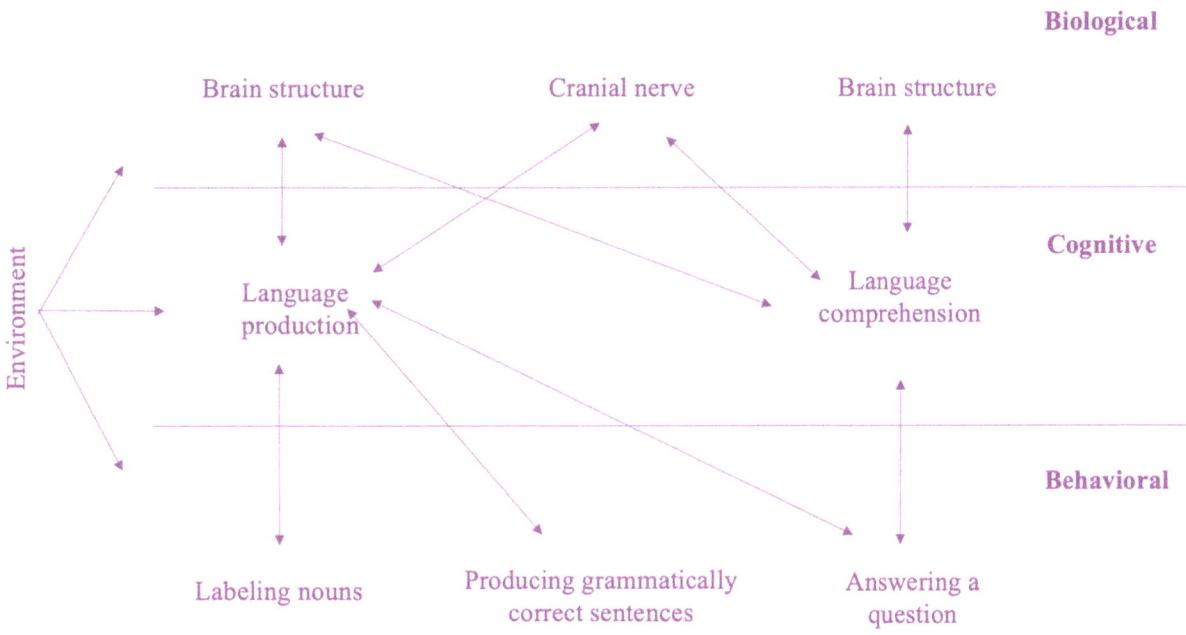

FIGURE 9–1. Causal model for language.

and production of language), and these cognitive components of language interact with the *behaviors* associated with language. That is, the cognitive ability of expressive language manifests behaviorally in many ways, such as asking for help, structuring sentences in grammatically correct ways, labeling nouns or attributes, and ordering a coffee with cream and sugar. And remember that the relationships between biology, cognition, and behavior are bidirectional (i.e., the interaction flows in both directions). So, to continue with our example, not only do brain structures affect expressive language, which impacts how we use language in our daily lives, but also these behaviors and skills contribute to the cognitive processes involved in language production because our cognitive processes are not fixed; they are malleable and can develop or deteriorate over time (consider a child developing language or a person who has a degenerative condition). These cognitive factors may indeed transform the biological structures, leading to changes in neuronal firing, connectivity between brain regions, activation of certain brain structures, and so on. And of course, we cannot forget the role that the environment plays at each level, including language modeling from others, environmental stressors, and so on. Are you starting to get a sense of why we care about anatomy and biology even though our focus is at (primarily) the behavioral and cognitive levels? We must understand the parts of the brain that are crucial to language because when one of these structures is damaged, language or communication will be affected, which has implications for how we approach the resulting language disorder. So, let's dive into the brain then, shall we?

The Brain

Many people associate the brain with intelligence. Consider the word *brainiac*, which means "a very intelligent person" (Merriam-Webster, n.d.). This narrow conceptualization of the brain forgoes the multi-dimensionality and comprehensiveness of the brain for everyday functioning. The brain consists of three main sections—the **cerebrum**, **cerebellum**, and **brainstem**; two main hemispheres—the right hemisphere and the left hemisphere; as well as four main lobes—the frontal lobe, parietal lobe, temporal lobe, and occipital lobe. The cerebellum is sometimes referred to as the "little brain" and sits underneath the cerebrum. Its primary functions include body positioning, maintaining balance, and fine motor coordination, although more recent studies suggest that the cerebellum plays a role in verbal fluency, receptive and expressive grammatical processing, identifying language mistakes, as well as reading and writing (Starowicz-Filip et al., 2017). The brainstem connects the brain to the spinal cord, and through it the brain communicates with the rest of the body. The cerebrum is the main part of the brain and what we tend to think of when we hear the word "brain." The cerebrum is divided into the left and right hemispheres and consists of four lobes (Figure 9–2).

Hemispheres of the Brain

As previously mentioned, the cerebrum is divided into two main hemispheres: the right hemisphere and the left hemisphere (Figure 9–3). In most people, the left hemisphere tends to be responsible for language and speech production, and the right hemisphere is responsible for nonverbal and paralinguistic skills and emotional processing (Kheirkhah et al., 2021). Although these are distinct entities, the hemispheres of your brain are connected by the corpus callosum, which allows both sides of the brain to communicate with one another. The corpus callosum is crucial because it allows the two hemispheres of the brain to operate contralaterally. This means that the right hemisphere controls the left side of your body, and the left hemisphere controls the right side of your body. So, when your right arm goes to scratch your leg, the movement is being controlled by the motor regions and processed by the sensory regions in your left hemisphere.

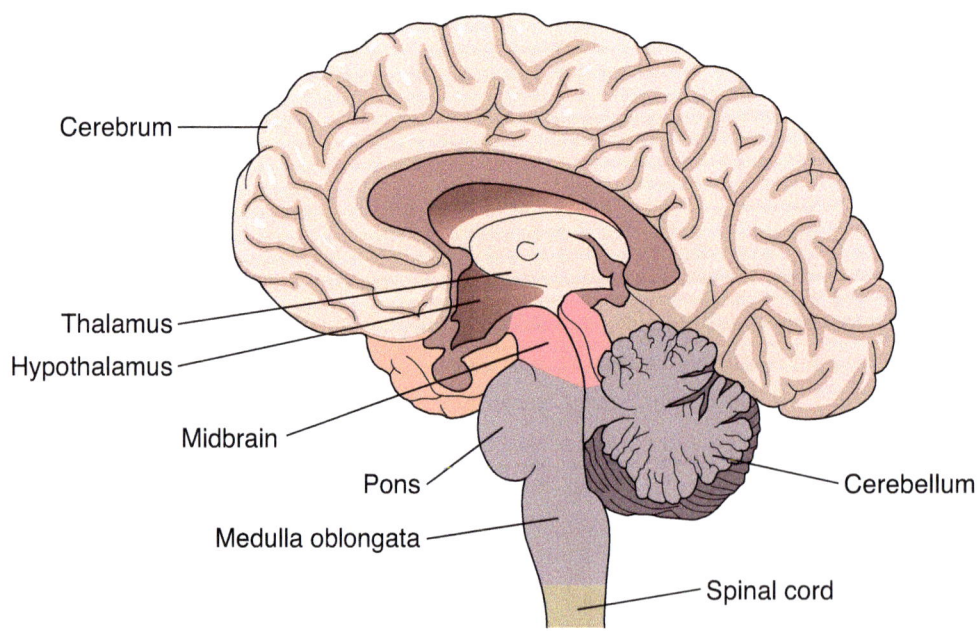

FIGURE 9–2. Cerebrum, cerebellum, and brainstem. *Source:* From *Motor Speech Disorders: Diagnosis and Treatment, Fourth Edition* by Freed, D. B. Copyright © 2025 Plural Publishing, Inc. All rights reserved.

Lobes of the Brain

The cerebrum consists of four lobes, which are symmetrical across the left and the right hemispheres (Figure 9–4). The frontal lobe, located in the front part of the brain, houses the prefrontal cortex and the motor cortex. The frontal lobe is important for **executive functions**, including planning and reasoning. Also located in the frontal lobe is **Broca's area**, which plays a role in the production of language. The

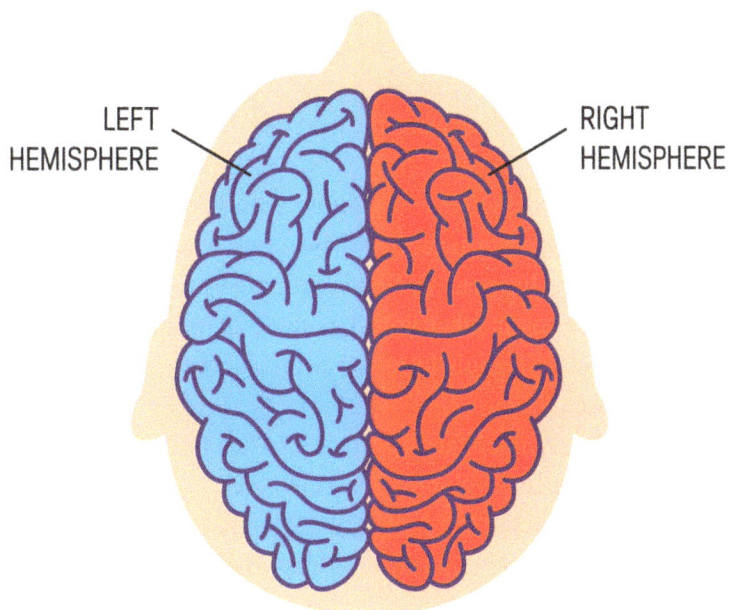

FIGURE 9–3. Hemispheres of the brain. *Source:* © Adobe Stock.

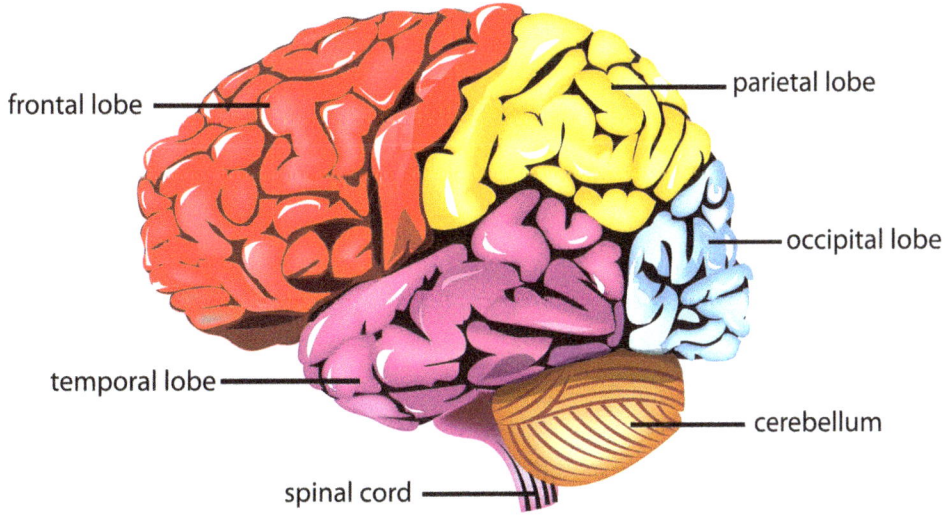

FIGURE 9–4. Lobes of the brain. *Source:* © Adobe Stock.

parietal lobe can be found behind the frontal lobe and includes the **somatosensory cortex**. The parietal lobe processes sensory information, such as perception of touch, as well as visuospatial information. The temporal lobe is located on the side and bottom of the cerebrum (near the "temples") and contains the **auditory cortex** and **Wernicke's area**. The auditory cortex is responsible for recognizing auditory information, and Wernicke's area is crucial for understanding language. The final lobe in the cerebrum, the occipital lobe, is located at the back of the brain, above the cerebellum. Housed in the occipital lobe is the **visual cortex**, which is necessary to decode incoming visual stimuli.

As you may have noticed, two of the lobes play a bigger role in language processing than the other two. That's right—the frontal and temporal lobes are particularly vital for how we understand and produce language, and that is because they contain Broca's area and Wernicke's area, both of which are in the left hemisphere. Let's take a closer look at what these structures do and how they interact with other brain structures.

First, auditory information is processed in the auditory cortex (in the temporal lobe) and gets sent to Broca's area (in the frontal lobe), where it is temporarily stored in working memory. At the same time, processing of linguistic information happens in Wernicke's area (also in the temporal lobe). Then, for language production, Broca's area sends what is being stored in working memory to the motor cortex (in the frontal lobe), which transmits signals to motor neurons responsible for speech. This is how we comprehend and produce language.

Now that we have a foundational understanding of the role that the brain plays in language processing, and we are familiar with what language development looks like in children through adults (see Chapter 7), we can dive into what abnormal language can look like in adults. In the following sections, we describe four acquired language and cognitive communication disorders in adults: aphasia, right hemisphere disorder, traumatic brain injury, and dementia.

Aphasia

One of the most common language disorders in adults is **aphasia**. When a person has an aphasia, they typically present with impairments in comprehending and/or producing written and spoken language (and their intellectual functioning is intact). One recent area of research has focused on a relatively new and common form of written communication (i.e., texting) and has found that although individuals with aphasia do text to communicate (and there are many advantages to this type of interaction), success with texting appears to be dependent on the severity of the aphasia (Lee & Cherney, 2022). Aphasia is most often caused by a stroke or brain damage that affects the specific language regions of the brain. In fact, one-third of stroke survivors have a resulting aphasia (Flowers et al., 2021), although the number varies depending on the socioeconomic status of the country, with higher income countries reporting aphasia resulting from stroke more often than middle-income countries; no data are available for low-income countries (Frederick et al., 2022).

Language consists of both comprehension and production. So, when injury results in damage to Broca's area, we see one type of aphasia, and when injury results in damage to Wernicke's area, we see another type of aphasia. And, you guessed it, when damage impacts both Wernicke's and Broca's areas, we see yet *another* type of aphasia. Because language processing is not confined neatly to these areas, aphasia can result from damage to other areas of the brain as well. Like other conditions, aphasia symptomology is widespread and ranges from mild to severe. Resulting severity is largely dependent on the site of the damage, the size of the lesion, as well as the age and health status of the person when they sustained the injury. Because of this, aphasia will look different for each person affected, despite there being commonalities that help characterize each aphasia type (e.g., Broca's aphasia, Wernicke's aphasia—more on this later). Although there is debate about the utility of the classification system of aphasia because not all aphasic language impairments fit nicely into these categories (Sheppard & Sebastian, 2021), we describe the aphasias in this way for the purpose of understanding, in general, how these aphasias present in clinical populations. That is, there are certain symptoms that tend to be representative of each type of aphasia. In addition to the type, aphasias are typically classified as fluent or nonfluent.

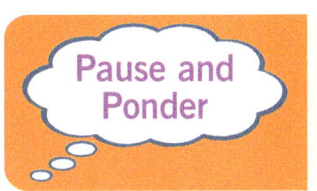 Can you recall which areas of the brain are primarily responsible for comprehension and production?

Fluent Aphasia

As the name implies, a person with a fluent aphasia has fluent speech. This means that in terms of the flow of verbal output, the speech stream of a person with a fluent aphasia sounds smooth and effortless. That is not to say that their verbal output is unaffected. In fact, it is quite the opposite. Although a person with a fluent aphasia may be loquacious (i.e., quite talkative) and follow the rules of syntax, their verbal (or written) output tends to be replete with word substitutions and novel/invented words (i.e., **neologisms**). Although fluent aphasias tend to have these main features in common, there are four types of fluent aphasia, each with its own unique characteristics: Wernicke's, anomic, conduction, and transcortical sensory aphasia.

Wernicke's aphasia results from damage to Wernicke's area in the temporal lobe and is primarily characterized by impaired auditory comprehension. Deficits in this area range from mild to severe. In addition, the language output of persons with Wernicke aphasia is impacted. Because Wernicke's aphasia is a fluent aphasia, expressive language is verbose, sounds smooth, and is grammatically appropriate. Moreover, individuals with Wernicke's aphasia speak confidently and effortlessly, with appropriate stress and intonation patterns. Although their language sounds smooth and effortless, it is often rife with neologisms, jargon, and word substitutions, often making their verbal messages incomprehensible (of course depending on the severity of the aphasia). People with Wernicke's aphasia are often described as having empty speech because despite using grammatically correct sentence structures and connecting words (e.g., articles, prepositions), content words are often replaced with words such as "thing" and "stuff." In addition, individuals with Wernicke's aphasia have little awareness of their errors.

Anomic aphasia is characterized primarily by difficulties with word retrieval (i.e., **anomia**) and occurs because of damage to the temporal and parietal lobes. Anomia involves the person knowing and understanding the word they want to say but not being able to retrieve the word in the moment (e.g., saying "cat" when intending to say "dog," pausing frequently to think of the correct word, correcting their own word productions). Although anomia is a core feature of all aphasia types, an anomic aphasia is classified as such when anomia is the only obvious deficit and there are no impairments in auditory comprehension or verbal speech production.

Conduction aphasia is another type of fluent aphasia that, unlike Wernicke's aphasia, is characterized by mild language comprehension with more severe impaired repetition, particularly repetition of multisyllabic and complex words. Whereas repetition is impacted, spontaneous speech tends to be preserved, although word-retrieval difficulties and word substitutions can also occur (e.g., saying "cup" for "bowl"). Conduction aphasia results primarily from damage to the upper temporal and lower parietal lobes.

Transcortical sensory aphasia results from damage to the upper parietal lobe, particularly the parietal–occipital–temporal junction. Some individuals with transcortical sensory aphasia appear like those with Wernicke's aphasia with regard to their comprehension of spoken language and obliviousness of their speech errors. Unlike Wernicke's aphasia, however, those with transcortical sensory aphasia demonstrate intact repetition skills and often will repeat words and phrases spontaneously (this is often described as echolalia).

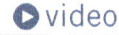

Check out the YouTube video **"Fluent Aphasia (Wernicke's Aphasia)"** featuring Byron, who presents with a fluent aphasia.

Nonfluent Aphasia

Contrasted with fluent aphasias, nonfluent aphasias are characterized by jolted and halting speech. The language output of persons with fluent aphasia is often slow and laborious, making speech sound production effortful. Nonfluent aphasias tend to have these main features in common; however, there are three main types of nonfluent aphasia, each with its own unique characteristics: Broca's, transcortical motor, and global aphasia.

Broca's aphasia results from damage to Broca's area in the frontal lobe. Many of the features of Broca's aphasia are in direct opposition of what we see in Wernicke's aphasia. As such, Broca's aphasia is characterized by slow and halted speech, and utterances are often limited to one or two words. Moreover, these utterances tend to be **agrammatical** (i.e., having incorrect grammatical structure). Remember how in Wernicke's aphasia connective words (e.g., articles, function words) are intact and content words are impacted? Well, in Broca's aphasia, we tend to see the opposite: Content words tend to be preserved, and connective words are often omitted. Comprehension of language is better than expressive language, and individuals with Broca's aphasia are often aware of their compromised language output.

Transcortical motor aphasia results from damage to the frontal lobe and is characterized by challenges initiating speech spontaneously, which results in reduced verbal output. Like transcortical sensory aphasia, repetition of words and sentences is intact; however, unlike transcortical sensory aphasia, individuals with transcortical motor aphasia have good language comprehension abilities.

Global aphasia is the final aphasia that we discuss. This type of aphasia results from damage to much of the left hemisphere and is characterized by widespread language difficulties in both receptive and expressive modalities. This type of aphasia resembles both fluent and nonfluent aphasias. Despite these challenges, individuals with global aphasia tend to be attentive and can perform nonverbal tasks.

▶ video

Check out the YouTube video **"Broca's Aphasia (Non-Fluent Aphasia)"** featuring Mike, who presents with a nonfluent aphasia.

Another type of aphasia that does not fall under any of these classifications is **primary progressive aphasia** (PPA). Unlike the aphasias discussed so far, PPA is a neurodegenerative condition that is not caused by a specific event or brain injury. In its initial presentation, symptoms associated with PPA are solely language-based, beginning with mild word-finding difficulties and progressing to more severe difficulties in word retrieval and comprehension. In addition, recent research suggests that almost half of individuals with PPA have a co-occurring motor speech disorder (Staiger et al., 2023). After an average of 5 years, and unlike individuals with other aphasias, persons with PPA tend to experience decline in other mental faculties, including memory, attention, and executive functioning.

Causes

As we described the classification system of aphasia, we noted which areas of the brain (generally) resulted in each kind of aphasia. Again, this way of classifying aphasia can be helpful for learning about the disorder, but keep in mind the limitations of such a system. Because the brain is so complex and the structures and neuronal pathways are so integrated with one another, it is highly likely that no two persons with any one type of aphasia will look entirely alike. Moreover, a person might present with symptoms that do not fall neatly into any of the aphasia types. Clinicians must take care to treat the person's symptoms instead of their classification.

As you may have guessed, there are many ways in which a person can sustain brain damage resulting in an aphasia. The leading cause of aphasia is brain damage because of a stroke. **Ischemic strokes** occur when blood flow to the brain is disrupted due to a complete or partial block in the artery. This blockage can occur from an embolism (e.g., blood clot, plaque buildup) or the thickening of the artery wall. **Hemorrhagic strokes** occur when arteries or blood vessels burst, which causes bleeding on the exterior of the brain or inside of the brain tissues. Another potential cause of aphasia is a brain injury if the injury is localized to one of the language domains in the brain. When the brain injury is more global, patients are often diagnosed with other clinical conditions (e.g., traumatic brain injury, discussed later), although they may still present with aphasia-like symptoms.

Impact of Aphasia Across the Lifespan

We hope that it is clear by this point that aphasia is a disorder of language and does not have any impact on a person's cognitive functioning or intellect (aside, of course, from PPA). However, damage to brain areas associated with language function may also result in total or partial weakness or paralysis, as well as dysphagia (see Chapter 12). In addition, aphasia may be accompanied by visual impairments and seizure disorders.

Because of the main causes of aphasia (e.g., stroke), this is a condition that occurs primarily in adults (as opposed to children and adolescents). When a person experiences a stroke, and they are aware that they are having one, medical help is usually solicited. Although mortality differs between ischemic and hemorrhagic stroke (Sennfält et al., 2018), people who survive their first stroke often have subsequent strokes that lead to further brain damage, resulting in greater chance of death, and undergo myriad changes in functioning. Some people who have a stroke experience a period of unconsciousness, and the length of time a person is unconscious is associated with overall prognosis and recovery. Those who remain or become conscious within a short period of time receive care for various aspects of functioning, including speech/language, mental health, and physical mobility.

In addition to potentially impacting one's ability to return to work, another consequence of aphasia is reduced or impaired social functioning. Language is one of the primary ways that we connect with others. When language functioning is intact one day and impaired the next, this can result in frustration and lead to disconnect with friends and family. A person with aphasia may have a reduced desire to interact with others and experience a sense of failure when their message is not communicated correctly. Moreover, old friends may not understand how the stroke and resulting aphasia have impacted the person and why they may be acting in ways that they had not before. This lack of social connection can result in increased loneliness and heightened psychological and emotional distress (Dalemans et al., 2010).

Furthermore, individuals with aphasia may experience an accompanying sense of concern for their loved ones who are also living with the effects of this abrupt shift in their lives (Baker et al., 2020). Because aphasia is a language disorder resulting from sudden onset, families must adjust to their loved one not having the same linguistic competencies as they once did. This can be confusing and frustrating to families and result in loneliness and decreased connection to their loved one. In addition, significant others of persons with aphasia report greater financial challenges, increased household responsibilities, more physical health-related problems, a reduction in time spent working, and less time available for leisure activities (either alone or with their spouse; Johansson et al., 2020). Consider, for example, a wife of a husband with a newfound diagnosis of aphasia. Perhaps the husband's household duties included managing the care of the property (e.g., hiring and calling a company to mow the lawn, plow the snow, and tend to flowers) and grocery shopping. In addition to the stroke negatively impacting his mobility and ability to drive, he is unable to make phone calls. Now, household responsibilities that were once shared fall primarily on the wife. Her social interactions with her husband have also changed. Where they once would chat and connect over morning coffee, they now are faced with feeding and dressing issues. Talking about current events, usually over dinner, is now a thing of the past, and the wife finds that her social network outside of her family has also diminished.

Right Hemisphere Disorder

As we have just learned, damage to the left hemisphere of the brain often results in language-specific deficits associated with aphasia. But what happens when the right hemisphere incurs damage? Recall that the left hemisphere is generally responsible for linguistic information, and the right hemisphere is generally responsible for nonlinguistic information (e.g., nonverbal and paralinguistic skills, emotional processing, pragmatic skills; Kheirkhah et al., 2021). Instead of deficits in language at the syntactic, morphological, and phonological levels, deficits from right hemisphere brain damage tend to be related to *how* the person communicates. Recall that although we communicate through linguistic processes, much of our communication relies on nonlinguistic information. This includes gestures, facial expressions, body language, prosody, and tone of voice. Individuals who have **right hemisphere disorder** (RHD) exhibit deficits in the appropriate use of these nonverbal skills, including prosody. In addition, persons with RHD exhibit breakdowns in linguistic processes of communication, particularly as it relates to discourse and comprehension (Parola et al., 2016). Estimates suggests that between 50% and 90% of people who sustain brain damage in the right hemisphere experience at least some deficits in their communicative abilities (Ferré & Joanette, 2016).

Discourse refers to the exchanging of ideas through either verbal or written means. Engaging in conversation with another person is considered conversational discourse. When engaging in conversational discourse, individuals with RHD are challenged to maintain the topic of conversation, often conversing in tangential and egocentric ways. They also may fail to suppress irrelevant information, which results in disorganized and sometimes repetitive communication. Moreover, context is important during conversations. That is, we modify our communication based on a variety of factors, including who we are talking to, where we are, and how familiar our listener is with the topic. Adapting communication based on contextual cues such as these may be challenging for those with RHD. Comprehension of language is also impaired, particularly as it relates to discourse. Determining the meaning of sentences and conversational utterances relies on understanding the context in which information is shared and often requires making inferences about the intended meaning of an utterance. Many words have multiple meanings, such as "bat," "date," and "novel," and the way that we figure out the meaning of the word is often through the context of the sentence. For example, if I were to say, "I saw a bat at the zoo," you would likely conclude that I was talking about the animal "bat" instead of the baseball "bat" because of the context in which I saw the bat (i.e., the zoo). The ability to use relevant contextual information in a sentence to determine the meaning of a multimeaning word is more challenging for those with RHD, impacting their ability to follow along during conversational discourse. Similarly, understanding nonliteral language, such as idioms, humor, and metaphors, can be a challenge in this population.

Communication is not the only area that is affected in those with RHD. Cognitive impairments include deficits in executive functioning skills such as attention, memory, inhibition, reasoning, and problem-solving. Attentional deficits include difficulty sustaining attention and reduced attention to detail, as well as difficulty attending to information on the left side. This is referred to as left-side neglect, which is evidenced by the individual being unable to attend to information or stimuli coming in from the left side. An example of this is presented in Figure 9–5.

Individuals with RHD may also have co-occurring **dysphagia**, **dysarthria**, and emotional disorders. They may present with flat affect or reduced emotional expression, as well as **aprosodia** (i.e., challenges with comprehending or using pitch and intonation to express emotional information).

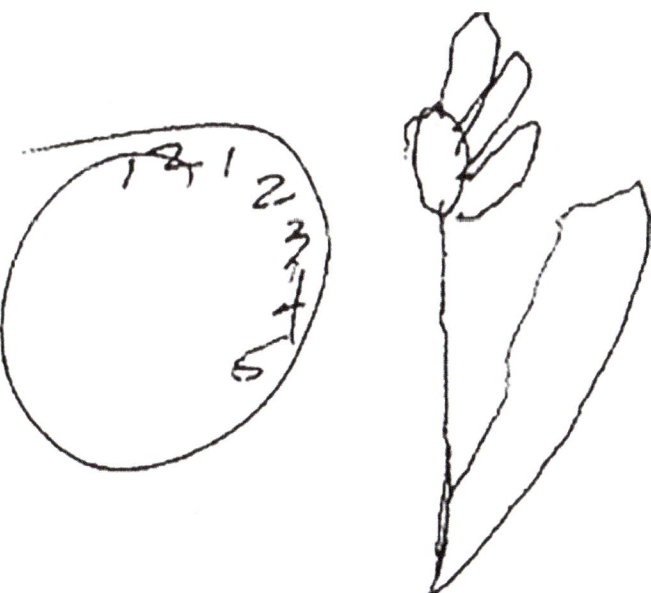

FIGURE 9–5. Left-side neglect. *Source:* © Elsevier.

Causes

Like aphasia, the primary cause of right hemisphere brain damage is stroke; however, it can result from other brain complications. This includes brain tumors and infections, brain surgery, seizures, as well as external insult to the brain (discussed further in the section on traumatic brain injury).

Impact of Right Hemisphere Brain Injury Across the Lifespan

Like aphasia, adults are more likely to experience RHD compared to children. This makes sense given the most common cause of RHD is stroke. Right hemisphere brain injury can impact more than just a person's ability to communicate. Because damage to the right hemisphere impacts more of the nonlinguistic processes associated with communication, a person with damage to this area may experience a variety of social challenges when interacting with others. Evidence suggests that persons with RHD have difficulty identifying facial emotions, particularly facial expressions other than happiness (Álvarez-Fernández et al., 2023). This may impact the ways in which the person interacts with and responds to others' emotions, such that they may not properly decode the nonverbal messages that another person is conveying and may respond inappropriately. Due to the cognitive communication deficits, as well as the visual–spatial neglect, associated with RHD, an individual might experience a loss of independence in their ability to hold a job and complete tasks of daily living. Moreover, individuals with RHD are at an increased risk for developing depression (Wei et al., 2015).

Although not much research has been done on the impacts of caring for an adult with RHD, it can be speculated that these caregivers face similar challenges to those of caregivers of adults with aphasia. To address this area of need, Davidson (2019) conducted a qualitative study examining the needs of primary caregivers (i.e., unpaid family members) in this population. Not surprisingly, results suggested that family members need different information during the various stages of recovery, including general information about RHD and the associated deficits, information about treatment and compensatory strategies, and clear and tangible medical information from health care providers.

Traumatic Brain Injury

So far, we have discussed the language and/or cognitive communication challenges associated with damage to specific and localized areas of the brain as seen in individuals with aphasia and RHD. But what about brain damage that is more global? Although the brain damage that occurs in aphasia and RHD is technically considered "brain injury," the term **traumatic brain injury** (TBI) is specific to more global and diffuse damage to the brain. In this sense, a TBI generally occurs from some external force to the head, such as a fall or an assault. We tend to think about TBI in two ways: closed-head injury and open-head injury. Closed-head injuries occur when the brain is jolted back and forth inside of the skull (and thus the skull remains closed and intact) and often result in swelling of the brain. Open-head injuries, as you might have guessed, occur when an external object strikes the skull and enters the brain tissue (e.g., a bullet or a weapon). Damage from an open-head injury tends to be more focused and localized to the specific area that was struck.

Not all head injuries result in the same severity of damage. TBIs are generally classified on a severity scale of mild, moderate, and severe; the majority of TBIs (roughly 90%) are mild (this includes concussions resulting from injury). A person who experiences a mild TBI will present in a clinically different way from someone who sustains a more severe TBI. The resulting severity of a TBI often has to do with the person's level of consciousness or post-traumatic amnesia. Four main levels of consciousness are described in the literature, and a person with a TBI may experience one or more of these states, depending on the extent of the injury: coma, vegetative state, minimally conscious state, and post-traumatic confusional state. Table 9–1 highlights the key features in various domains at each consciousness level.

Because of the diffuse damage resulting from a TBI, the person usually experiences a variety of changes in their functioning. These include disruptions in behavioral/psychological, physical/sensory, and cognitive functioning. People with a TBI may experience changes in mood and have increased feelings of anger, anxiety, and/or depression. They may experience episodes of dizziness, fainting, or seizures, as well as reduced balance and sensitivity to lights or sounds. A person with a TBI may also experience a co-occurring motor speech and/or swallowing disorder. The language impairments associated with TBI are often secondary to deficits in cognitive skills, such as attention and memory. For this reason, TBI is not considered to result in a language disorder but, rather, a cognitive communication disorder. A person who sustains a TBI generally experiences cognitive deficits associated with executive functioning, including attention, memory, planning, self-monitoring, inhibitory control, and goal-directed behaviors.

TABLE 9–1. Characteristics of Levels of Consciousness Resulting From a Traumatic Brain Injury

Level of Consciousness	Attention/Arousal	Cognition	Language	Motor
Coma	No sleep–wake cycles Eyes closed	—	—	Primary reflexes
Vegetative state	Periodic bouts of wakefulness	—	—	Involuntary movement
Minimally conscious state	Periodic bouts of wakefulness	Some awareness of self and environment	Inconsistency in following one-step directions Production of single words or short phrases	Nonreflexive responses to certain environmental stimuli Manipulation of objects
Post-traumatic confusional state	Extended bouts of wakefulness	Confusion Disorientation	Consistency in following one-step directions Production of sentences (albeit often confused and perseverative) Appropriate responses to yes/no questions	Functional use of objects

Source: Adapted from Giacino et al. (2014).

The secondary language challenges tend to be in areas that rely on executive functions, such as difficulties with word retrieval and auditory/reading comprehension. Moreover, deficits in inhibitory control often result in social cognitive impairments particularly related to conversational discourse. These challenges are similar to those seen in persons with RHD and include disorganized language output, difficulty with turn-taking during conversations, challenges with facial emotion recognition and using and understanding prosody and other nonverbal cues, as well as an overall impaired ability to navigate social interactions. Evidence also suggests that those with severe TBI may have difficulty assessing their communication partner's knowledge, as well as adjusting their verbal output based on the communication partner's verbal or nonverbal feedback (Rousseaux et al., 2010).

Causes

The most common causes of TBI are falls and motor vehicle accidents, as well as hits to the head (as happens in sports) and assaults. According to U.S. data, in 2020, more than 200,000 individuals were hospitalized after sustaining a TBI, and roughly 70,000 people died from TBI-related injuries. Hospitalization- and death-related TBIs were most prevalent in individuals older than age 75 years. Note, however, that these data do not account for TBIs that did not result in hospitalization or death. Children aged 0 to 4 years and adults older than age 75 years tend to experience TBIs at a higher rate than the rest of the population. This is because young children and older adults are more vulnerable to falling. Adolescents and young adults (ages 15–24 years) tend to have TBIs related to motor vehicle accidents, and males are more likely to get a TBI in their lifetime compared to females (Faul & Coronado, 2015). In addition, it is important to note that a concussion is a form of a TBI.

Impact of Traumatic Brain Injury Across the Lifespan

The effects of TBI can be far-reaching and pervasive throughout a person's lifetime and experiences. The accompanying social cognitive challenges can significantly impact a person's relationships with others, including family, friends, and employers and colleagues, which can directly impact their ability to get or keep a job, enjoy recreational activities, and connect with loved ones. This reduction in the ability to socially connect has negative consequences, such as increased loneliness and depression, negative beliefs about oneself, and more social withdrawal. Evidence suggests that these negative consequences can last for 10 to 20 years (or more) after the person's injury (Finch et al., 2016). The negative consequences of a TBI also impact the person's loved ones, who have described the changes associated with a TBI to be challenging and often tiring to manage. Loved ones may also feel embarrassed by the newfound social inappropriateness of the person with a TBI (Wiseman-Hakes et al., 2020) and must learn to cope with changes in the family dynamic and roles and responsibilities.

Dementia

Language functioning can be negatively impacted by direct trauma to specific brain structures, but that's not all. Adults who experience a slow decline in cognitive functioning over time endure language losses that may be commensurate with those described already. **Dementia**, which has been relabeled in the fifth edition of the *Diagnostic and Statistical Manual of Mental Disorders* (American Psychiatric Association, 2013) as major neurocognitive disorder, is diagnosed when a person has significant decline in one or more of the following cognitive functions: complex attention, executive ability, learning and memory, language, perceptual–motor–visual perception, praxis, and/or social cognition. If the patient's decline in these skills is significant and interferes with their daily functioning and independence, they are diagnosed with a major neurocognitive disorder (also known as dementia); if their decline in these skills is mild to moderate and does not interfere with daily functioning and independence, they receive a slightly lesser diagnosis of minor neurocognitive disorder (also referred to as mild cognitive impairment). Of note, these symptoms cannot be due to any other mental health condition.

Causes

Dementia affects roughly 35 million people throughout the world (Prince et al., 2013), and there is no single cause of dementia. Despite this, the location in the brain where neurological changes occur can help determine the type of dementia—**Alzheimer's disease, frontotemporal dementia, Lewy body dementia, Parkinson's disease, Huntington's disease**, and so on. Numerous risk factors are also associated with dementia, including old age, lower socioeconomic status, certain medical (e.g., cardiovascular disease, stroke) and psychiatric (e.g., depressions, post-traumatic stress disorder) conditions, smoking, and excessive consumption of alcohol. Furthermore, there is also a genetic component to dementia (Hugo & Ganguli, 2014), as well as family history. The most common type of dementia is Alzheimer's disease (AD); as such, we focus on describing the symptoms associated with AD for this chapter.

Alzheimer's Disease

Alzheimer's disease has been reported to be the most common neurodegenerative disease and is responsible for the most hospital, skilled nursing facility, and home health care admissions (Hugo & Ganguli, 2014). In addition, in 2010, AD was among the top 10 leading causes of death in the United States (Murphy et al., 2013). Because AD is a progressive neurodegenerative condition, a person's symptoms change as the disease progresses. Individuals with early stage AD may present with some mild cognitive deficits (particularly regarding memory) and social communicative challenges (e.g., repeating information, veering off topic, offering irrelevant information in a conversation), but their language is usually relatively intact or only mildly impacted. A person in this stage may present with some word-finding difficulties and have reduced comprehension of complex language, but their grammatical structures tend to be preserved. Individuals with middle-stage AD tend to present with more severe memory loss and language and conversational difficulties, including more severe word-finding challenges and an increase in agrammatical and fragmented utterances. It is at this stage that individuals start to withdraw from conversations and let others take the lead in interactions. They also have more difficulty following the "rules" of conversation, particularly as it relates to turn-taking. Finally, when a person enters the late stage of AD, their deficits in memory significantly impact their functioning. Their communication consists of empty speech, single-word utterances, and incoherent phrases. In the very late stages, the person stops using language altogether. In addition to memory and language losses, a person in this stage of AD presents with emotional and personality changes. They may have overall mood changes, such as increased agitation and anxiety, and these behavioral manifestations are commonly associated with caregiver burden.

Impact of Dementia Across the Lifespan

Having a diagnosis of a dementia not only impacts the person with the disorder but also significantly affects family members and loved ones (Savundranayagam et al., 2005). Spouses and adult children often experience a shift in their familial role as the relationship drastically changes over time. Spouses often report that they miss the rich and meaningful conversations that they had with their partner pre-dementia, such as sharing about their day or talking about current events. Moreover, there is usually less reciprocity in the conversations, especially as the disease progresses, and caregivers and loved ones may find themselves responsible for initiating and maintaining conversations. To further complicate the shift in the relationship, family members are now unable to seek guidance or comfort from their loved one with dementia.

Assessment

Assessment is crucial for designing an individualized intervention plan for each client with an adult language or cognitive communication disorder. Many assessment components will look the same regardless of the exact language or cognitive communication disorder. For this reason, we discuss the general components for assessment that are crucial regardless of whether the person has aphasia, RHD, TBI, or dementia (or any other adult disorder of communication). Along the way, we describe parts of the assessment that are specific to aphasia, RHD, TBI, and dementia.

Assessment and treatment of a person who presents with an acquired language or cognitive communication disorder are best completed by a team of professionals spanning numerous disciplines. The team may include a neurologist, SLP, physical therapist, occupational therapist, nutritionist, and psychologist or social worker. These team members will play valuable roles throughout the person's recovery or decline. An SLP will be a vital member of the assessment team because they can screen and assess information related to speech, language, swallowing function, and certain areas of cognition. As always, it is important to collect assessment data before beginning any treatment because this will provide important information on the client's baseline functioning and which treatment approaches will be the most appropriate. An SLP's assessment may depend on the severity of the language disorder and co-occurring conditions. However, a thorough assessment should be completed using the *International Classification of Functioning, Disability and Health* (ICF) framework (World Health Organization, 2001). This framework considers not only the person's impairments but also how their health condition interacts with other co-occurring conditions, the person's environment, and personal factors to offer a comprehensive picture of the person's functional limitations to participating in meaningful and purposeful communicative activities. The overall goal of assessment through the ICF framework is to support the person's quality of life.

Two crucial components of the assessment process that are always necessitated are a patient/caregiver interview and observation. A background of the patient's medical history can also be useful for determining treatment because it will likely offer information about prior medical concerns (e.g., previous strokes) that could impact prognosis and success of any intervention. A thorough medical history should also include information about the patient's past or present mental health conditions; cognitive, linguistic, physical, or motor speech impairments; and chronic pain. This information provides the SLP with an overview of the patient's strengths and challenges at the current moment, as well as prior to their injury, so that realistic expectations for recovery are ensured. The interview with the client and family is necessary to understand their goals and priorities and what they value most in terms of communicating and interacting with their loved one. During this time, the SLP should also provide guidance to the patient and family regarding what to expect in terms of speech, language, communication, and swallowing abilities in both the short-term and long-term recovery.

As previously mentioned, another important component of an assessment involves gathering data on factors unrelated to the language or cognitive communication disorder that may impact recovery, including environmental or personal factors (World Health Organization, 2001). This includes the external support (e.g., family members, friends, community) the client has outside of the medical team, as well as their communication partners' willingness and ability to accept and use the recommended facilitating strategies to support communication.

Aphasia

Recall that aphasia results from localized brain damage, often due to a stroke for which a person (it is hoped) receives medical assistance right away. The aftermath of a stroke can leave a person with a variety of diminished levels of functioning. Although an SLP cannot diagnose stroke, through careful assessment, they can provide a clinical diagnosis of aphasia. After interviewing the patient and their caregiver(s) and careful observation of residual speech and language skills, the SLP must perform an oral mechanism exam to determine strengths and weaknesses of the client's muscles involved in speech production. Although aphasia is purely a disorder of language, an oral mechanism exam can help provide information regarding any co-occurring speech disorders that are common with aphasia, including motor speech disorders (see Chapter 6); this will aid in the SLP's differential diagnosis, which ultimately supports treatment planning.

Spontaneous recovery of skills is common within the time frame directly following the stroke (Sheppard & Sebastian, 2021), which can make formalized assessment tricky. Patients may make substantive improvements in language skills without any intervention at all during the acute (the first 2 weeks post-stroke) and subacute (3–11 weeks post-stroke) stages of recovery compared to the chronic phase (often defined as 6 months post-stroke; Sheppard & Sebastian, 2021; Wu et al., 2015). Because of this, formalized assessment should be delayed until the patient's speech/language skills have stabilized; however, the SLP can gather informal data on the client's receptive and expressive language skills daily. When the client's skills appear to stabilize after a period (this can be as soon as a few days), the SLP can begin a more formal assessment of their language abilities. As you might imagine based on the symptoms associated with aphasia, a formal aphasia assessment will provide insight into the patient's expressive and receptive language, including abilities related to word finding, labeling, repetition of words and sentences, spontaneous language output, and following directions. Literacy skills (i.e., reading and writing) are also typically assessed, as are social communication skills (e.g., greetings, turn-taking in conversations). It is best if these skills are assessed across contexts.

Two common formalized assessment methods used to diagnose aphasia are the Western Aphasia Battery–Revised (WAB-R; Kertesz, 2006) and the Boston Diagnostic Aphasia Examination–Third Edition (BDAE-3; Goodglass et al., 2000). These standardized assessments are useful in determining aphasia type, highlighting which areas of language are preserved and impaired, and differentially diagnosing aphasia from other related conditions.

As with all assessments, interpretation of results is key. That is, the SLP should not simply take the patient's responses at face value and attribute them to their language disorder. The SLP must decide if the patient's response was a result of the aphasia or perhaps something else. For example, did the patient fail to verbally repeat the sentence correctly because of deficits in repetition or did they mishear the sentence?

Right Hemisphere Disorder

As with aphasia, assessment of RHD relies on an interprofessional team, which includes (but is not limited to) neurology, SLP, and physical therapy. In addition to the common evaluation techniques described previously (e.g., case history), SLP assessment will include an oral mechanism exam, a language and cognitive communication skills evaluation, and assessment of swallowing. Language assessment will specifically include expressive and receptive skills related to discourse; use and understanding of prosody, intonation, and nonverbal behaviors; as well as more general social communication abilities. Assessment of cognitive communication skills includes gathering information about a person's executive functioning abilities, including attention, memory, inhibition, and problem-solving. Some formal assessment measures have been designed to assess the broad range of pragmatic skills in RHD. The Assessment Battery for Communication (ABaCo; Sacco et al., 2008) includes subscales measuring the comprehension and production of facial expressions and gestures, prosody, discourse, and nonliteral language. Other assessments have been used to examine discourse skills in persons with right hemisphere damage, including the Discourse Comprehension Test (DCT; Brookshire & Nicholas, 1993).

Traumatic Brain Injury

Assessment of TBI is completed by a similar interprofessional team as described for the previous disorders in that it includes physicians, neurologists, psychologists, physical therapists, and SLPs. Typically, gathering information on the person's level of consciousness and post-traumatic amnesia is one of the first areas of assessment. This assessment provides information about the client's current state of functioning, and measures of post-traumatic amnesia have been found to be predictive of long-term cognitive outcomes (Tenovuo et al., 2021). The SLP's role in assessment of TBI includes the assessment of language, cognitive communication, social communication, and swallowing abilities. Because those with TBI generally follow stages of recovery and move through levels of consciousness, it is paramount that assessment be continuous and ongoing. This will ensure that any intervention matches the patient's current level of functioning to support optimal recovery. When conducting a communication assessment, the SLP must consider all aspects of language and cognitive communication abilities. For this reason, a comprehensive battery of tests is crucial, as is observation of skill in naturalistic contexts. Recall that social communication abilities tend to be the most severely affected part of language in persons with TBI. For this reason, SLPs must perform a thorough assessment of social communication so that intervention can lead to functional outcomes. This includes discourse analysis, the Montreal Evaluation of Communication (MEC; Joanette et al., 2015), the La Trobe Communication Questionnaire (Douglas et al., 2007), and the Adapted Kagan Scales (Togher et al., 2010; for a description of each assessment method, see Moore Sohlberg et al., 2019).

Dementia

Assessment of dementia is also done by an interprofessional team. To determine cognitive functioning, physicians take into consideration medical history and perform a variety of tests, including neurological exams, brain imaging, cognitive tests, and sometimes even blood or cerebrospinal fluid tests (Alzheimer's Association, 2023). Although unable to diagnose dementia, SLPs are also members of the interprofessional team who help determine the language functioning of the patient. It is important for SLPs to monitor language skills and deterioration over time because language and communication abilities decline as the dementia becomes more severe. To determine language skills in a patient with dementia, SLPs might use observational techniques, rating scales, caregiver interviews, as well as language-specific assessments that are designed for aphasia. Because the language assessments for aphasia cover various components of language, they are well suited to provide language-related information about a client with dementia. Note, however, that if a person with dementia scores in the clinical range on an assessment designed to detect aphasia, this does not mean that they have aphasia. These assessments are merely useful in detecting language skills throughout the person's dementia experience. There are also a few assessments that are designed to measure cognitive communication skills in dementia, including the Severe Impairment Battery–Language Scale (SIB; Saxton et al., 1993), the Arizona Battery for Communication Disorders–Second Edition (ABCD-2; Bayles & Tomoeda, 2020b), the Functional Linguistic Communication Inventory–Second Edition (FLCI-2; Bayles & Tomoeda, 2020a), and the Cognitive Linguistic Quick Test (CLQT: Helm-Estabrooks, 2001). However, these tools are not designed to measure a person's skills at different stages of dementia. In addition, not all assessment methods examine a person's functional communication skills, which is important for prioritizing goals that support the person's communication skills in real life (Dooley & Walshe, 2019). Moreover, assessment should include the communication and interaction skills of the caregiver because intervention for dementia often includes educating and training caregivers on how to interact with and support their loved one with dementia.

Cultural Considerations

Assessment of adult language and/or cognitive communication disorders must be sensitive to the patient's cultural background. Many of the standardized assessments discussed in this chapter incorporate pictures, topics, and specific questions that might not always be relevant to the patient's cultural experiences. When these tools are used without the knowledge that they may be culturally biased, it will be difficult to discern if the client has a communication disorder or if their performance is due to cultural differences. However, much of the assessment of language and cognitive communication disorders involves observation of the patient's abilities and social interactions in various environments. For this reason, it is paramount that the SLP have awareness of the social rules and nuances that are part of their client's cultural experiences and collaborate with the client's family so that the SLP does not provide treatment for a behavior that is socially appropriate in the client's culture. As such, some evidence suggests that when clinicians and clients come from different backgrounds, SLPs are more likely to rate a client's behavior as "inappropriate" when family members rate the behavior as "appropriate" (Baron et al., 2005). Care should be taken to incorporate family perspectives in the assessment process.

Intervention

Regardless of the communication disorder, the goal of intervention is most often to support the patient's participation in activities and with people who are important to them. This is true for adults with acquired language disorders too, although the approaches to supporting communication and participation will vary depending on the condition. In addition, as with intervention for all communication disorders, SLPs should adopt a patient-/family-centered approach to providing treatment. This means that the patient's/family's values and goals for intervention are incorporated and respected. Again, the key to designing the most appropriate intervention is conducting a thorough assessment. For adult language disorders, the two primary approaches to intervention are restorative and compensatory. **Restorative approaches** to intervention, also called **impairment-based approaches**, focus on improving skills that have been negatively affected, whereas **compensatory strategies** involve teaching strategies to help the patient compensate for any resulting deficits. Another type of approach to intervention is called **functional communication training**, which focuses on teaching communication that is most personally relevant and can include reducing barriers to communication and training caregivers to support their loved one's communication (Martin et al., 2008). Although clinicians and patients may prefer one method over the other, some conditions (particularly degenerative ones) may require more compensatory strategies due to the nature of the disorder. Using both restorative and compensatory strategies is usually optimal to support the person's overall functioning.

Aphasia

Remember how people who have a stroke usually have a period of spontaneous recovery and how SLPs should hold off on more formal assessments until the person's language abilities stabilize? The same is true for intervention. It is unclear whether language intervention in acute aphasia results in meaningful gains in language skills; however, once the patient's language skills post-stroke have stabilized, and the person is classified as having chronic aphasia, evidence suggests more positive effects resulting from targeted language intervention (Johnson et al., 2019). Intervention should be tailored to each client because each person with aphasia will have their own strengths and challenges. Moreover, it is unclear how success of intervention interacts with a patient's age, health status, education, or aphasia type, but recent evidence suggests that two factors are associated with language outcomes: age and severity of the aphasia. To elaborate, Kristinsson et al. (2023) found that younger adults with aphasia responded to language treatment better than older people with aphasia. It is also reported that the more severe the aphasia, the less positive language treatment outcomes are realized, either spontaneous or treatment-induced (Fridriksson & Hillis, 2021; Kristinsson et al., 2023). Several restorative therapy options exist depending on the person's challenges. For example, many treatment approaches designed for use with people with aphasia target word-finding difficulties (e.g., semantic feature analysis, verb network strengthening treatment), producing grammatically correct sentences (e.g., treatment of underlying forms), and increasing fluency of speech (e.g., melodic intonation therapy). Therapies designed to support auditory comprehension can also be effective; however, the exact protocols for intervention remain unclear (Wallace et al., 2022).

From the lens of family- and patient-centered care, intervention should focus on what language and discourse skills are most important to the client. That is, if the client's goal is to be a better conversation partner, then targeting conversational discourse during therapy would be beneficial. Or perhaps the client's goal is to regain skills in sharing stories with others, in which case working on narrative discourse would be a prime target. For a more in-depth discussion of different types of discourse and how to support these areas in aphasia, we refer you to a clinical discussion by Leaman and Archer (2023).

Explore and Find Out!

Leaman, M., & Archer, B. (2023). Choosing discourse types that align with person-centered goals in aphasia rehabilitation: A clinical tutorial. *Perspectives of the ASHA Special Interest Groups, 8*, 254–273.

In addition to restorative practices, people with aphasia will benefit from compensatory strategies to support their language and communication. This includes, but is not limited to, using gestures, writing, and other visual supports instead of relying on purely verbal language output. Using augmentative and alternative communication (AAC) methods can be an excellent way to support the communication abilities of a person with aphasia. We discuss this in more depth in Chapter 14.

Individual, face-to-face therapy is not the only option for people who experience chronic aphasia. New modes of intervention are emerging, including group therapy, telehealth, and computerized therapy. Group therapy is often a component of the Life Participation Approach to Aphasia, which "focuses on increasing participation and re-engagement in life activities [and] empowers those affected by aphasia to be more actively involved in choosing how to participate in their recovery process" (Edmonds & Morgan, 2022, p. 2379). Group therapy provides a social network for people with aphasia where they can engage with others who have similar experiences. These group sessions may be guided by an SLP but led by and tailored to the needs of the members. In addition, caregivers may also attend these group sessions to support their loved ones or to find community themselves. Group models of intervention are useful not only for supporting language outcomes but also for increasing social interaction and supporting integration back into the community (Edmonds & Morgan, 2022; Elman, 2016). Another promising avenue for increasing access to therapy (either individualized or group) for persons with chronic aphasia is language therapy provided electronically through telehealth (Pitt et al., 2019; Woolf et al., 2016). Although more research is needed in this area, current evidence suggests that telehealth services for people with aphasia are comparable to face-to-face intervention and effective in supporting language outcomes (Teti et al., 2023). Computerized therapy can be a useful avenue for individuals who do not have access to clinics or telehealth services. Evidence suggests that self-administered computerized therapy can help support an individual's ability to correctly label items, their auditory comprehension, and general language outcomes, although more research is needed to understand the impacts of computerized therapy on functional communication (for a review, see Fridriksson & Hillis, 2021). Another newer area of research suggests that noninvasive brain stimulation, when paired with speech-language therapy, can also support language outcomes, including naming, repetition, comprehension, and response time (for a review, see Fredriksson & Hills, 2021).

Right Hemisphere Disorder

Despite being diagnosed with a cognitive communication disorder, only approximately half of persons with RHD are referred for speech-language intervention, and those who do receive services are treated primarily for swallowing and executive functioning challenges. Data suggest that services for language and social communication are far less prevalent despite social communication being a primary deficit in RHD (Lehman Blake et al., 2013). However, current evidence suggests that intervention to support prosody, discourse, and social communication may be promising for persons with RHD (for reviews, see Lehman Blake et al., 2013; Tompkins, 2012).

To target prosody in communication, two types of intervention have been used: motoric-imitative and cognitive-affective. Motoric-imitative treatment uses a motor planning approach in which the client produces an utterance in unison with the clinician. Cognitive-affective therapy involves photographs of emotions with descriptions of the verbal qualities associated with those emotions. A few studies have also examined the use of contextual training to support comprehension of sentence- and discourse-level production, particularly those involving multimeaning words (i.e., contextual prestimulation training; Thompkins et al., 2011). Moreover, narrative production training (including story retell and generation) has been used to facilitate narrative discourse (expressive language; Cannizzaro & Coelho, 2002). In addition, researchers have examined the effects of social skills interventions on persons with RHD. These interventions include video feedback, modeling, coaching, and rehearsal strategies to support attention and conversational discourse (Youse & Coelho, 2009). Because only a few studies have examined each of these interventions, more research is needed to determine their effectiveness.

Traumatic Brain Injury

Recall that individuals who sustain a TBI tend to progress through stages of recovery in which they experience periods of improvement as well as periods of no improvement. For this reason, intervention will look different at each stage of recovery. Treatment for someone in the earlier stages of recovery might focus on orienting and attending to familiar people and objects, whereas later intervention might focus on following directions, word learning/recall, cohesiveness of expressive language, and conversational turn-taking. Final stages of intervention support functional independence, which includes various aspects of social communication and cognitive skills associated with communication (e.g., attention, memory), as well as self-monitoring.

During intervention, the SLP must explore and consider the values and goals of the client and their caregivers. Patient and family collaboration is important in developing treatment plans, as is education about TBI and the recovery process (Hardin et al., 2021). Because patients with TBI progress through phases of improvement, SLPs may use restorative intervention approaches to increase functioning in certain skill areas. This may include strategies to improve attention and memory to support language and communication gains. Compensatory strategies are also used to aid in recovery, and these include supports such as memory logs (Barman et al., 2016).

One primary area of intervention for persons with TBI is social communication training. Sustaining a TBI negatively impacts a person's social skills and reduces the number of social interactions that a person has, which can lead to loneliness and depression. Incorporating social communication training into the treatment plan is a priority for SLPs. Evidence suggests that these types of interventions are most successful when they incorporate the following: goals and skills that are important to the client, inclusion of family members/communication partners, and activities for skill generalization in various settings (Togher et al., 2014). Moreover, Togher et al. (2016) found that training communication partners results in improved conversational performance of persons with TBI compared to intervention just targeting the person with the TBI. These conversational gains were found to be maintained 6 months following the training.

Based on the current science, an international group of clinicians and researchers compiled a list of seven recommendations for intervention of persons with TBI who experience cognitive communication challenges (Togher et al., 2014):

1. Clinicians must recognize that communication skills may vary depending on a variety of factors (including communication priorities, communication partner, environment, fatigue, and personal factors).
2. Patients with TBI should be offered interventions to support communication by an SLP.
3. Intervention should consider the patient's profile prior to the TBI: language, literacy, cognitive, communication style, and culture.
4. Intervention should support skills in contexts that are important to the individual (e.g., home, work, community).

5. Intervention should aim to provide education and training to caregivers.
6. Augmentative and alternative communication methods should be provided to individuals with severe communication deficits.
7. Social communication goals that are important to the client should be incorporated into the intervention plan.

Dementia

Because dementia is a progressive neurodegenerative condition, you might be wondering how intervention in this population works. Currently, there is very little (and inconsistent) evidence for pharmaceutical interventions that reverse the effects of dementia. As such, behavioral interventions that focus on preventing and slowing the rate of cognitive decline, as well as managing symptoms associated with cognitive decline and language loss, are of utmost importance (Chow et al., 2021; Loprinzi et al., 2019; Yang et al., 2020). Of course, these behavioral interventions should begin as soon as possible, even before the individual experiences any cognitive declines. Interventions of this sort may simply be considered lifestyle changes and include diet modifications, exercise, and cognitive stimulation. Once an individual begins experiencing mild (or greater) cognitive decline, SLPs provide **cognitive communication training** (supporting the domains of attention, memory, and language) to help clients maintain their current skills and improve their quality of life. Cognitive communication training includes approaches such as spaced retrieval, errorless learning, computer-based interventions, virtual reality training, and reminiscence therapy. Evidence suggests that clients who receive spaced retrieval training demonstrate improved recollection of facts as well as performance on tasks associated with activities of daily living, and those who receive errorless learning training demonstrate gains on word and picture recall, but not necessarily participation in activities of daily living (Hopper et al., 2013). It is suggested that computer-based interventions help support memory functions, but not necessarily overall cognition or language, in community-dwelling individuals with mild cognitive impairment, and more research is needed to see the effects of these interventions on the cognitive and communicative skills of individuals with dementia (Zuschnegg et al., 2023). Virtual reality interventions have been shown to support overall cognition, as well as attention, memory, and executive functions more broadly, in individuals with mild cognitive impairment and those with dementia (Papaioannou et al., 2022). Another finding suggests that individuals with dementia who engage in arts-based programs, such as painting, demonstrate increased engagement and conversational interactions during those activities. More research, however, is needed to determine if these improvements are sustained and generalize after the therapy ends (Jeppson et al., 2022). Another promising avenue for dementia intervention is reminiscence therapy, in which the person with dementia reminisces about their past personal experiences, often with visual supports (e.g., photographs, videos, artifacts). Implementation of this type of intervention varies in terms of delivery (e.g., group vs. individual), setting (e.g., home, community, care setting), reminiscing partner (e.g., loved one vs. therapist), and type of memory (e.g., recent vs. remote, positive vs. negative). This makes it somewhat challenging to determine the effectiveness of reminiscence therapy; however, evidence suggests that this type of intervention can support cognition, communication, mood, and quality of life in persons with dementia (Woods et al., 2018).

SLPs also work with clients and their loved ones in an educational capacity to prepare them for upcoming changes in cognition and language functioning. Evidence suggests that these interventions support quality of life in patients with mild cognitive decline (Chandler et al., 2019) and lead to improvements in caregivers' knowledge, depression/anxiety, and burden (Pleasant et al., 2020). In addition, digital technologies, including social robots and smart home technologies, have also been shown to reduce caregiver burden of caring for a loved one with dementia. These technologies help reduce caregiver burden by providing social and daily life support to those with dementia (Sohn et al., 2023).

Cultural Considerations

When selecting the most appropriate intervention for each individual patient, clinicians must ensure that they are carefully considering cultural factors that may impact the client–clinician relationship, the client's outcomes, and how the current evidence fits with each unique client's demographics. For example, if the person with aphasia speaks more than one language, the SLP must consider the age at which the person acquired each language, as well as how much each language was used prior to their aphasia diagnosis. An important factor for a well-designed intervention plan is how much the person will use each of their languages during and after recovery. Moreover, SLPs working with bilingual or multilingual persons with language or cognitive communication disorders may face barriers if they themselves are monolingual and specifically if their clients require augmentative and alternative methods of communication. In fact, many SLPs note that they face barriers to delivering good intervention to clients with aphasia who require AAC, including lack of training in bilingual AAC (Hung et al., 2023).

Clinicians must also keep in mind how (and if) their specific clients are demographically like those who are represented in research. For example, although almost all intervention research in aphasia reports on the age and sex of their participants, fewer than 30% of studies report on information regarding race and ethnicity. This can be problematic because, due to challenges recruiting participants, research on aphasia often relies on **convenience sampling** (i.e., easily accessible to the researchers). This means that people with aphasia who participate in research studies are those who are readily available to the researchers and are not representative of the general population of people living with aphasia (Nguy et al., 2022).

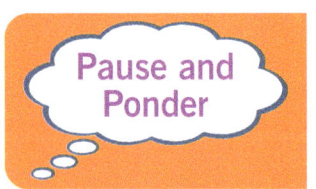 What do you think the clinical implications of this are? Why do you think this would be important when providing clinical services to those with aphasia, RHD, TBI, and dementia?

Why Is This Topic Important?

Although children can (and do) experience language and/or cognitive communication disorders, adults are faced with unique life challenges when they acquire a communication disorder. Many adults who are diagnosed with a language or cognitive communication disorder later in life are suddenly faced with challenges that they had never experienced or likely even thought about prior to their stroke or injury. This means that they very likely were successful communicators with established relationships and educational or vocational experiences. The sudden onset of communication deficits, along with other co-occurring challenges, leaves the patient and their loved ones to navigate a whole new lifestyle that they had likely not prepared for. It is important, therefore, that we not only adequately assess acquired disorders like those discussed in this chapter but also educate both the patient and their family about the likely implications of the patient's language and cognitive changes. The importance of an interprofessional team that understands the various needs of each individual client and family in this process cannot be stressed enough. Furthermore, training and educating family members on the changes in their loved one's skills and behaviors will help them prepare for a new environmental context and adjusted expectations for quality of life.

Finally, recall the ICF model (World Health Organization, 2001) discussed in Chapter 2. Let's apply the ICF framework to an adult (Joe) with aphasia (Figure 9–6). To get a better sense of the how Joe's disability interacts with various environmental and personal factors to support or hinder his participation in activities throughout his day, let's look at a completed ICF diagram. Here, we want to know about Joe's ability to participate in a common activity in his daily life: going to the grocery store. We consider the factors that are both supportive of and barriers to his participation in this activity. Several factors contribute to Joe's ability to go to the grocery store. Five years ago, Joe had a stroke that resulted in a nonfluent aphasia as well as difficulty using his right arm and leg. These physical mobility challenges (body functions and structure) impact his ability to drive and thus his independence in getting to the grocery store. He relies on the help of neighbors and public transportation to bring him to the store. Because he has a nonfluent aphasia, significant word-finding difficulties impact his ability to verbally communicate quickly. E-mailing and texting help Joe set up his weekly grocery store outings. Environmental factors that may impact his participation in this activity include the people he engages with on public transportation as well as at the grocery store. Drivers and cashiers who are familiar with Joe understand the importance of allowing him extra time to speak as well as to use writing/drawing to support his verbal speech. In addition, if the grocery store is busy with other customers, cashiers might feel they have less time to interact with Joe, and Joe might feel pressured to communicate quickly, which may

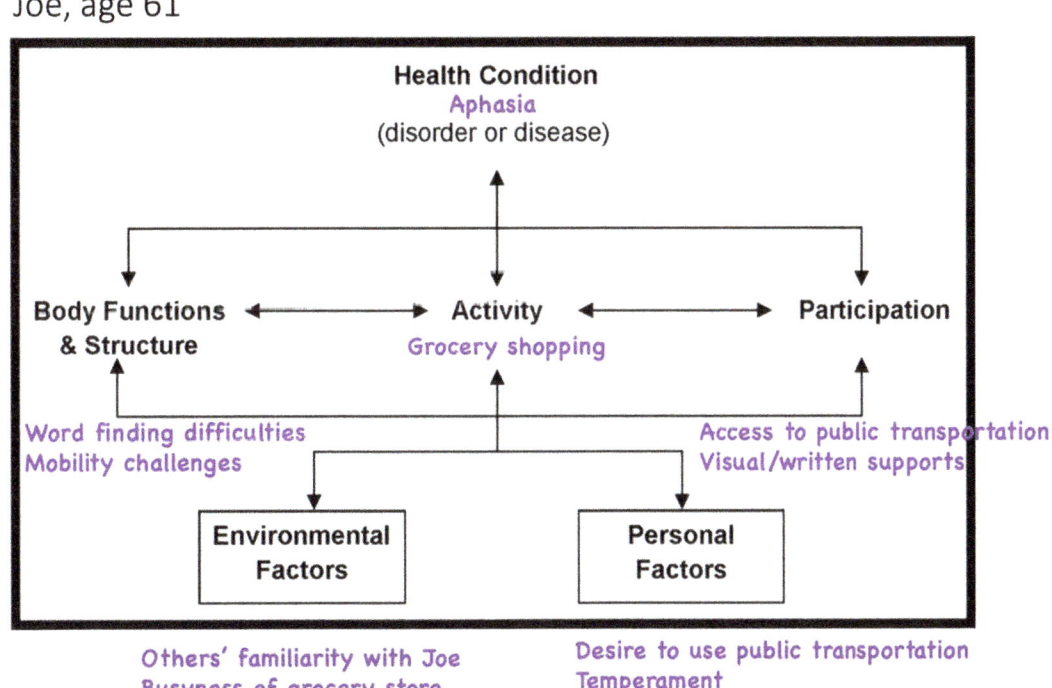

FIGURE 9–6. ICF model example. *Source:* Adapted from the World Health Organization (2001).

negatively impact his ability to get his message across. Personal factors may also impact Joe's ability to go to the grocery store, including his desire or reluctance to use public transportation when a neighbor is unable to drive him to the store (or vice versa) on any given day. Moreover, Joe's temperament and how he interacts with others may impact their desire to support him.

Application to an Adult

Claudia Gosling is a 68-year-old retired university librarian who suffered a stroke earlier this year while on a beach vacation with her husband. Claudia was referred to an SLP after her stroke. The SLP's assessment revealed that Claudia presents with a fluent aphasia (i.e., anomic aphasia), characterized by lengthy and complex speech utterances with some use of nonword fillers, such as "um" or "uh." Claudia's frequent use of nonword fillers suggests that she presents with anomia. She also acknowledges that she has trouble finding the words she wants to say. Claudia demonstrates good auditory comprehension and relatively good expressive discourse in terms of telling a story from start to finish. Due to her anomia, however, her expressive speech is somewhat slowed in complex discourse. Claudia's use of syntax during the assessment tasks was within normal range, which was evidenced by her use of subject–verb agreement, correct pronoun usage, use of prepositions, and use of appropriate verb tense. Claudia does not present with apraxia, agrammatic language, jargon, neologisms, perseverations, or stereotypic utterances. On an assessment of narrative retell, Claudia demonstrated good topic maintenance, provided accurate information, used appropriate vocabulary and accompanying details to discuss events, her ideas were organized logically and sequentially, and she used appropriate grammar (e.g., sentence structure and word order). Claudia also clearly introduced the topic at hand and conveyed her intended message despite some word-finding difficulties. Some pauses, phrase repetitions (e.g., "Um the phone was um . . . the phone was . . . the phone was ringing"), and paraphasias were noted in her speech in conversation and during the picture description task. These impact her ability to speak efficiently, causing breakdowns in her discourse.

Claudia's aphasia impacts her communication in daily life. She takes slightly longer to convey her messages than she had previously; however, the messages she does convey are complete, grammatical, and organized. In addition, Claudia has trouble coming up with the correct words in daily communication, which may contribute to her slowed expressive speech and use of pauses, thus leading to her frustration with communication. Despite these challenges, her communication partners usually understand her messages.

Intervention to support Claudia's communication includes reducing word-finding deficits that result in slow and halting speech and are quite frustrating for Claudia. Using a combination of restorative and compensatory strategies, the SLP will implement opportunities for Claudia to make associations between words to facilitate word retrieval. In addition, the SLP will work with Claudia to decrease the frequency of her dysfluent characteristics, including using fillers, repetitions, and sound revisions, because this will help Claudia communicate information in a more productive manner. Finally, the SLP will continue to educate Claudia's husband on aphasia and how to support Claudia in her recovery process.

Chapter Summary

Aphasia is a common language disorder in adults that affects spoken and written language comprehension and production while leaving intellectual functioning intact. Those with a fluent aphasia tend to exhibit smooth but often incomprehensible speech filled with neologisms and word substitutions, as well as word retrieval difficulties and deficits in comprehension. Those with a nonfluent aphasia tend to have halted, effortful, and agrammatical speech and usually preserved comprehension. Whereas damage to the left hemisphere of the brain often leads to aphasia, damage to the right hemisphere results in challenges related to communication rather than language-specific skills. Individuals with right hemisphere damage experience deficits in cognitive skills, such as attention and memory, which in turn impact their social communication. TBI refers to global and diffuse brain damage usually resulting from the brain shifting in the skull or the external force of an object on the skill. TBI disrupts behavioral, physical, and cognitive functioning, leading to mood changes and language difficulties secondary to cognitive deficits. The primary communicative challenges seen in individuals with TBI are related to social interaction. Dementia is an impairment associated with progressive cognitive decline. AD, the most common form of dementia, impacts memory, language, and conversational skills.

Assessment of communication disorders in adults is often completed by an interdisciplinary team of professionals, caregivers, and the individuals themselves. For aphasia, assessment involves evaluating expressive and receptive language abilities, word finding, repetition, reading, writing, and social communication skills across different contexts. Assessment of RHD focuses on evaluating discourse, prosody, nonverbal behaviors, and social communication skills. For those with TBI, SLPs assess the client's language, cognitive communication, social communication, and swallowing abilities. For those with dementia, assessment involves language-specific measures, as well as measures of cognitive communication. In all cases, assessments should be culturally sensitive, recognizing potential biases in standardized tools and acknowledging diverse cultural backgrounds. Awareness of cultural norms and collaboration with families ensure that assessment procedures align with the patient's cultural experiences. Overall, an interdisciplinary approach to assessment enables a comprehensive understanding of the individual's needs, ensuring tailored interventions for improving communication and quality of life.

The primary goal of intervention for adults with communication disorders, regardless of the specific condition, is to facilitate their participation in meaningful activities and interactions. This involves adopting a patient- and family-centered approach that integrates the values and goals of the patient and their family into the treatment plan. Intervention strategies include restorative or compensatory strategies, and it is often beneficial to employ a combination of both for optimal outcomes. Interventions for aphasia have shown improvements in language skills and include approaches that target word finding, sentence production, fluency, and auditory comprehension. Group therapy, telehealth, and computerized therapy are emerging options, promoting social interaction and providing access to therapy beyond traditional face-to-face settings. Persons with RHD benefit from interventions targeting prosody, discourse, and social communication. Techniques involving motoric-imitative and cognitive-affective approaches address prosody, whereas contextual training aids in comprehension. Narrative production training and social skills interventions show potential, although more research is required to determine their effectiveness. For TBI, intervention at various stages of recovery focuses on orienting, attention, memory, and social communication skills. Social communication training involving family members leads to improved conversational performance for those with TBI. Intervention for persons with dementia focuses on lifestyle changes, cognitive communication training, and reminiscence therapy. Approaches such as spaced retrieval, errorless learning, computer-based interventions, virtual reality training, and arts-based programs show promise in maintaining cognition, communication, and quality of life. Educating clients and caregivers about the condition also contributes to improving the well-being of individuals with dementia and their caregivers.

As with assessment, clinicians delivering intervention to adults with communication disorders must consider the cultural factors that may impact the client–clinician relationship and the client's outcomes. To provide better care, clinicians must understand cultural influences as well as incorporate family members into the intervention process as necessary steps to creating more inclusive and effective intervention plans for individuals with communication disorders.

Chapter Review Questions

1. Describe the functions of the frontal, occipital, parietal, and temporal lobes.
2. What is the difference between fluent and nonfluent aphasia? Which types of aphasias are generally categorized under each?
3. What are the primary areas of language that are affected in aphasia, RHD, TBI, and dementia?
4. How is an RHD different than a TBI?
5. How are language disorders different from cognitive communication disorders?
6. Why is it important to incorporate the family's perspective into assessment and intervention of adults with language and/or cognitive communication disorders?
7. What is the primary objective of intervention for individuals with communication disorders?
8. What is the difference between compensatory and restorative approaches to intervention?
9. Name one intervention approach for each of the following: Aphasia, RHD, TBI, and dementia.
10. What is an important factor to consider when distinguishing a communication disorder in an adult compared to a child?

Learning Activities

1. In small groups or individually, create an informational brochure that educates people about aphasia, RHD, TBI, or dementia. Include information about the symptoms, causes, and implications of the condition. Discuss implications for the person with the disorder as well as how the disorder can affect loved ones.
2. Watch the 2014 film *Still Alice*, which depicts the real-life story of a woman with early onset dementia. Compare and contrast the information in the film with what you learned about dementia in this chapter. What intervention strategies might be useful for Alice and her family?
3. Watch the 2013 documentary *The Crash Reel*, which follows the story of snowboarder Kevin Pearce, who sustained a TBI during his training for the 2010 Winter Olympics. Compare and contrast the information in the documentary with what you learned about TBI in this chapter. What do you notice about Kevin's TBI and how it affected him and his family?

Suggested Reading

Álvarez-Fernández, A., Andrade-González, N., Simal, P., Matias-Guiu, J., Gómez-Escalonilla, C., Rodriguez-Jiminez, R., . . . Lahera, G. (2023). Emotional processing in patients with single brain damage in the right hemisphere. *BMC Psychology, 11*(8), 3–11.

This study examined the emotional processing abilities of individuals who sustained brain damage in the right hemisphere. The authors were interested in how individuals with damage to the right hemisphere perform on tasks of emotional face recognition and subjective emotional response. Forty-one adults with brain damage resulting from stroke and 45 healthy controls participated in this study. All participants were presented with an emotion recognition task in which they were instructed to identify the following emotions in a series of photographs: happiness, sadness, anger, surprise, disgust, and fear. Participants also completed a subjective emotional response task in which they were shown photographs ranging from neutral to disturbing in content and asked to rate each picture on a scale from *very unpleasant* to *very pleasant*. Results suggest that those with right hemisphere damage performed worse on the emotion recognition task compared to healthy controls and that participants in both groups recognized "happiness" with greater accuracy than the other emotions. Findings also reveal that individuals with right hemisphere damage performed similarly to healthy controls on the subjective emotional response task. The authors indicate that these findings are important when considering the social communication abilities of individuals with damage to their right hemispheres. Challenges with emotional facial recognition may impact a person's ability to respond appropriately during social interactions, which may lead to reduced social interactions, social withdrawal, and isolation.

Edmonds, L., & Morgan, J. (2022). Two-year longitudinal evaluation of community aphasia center participation on linguistic, functional communication, and quality of life measures across people with a range of aphasia presentations. *American Journal of Speech-Language Pathology, 31*, 2378–2394.

This study examined a variety of language and communication abilities, as well as quality of life, in a group of 27 adults with aphasia who attended a rehabilitation aphasia center for 2 years. The authors highlight that a key component of this study was that the participants were able to attend the center and the groups at their leisure and that the events fostered friendship, community, and peer support. Language, communication, and quality of life were measured prior to attendance at the rehabilitation center, after 1 year of participation at the center, and again after 2 years of participation at the center. In addition to each participant completing questionnaires designed to measure their language, communication, and quality of life, communication partners also completed a questionnaire regarding the functional communication skills of the person with aphasia.

Findings revealed that after being at the aphasia center for 1 year, persons with aphasia demonstrated improvements in all areas except self-reported functional communication, and these effects were maintained after the second year. This study was important because minimal research has been conducted on the benefits of aphasia centers and the group interactions that they inherently provide.

Jeppson, T., Nudo, C., & Mayer, J. (2022). Painting for a purpose: A visual arts program as a method to promote engagement, communication, cognition, and quality of life for individuals with dementia. *American Journal of Speech-Language Pathology, 31*, 1687–1701.

This study examined the quality of life and communication skills of individuals with dementia after a free-form painting intervention. Researchers gathered information about the patients' engagement in conversational interactions during the program, their cognitive communicative functioning following the intervention, whether effects were maintained over time, and the patient's quality of life following the intervention.

Three non-Hispanic, White females participated in this study. Each participant was paired with a trained undergraduate student to maximize social interaction. Free-form painting was used to promote self-efficacy. Reminiscence was a key aspect of the intervention because participants were asked to generate titles for their works of art. Both intervention and control (i.e., cooking) conditions took place over 4 weeks. Measures for quality of life and cognitive communication skills were administered before and after intervention.

All three participants were able to engage in the activity over the intervention period and produced several paintings. At the end of the intervention period, two of the three participants showed an increase in utterances compared to baseline. Participants demonstrated mixed skill improvement on the cognitive linguistic measures. Although there was not a significant difference in quality of life pre- and post-intervention, there was a positive trend for each participant. The authors suggest that SLPs should advocate for more holistic approaches to intervention that include cognitive stimulation such as communication and memory. More research and a larger sample size are necessary to determine the success of this intervention.

Togher, L., McDonald, S., Tate, R., Rietdijk, R., & Power, E. (2016). The effectiveness of social communication partner training for adults with severe chronic TBI and their families using a measure of perceived communication ability. *NeuroRehabilitiation, 38*, 243–255.

This study examined the effects of communication partner training on the communication skills of adults with TBI. Forty-one patients with severe brain injuries and their caregivers participated in this study and were allocated to one of three groups: social communication training for the patient with TBI, social communication training for the patient with TBI and their caregiver, or delayed treatment control group. Participants in the delayed treatment control group were offered the intervention at the close of the study. Participants in the social communication groups (TBI-only and TBI + caregiver) received the same social communication skills training program for 10 weeks. Assessment of the patient's cognitive and communication skills was completed pre- and post-intervention. Training sessions included teaching the participants about how brain injury impacts communication and how to be more successful in social interactions, including initiating new topics and extending conversational interactions.

Findings suggest that participants in the TBI + caregiver group demonstrated greater improvements in perceived communication abilities compared to those in the TBI-only and control groups, and these effects were maintained 6 months post-intervention. This suggests that training caregivers can be a powerful tool in supporting the perceived communication abilities of those with TBI. It was also noted that participants in the TBI-only intervention group noted improvements in their own communication skills compared to those in the control group. The authors suggest that social communication training can still be beneficial when caregivers are not available to participate in an intensive training.

References

Álvarez-Fernández, A., Andrade-Gonzalez, N., Simal, P., Matias-Guiu, J., Gómez-Escalonilla, C., Rodriguez-Jiminez, R., . . . Lahera, G. (2023). Emotional processing in patients with single brain damage in the right hemisphere. *BMC Psychology, 11*(8), 3–11.

Alzheimer's Association. (2023). *Medical tests for diagnosing Alzheimer's.* https://www.alz.org/alzheimers-dementia/diagnosis/medical_tests

American Psychiatric Association. (2013). *Diagnostic and statistical manual of mental disorders* (5th ed.).

Baker, C., Worrall, L., Rose, M., & Ryan, B. (2020). "It was really dark": The experiences and preferences of people with aphasia to manage mood changes and depression. *Aphasiology, 34*(1), 19–46.

Barman, A., Chatterjee, A., & Bhide, R. (2016). Cognitive impairment and rehabilitation strategies after traumatic brain injury. *Indian Psychiatric Society, 38*, 172–181.

Baron, C., Hatfield, B., & Georgeadis, A. (2005). Management of communication disorders using family member input, group treatment, and telerehabilitation. *Topics in Stroke Rehabilitation, 12*(2), 49–56.

Bayles, K., & Tomoeda, C. (2020a). *Functional Linguistic Communication Inventory–Second Edition (FLCI-2)*. Pro-Ed.

Bayles, K., & Tomoeda, C. (2020b). *Arizona Battery for Communication Disorders of Dementia–Second Edition (ABCD-2)*. Pro-Ed.

Brookshire, R., & Nicholas, L. (1993). *Discourse Comprehension Test (DCT)*. Communication Skill Builders.

Cannizzaro, M., & Coelho, C. (2002). Treatment of story grammar following traumatic brain injury: A pilot study. *Brain Injury, 16*, 1065–1073.

Chandler, M., Locke, D., Crook, J., Fields, J., Ball, C., Phatak, V., . . . Smith, G. (2019). Comparative effectiveness of behavioral interventions on quality of life for older adults with mild cognitive impairment: A randomized clinical trial. *JAMA Network Open, 2*(5), Article e193016.

Chow, G., Gan, J., Chan, J., Wu, X., & Klainin-Yobas, P. (2021). Effectiveness of psychosocial interventions among older adults with mild cognitive impairment: A systematic review and meta-analysis. *Aging & Mental Health, 25*(11), 1986–1997.

Dalemans, R., Witte, L., Beurskens, A., Van Den Heuvel, W., & Wade, D. (2010). An investigation into the social participation of stroke survivors with aphasia. *Disability Rehabilitation, 32*(20), 1678–1685.

Davidson, C. (2019). *Information needs for carers following a family member's right hemisphere stroke* [Master's thesis]. Duquesne University. https://core.ac.uk/download/pdf/270177929.pdf

Dooley, S., & Walshe, M. (2019). Assessing cognitive communication skills in dementia: A scoping review. *International Journal of Language & Communication Disorders, 54*(5), 729–741.

Douglas, J. M., Bracy, C. A., & Snow, P. C. (2007). Exploring the factor structure of the La Trobe Communication Questionnaire: Insights into the nature of communication deficits following traumatic brain injury. *Aphasiology, 21*, 1181–1194.

Edmonds, L., & Morgan, J. (2022). Two-year longitudinal evaluation of community aphasia center participation on linguistic, functional communication, and quality of life measures across people with a range of aphasia presentations. *American Journal of Speech-Language Pathology, 31,* 2378–2394.

Elman, R. (2016). Aphasia centers and the life participation approach to aphasia. *Topics in Language Disorders, 36,* 154–167.

Faul, M., & Coronado, V. (2015). Epidemiology of traumatic brain injury. In J. Grafman & A. M. Salazar (Ed.), *Handbook of clinical neurology* (pp. 3–13). Elsevier.

Ferré, P., & Joanette, Y. (2016). Communication abilities following right hemisphere damage: Prevalence, evaluation, and profiles. *Perspectives of the ASHA Special Interest Groups, 1*(2), 106–115.

Finch, E., Copley, A., Cornwell, P., & Kelly, C. (2016). Systematic review of behavioral interventions targeting social communication difficulties after traumatic brain injury. *Archives of Physical Medicine and Rehabilitation, 97*(8), 1352–1356.

Flowers, H., Skoretz, S., Silver, F., Rochon, E., Fang, J., Flamand-Roze, C., & Martino, R. (2021). Poststroke aphasia frequency, recovery, and outcomes: A systematic review and meta-analysis. *Archives of Physical Medicine and Rehabilitation, 97*(12), 2188–2201.

Frederick, A., Jacobs, M., Adams-Mitchell, C., & Ellis, C. (2022). The global rate of post-stroke aphasia. *Perspectives of the ASHA Special Interest Groups, 7,* 1567–1572.

Giacino, J., Fins, J., Laureys, S., & Schiff, N. (2014). Disorders of consciousness after acquired brain injury: The state of the science. *Nature Reviews Neurology, 10*(2), 99–114.

Goodglass, H., Kaplan, E., & Barresi, B. (2000). *BDAE-3: Boston Diagnostic Aphasia Examination–Third Edition.* Pro-Ed.

Hardin, K., Black, C., Caldbick, K., Kelly, M., Malhotra, A., Tidd, C., . . . Turkstra, L. (2021). Current practices among speech-language pathologists for mild traumatic brain injury: A mixed methods modified Delphi approach. *American Journal of Speech-Language Pathology, 30*(4), 1625–1655.

Helm-Estabrooks, N. (2001). *Cognitive Linguistic Quick Test.* Pearson.

Hopper, T., Bourgeois, M., Pimentel, J., Dean Qualls, C., Hickey, E., Frymark, T., & Schooling, T. (2013). An evidence-based systematic review on cognitive interventions for individuals with dementia. *American Journal of Speech-Language Pathology, 22*(1), 126–145.

Hugo, J., & Ganguli, M. (2014). Dementia and cognitive impairment: Epidemiology, diagnosis, and treatment. *Clinics in Geriatric Medicine, 30*(3), 421–442.

Hung, P., Brock, K., Sun, L., Hanson, J., Larsen, S., & Small, C. (2023). Perceived factors that facilitate or prevent the use of speech-generating devices in bilingual individuals with aphasia. *American Journal of Speech-Language Pathology, 32,* 1644–1664.

Jeppson, T., Nudo, C., & Mayer, J. (2022). Painting for a purpose: A visual arts program as a method to promote engagement, communication, cognition, and quality of life for individuals with dementia. *American Journal of Speech-Language Pathology, 31,* 1687–1701.

Joanette, Y., Ska, B., Cote, H., Ferre, P., LaPointe, L., Coppens, P., & Small, S. (2015). *Montreal Protocol for the Evaluation of Communication.* ASSBI Resources.

Johansson, M., Carlsson, M., Östeberg, P., & Sonnander, K. (2020). Self-reported changes in everyday life and health of significant others of people with aphasia: A quantitative approach. *Aphasiology, 36*(1), 76–94.

Johnson, L., Basilakos, A., Yourganov, G., Cai, R., Bonilha, L., Rorden, C., & Fridriksson, J. (2019). Progression of aphasia severity in the chronic stages of stroke. *American Journal of Speech Language Pathology, 28,* 639–649.

Kertesz, A. (2006). *Western Aphasia Battery–Revised (WAB-R)*. Pearson.

Kheirkhah, M., Baumbach, P., Leistritz, L., Witte, O., Walter, M., Gilbert, J., . . . Klingne, C. (2021). The right hemisphere is responsible for the greatest difference in human brain response to high-arousing emotional versus neutral stimuli: A MEG study. *Brain Science, 11*(8), 1–15.

Kristinsson, S., Basilakos, A., den Ouden, D., Cassarly, C., Spell, L., Bonilha, L., . . . Fredriksson, J. (2023). Predicting outcomes of language rehabilitation: Prognostic factors for immediate and long-term outcomes after aphasia therapy. *Journal of Speech, Language, and Hearing Research, 66*, 1068–1084.

Leaman, M., & Archer, B. (2023). Choosing discourse types that align with person-centered goals in aphasia rehabilitation: A clinical tutorial. *Perspectives of the ASHA Special Interest Groups, 8*, 254–273.

Lee, J., & Cherney, L. (2022). Transactional success in the texting of individuals with aphasia. *American Journal of Speech-Language Pathology, 31*, 2348–2365.

Lehman Blake, M., Frymark, T., & Venedictov, R. (2013). An evidence-based systematic review on communication treatments for individuals with right hemisphere brain damage. *American Journal of Speech-Language Pathology, 22*, 146–160.

Loprinzi, P., Blough, J., Ryu, S., & Kang, M. (2019). Experimental effects of exercise on memory function among mild cognitive impairment: Systematic review and meta-analysis. *The Physician and Sportsmedicine, 47*(1), 21–26.

Martin, N., Thompson, C., & Worrall, L. (2008). *Aphasia rehabilitation: The impairment and its consequences*. Plural Publishing.

Merriam-Webster. (n.d.). Brainiac. In *Merriam-Webster.com dictionary*. https://www.merriam-webster.com/dictionary/brainiac

Moore Sohlberg, M., MacDonald, S., Byom, L., Iwashita, H., Lemoncello, R., Meulenbroek, P., . . . O'Neil-Pirozzi, T. (2019). Social communication following traumatic brain injury Part 1: State-of-the-art review of assessment tools. *International Journal of Speech-Language Pathology, 21*, 115–127.

Murphy, S., Xu, J., & Kochanek, K. (2013). Deaths: Final data for 2010. *National Vital Statistics Reports, 61*(4), 1–118.

Nguy, B., Quique, Y., Cavanaugh, R., & Evans, W. (2022). Representation in aphasia research: An examination of U.S. treatment studies published between 2009 and 2019. *American Journal of Speech-Language Pathology, 31*, 1424–1430.

Papaioannou, T., Voinescu, A., Petrini, K., & Stanton Fraser, D. (2022). Efficacy and moderators of virtual reality for cognitive training in people with dementia and mild cognitive impairment: A systematic review and meta-analysis. *Journal of Alzheimer's Disease, 88*(4), 1341–1370.

Parola, A., Gabbatore, I., Bosco, F., Bara, B., Cossa, F., Gindri, P., & Sacco, K. (2016). Assessment of pragmatic impairment in right hemisphere damage. *Journal of Neurolinguistics, 39*, 10–25.

Pitt, R., Theodoros, D., Hill, A., & Russell, T. (2019). The impact of the telerehabilitation group aphasia intervention and networking programme on communication, participation, and quality of life in people with aphasia. *International Journal of Speech-Language Pathology, 21*, 513–523.

Pleasant, M., Molinari, V., Dobbs, D., Meng, H., & Hyer, K. (2020). Effectiveness of online dementia caregivers training programs: A systematic review. *Geriatric Nursing, 41*(6), 921–935.

Prince, M., Bryce, R., Albanese, E., Wimo, A., Ribeiro, W., & Ferri, C. (2013). The global prevalence of dementia: A systematic review and meta-analysis. *Alzheimer's and Dementia, 9*(1), 63–75.

Rousseaux, M., Vérigneaux, C., & Kozlowski, O. (2010). An analysis of communication in conversation after severe traumatic brain injury. *European Journal of Neurology, 17*, 922–929.

Sacco, K., Angeleri, R., Bosco, F., Colle, L., Mate, D., & Bara, B. (2008). Assessment Battery for Communication—ABaCo: A new instrument for the evaluation of pragmatic abilities. *Journal of Cognitive Science, 9*, 111–157.

Savundranayagam, M., Hummert, M., & Montgomery, R. (2005). Investigating the effects of communication problems on caregiver burden. *Journals of Gerontology: Series B: Psychological Sciences and Social Sciences, 60*(1), S48–S55.

Saxton, J., McGonigle-Gibson, K., Swihart, A., & Boller, F. (1993). *The Severe Impairment Battery (SIB) manual*. Pearson.

Sennfält, S., Noorving, B., Petersson, J., & Ullberg, T. (2018). Long-term survival and function after stroke: A longitudinal observational study from the Swedish Stroke Register. *Stroke, 50*(1), 53–61.

Sheppard, S., & Sebastian, R. (2021). Diagnosing and managing post-stroke aphasia. *Expert Review of Neurotherapeutics, 21*(2), 221–234.

Sohn, M., Yang, J., Sohn, J., & Lee, J. (2023). Digital healthcare for dementia and cognitive impairment: A scoping review. *International Journal of Nursing Studies, 140*, Article 104413.

Staiger, A., Schroeter, M., Ziegler, W., Pino, D., Frank, R., Schölderle, T., . . . Diehl-Schmid, J. (2023). Speech motor profiles in primary progressive aphasia. *American Journal of Speech-Language Pathology, 32*, 1296–1321.

Starowicz-Filip, A., Chrobak, A., Moskała, M., Kryżewski, R., Kwinta, B., Kwiatkowski, S., . . . Zielińska, D. (2017). The role of the cerebellum in the regulation of language functions. *Psychiatria Polska, 51*(4), 661–671.

Tenovuo, O., Diaz-Arrastia, R., Goldstein, L., Sharp, D., van der Naalt, J., & Zasler, N. (2021). Assessing the severity of traumatic brain injury—Time for a change? *Journal of Clinical Medicine, 10*(148), 1–12.

Teti, S., Murray, L., Orange, J., Page, A., & Kankam, K. (2023). Telehealth assessments and interventions for individuals with poststroke aphasia: A scoping review. *American Journal of Speech-Language Pathology, 32*, 1360–1375.

Togher, L., McDonald, S., Tate, R., Rietdijk, R., & Power, E. (2016). The effectiveness of social communication partner training for adults with severe chronic TBI and their families using a measure of perceived communication ability. *NeuroRehabilitiation, 38*, 243–255.

Togher, L., Power, E., Tate, R., McDonald, S., & Rietdijk, R. (2010). Measuring the social interactions of people with traumatic brain injury and their communication partners: The Adapted Kagan scales. *Aphasiology, 24*, 914–927.

Togher, L., Wiseman-Hakes, C., Douglas, J., Stergiou-Kita, M., Posnford, J., Teasell, R., . . . Turkstra, L. (2014). INCOG recommendations for management of cognition following traumatic brain injury, Part IV: Cognitive communication. *Journal of Head Trauma Rehabilitation, 29*(4), 353–368.

Tompkins, C. (2012). Rehabilitation for cognitive-communication disorders in right hemisphere brain damage. *Archives of Physical Medicine and Rehabilitation, 93*(1), S61–S69.

Wallace, S., Patternson, J., Purdy, M., Knollman-Porter, K., & Coppens, P. (2022). Auditory comprehension interventions for people with aphasia: A scoping review. *American Journal of Speech-Language Pathology, 31*, 2404–2420.

Wei, N., Yong, W., Li, X., Zhou, Y., Deng, M., Zhu, H., & Jin, H. (2015). Post-stroke depression and lesion location: A systematic review. *Journal of Neurology, 262,* 81–90.

Wiseman-Hakes, C., Ryu, H., Lightfoot, D., Kukreja, G., Colantonio, A., & Matheson, F. (2020). Examining the efficacy of communication partner training for improving communication interactions and outcomes for individuals with traumatic brain injury: A systematic review. *Archives of Rehabilitation Research and Clinical Translation, 2*(1), Article 100036.

Woods, B., O'Philbin, L., Farrell, E., Spector, A., & Orrell, M. (2018). Reminiscence therapy for dementia. *Cochrane Database of Systematic Reviews, 2018*(3), Article CD001120.

Woolf, C., Caute, A., Haigh, Z., Galliers, J., Wilson, S., Kessie, A., . . . Marshall, J. (2016). A comparison of remote therapy, face to face therapy and an attention control intervention for people with aphasia: A quasi-randomised controlled feasibility study. *Clinical Rehabilitation, 30,* 359–373.

World Health Organization. (2001). *International classification of functioning, disability and health (ICF).*

Wu, P., Zeng, F., Li, Y., Yu, B., Qui, L., Qin, W., . . . Liang, F. (2015). Changes of resting cerebral activities in subacute ischemic stroke patients. *Neural Regeneration Research, 10*(5), 760–765.

Yang, C., Moore, A., Mpofu, E., Dorstyn, D., Li, Q., & Yin, C. (2020). Effectiveness of combined cognitive and physical interventions to enhance functioning in older adults with mild cognitive impairment: A systematic review of randomized controlled trials. *The Gerontologist, 60*(8), e633–e642.

Youse, K., & Coelho, C. (2009). Treating underlying attention deficits as a means for improving conversational discourse in individuals with closed head injury: A preliminary study. *Neurorehabilitation, 24,* 355–364.

Zuschnegg, J., Schoberer, D., Häussl, A., Herzog, S., Russegger, S., Ploder, K., . . . Schüssler, S. (2023). Effectiveness of computer-based interventions for community dwelling people with cognitive decline: A systematic review with meta-analyses. *BMC Geriatrics, 23*(1), Article 229.

Chapter 10

Fluency Disorders

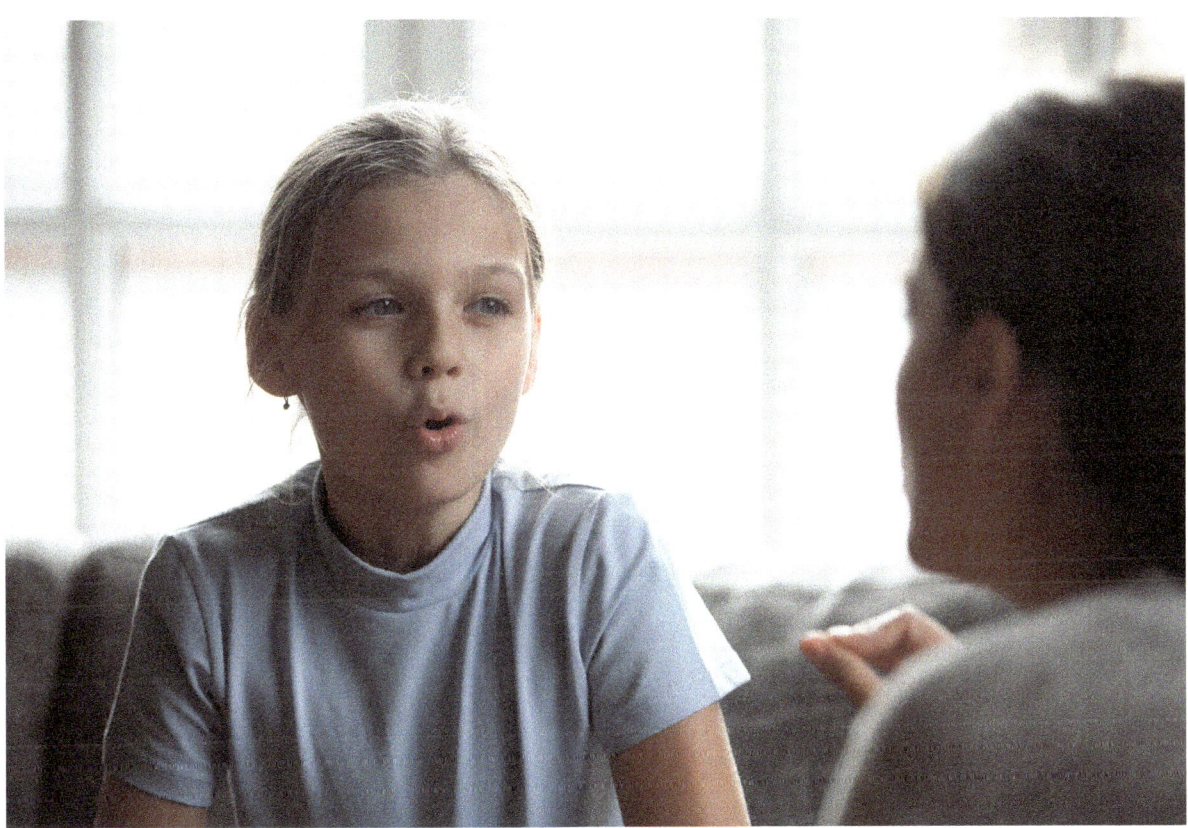

Learning Objectives

After reading this chapter, you will be able to:

- Describe the onset and development of a stuttering disorder.
- Differentiate between stuttering and cluttering.
- Identify ways to recognize and assess a fluency disorder.
- Explain strategies that help young children through adults address the challenges a fluency disorder presents.

Key Terms

- ableist language
- acceptance and commitment therapy
- awareness
- cognitive–behavioral therapy
- continuous phonation
- covert stuttering behaviors
- desensitization
- Down syndrome
- easy onset
- effortful control
- fluency
- fluency disorder
- fragile X
- gray matter
- incidence
- mindfulness
- overt stuttering behaviors
- prevalence
- secondary behaviors
- self-disclosure
- stimulability testing
- support
- Tourette syndrome
- white matter

Introduction

Did you know that Emily Blunt (Golden Globe award-winning actress), James Earl Jones (the voice of Darth Vader and Mufasa), Ed Sheeran (Grammy award-winning singer and songwriter), Tiger Woods (professional golfer), and President Joe Biden are just some of the successful people you may know who

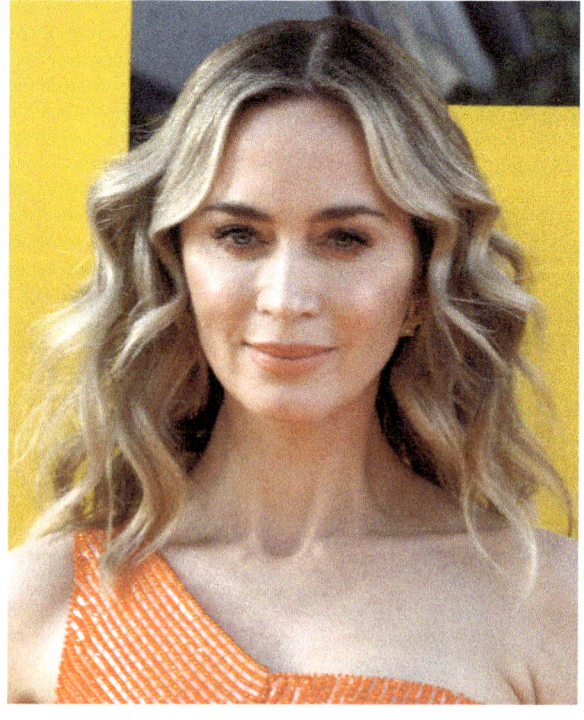

Emily Blunt

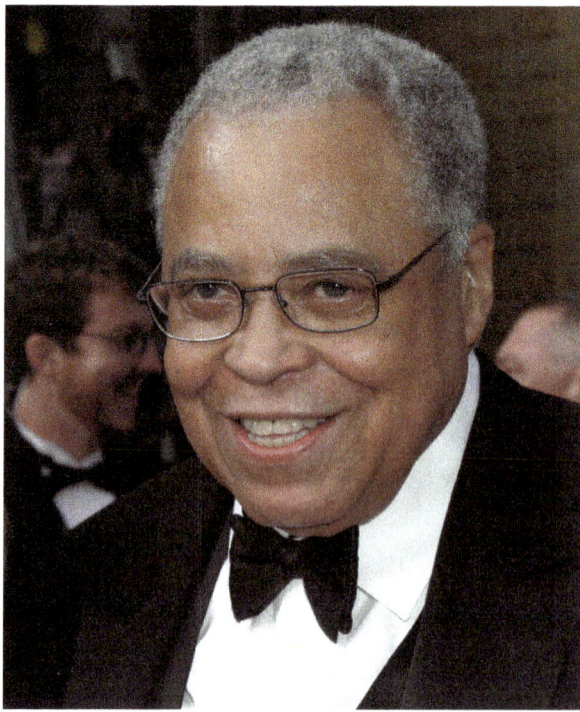

James Earl Jones

stutter? Each of these individuals found ways to navigate the barriers they faced as a stutterer to create opportunities to communicate their message. If you have not seen the movie *The King's Speech*, you might want to check it out. It is the story of King George VI (played by actor Colin Firth), a well-known figure

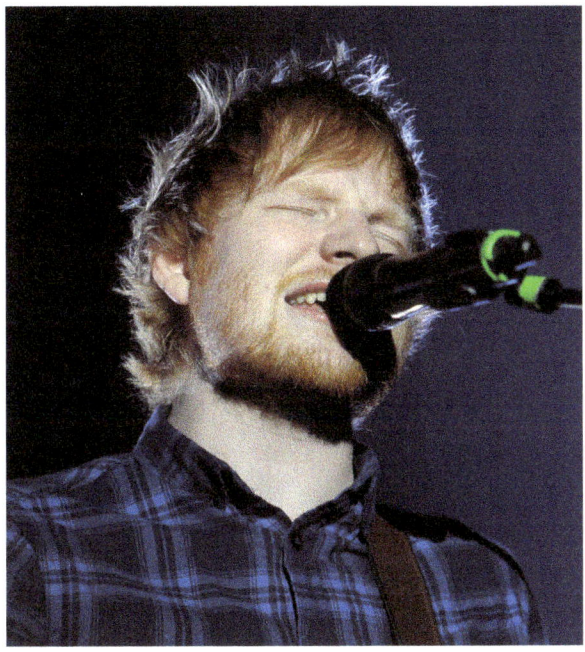

Ed Sheeran

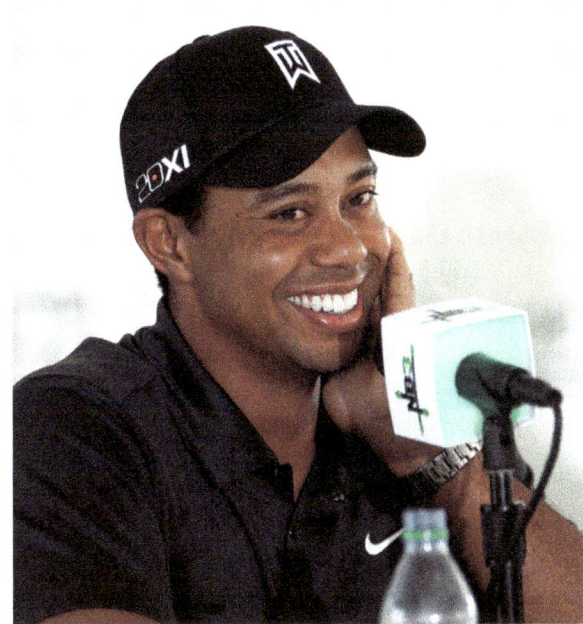

Tiger Woods

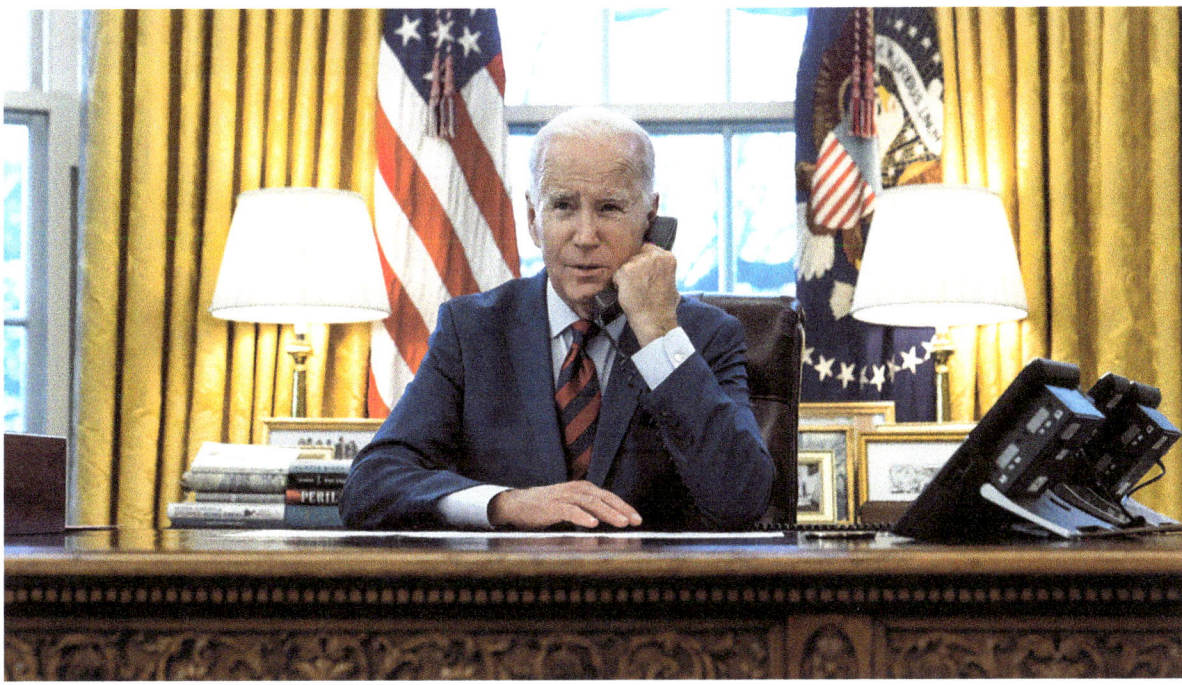

President Joe Biden

in history who worked with a speech therapist in London to address his stuttering as he delivered one of the most impactful radio speeches during World War II.

What *The King's Speech* Can Teach Us About Stuttering

Fluency is how we describe the effort, rate, and smoothness of one's speech. A **fluency disorder** suggests a disruption to the flow of one's speech, including hesitations; repetitions of sounds, syllables, and words; and significant tension when speaking. Many of us experience typical disfluencies when we speak. For example, when giving a talk in class, you might pause as you are formulating a thought, say "uh" in between your thoughts, or interject a filler word (e.g., like; "He 'like' runs fast") as you speak. You might even repeat a word (e.g., "This, this is the reason I run") or a phrase (e.g., "I want to, I want to finish this first"; Prelock & Hutchins, 2018). Stuttering, which is a type of fluency disorder, is characterized by more significant disruptions of speech, including repetitions of sounds, syllables, words, and phrases (e.g., "See the p – p – p picture"), sound prolongations (e.g., "*I would like sssssssssssssome cheese*"), blocks (i.e., an inability to produce audible sounds), and interjections and revisions, all of which may affect the individual's speech rate and rhythm. Stuttering may also be accompanied by **secondary behaviors**, such as eye blinking or excessive arm movements.

Although the range of onset generally occurs between ages 2 and 7 years, stuttering is usually seen prior to age 6 years, and onset can be gradual or occur suddenly (American Psychiatric Association [APA], 2022). It is also common for stuttering to occur with other disorders such as speech-sound and language disorders or intellectual disabilities. Interestingly, between 65% and 85% of young children who stutter

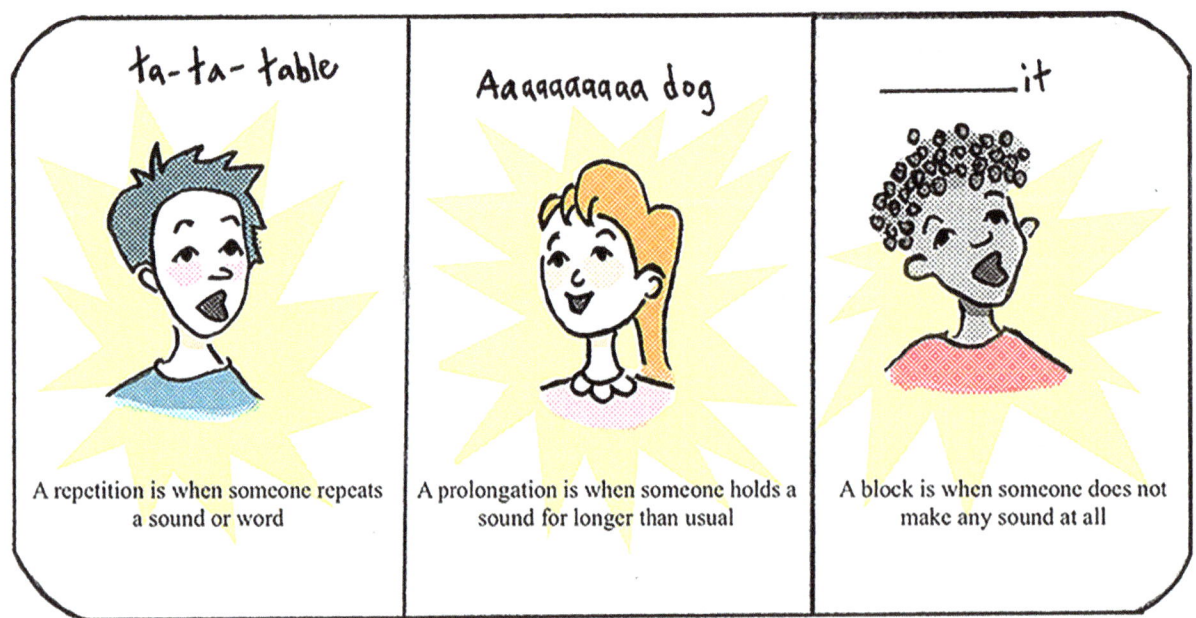

Repetitions, prolongations, and blocks are examples of different types of stuttering. *Source:* Frontiers for Young Minds.

will stop stuttering whether or not they have intervention, and the severity of their stuttering at age 8 years predicts stuttering persistence later on (APA, 2022). Importantly, however, persistent stuttering can lead to social, emotional, and psychological impacts that include, but are not limited to, negative self-thoughts, anxiety in social situations, and feelings of little control over one's communication (Boyle, 2015; Craig & Tran, 2014; Iverach et al., 2016; Iverach & Rapee, 2014). In fact, recent research suggests that children and adolescents who stutter and have repetitive negative thoughts have greater social anxiety (Tichenor et al., 2023).

In the following sections, you will learn more about the signs and symptoms of stuttering, why people might stutter, and how fluency disorders are assessed and treated. You will also learn about the difference between stuttering and cluttering and how these disorders impact an individual's day-to-day experiences. Finally, you will gain additional insights into fluency disorders through both a child and an adult case study.

See the **ASHA Fluency Disorders Practice Portal** for more information.

What We Know About This Topic

In this section, you will learn about both stuttering and cluttering, two types of fluency disorders that you might encounter. You will learn about the incidence and prevalence of fluency disorders and also the characteristics and known causes of stuttering and cluttering. Ways to assess fluency disorders and the most common intervention approaches to address the challenges associated with stuttering and cluttering are highlighted.

Incidence and Prevalence

The **incidence** (number of identified new cases) and **prevalence** (number of those who are living with a specific condition) of stuttering vary due to how it is defined and identified (e.g., younger children vs. older children and adults). Reported incidence of stuttering for children ranges from 5% to 8% (Yairi & Ambrose, 2013), with a prevalence of approximately 0.72% (Craig et al., 2002). Overall, it is a low prevalence disorder, although incidence rates (11%) and prevalence rates (2.2–5.6%) for preschool children are much higher (Craig et al., 2002; Yairi & Ambrose, 2013). A more recent study indicated that approximately 2% of children between ages 3 and 17 years stutter (Zablotsky et al., 2019) and that the rate of stuttering in adults is much lower (0.78% for adults aged 21–50 years and 0.37% for those older than age 50 years; Craig et al., 2002).

Nearly 5% of all people will stutter during some part of their lives. Maybe you have had this experience when you were first learning to talk. There is evidence that having a parent or sibling who stutters increases the likelihood that you will also stutter (Kraft & Yairi, 2011; Singer et al., 2020), and this likelihood increases if the sibling is a twin. Notably, rates of stuttering incidence are highest for preschool children and males (Singer et al., 2020).

Stuttering prevalence in African American preschool children is not significantly different from that in European American preschoolers, with estimates around 2.52% (Proctor et al., 2008). Similar rates are reported for English-speaking versus non–English-speaking countries, with estimates slightly more than 1% but some as high as 8% (Abou et al., 2015; Al-Jazi & Al-Khamra, 2015; Oyono et al., 2018). There are also increased rates of stuttering for children with other conditions, such as learning disorders, attention-deficit/hyperactivity disorder (ADHD), hearing loss, autism, and genetic disorders such as **fragile X** and **Down syndrome** (Arenas et al., 2017; Briley & Ellis, 2018).

Characteristics of Stuttering

Individuals who stutter may exhibit both overt and covert stuttering behaviors. **Overt stuttering behaviors** are speech behaviors and patterns that you can see or hear, such as sound prolongations, syllable or word repetitions, and blocking on words. You might also observe some secondary behaviors, such as arm or other body movements, which are often used to try to stop stuttering or help get the words out (Guitar, 2019). Table 10–1 summarizes the key characteristics of stuttering. Overt stuttering varies across speaking situations and often increases with the pressure to talk, such as might be expected if giving a presentation at school or talking on the phone.

In contrast, **covert stuttering behaviors** are used to mask or hide a person's stuttering. Stutterers will avoid certain situations or find a way to escape from speaking situations to keep from stuttering (Tichenor & Yaruss, 2018, 2019a, 2019b). Notably, however, concealing stuttering may impact the person's quality of life (Boyle et al., 2018) and lead to embarrassment, low self-esteem, and increased anxiety. Several impacts of covert stuttering have been identified in the literature, including, but not limited to, the following:

- Social anxiety
- Negative thoughts about one's ability to communicate
- Feeling less in control
- Decreased self-confidence and self-worth

TABLE 10–1. Primary and Secondary Stuttering Behaviors

Primary Behaviors	Secondary, Avoidance, or Accessory Behaviors
• Single syllable/word repetitions (e.g., "When-when-when will you get home?")	• Producing distracting sounds (e.g., throat clearing)
• Sound/syllable repetitions (e.g., "See the t-t-toy")	• Using facial grimaces (e.g., eye blinks, tics, lip or facial tremors)
• Sound prolongations ("Sssssee the picture")	• Making head movements (e.g., nodding)
• Audible or silent blocking (filled or unfilled pauses when speaking)	• Moving other parts of the body (e.g., fist clinching)
• Words produced with excess struggle or physical tension	• Avoiding certain sounds or words
• Pauses within words	• Limiting speaking especially in social situations
• Circumlocutions (substituting words for difficult-to-produce words)	

- Depression and suicidal ideation
- Avoiding speaking opportunities, social interactions, and using specific words and sounds

In a qualitative study with 30 participants who stuttered, Gerlach-Houck and colleagues (2023) learned that adults who were exposed to repeated instances of both implicit and explicit **ableist language** (see Chapter 2) about stuttering in conjunction with challenging social encounters tended to hide their disfluencies. This concealment became a strategy to escape the stigma they felt and experienced as children and adolescents in school. The adults interviewed indicated speech-language pathologists (SLPs) could best support them by creating a safe and supportive educational environment and by attending to the social and emotional problems that often occur when a student communicates differently.

Although adults who stutter report a range of negative personal–social experiences related to their stuttering, there are also reports of positive experiences, such as the opportunity to develop self-improvement and introspection skills, as well as the ability to manage their speech challenges (Manivannan et al., 2023). These psychosocial benefits may evolve from a recognition that the stutterer is, in fact, able to face challenges and be successful (Boyle et al., 2019).

▶ video

Check out the YouTube video **"For Parents of a Child Who Stutters: Causes of Concern"** to see what multiple repetitions, prolongations, and blocks look like.

Characteristics of Cluttering

Cluttering is a type of fluency disorder that is characterized by an irregular or rapid rate of speech. A person who clutters will omit syllables or word endings, which makes their connected speech difficult to understand. They will also use filler words such as "uh" or "um" more excessively than is typical in normal disfluency. Because cluttering is characterized by unusual pauses within sentences, it leads to an atypical prosody that interferes with the natural rhythm of speech.

Like stuttering, cluttering can co-occur with other disorders, such as learning disabilities, **Tourette syndrome**, and ADHD. A small percentage of individuals who stutter also exhibit the characteristics of cluttering. Table 10–2 compares the characteristics of stuttering and cluttering.

Causes of Stuttering

Several genetic and neurophysiological factors have been described in the literature as potential causes of stuttering (Smith & Weber, 2017). Furthermore, the demands for speaking and other environmental conditions, such as family stress and anxiety, may increase the occurrence of stuttering behavior and influence how an individual reacts to their stuttering. Temperamental styles might also be related to stuttering in children such that their emotional regulation may impact their ability to manage their stuttering behaviors (Choi et al., 2013; Guttormsen et al., 2015) and may have an adverse impact on their stuttering across their lifespan (Tichenor, Walsh, et al., 2022). Notably, bilingual children may experience an onset of stuttering or an increase in stuttering when placed in unfamiliar situations, when language input is mixed, or when a new language is being learned (Shenker, 2013); however, note that stuttering is not caused by exposure to or learning another language (Byrd, 2018).

TABLE 10–2. Comparison of Stuttering and Cluttering Characteristics

Stuttering	Cluttering
• Repetitions (sounds, syllables, words, phrases) (e.g., "See the *b-b*-ball")	• Irregular speech rate leading to breakdowns in the clarity of one's speech
• Sound prolongations (e.g., "*Ssssss*see the ball")	• Omission of syllables (e.g., "I hear tephone" for "I hear the telephone") and/or word endings (e.g., "Turn the move off" for "Turn the movie off")
• Blocks (i.e., difficulty initiating sounds leading to silence)	
• Revisions, which may affect the rate and rhythm of speech	• Excessive common disfluencies (e.g., revisions, interjections)
• Physical tension leading to the avoidance of certain sounds, words, or speaking situations	• Unexpected pauses in sentences (e.g., "I will go to the [pause] park and play with my [pause] friends")

Although there are no definitive expressions of genes and chromosomes or sex factors to explain the occurrence of stuttering in the general population, there are some gene mutations linked to stuttering in approximately 10% of families affected (Drayna & Kang, 2011; Frigerio-Domingues & Drayna, 2017; Kraft & Yairi, 2011). There is also some suggestion that genetic factors may predict whether a person's stuttering persists and how an individual might respond to treatment (Frigerio-Domingues et al., 2019; Han et al., 2014). Research also shows that children who stutter have functional and structural differences (Chang, 2014; Chang et al., 2019), including **gray and white matter** differences (Chang et al., 2015) and reduced neural connectivity (Chang & Zhu, 2013). In addition, neurological studies show differences between children and adults who stutter.

It is difficult to know which children will stutter and in which children stuttering will persist. Some factors that are associated with children who continue to stutter include gender (boys have an increased risk compared to girls), family history, duration of initial stuttering period (greater than 6–12 months), age of onset (age 3½ years or later), and delayed language development or language impairment (Kraft & Yairi, 2011; Leech et al., 2017, 2019; Yairi & Ambrose, 2005, 2013).

Causes of Cluttering

Currently, there is insufficient research to identify the specific causes of cluttering. There is some evidence that there are differences in cortical and subcortical activity for adults who clutter versus those who do not (Ward et al., 2015), but little genetic information is available. There are some connections of cluttering with other neurodevelopmental and neurobiological disorders, such as ADHD, autism, and Tourette syndrome. There are insufficient data to identify risk factors for cluttering because there are no good data on age of onset or long-term outcomes. Interestingly, approximately one-third of those who stutter also exhibit some characteristics of cluttering (Ward, 2006).

Assessment

An SLP has an important role in screening and assessing children, youth, and adults who stutter (see the ASHA "Scope of Practice for Speech-Language Pathology"). Individuals who stutter should be referred to an SLP, who can perform a comprehensive assessment that consists of several components.

See the **ASHA Scope of Practice for Speech-Language Pathology.**

A first step in the assessment is an interview with the family and/or the individual who stutters (when appropriate) about their overall development, medical history and status, development of speech and language, exposure to other languages, and any family history of fluency disorders. In addition, individuals who stutter and their families are asked to describe the stutterers' disfluent characteristics, when the disfluencies were first observed, how the family responds to the disfluencies, any previous intervention, and the family's overall perception of how stuttering impacts the individual and the family.

The next step is to consult with the family, the child's teachers, and any other professionals who work with the child who stutters to get a sense of the stability or variability of the child's stuttering. The SLP wants to understand in what situations disfluencies occur most and least often and what the impact of the child's stuttering is in these situations. The SLP also spends time reviewing any previous educational and fluency assessments.

An SLP usually requests an audio and video recording of a speech sample so they can hear and see the child's stuttering in contexts beyond the clinical setting. In addition, the SLP records a real-time speech sample and conducts an analysis of the child's stuttering during the assessment visit. When assessing a child's fluency, the clinician will usually consider the following:

- Frequency, type, and duration of disfluencies
- Rate of speech
- Intelligibility of speech
- Evidence of secondary behaviors across communication contexts

The clinician might also examine the child's awareness of their disfluencies and their sense of difficulty communicating orally. **Stimulability testing** is a type of diagnostic intervention that is frequently done; it involves the child purposefully decreasing their rate of speech or increasing the amount of pausing to reduce any symptoms of cluttering. Because both stuttering and cluttering have a potential impact on social–emotional, language, and cognitive development, these areas of development are also assessed. Furthermore, the assessment usually identifies the child's individual strengths and ability to cope with their fluency disorder.

Because the severity and specific symptoms of fluency disorders can vary, it is important to assess both overt and covert stuttering behaviors (Davidow & Scott, 2017; St. Louis & Schulte, 2011). For example, more formal assessments might result in increased self-monitoring and lead to fewer observed symptoms, whereas less formal situations might allow for a more accurate and representative picture of the individual's observed symptoms. Clinicians must be aware of more subtle behaviors associated with stuttering, such as avoiding speaking situations (Boyle, 2013).

Results of an Assessment

Once an assessment is completed, there may be several possible outcomes, including a diagnosis of a fluency disorder, a differential diagnosis between a language disorder and a fluency disorder, or other neurodevelopmental disorders. A comprehensive assessment should also provide the clinician with a fluency profile that describes the characteristics of the individual's fluency, the severity of their stuttering and/or cluttering, and the impact on the individual's quality of life. Assessment also leads to a determination of whether treatment is recommended, what type of treatment might be most beneficial, the value of family counseling to ensure appropriate responses to the child's stuttering, and if engagement with other professionals is needed.

Assessment approaches and outcomes will likely be different for preschool children, school-age children and adolescents, and adults. For example, when assessing a preschool child, the first step is to determine if the child's disfluencies are what we typically see at this age or if they are more representative of a fluency disorder. If the latter is determined, then the child's speech will be monitored or treatment will be initiated. When assessing a school-age child or adolescent, the clinician observes the presence and severity of the fluency disorder and how it impacts the student. Because older students who stutter often learn to avoid certain words and situations that increase their stuttering, an assessment might reveal few stuttering behaviors. Clinicians know, however, that these strategies can lead to negative experiences for the student that might indeed warrant intervention. For a child at this age, it is often recommended that a self-assessment of the student's experience with stuttering be completed and that the clinician ask open-ended questions about the student's engagement in class discussions, talking with people they do not know very well, and how comfortable they are speaking in situations outside of their home. For adults who stutter, it is likely they have been managing their stuttering for some time, so the assessment is less about a diagnosis and more about a determination of the severity and impact of the fluency disorder on the adult and their desire for help to change their approach to communication. In the adult assessment, it is important to examine the lived experiences of the stutterer, their perception of the impact of these experiences, and why they are seeking to engage in intervention.

Cultural and Linguistic Considerations for Assessment

To assess a bilingual child for stuttering, the assessment should occur in both languages. Certainly, how proficient a child is in each language and the social context will likely influence how much and when a child stutters (Foote, 2013). Typically, children who stutter and speak multiple languages have higher rates of sound, syllable, and word repetitions than those who speak only one language, and they are less self-aware of their struggles with getting their words out to communicate their message (Byrd, 2018). Having access to a fluent speaker in the language a child speaks and engaging the parents in the assessment are beneficial strategies for identifying whether the communication difficulties are related to stuttering versus managing the linguistic input of more than one language (Shenker, 2011, 2013).

See the **ASHA Multilingual Service Delivery in Audiology and Speech-Language Pathology Practice Portal** and the **ASHA Collaborating With Interpreters, Transliterators, and Translators Practice Portal** for more information.

See the **ASHA Fluency Disorders Evidence Map**, which highlights the research for stuttering intervention.

What Do We Do to Address This Communication Challenge?

Intervention for fluency disorders is variable and considers an individual's needs based on a comprehensive assessment of not only their fluency but also their language, co-occurring conditions, and other emotional and life circumstances (Byrd & Donaher, 2018). When creating a treatment plan, the SLP considers the preferences, values, beliefs, and motivation of the individual as well as the support of the individual's family to determine the most appropriate materials and approaches to developing a plan for intervention (Sisskin, 2018). Ultimately, the clinician wants to create an intervention plan that will help the individual with a fluency disorder react more positively to their disfluencies and take command of their disfluencies when they occur. Counseling is typically a part of the intervention plan to support the person who stutters and to help lessen the challenge of having a communication disorder.

See ASHA's resources titled **"Person-Centered Focus on Function: Preschool Stuttering"** (PDF), **"Person-Centered Focus on Function: School-Age Stuttering"** (PDF), and **"Person-Centered Focus on Function: Adult Stuttering"** (PDF) for more information.

Interventions for Stuttering

When initiating planning for intervention, it is most effective to use a team approach. This approach ensures that the priorities and desired outcome for the child, adolescent, and/or adult and those of their families are addressed. Certainly, intervention planning should consider goals that are responsive to the larger impact of stuttering on the individual's day-to-day activities and lessen the difficulties experienced. The assessment profile obtained guides what intervention is appropriate for the individual. For the youngest children who stutter, engaging their families in implementing the selected intervention techniques is critical, especially for those who are second language learners. A person- and family-centered approach to intervention should be taken, in which the SLP engages in conversations with the child who stutters and their family about expectations for effective communication, their experiences with stuttering, and how best to support communication to achieve their communication goals (Berquez & Kelman, 2018; Millard et al., 2018; Rocha et al., 2020). Communicators who participate in the development and implementation of their intervention goals are usually more motivated to receive intervention (Sønsterud et al., 2019). Counseling is also an essential part of the intervention plan to help those who stutter ease the challenge of dealing with a communication disorder daily.

Some special considerations may be needed depending on the age of the individual. For preschool children, intervention not only is based on the needs of the child but also considers the communication patterns of the family. Goals for treatment generally emphasize ways to minimize the child's stuttering and help the child manage their stuttering moments without developing negative reactions (Yaruss et al., 2006). A home component to the intervention plan is critical (Kelman & Nicholas, 2020), and a variety of parent- and child-focused approaches are typically used, such as the following:

- Indirect treatment: Working with families to adjust their own speech, such as modeling fluent speech and limiting direct questions, as well as changing the child's environment (Millard et al., 2008). Building child and family resilience (the ability to adjust and cope with adversity) is key (Berquez & Kelman, 2018) and may protect the child from the negative impact of ongoing stuttering (Freud & Amir, 2020).
- Direct treatment: Working directly with the child to modify their speech to reduce disfluencies. In addition, resilience is built within the family to lessen the negative impact of stuttering (Caughter & Crofts, 2018; Coifman & Bonanno, 2010; Druker et al., 2019; Kraft et al., 2019; Yaruss et al., 2006).
- Operant treatment: A combination of working directly with the child and their family. The clinician reinforces fluent speech, redirects disfluency, and intermittently asks for corrections to disfluency; parents provide the child with feedback related to fluent versus nonfluent speech (e.g., Palin Parent–Child Interaction Therapy [Kelman & Nicholas, 2020], Lidcombe Program [Onslow et al., 2003]).

For older children and adolescents who stutter, intervention considerations are likely to be adjusted because they may require multiple goals addressing several facets of the stuttering experience. These include acceptance of stuttering, minimizing secondary behaviors, and increasing confidence in managing their communication differences with peers (Yaruss et al., 2012). By adolescence, stuttering often becomes more complex, and tendencies to avoid communication and anxiety around communicating increase. Intervention focuses on reducing the individual's negative reactions to their stuttering as well as educating others about stuttering (Murphy et al., 2007a, 2007b; Yaruss et al., 2012).

Strategies include the following:

- Modification of speech: Changing the pausing between syllables and words and decreasing the tension of speech production (Guitar, 2019). This might include teaching **easy onset** (gradual voicing of initial vowels), **continuous phonation** (voicing throughout an utterance), reducing rate of speech, or stretching out syllables.
- Reduction of physical tension: Locating where physical tension is occurring during disfluent moments and adjusting that tension.
- Increased communication efficiency: Reducing the avoidance of words that create moments of struggle.
- Integrated treatment: Supporting self-regulation, including **effortful control**, and engaging families in intervention (Druker et al., 2019; Kraft et al., 2019).
- Reduction of negative responses: Using several cognitive–behavioral strategies such as mindfulness, awareness, desensitization, cognitive–behavioral therapy, acceptance and

commitment therapy, self-disclosure, and support, which are further explained by Tichenor, Herring et al. (2022).

Reducing negative reactions to stuttering is an important part of the overall intervention plan for school-age children, adolescents, and adults who stutter. One strategy that has been used to decrease such negative reactions is **mindfulness** or "increasing awareness and responding skillfully to mental processes that contribute to emotional distress and maladaptive behavior" (Bishop et al., 2004, p. 230). Mindfulness is used to help an individual who stutters focus on what is happening in the moment of stuttering instead of reacting to the stutter by increasing muscle tension (Tichenor, Herring et al., 2022). The clinician guides the individual to (a) think about what they are doing and feeling (Guitar, 2019), which leads to a greater understanding of the stuttering behaviors; and (b) practice nonjudgment so that stuttering moments become less uncomfortable. Mindfulness is often a complementary strategy to traditional stuttering therapy, and there is some evidence that when used, persons who stutter notice positive changes in their personal lives (Medina, Mead, et al., 2023).

Awareness is a strategy designed to educate the person who stutters about the systems that are important to understanding communication (i.e., respiration, phonation, articulation, and resonance). This education also includes understanding both the verbal and nonverbal components of language and the use of language in social situations.

Another strategy used in addressing stuttering is **desensitization** or limiting negative personal reactions through gradual exposure to stimuli that are uncomfortable (Guitar, 2019). An example of how this might work is the use of voluntary stuttering. This occurs when a person intentionally stutters in a safe environment, allowing them to deliberately experience the discomfort that usually occurs when they do stutter. Experiencing repeated intentional stuttering opportunities helps increase tolerance and decrease the distress and tension associated with actual stuttering moments (Tichenor, Herring et al., 2022).

Cognitive therapy is also a frequently used strategy and includes both **cognitive–behavioral therapy** (CBT) and **acceptance and commitment therapy** (ACT; Beilby et al., 2012; Gupta et al., 2016; Helgadóttir et al., 2014; Palasik & Hannan, 2013). CBT helps limit an individual's negative thoughts about their stuttering by identifying those thoughts, obtaining evidence that those thoughts are unwarranted (e.g., "Your stuttering doesn't bother your peers"), and substituting with more helpful thoughts. CBT is an evidence-based intervention that helps decrease negative and increase positive thoughts associated with stuttering. In contrast, ACT helps the individual recognize their thoughts (without requiring changing them) and learn that negative thoughts do not have to determine how one feels (Fletcher & Hayes, 2005; Hayes et al., 2006).

Self-disclosure is a strategy in which the individual who stutters tells others about their stuttering. In the self-disclosure process, the individual not only talks about their stuttering and how they manage it but also shares ways that others can respond to someone who stutters. The ability to disclose has notable benefits for both the person who stutters and their communication partner because it often eases the communication exchange (Boyle et al., 2018; Boyle & Gabel, 2020; Byrd et al., 2017; Mancinelli, 2019). In fact, Young and colleagues (2022) found that adults who stutter believe self-disclosure is an effective strategy for them as a speaker and for their listener and that clinicians should provide opportunities to practice personal disclosure and discuss the timing and context in which that disclosure might occur.

Support is another strategy frequently used to facilitate self-confidence and decrease isolation for persons who stutter (Yaruss et al., 2007). This includes participating in activities in environments in which it is safe to stutter, such as group therapy and self-help groups (Trichon & Raj, 2018). For example, groups such as the National Association of Young People Who Stutter, the National Stuttering Association, and the Stuttering Association for the Young are available, as are various online platforms.

There are additional considerations for adults who stutter because they have experienced years of disfluency and likely a variety of interventions that had variable outcomes. Some adults may show little confidence in their communication because of the stereotypes that others associate with stuttering or because of their own negative perceptions of stuttering (Beilby et al., 2012; Boyle, 2013). Some adults who stutter might have increased social anxiety and a greater tendency to avoid opportunities for social engagement (Blumgart et al., 2010), and others have experienced discrimination in their job settings (Gerlach et al., 2018). As is true for children and adolescents who stutter, intervention for adults should always be individualized and responsive to the changing needs of the individual. SLPs provide information about stuttering and the stuttering process, work hard to build a relationship with the adult, talk about treatment options, and create a flexible plan responsive to the individual's needs and goals (Amster & Klein, 2018).

Indicators of Positive Change

Research has identified several positive outcomes following the therapeutic experience for children and adolescents who stutters. These outcomes include the following (Manning & DiLollo, 2018):

- Increased comfort with stuttering
- Ability to talk about their stuttering
- Ability to advocate for their individual needs
- Decreased anxiety when speaking
- Decreased social–emotional impacts
- Increased social engagement and enjoyment when speaking

In addition, a successful plan for managing stuttering in adults results in the following (Plexico et al., 2005):

- Reduced fear and increased self-acceptance
- Increased participation in several types of communicative interactions
- Increased optimism about stuttering and how to manage disfluent behavior

Interventions for Cluttering

Because cluttering often involves a rate of speech that is too rapid and difficult for the communication system to manage, intervention that incorporates pausing is frequently used. Research suggests that pausing, in fact, may increase intelligibility (Scaler Scott et al., 2013). Stressing multisyllabic words and word endings can also be used to treat cluttering. In addition, observing the reactions of a communication partner can let the individual who clutters know that a communication breakdown has occurred, and they can work to improve the regulation of the speech rate and clarity. Stuttering strategies, such as easy onset and continuous phonation, may not be appropriate for clutterers.

Cultural and Linguistic Considerations for Stuttering Intervention

There are a range of beliefs that people of different cultures and backgrounds have about how to manage disfluency. Therefore, clinicians must attend to these varying beliefs and understand that what is being asked of the stutterer and their family might be stressful.

See the **ASHA Cultural Responsiveness Practice Portal** for more information.

Generally, behavioral interventions are effective across cultures, and improved fluency will likely generalize from one language to another for those who are bilingual (Roberts & Shenker, 2007). Furthermore, similar outcomes are observed for both bilingual and monolingual individuals (Shenker, 2011); however, some adjustments in intervention protocols may be needed, such as the following:

- Changing instructions so they are available in the individual's first language
- Providing examples using media formats in the individual's first language
- Giving practice opportunities in relevant cultural and linguistic environments

Engaging parents is also effective for achieving generalized use of strategies learned to manage stuttering across languages (Shenker, 2013). Medina, Pareja, et al. (2023) conducted a qualitative study of 36 racially and ethnically diverse individuals who stuttered and identified the types of support they perceived as being positive and negative from their families. Families that were patient, listened with empathy, and sought outside support were viewed positively, whereas families that were judgmental, teased, and punished the family member who stuttered were viewed negatively. Negative perceptions included family members finishing the individual's sentences, telling them to slow their speech, and refusing to talk openly about the fluency disorder. This has important implication for clinicians. Providing culturally appropriate family education regarding the types of support related to stuttering is a necessary step to meet the individualized needs of the person who stutters.

SLPs are expected to provide the services needed by an individual who stutters no matter what their cultural and linguistic background unless the family or individual does not want those services. Bilingual SLPs have the background to provide these services, but an interpreter can be used if the SLP does not speak the client's language.

Why Is This Topic Important?

A fluency disorder impacts day-to-day activities and can interfere with a child's play with peers or performance in school. For adults, a fluency disorder can interfere with the individual's work and social interactions (Yaruss & Quesal, 2004). Because fluency disorders can impact all aspects of an individual's ability to fully participate in their environment, it is important to consider the range of interventions and support systems described previously.

Examples of the social–emotional impacts of fluency disorders include challenges with expressing an individual's wants and needs, telling stories and engaging in conversations, managing emotions, exhibiting confidence, and developing friendships. Academic impacts might be seen when asked to read aloud or answer questions, as well as when giving presentations. Because of the anxiety often associated with speaking and the effort it takes to communicate, it is important to understand the daily challenges the stutterer experiences. In fact, there is increased risk of bullying for children who stutter (Blood & Blood, 2004). The SLP has a responsibility to support the development of an Individualized Education Plan when stuttering impacts the student's academic and social development. Eligibility for public school services is determined by a documented "adverse educational impact" of the fluency disorder using standardized measures as well as a communication profile gathered across school and home contexts (Coleman & Yaruss, 2014).

Vocational impacts may be seen when a person who stutters is being interviewed for a job or the work environment requires frequent interactions and communication exchanges, whether face-to-face or via the telephone. Such challenges often determine the career options for the person who stutters (Klein & Hood, 2004). Furthermore, individuals with whom the stutterer works may associate a less than positive attitude about their coworker—often leading to a sense of isolation and exclusion for the person who stutters. It is important, therefore, that SLPs help individuals who stutter learn more about their stuttering, be able to talk about their stuttering, and accept their stuttering so they can advocate for their needs and create workplace support systems (Plexico et al., 2019).

Application to a Child

Antonia is a 4-year-old African American child who has a father and uncle who stutter. She started exhibiting typical disfluencies as she was developing language and putting words together at approximately age 2 years. These disfluencies were generally word repetitions. The pediatrician told the family that this type of disfluency is expected for young children learning language and not to worry. Antonia's disfluency, however, persisted. She is now prolonging initial consonant sounds and repeating syllables within words. Her parents are becoming anxious about Antonia's increased disfluency and are asking her to slow down when she talks. Antonia is becoming frustrated and is starting to block on certain words and consonants. The preschool SLP completed a comprehensive assessment and found that Antonia's receptive language is age appropriate but that there is a 1-year delay in her expressive language. Her cognitive abilities are within normal limits. An interview with Antonia's parents indicated that she has started to avoid speaking situations, which impacts her interactions with peers at her preschool. A speech assessment revealed that Antonia struggles with initial consonant sounds, especially those beginning with [p, t, s], as well as some vowel sounds, including the first vowel sound in her name. After speaking with Antonia and her parents, the SLP decided that an appropriate goal was to minimize Antonia's stuttering and help her manage her stuttering moments. In addition to direct therapy, the SLP decided to implement a home-based intervention plan so that the parents could carry over what Antonia was learning in therapy in the home. The home-based intervention plan includes working with Antonia's family members to adjust their speech, model fluent speech, and limit questions directed at Antonia. The SLP also began working with Antonia to modify her speech to lessen the negative impact of her stuttering, as well as employing some operant treatment strategies to reinforce Antonia's fluent speech and intermittently correct her disfluency. Antonia's parents also learned to provide Antonia feedback when she was fluent and nonfluent.

As you think about Antonia's initial disfluencies and the recommendation for a wait-and-see approach, what about her background suggested she was at greater risk than other young children with early disfluencies? Was the SLP's assessment sufficiently comprehensive to get a clear picture of Antonia's difficulties across settings? What other information could or should the SLP have gathered? The SLP used indirect, direct, and operant intervention strategies to address Antonia's disfluencies. Do you agree with her approach? Are there any other strategies you believe might have helped Antonia and her family?

Application to an Adolescent or Adult

Billy is a 22-year-old young man who has been stuttering since he was 6 years old. He has received therapy from several SLPs with intermittent success. Generally, he knows how to manage his stuttering by using an easy onset approach as well as continuous phonation—strategies he learned early on—but he often finds himself avoiding speaking situations where he knows that his stuttering might be exacerbated. Because his family moved frequently, he has not had a chance to build a support system that understands what it is like to be a person who stutters and how best to navigate the next steps in his life. He just graduated from college with a dual degree in business and computer science and is now searching for a job. He has had several interviews but does not ever make it to the final selection. He believes that his stuttering is the reason that he is not getting the jobs that he believes he is highly qualified for. His friends have moved since graduating from college, which has left him feeling isolated and with an increase in negative thoughts about his stuttering, his life, and his ability to have a successful future. He has a girlfriend who is encouraging him to return to speech-language therapy. He is considering this but does not want to be disappointed, yet again, when the interventions do not eliminate his stuttering or the associated negative feelings. Billy decides to call the local university-based speech and language clinic to find out if the clinic is taking patients and what experience the clinic has working with adults who stutter. The clinic currently has a waiting list for individual treatment sessions, but there is availability in an adult stuttering support group that meets each Monday evening. Billy is hesitant to take this step because his stuttering is still an embarrassment to him, and he would prefer individual therapy.

Knowing what you learned about stuttering reading this chapter, consider how you would address the following questions.

- Would you recommend that Billy attend the adult support group?
- How might this support group be helpful to Billy?

- Considering the strategies described in this chapter to support those who experience continuous stuttering, what approaches do you think might be helpful to Billy and why?
- How might you help Billy decrease his negative attitude about his stuttering and his future career?

Chapter Summary

This chapter describes two fluency disorders: stuttering and cluttering. Stuttering is characterized by repetitions, prolongations, blocks, and physical tension. In contrast, cluttering is characterized by an irregular speech rate, syllable omissions, and unexpected pauses in sentences that lead to breakdowns in speech clarity. Both types of fluency disorders can have a significant impact on the daily functioning of an individual. Furthermore, although the overall prevalence of fluency disorders is less than 1%, the incidence is higher, particularly in the preschool population. Factors such as a family history of stuttering, gender, and co-occurring conditions can increase the risk of stuttering in a child.

Stuttering assessment has many steps. An interview with the family and the individual who stutters should be completed to gather information about the person's overall development and any family history of stuttering or cluttering. In addition, the family should be asked to describe the disfluent characteristics, when the disfluencies first occurred, what the response was to those disfluencies, and how stuttering impacts the individual and the family. Teachers and other professionals who work with the individual who stutters are also interviewed to get a sense of how stable or variable the stuttering is across different environments. Speech samples from the child's home environment and during the assessment are obtained. The clinician's goal is to gather information on the individual's frequency, type, and duration of disfluencies; their speech rate and intelligibility; and any evidence of secondary behaviors.

Intervention for fluency disorders is variable and considers an individual's needs. When developing an intervention plan, the SLP considers the preferences, values, beliefs, and motivation of the person who stutters and the available family support. There are a range of interventions that may look different for preschoolers versus school-age children, adolescents, and adults. The goal of any intervention plan, however, is to help the stutterer react more positively to their disfluencies and use the strategies they have learned to manage the disfluencies when they occur. Counseling is often part of the intervention to provide additional support and lessen the burden of living with a communication disorder.

Chapter Review Questions

1. Identify the risk factors for a fluency disorder.
2. Compare and contrast the signs and symptoms of cluttering versus stuttering.
3. What types of disfluencies do not require intervention?
4. What is the prevalence and incidence of stuttering?
5. Describe the elements of an assessment for a fluency disorder.

6. How is mindfulness used to support those impacted by stuttering?
7. Describe direct, indirect, and operant intervention strategies for young children who stutter?
8. How is desensitization used to support the individual who stutters?
9. What is the difference between cognitive–behavior therapy and acceptance commitment therapy?
10. Describe the additional intervention considerations that should be made for adults who stutter.

Learning Activities

1. Parents bring their 3-year-old child in for her annual visit to the pediatrician. The parents describe some concerns with their daughter's speech fluency. She is repeating words and phrases when she communicates while telling a story. Which of the following would you recommend and why?
    a. Make an immediate referral to an SLP because these signs are symptomatic of stuttering.
    b. Tell the parents that their daughter is stuttering and that they should correct her speech when she does stutter.
    c. Explain these are typical disfluencies that often occur when a child is in a period of language explosion and that you will keep an eye on it.
    d. Tell the parents that their daughter is really demonstrating symptoms of cluttering.

2. Watch and listen to the YouTube video "For Parents of a Child Who Stutters: Causes of Concern" to see what multiple repetitions, prolongations, and blocks look like. Then watch and listen to the YouTube video "Kids Talk About Stuttering" and identify when you hear repetitions, blocks, and prolongations on sounds, words, and phrases.

"For Parents of a Child Who Stutters: Causes of Concern"

"Kids Talk About Stuttering"

3. Find and read about a personal account of someone who stutters in the entertainment industry and learn about their struggles with stuttering, how they manage their stuttering, and the support they received to be successful in their career.

4. Read the following article:

    Gerlach-Houck, H., & Constantino, C. D. (2022). Interrupting ableism in stuttering therapy and research: Practical suggestions. *Perspectives of the ASHA Special Interest Groups, 7*, 357–374.

    After reading this article, reflect on the following questions:

    - How has your view of a person who stutters changed, if at all, after reading this article?
    - In what ways have you contributed to ableism in stuttering?
    - What steps will you take in any future interactions you might have with a person who stutters that are responsive to the suggestions in this article?

Suggested Reading

O'Brian, S., Jones, M., Packman, A., Onslow, M., Menzies, R., Lowe, R., . . . Briem, A., (2022). The complexity of stuttering behavior in adults and adolescents: Relationship to age, severity, mental health, impact of stuttering, and behavioral treatment outcome. *Journal of Speech, Language, and Hearing Research, 65*, 2446–2458.

This study discusses the unique differences and complexities of stuttering by examining individual stuttering moments using the Lidcombe Behavioral Data Language, which is a measure that describes the speech behavior of stuttering. Stuttering behaviors have been seen as early as preschool age, and addressing stuttering earlier in life may be beneficial to mental health later in life.

This study examined the influence of age, gender, behavioral treatment, severity, and comorbidities of anxiety on stuttering behaviors. There were 84 adolescents and adults who participated in behavioral treatment (17 females and 67 males), with a mean age of 26.9 years and a range of 11 to 74 years. The behavioral treatment ran for 8 hours a day, 5 days a week, for 7 weeks. There was also a 90-minute weekly follow-up. Each participant had a 10-minute video recording made before and after intensive treatment.

In the 147 videos, 3,100 stuttering moments were used for analysis. Approximately half of the moments included repeated movement and superfluous verbal (e.g., grunting or adding words such as "oh well") or nonverbal behaviors (e.g., tics, facial grimaces). Fixed posture with (e.g., "mmmmmy little kkkkkitty played!") or without (e.g., "I [no sound] built . . . ") audible airflow was identified during two-thirds of the moments. The most common type of stuttering was a combination of fixed posture and extraneous behaviors. This combination did not change significantly prior to or following treatment, and it was not associated with mental health disorders, self-reported stuttering, anxiety, and depression. Percentage of stuttered syllables, gender, and Overall Assessment of the Speaker's Experience of Stuttering (OASES) were not statistically significant when paired with a combination of fixed posture and superfluous behaviors.

The authors found that severity of stuttering may change throughout a person's lifetime. The complexity of behavioral stuttering types assigned by SLPs was related to the severity of stuttering that SLPs rated for each video. The complexity of stuttering did not change with intensive speech therapy.

Walsh, B. W., Grobbel, H., Christ, S. L., Tichenor, S. E., & Gerwin, K. L. (2023). Exploring the relationship between resilience and the adverse impact of stuttering in children. *Journal of Speech, Language, and Hearing Research, 66*, 2278–2295.

In this study, the authors investigated the relationship between resilience (the ability to carry on when confronted with difficult circumstances) and the impact of stuttering on a child who stutters. Participants in the study included 148 children aged 5 to 18 years who stutter. The children were asked to complete two measures: the Child and Youth Resilience Measure (CYRM) and OASES. The children's parents also completed a behavioral checklist as well as the parent form of the CYRM. The authors found that children who identified more external and/or personal resilience often had fewer reports of adverse impact regarding their stuttering. With variable experiences and responses to stuttering in relation to personal and external resilience factors, the authors describe the importance of a strengths-based approach to therapy.

Additional Resources

- American Speech-Language-Hearing Association, "ASHA Digital Toolkit: Stuttering 101" https://www.asha.org/public/stuttering-toolkit
- *The ASHA LeaderLive*, "How Can You Tell if Childhood Stuttering Is the Real Deal?" https://leader.pubs.asha.org/do/10.1044/how-can-you-tell-if-childhood-stuttering-is-the-real-deal/full
- The Stuttering Foundation https://www.stutteringhelp.org
- "The Stuttering Homepage" https://web.mnsu.edu/comdis/kuster/stutter.html
- "Stuttering vs. Cluttering" [PDF] https://d2r0txsugik6oi.cloudfront.net/neon/resource/nsa/File/Brochures/StuttervsClutter.pdf

References

Abou, E. M., Saleh, M., Habil, I., El Sawy, M., & El Assal, L. (2015). Prevalence of stuttering in primary school children in Cairo-Egypt. *International Journal of Speech-Language Pathology*, *17*(4), 367–372.

Al-Jazi, A. B., & Al-Khamra, R. (2015). Prevalence of speech disorders in elementary school students in Jordan. *Education*, *136*(2), 159–168.

American Psychiatric Association. (2022). *Diagnostic and statistical manual of mental disorders* (5th ed., text rev.).

Amster, B. J., & Klein, E. R. (2018). Introduction: The importance of the social, emotional, and cognitive dimensions of stuttering. In B. J. Amster & E. R. Klein (Eds.), *More than fluency: The social, emotional, and cognitive dimensions of stuttering* (pp. 1–5). Plural Publishing.

Arenas, R. M., Walker, E. A., & Oleson, J. J. (2017). Developmental stuttering in children who are hard of hearing. *Language, Speech, and Hearing Services in Schools*, *48*(4), 234–248.

Beilby, J. M., Byrnes, M. L., & Yaruss, J. S. (2012). Acceptance and commitment therapy for adults who stutter: Psychosocial adjustment and speech fluency. *Journal of Fluency Disorders*, *37*(4), 289–299.

Berquez, A., & Kelman, E. (2018). Methods in stuttering therapy for desensitizing parents of children who stutter. *American Journal of Speech-Language Pathology*, *27*(3S), 1124–1138.

Bishop, S. R., Lau, M., Shapiro, S., Carlson, L., Anderson, N. D., Carmody, J., . . . Devins, G. (2004). Mindfulness: A proposed operational definition. *Clinical Psychology: Science and Practice*, *11*(3), 230–241.

Blood, G. W., & Blood, I. M. (2004). Bullying in adolescents who stutter: Communicative competence and self-esteem. *Contemporary Issues in Communication Science and Disorders*, *31*, 69–79.

Blumgart, E., Tran, Y., & Craig, A. (2010). Social anxiety disorder in adults who stutter. *Depression & Anxiety*, *27*(7), 687–692.

Boyle, M. P. (2013). Assessment of stigma associated with stuttering: Development and evaluation of the Self-Stigma of Stuttering Scale (4S). *Journal of Speech, Language, and Hearing Research*, *56*(5), 1517–1529.

Boyle, M. P. (2015). Identifying correlates of self-stigma in adults who stutter: Further establishing the construct validity of the Self-Stigma of Stuttering Scale (4S). *Journal of Fluency Disorders, 43,* 17–27.

Boyle, M. P., Beita-Ell, C., & Milewski, K. M. (2019). Finding the good in the challenge: Benefit finding among adults who stutter. *Perspectives on Fluency and Fluency Disorders, 4*(6), 1316–1326.

Boyle, M. P., & Gabel, R. (2020). Toward a better understanding of the process of disclosure events among people who stutter. *Journal of Fluency Disorders, 63,* Article 105746.

Boyle, M. P., Milewski, K. M., & Beita-Ell, C. (2018). Disclosure of stuttering and quality of life in people who stutter. *Journal of Fluency Disorders, 58,* 1–10.

Briley, P. M., & Ellis, C. (2018). The coexistence of disabling conditions in children who stutter: Evidence from the National Health Interview Survey. *Journal of Speech, Language, and Hearing Research, 61*(12), 2895–2905.

Byrd, C. T. (2018). Assessing bilingual children: Are their disfluencies indicative of stuttering or the by-product of navigating two languages? *Seminars in Speech and Language, 39*(4), 324–332.

Byrd, C. T., Croft, R., Gkalitsiou, Z., & Hampton, E. (2017). Clinical utility of self-disclosure for adults who stutter: Apologetic versus informative statements. *Journal of Fluency Disorders, 54,* 1–13.

Byrd, C. T., & Donaher, J. (2018). Best practice for developmental stuttering: Balancing evidence and expertise. *Language, Speech, and Hearing Services in Schools, 49*(1), 1–3.

Caughter, S., & Crofts, V. (2018). Nurturing a resilient mindset in school-aged children who stutter. *American Journal of Speech-Language Pathology, 27*(3S), 1111–1123.

Chang, S.-E. (2014). Research updates in neuroimaging studies of children who stutter. *Seminars in Speech and Language, 35*(2), 67–79.

Chang, S.-E., Garnett, E. O., Etchell, A., & Chow, H. M. (2019). Functional and neuroanatomical bases of developmental stuttering: Current insights. *The Neuroscientist, 25*(6), 566–582.

Chang, S.-E., & Zhu, D. C. (2013). Neural network connectivity differences in children who stutter. *Brain, 136*(12), 3709–3726.

Chang, S.-E., Zhu, D. C., Choo, A. L., & Angstadt, M. (2015). White matter neuroanatomical differences in young children who stutter. *Brain, 138*(3), 694–711.

Choi, D., Conture, E. G., Walden, T. A., Lambert, W. E., & Tumanova, V. (2013). Behavioral inhibition and childhood stuttering. *Journal of Fluency Disorders, 38*(2), 171–183.

Coifman, K. G., & Bonanno, G. A. (2010). When distress does not become depression: Emotion context sensitivity and adjustment to bereavement. *Journal of Abnormal Psychology, 119*(3), 479–490.

Coleman, C., & Yaruss, J. S. (2014). A comprehensive view of stuttering: Implications for assessment and treatment. *SIG 16 Perspectives on School-Based Issues, 15*(2), 75–80.

Craig, A., Hancock, K., Tran, Y., Craig, M., & Peters, K. (2002). Epidemiology of stuttering in the community across the entire life span. *Journal of Speech, Language, and Hearing Research, 45*(6), 1097–1105.

Craig, A., & Tran, Y. (2014). Trait and social anxiety in adults with chronic stuttering: Conclusions following meta-analysis. *Journal of Fluency Disorders, 40,* 35–43.

Davidow, J. H., & Scott, K. A. (2017). Intrajudge and interjudge reliability of the Stuttering Severity Instrument–Fourth Edition. *American Journal of Speech-Language Pathology, 26*(4), 1105–1119.

Drayna, D., & Kang, C. (2011). Genetic approaches to understanding the causes of stuttering. *Journal of Neurodevelopmental Disorders*, *3*(4), 374–380.

Druker, K., Mazzucchelli, T., Hennessey, N., & Beilby, J. (2019). Parent perceptions of an integrated stuttering treatment and behavioral self-regulation program for early developmental stuttering. *Journal of Fluency Disorders*, *62*, Article 105762.

Fletcher, L., & Hayes, S. C. (2005). Relational frame theory, acceptance and commitment therapy, and a functional analytic definition of mindfulness. *Journal of Rational Emotive and Cognitive Behavior Therapy*, *23*(4), 315–336.

Foote, G. (2013). Overheard: Bilingual and disfluent: A unique treatment challenge. *The ASHA Leader*, *18*(3), 14–15.

Freud, D., & Amir, O. (2020). Resilience in people who stutter: Association with covert and overt characteristics of stuttering. *Journal of Fluency Disorders*, *64*, Article 105761.

Frigerio-Domingues, C. E., & Drayna, D. (2017). Genetic contributions to stuttering: The current evidence. *Molecular Genetics & Genomic Medicine*, *5*(2), 95–102.

Frigerio-Domingues, C. E., Gkalitsiou, Z., Zezinka, A., Sainz, E., Gutierrez, J., Byrd, C., . . . Drayna, D. (2019). Genetic factors and therapy outcomes in persistent developmental stuttering. *Journal of Communication Disorders*, *80*, 11–17.

Gerlach, H., Totty, E., Subraminian, A., & Zebrowski, P. (2018). Stuttering and labor market outcomes in the United States. *Journal of Speech, Language, and Hearing Research*, *61*(7), 1649–1663.

Gerlach-Houck, H., Kubart, K., & Cage, E. (2023). Concealing stuttering at school: When you can't fix it . . . the only alternative is to hide it. *Language, Speech, and Hearing Services in Schools*, *54*, 96–113.

Guitar, B. (2019). *Stuttering: An integrated approach to its nature and treatment* (5th ed.). Wolters Kluwer.

Gupta, S., Yashodharakumar, G. Y., & Vasudha, H. H. (2016). Cognitive behavior therapy and mindfulness training in the treatment of adults who stutter. *International Journal of Indian Psychology*, *3*(3), 78–87.

Guttormsen, L. S., Kefalianos, E., & Næss, K. A. B. (2015). Communication attitudes in children who stutter: A meta-analytic review. *Journal of Fluency Disorders*, *46*, 1–14.

Han, T.-U., Park, J., Domingues, C. F., Moretti-Ferreira, D., Paris, E., Sainz, E., . . . Drayna, D. (2014). A study of the role of the *FOXP2* and *CNTNAP2* genes in persistent developmental stuttering. *Neurobiology of Disease*, *69*, 23–31.

Hayes, S. C., Luoma, J. B., Bond, F. W., Masuda, A., & Lillis, J. (2006). Acceptance and commitment therapy: Model, processes, and outcomes. *Behaviour Research and Therapy*, *44*(1), 1–25.

Helgadóttir, F. D., Menzies, R. G., Onslow, M., Packman, A., & O'Brian, S. (2014). A standalone internet cognitive behavior therapy treatment for social anxiety in adults who stutter: CBTpsych. *Journal of Fluency Disorders*, *41*(C), 47–54.

Iverach, L., Jones, M., McLellan, L. F., Lyneham, H. J., Menzies, R. G., Onslow, M., & Rapee, R. M. (2016). Prevalence of anxiety disorders among children who stutter. *Journal of Fluency Disorders*, *49*, 13–28.

Iverach, L., & Rapee, R. M. (2014). Social anxiety disorder and stuttering: Current status and future directions. *Journal of Fluency Disorders*, *40*, 69–82.

Kelman, R., & Nicholas, A. (2020). *Palin Parent–Child Interaction Therapy for early childhood stammering*. Routledge.

Klein, J. F., & Hood, S. B. (2004). The impact of stuttering on employment opportunities and job performance. *Journal of Fluency Disorders, 29*(4), 255–273.

Kraft, S. J., Lowther, E., & Beilby, J. (2019). The role of effortful control in stuttering severity in children: Replication study. *American Journal of Speech-Language Pathology, 28*(1), 14–28.

Kraft, S. J., & Yairi, E. (2011). Genetic bases of stuttering: The state of the art, 2011. *Folia Phoniatrica et Logopaedica, 64*(1), 34–47.

Leech, K. A., Bernstein Ratner, N., Brown, B., & Weber, C. M. (2017). Preliminary evidence that growth in productive language differentiates childhood stuttering persistence and recovery. *Journal of Speech, Language, and Hearing Research, 60*(11), 3097–3109.

Leech, K. A., Bernstein Ratner, N., Brown, B., & Weber, C. M. (2019). Language growth predicts stuttering persistence over and above family history and treatment experience: Response to Marcotte. *Journal of Speech, Language, and Hearing Research, 62*(5), 1371–1372.

Mancinelli, J. M. (2019). The effects of self-disclosure on the communicative interaction between a person who stutters and a normally fluent speaker. *Journal of Fluency Disorders, 59*, 1–20.

Manivannan, V., Medina, A. M., Maruthy, S., Singhal, M., Agarwal, A., & Manchaiah, V. (2023). Positive experiences related to stuttering in adults who stutter. *Perspectives of the ASHA Special Interest Groups, 8*, 932–942.

Manning, W. H., & DiLollo, A. (2018). *Clinical decision making in fluency disorders.* Plural Publishing.

Medina, A. M., Mead, J. S., Comas, K., Perez, G., Prieto, J., & Valencia, I. (2023). Outcomes of a remote mindfulness program for adults who stutter: Five case studies. *Perspectives of the ASHA Special Interest Groups, 8*, 897–912.

Medina, A. M., Pareja, D., Berlanga, E., Crawford, C., & Tormo, A. (2023). Concepts of family support in stuttering: A multicultural perspective. *Perspectives of the ASHA Special Interest Groups, 8*, 343–357.

Millard, S. K., Nicholas, A., & Cook, F. M. (2008). Is parent–child interaction therapy effective in reducing stuttering? *Journal of Speech, Language, and Hearing Research, 51*(3), 636–650.

Millard, S. K., Zebrowski, P., & Kelman, E. (2018). Palin Parent–Child Interaction Therapy: The bigger picture. *American Journal of Speech-Language Pathology, 27*(3S), 1211–1223.

Murphy, W. P., Yaruss, J. S., & Quesal, R. W. (2007a). Enhancing treatment for school-age children who stutter: I. Reducing negative reactions through desensitization and cognitive restructuring. *Journal of Fluency Disorders, 32*(2), 121–138.

Murphy, W. P., Yaruss, J. S., & Quesal, R. W. (2007b). Enhancing treatment for school-age children who stutter: II. Reducing bullying through role-playing and self-disclosure. *Journal of Fluency Disorders, 32*(2), 139–162.

Onslow, M., Packman, A., & Harrison, E. (Eds.). (2003). *The Lidcombe Program of early stuttering intervention: A clinician's guide.* Pro-Ed.

Oyono, L. T., Pascoe, M., & Singh, S. (2018). The prevalence of speech and language disorders in French-speaking preschool children from Yaoundé (Cameroon). *Journal of Speech, Language, and Hearing Research, 61*(5), 1238–1250.

Palasik, S., & Hannan, J. (2013). The clinical applications of acceptance and commitment therapy with clients who stutter. *Perspectives on Fluency and Fluency Disorders, 23*(2), 54–69.

Plexico, L. W., Hamilton, M. B., Hawkins, H., & Erath, S. (2019). The influence of workplace discrimination and vigilance on job satisfaction with people who stutter. *Journal of Fluency Disorders, 62*, Article 105725.

Plexico, L. W., Manning, W. H., & DiLollo, A. (2005). A phenomenological understanding of successful stuttering management. *Journal of Fluency Disorders, 30*(1), 1–22.

Prelock, P. A., & Hutchins, T. (2018). Children with speech disorders. In *Clinical guide to assessment and treatment of communication disorders* (pp. 75–88). Springer.

Proctor, A., Yairi, E., Duff, M., & Zhang, J. (2008). Prevalence of stuttering in African American preschool children. *Journal of Speech, Language, and Hearing Research, 51*(6), 1465–1479.

Roberts, P., & Shenker, R. (2007). Assessment and treatment of stuttering in bilingual speakers. In E. Conture & R. F. Curlee (Eds.), *Stuttering and related disorders of fluency* (pp. 297–325). Thieme.

Rocha, M., Yaruss, J. S., & Rato, J. R. (2020). Stuttering impact: A shared perception for parents and children. *Folia Phoniatrica et Logopaedica, 72*(6), 478–486.

Scaler Scott, K., & Ward, D. (2013). *Managing cluttering: A comprehensive guidebook of activities*. Pro-Ed.

Shenker, R. C. (2011). Multilingual children who stutter: Clinical issues. *Journal of Fluency Disorders, 36*(3), 186–193.

Shenker, R. C. (2013). Bilingual myth-busters series when young children who stutter are also bilingual: Some thoughts about assessment and treatment. *Perspectives on Communication Disorders and Sciences in Culturally and Linguistically Diverse (CLD) Populations, 20*(1), 15–23.

Singer, C. M., Hessling, A., Kelly, E. M., Singer, L., & Jones, R. M. (2020). Clinical characteristics associated with stuttering persistence: A meta-analysis. *Journal of Speech, Language, and Hearing Research, 63*(9), 2995–3018.

Sisskin, V. (2018). Avoidance Reduction Therapy for Stuttering (ARTS). In B. J. Amster & E. R. Klein (Eds.), *More than fluency: The social, emotional, and cognitive dimensions of stuttering* (pp. 157–186). Plural Publishing.

Smith, A., & Weber, C. (2017). How stuttering develops: The multifactorial dynamic pathways theory. *Journal of Speech, Language, and Hearing Research, 60*(9), 2483–2505.

Sønsterud, H., Feragen, K. B., Kirmess, M., Halvorsen, M. S., & Ward, D. (2019). What do people search for in stuttering therapy: Personal goal-setting as a gold standard? *Journal of Communication Disorders, 85*, Article 105944.

St. Louis, K. O., & Schulte, K. (2011). Defining cluttering: The lowest common denominator. In D. Ward & K. Scaler Scott (Eds.), *Cluttering: Research, intervention and education* (pp. 233–253). Psychology Press.

Tichenor, S. E., Gerwin, K. L., & Walsh, B. (2023). Repetitive negative thinking in adolescents who stutter. *Journal of Speech, Language, and Hearing Research, 66*, 3290–3306.

Tichenor, S. E., Herring, C., & Yaruss, J. S. (2022). Understanding the speaker's experience of stuttering can improve stuttering therapy. *Topics in Language Disorders, 42*(1), 57–75.

Tichenor, S. E., Walsh, B. M., Gerwin, K. L., & Yaruss, J. S. (2022). Emotional regulation and its influence on the experience of stuttering across the life span. *Journal of Speech, Language, and Hearing Research, 65*, 2412–2430.

Tichenor, S. E., & Yaruss, J. S. (2018). A phenomenological analysis of the moment of stuttering. *American Journal of Speech-Language Pathology, 27*(3S), 1180–1194.

Tichenor, S. E., & Yaruss, J. S. (2019a). Group experiences and individual differences in stuttering. *Journal of Speech, Language, and Hearing Research, 62*(12), 4335–4350.

Tichenor, S. E., & Yaruss, J. S. (2019b). Stuttering as defined by adults who stutter. *Journal of Speech, Language, and Hearing Research, 62*(12), 4356–4369.

Trichon, M., & Raj, E. X. (2018). Peer support for people who stutter: History, benefits, and accessibility. In B. J. Amster & E. R. Klein (Eds.), *More than fluency: The social, emotional, and cognitive dimensions of stuttering* (pp. 187–214). Plural Publishing.

Ward, D. (2006). *Stuttering and cluttering: Frameworks for understanding and treatment.* Psychology Press.

Ward, D., Connally, E. L., Pliatsikas, C., Bretherton-Furness, J., & Watkins, K. E. (2015). The neurological underpinnings of cluttering: Some initial findings. *Journal of Fluency Disorders, 43,* 1–16.

Yairi, E., & Ambrose, N. (2005). *Early childhood stuttering for clinicians by clinicians.* Pro-Ed.

Yairi, E., & Ambrose, N. (2013). Epidemiology of stuttering: 21st century advances. *Journal of Fluency Disorders, 38*(2), 66–87.

Yaruss, J. S., Coleman, C., & Hammer, D. (2006). Treating preschool children who stutter: Description and preliminary evaluation of a family-focused treatment approach. *Language, Speech, and Hearing Services in Schools, 37*(2), 118–136.

Yaruss, J. S., Coleman, C. E., & Quesal, R. W. (2012). Stuttering in school-age children: A comprehensive approach to treatment. *Language, Speech, and Hearing Services in Schools, 43*(4), 536–548.

Yaruss, J. S., & Quesal, R. W. (2004). Stuttering and the International Classification of Functioning, Disability and Health (ICF): An update. *Journal of Communication Disorders, 37*(1), 35–52.

Yaruss, J. S., Quesal, R. W., & Reeves, L. (2007). Self-help and mutual aid groups. In E. G. Conture & R. F. Curlee (Eds.), *Stuttering and related disorders of fluency* (pp. 256–276). Thieme.

Young, M. M., Byrd, C. T., Gabel, R., & White, A. Z. (2022). Self-disclosure experiences of adults who stutter: An interpretative phenomenological analysis. *American Journal of Speech-Language Pathology, 31,* 2045–2060.

Zablotsky, B., Black, L. I., Maenner, M. J., Schieve, L. A., Danielson, M. L., Bitsko, R. H., . . . Boyle, C. A. (2019). Prevalence and trends of developmental disabilities among children in the United States: 2009–2017. *Pediatrics, 144*(4), Article e20190811.

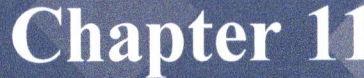

Chapter 11

Voice Disorders

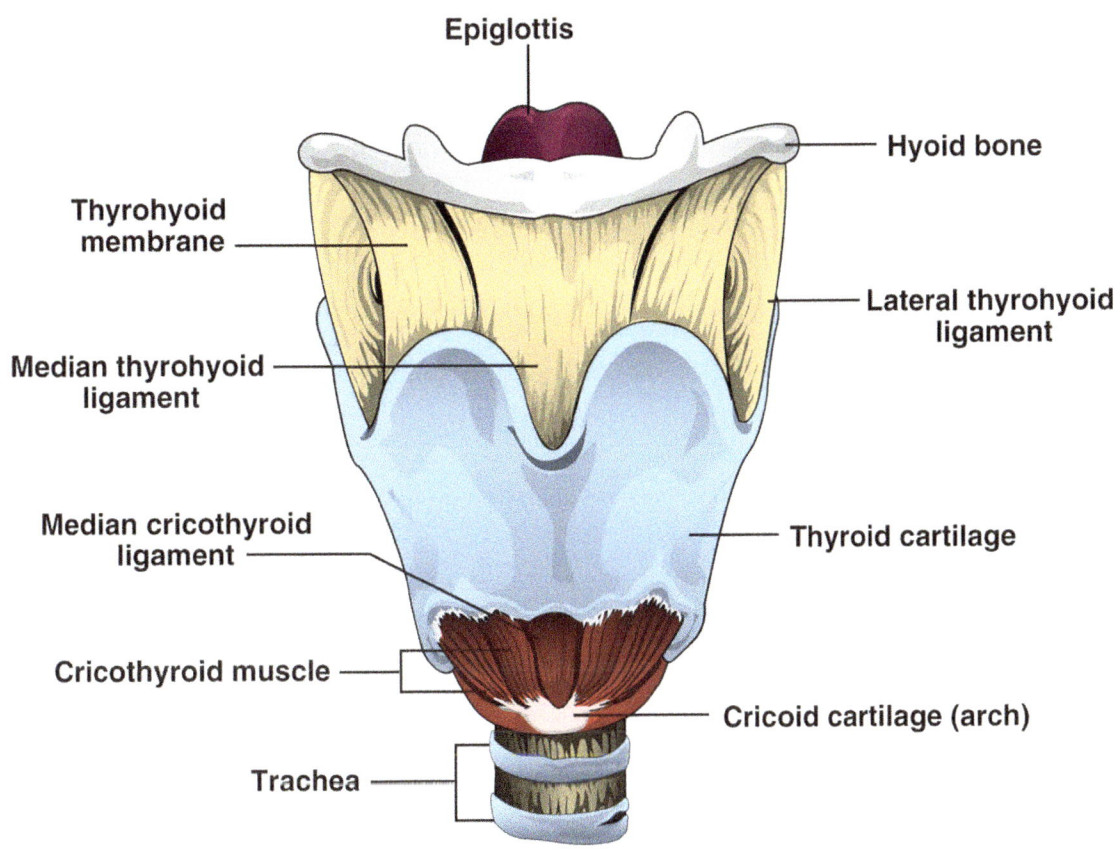

Learning Objectives

After reading this chapter, you will be able to:

- Explain the impact of voice disorders on children and adults.
- Describe the causes and characteristics of voice disorders, including vocal nodules and vocal fold paralysis.
- Identify the impact of laryngeal cancer on the ability to communicate.
- Explain the importance of voice therapy in gender transition.

Key Terms

- adduction
- aphonia
- cul-de-sac resonance
- dysphonia
- dysphoria
- dyspnea
- edema
- exercise-induced laryngeal obstruction (EILO)
- expiratory pressure device
- functional voice disorder
- gender-affirming voice therapy
- gender dysphoria
- glottal stop
- glottic stenosis
- human papillomavirus
- hypernasality
- hyponasality
- laryngeal cleft
- laryngeal nerve
- laryngeal webbing
- laryngomalacia
- multiple sclerosis
- neurogenic voice disorders
- organic voice disorders
- papilloma
- paradoxical vocal fold movement (PVFM)
- Parkinson disease
- presbyphonia
- pseudobulbar palsy
- psychogenic aphonia/dysphonia
- psychogenic conversion aphonia/dysphonia
- puberphonia
- sarcopenia
- spasmodic dysphonia
- stridor
- structural voice disorders
- tracheostomy
- vocal fold paralysis
- ventricular phonation
- videoendoscopy
- videostroboscopy
- vocal cords or vocal folds
- vocal cyst
- vocal fatigue
- vocal nodules
- vocal polyps

Introduction

Have you ever been at a football game cheering for your team with such energy that you have lost your voice? Do you know a singer who had to cancel a show because they lost their voice? In this chapter, we discuss the voice and voice disorders. A voice disorder is characterized by a person identifying that their voice does not meet their needs and that there is a notable difference in their vocal quality, loudness, or pitch that is different than what might be expected for their gender, age, area in which they live, or their cultural background (American Speech-Language-Hearing Association [ASHA], 2023; Aronson & Bless, 2009; Boone et al., 2010; Colton et al., 2011; Stemple et al., 2010).

Many occupations require the use of one's voice, such as a teacher, singer, coaches, professional speakers, and so on. Teachers, for example, are at particular risk for voice disorders, with an estimated occurrence of two or three times that of the general population, because they talk to students for 5 or 6 hours a day (Byeon, 2019; Martins et al., 2014). Singers are another at-risk population, with a voice disorder estimate of 46% (Pestana et al., 2017). To avoid developing vocal fatigue and a possible voice disorder, education on vocal hygiene is often recommended for both teachers and singers, in addition to home-based relaxation and breathing exercises (Lin et al., 2023).

In the United States, almost 18 million adults exhibit voice disorders or report difficulty phonating (making sound), which certainly impacts their ability to communicate and engage effectively in social interactions (Bhattacharyya, 2014; Fujiki & Thibeault, 2023). When surveyed, slightly fewer than 10 million people reported a voice problem in the previous 12 months that lasted a week or longer (Bhattacharyya, 2014; Hoffman et al., 2014; Morris et al., 2016). The prevalence of voice disorders in adults varies, with 6% noted for 24- to 34-year-olds and no real difference across diverse categories (Bainbridge et al., 2017). Between ages 19 and 60 years, the most commonly occurring voice disorders include functional dysphonia (20.5%), acid laryngitis (12.5%), and vocal polyps (12%) (Martins et al., 2015). The occurrence of voice disorders increases with age, as estimates range from 4.8% to 29.1% for adults older than age 60 years (de Araújo Pernambuco et al., 2014). Vocal changes in older adults are most often the result of an aging voice (**presbyphonia**), as well as reflux/inflammation, vocal cord paralysis, and functional dysphonia (Martins et al., 2015). For adults between ages 75 and 79 years, voice disorders are most often due to laryngeal cancers (Roy et al., 2016). Voice disorders also seem to occur more often in adult females than males (Martins et al., 2015).

The exact occurrence of voice disorders in children is unknown because many children are not diagnosed, but researchers hint at a wide range from 1.4% to 23.9% (Bhattacharyya, 2014; Johnson et al., 2020). It appears that premature infants who are hospitalized for more than 28 days experience **dysphonia** often related to the intubation they need while in the neonatal intensive care unit (Hseu et al., 2018). Vocal nodules, also resulting in dysphonia, are a common voice disorder in children (41–73%) because of vocal misuse (Martins et al., 2015). Male children also seem to exhibit more voice disorders than females (Martins et al., 2015). Notably, adverse childhood experiences and other social determinants of health (e.g., discrimination) can create situations of extreme stress that impacts the health of the individual, including the occurrence of some voice disorders (Mayne & Namazi, 2023).

Typically, speech-language pathologists (SLPs) and laryngologists manage the assessment and treatment of voice disorders. In some cases, surgery might be needed, but often the SLP is the initial intervention path (Desjardins et al., 2017). Even when surgery is needed for specific voice problems, the SLP partners with the surgeon and the patient to ensure that the individual learns to use their voice appropriately so additional damage to the voice does not occur (Tang & Thibeault, 2017; Tibbetts et al., 2018). Often, patients report positive outcomes following voice therapy, and objective measures are used to verify outcomes (Schindler et al., 2013).

Several direct and indirect strategies may be used to address a voice disorder. Vocal exercises to improve resonance, vocal function, and phonation are just some of the direct approaches used (Meerschman et al., 2019; Verdolini & Li, 2019). Vocal hygiene education is an example of an indirect approach. The number of sessions in voice therapy also varies, but many patients need five or six sessions to achieve positive outcomes (Fujiki & Thibeault, 2023).

In the next sections, you will learn about several different types of voice disorders, their symptoms and causes, the approach to assessing voice disorders, and strategies that are frequently used to address different voice disorders. You will also apply what you learn by reviewing case studies of a child and a young adult with voice disorders.

What We Know About This Topic

A voice disorder is identified when an individual shares concern about having a voice that is different than the voice they expect to meet their daily communication needs (ASHA, 2023). It also appears that as one ages, the bodily structures that are involved in making sounds are also aging, which leads to changes in the voice (Gois et al., 2018). Having a voice disorder may also lead to other mental health conditions such as depression and withdrawing from social situations, which may negatively impact a person's quality of life (Etter et al., 2013; Gregory et al., 2012).

Voice disorders are described as either **organic** or **functional**. An organic voice disorder suggests that there are changes in the mechanisms used to speak, whether it is the laryngeal area, the vocal tract, or the respiratory function. An organic voice disorder can be **structural** (i.e., the vocal mechanism has physical changes), such as the presence of **vocal nodules**, or **neurogenic** (i.e., there are problems in the nervous system that affect vocal mechanism functioning), such as **vocal fold paralysis** or **spasmodic dysphonia** (ASHA, 2023).

Vocal folds are the elastic-like bands that vibrate to make sound and open and close to direct airflow. Changes to the vocal folds are structural, sometimes occurring in pediatric populations when children engage in excessive screaming, loud talking, and other activities that might strain the voice. Such changes can also occur for cheerleaders, coaches, teachers, singers, and others who use their voice a great deal and do not engage in proper vocal hygiene (e.g., breathing from the diaphragm, staying hydrated, decreasing muscle tension). Repeated screaming and excessive talking result in the vocal folds (or cords) slamming together. Just as too much pressure on a finger or a foot causes callouses to form, the same can happen with the vocal folds. Swelling (i.e., **edema**) might occur, and vocal nodules may form on both sides of the folds (bilaterally; Figure 11–1) or vocal polyps may form on one (unilateral) of the folds. This is a common occurrence for young people who use their voice excessively with pitch breaks and increased loudness levels. This often leads to a voice that sounds hoarse, low-pitched (because the vocal fold muscles have thickened), and sometimes breathy with frequent throat clearing as if something is in the throat. Throat clearing can further damage the vocal folds because it causes rapid closure of the vocal folds and then a quick release of air to make a sound (i.e., **glottal stop**).

In a functional voice disorder, there are no differences or anomalies in the physical mechanism used to speak, but there is inefficient use of the vocal mechanism. **Vocal fatigue** is a decline in vocal function characterized by limited voice projection, reduced range of pitch and vocal flexibility, and a change

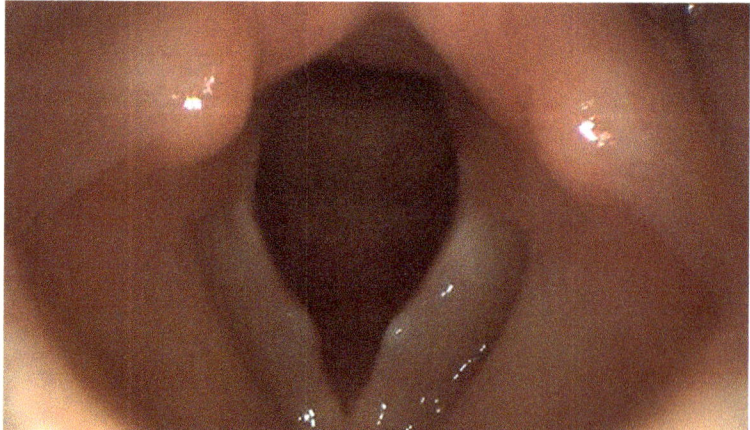

FIGURE 11–1. Image of bilateral vocal nodules. *Source:* Weill Cornell Medicine (https://voice.weill.cornell.edu/voice-disorders/nodules).

in voice quality (Acevedo et al., 2023; Hunter et al., 2020; Nanjundeswaran et al., 2015). People who experience vocal fatigue often have a sensation of tightness in their laryngeal area or soreness and dryness (Welham & Maclagan, 2003). **Aphonia** is when there is a loss of voice, which can be partial or total, and this can occur suddenly or gradually.

There are also rare voice disorders known as **psychogenic voice disorders** or **psychogenic conversion aphonia/dysphonia** (Stemple et al., 2010). These voice disorders affect a person's vocal quality but have no structural or neurogenic explanation. Instead, the loss of phonatory control is the result of anxiety or depression, or in the case of conversion aphonia, there is a loss of voice due to a traumatic event. Although the causal mechanism is unclear, clients who exhibit voice disorders also report increased stress, anxiety, and depression (Marmor et al., 2016; Martinez & Cassol, 2015). Psychological stress can affect the quality of an individual's voice, and with repeated stress, dysphonia or aphonia might occur. In addition, some people just do not like how they sound when they talk. **Dysphoria** occurs when there is a disparity between how someone views themself and how they communicate or how their voice sounds. The differences between identity and the sound of voice occur on a spectrum and often lead to a dysregulated emotional state (DeYoung, 2015). The incompatibility that an individual experiences between the voice they hear and how they view themself has relevance to SLPs, although research is limited in this area (Welch & Helou, 2022).

Voice disorders affect one's communication ability, but the occurrence of voice disorders has not been fully examined in older adults. There are several factors and conditions that might affect the voice of older adults, and a systematic review of voice disorders in older adults suggests the need to both create an assessment protocol and refer for treatment older adults who experience dysphonia (impaired voice production usually characterized by hoarseness or some other changes in voice quality such as pitch and loudness level) (Wang et al., 2023).

There are also two conditions that are not classified as voice disorders but that affect the laryngeal mechanism: **paradoxical vocal fold movement** (PVFM) and **exercise-induced laryngeal obstruction** (EILO). In PVFM, **adduction** (i.e., the bringing together of the vocal folds) is intermittent, and this affects breathing. EILO, often seen in adolescents, occurs when an obstruction occurs during exercise (Halvorsen et al., 2017; Murry & Milstein, 2016; Patel et al., 2015; Traister et al., 2016). The vocal cords come together (adduct) involuntarily and intermittently restrict one's airway when inhaling and exhaling (Fujiki et al., 2023; Guglani et al., 2014; Patel et al., 2015). This is also known as **dyspnea** (i.e., the sensation of running out of air and not being able to breathe during physical activity). In addition, an individual experiencing EILO might also have a feeling of tightness in their throat or chest, a cough, lightheadedness, or even a tendency to hyperventilate (Fujiki et al., 2023; Hseu et al., 2018; Vance et al., 2021; Yi et al., 2021). A person might experience EILO during a period of stress, excessive physical exercise, or if they have gastroesophageal reflux disease (Fujiki et al., 2023; Smith et al., 2017). A decrease in symptoms usually occurs when the physical exercise stops and whatever is causing the symptoms is removed (Fujiki et al., 2023; Wilson et al, 2009). Although the actual prevalence of EILO is unknown, it has been suggested that it occurs in up to 30% of children and adolescents (Zalvan et al., 2021). The prevalence for elite athletes is approximately 5% (Rundell & Spring, 2003), and for those exercising for recreational purposes the occurrence ranges between 5.7% and 8.1%, with young female athletes affected the most (Christensen et al., 2011; Ersson et al., 2020, Johansson et al., 2015). As you might expect, EILO has implications for the performance of athletes and might even lead to burnout and a need to discontinue athletic competitions and other high-intensity performances (Nascimento & Tenenbaum, 2013).

Voice Disruption in Voice Disorders

When you speak, your voice is powered by several factors that support your airflow to make sound. Voicing requires a healthy respiratory system, activation of the laryngeal muscles, coordination of several subsystems (i.e., respiratory, resonance, and phonatory), and the engagement of the pharynx, oral cavity, and nasal cavity to achieve voice production (for more information about the vocal mechanism, see Chapter 4).

When the voice is impacted by a voice disorder, this is referred to as dysphonia, which can include changes in the individual's vocal quality, pitch, loudness level, and vocal effort. There are several symptoms that characterize dysphonia, as described in the ASHA Voice Disorders Practice Portal. See Table 11–1 for a description of the voice quality symptoms considered in a comprehensive voice assessment.

See the **ASHA Voice Disorders Practice Portal.**

You might also notice other signs of a voice disorder such as increased effort when speaking or fatigue when there is a long period of vocal use. Other signs include a change in voice quality or an individual seeming to run out of breath while speaking. In addition, you might notice throat clearing, coughing, laryngeal tension, and/or noticeable discomfort. Voice quality varies in those with voice disorders, and

TABLE 11–1. Description of Voice Quality Symptoms Often Considered in Assessment

Voice Quality Symptom	Description
Rough voice quality	Raspy; irregular sound production
Breathy	Air escapes when making sound
Strained	Harsh and tense voice; increased effort to speak
Strangled	Talking as if holding one's breath
Atypical pitch	Too high or too low or uneven
Atypical loudness	Too loud or too soft or uneven
Atypical resonance	Hyper- or hyponasal
Aphonia	No voice
Phonation breaks	A pause in sound
Asthenia	Weak
Gurgly	Wet-sounding
Pulsed	Creaks or pulses when making sound
Shrill	High pitched, piercing
Tremorous	Shaky

Source: Adapted from the ASHA Practice Portal on Voice Disorders: https://www.asha.org/practice-portal/clinical-topics/voice-disorders/

severity is often determined by structural differences that have occurred in the vocal mechanism or an imbalance in the respiratory, resonance, or phonatory systems.

Causes of Voice Disruption

As described previously, disruptions to the voice may be structural, functional, or psychogenic. As a reminder, structural disruptions can be either organic or neurologic. Organic causes include differences in the vocal folds, such as the following:

- Vocal nodules (callus-like formation on the vocal cords), **cysts** (benign growth on vocal cord), or **polyps** (lesion on only one vocal cord) usually due to vocal misuse (and will disappear when misuse stops)
- **Edema**: Swelling of the vocal folds
- **Glottic stenosis**: Narrowing of the larynx at the vocal folds due to scarring, webbing, and so on
- Recurrent respiratory **papilloma**: Benign wart-like growths on the voice box caused by **human papillomavirus**
- **Sarcopenia**: Muscle atrophy that occurs with aging

There might also be some laryngeal edema or inflammation because of laryngitis, reflux, or arthritis of the laryngeal muscles or joints; or laryngeal trauma due to intubation, exposure to chemicals, or some type of external trauma. A neurologic-based structural cause may be the result of paralysis of the **laryngeal nerve**, **Parkinson's disease**, **multiple sclerosis**, **pseudobulbar palsy**, or spasmodic dysphonia.

Check out the YouTube videos "**Singing With Nodules**" and "**Let's Talk Vocal Injuries: My Experience With Vocal Nodules**" that explain the impact of vocal nodules for singers.

There are also functional causes of voice disruption, such as the phonation changes that occur with yelling or screaming, throat clearing, or coughing, as well when an individual consistently speaks at a pitch that is either too high or too low. Functional causes might also be seen with vocal fatigue from increased effort or overuse or muscle tension. **Ventricular phonation** might also be a functional cause. This occurs when false vocal folds compress over the true vocal folds with insufficient capacity to vibrate to make sufficient sound. Psychogenic causes are due to several emotional factors, such as chronic stress, depression, and anxiety, as well as a conversion reaction to a traumatic event with either a total loss of voice (aphonia) or a disruption in vocal quality (dysphonia).

Notably, although similar voice disorders occur for children and adults, there are some unique pediatric conditions that clinicians need to be aware of when completing a voice assessment (Sapienza & Ruddy, 2009). For example, **laryngomalacia** is a congenital laryngeal condition that is a frequent cause of **stridor** (high-pitched or noisy sound made when breathing) in infants, which may indicate that the upper airway is partially blocked. **Laryngeal webbing** occurs when a web of tissues connects the vocal folds, which may also block the airway, potentially leading to stridor or dyspnea (a sense of running out of air). Although a rare condition, it is a frequent occurrence in infants during the 4th to 10th week of gestation. A **laryngeal cleft** is a rare condition that results in an opening between the larynx and the esophagus accompanied by hoarseness, stridor, dysphagia, and coughing (Rahbar et al., 2006). Finally, **puberphonia** is a functional voice condition usually affecting adolescent males following their voice change during puberty in which they maintain a high-pitched voice.

See the **ASHA Aerodigestive Disorders Practice Portal** for more information regarding laryngomalacia and laryngeal cleft.

What Do We Do to Address This Communication Challenge?

It is important that SLPs who work with individuals with voice disorders are knowledgeable about the disorders and are trained to assess them and provide intervention if warranted (see ASHA Code of Ethics; ASHA, 2016). An SLP will have several roles in the assessment and treatment of voice disorders, including making appropriate referrals to other health professions if a surgical procedure or pharmacological approach is needed and making decisions in collaboration with the patient and their family about the intervention plan that is culturally responsive to the individual's and the family's unique cultural values, beliefs, and desires. The assessment and intervention process will involve both counseling and educating the patient and their family about the vocal mechanism and the causes of the observed voice disruption.

To provide the best possible assessment and intervention planning, the SLP must be a member of an interdisciplinary, collaborative team of professionals that includes, but is not limited to, otolaryngologists (i.e., ear, nose, and throat specialists), pulmonologists (who provide input on the respiratory system), allergists, neurologists, mental health professionals, and voice coaches. SLPs are skilled at evaluating the function and use of the voice and using this information to identify appropriate intervention methods. They can diagnose a voice disorder and refer patients to an appropriate physician if a medical diagnosis is needed.

See the **ASHA Intellectual Disability Practice Portal** and **ASHA's Interprofessional Education/Interprofessional Practice (IPE/IPP) Practice Portal** for more information on collaboration, teaming, and interprofessional education/interprofessional practice.

Assessment of Voice Disorders

The first step to assessment may be a screening of the individual's voice to determine if there are sufficient concerns identified by the individual, their parents, or providers or that there are noticeable differences in voice production than might be expected. Screening measures often examine an individual's voice in terms of the respiratory, phonatory, and resonance systems and consider the individual's vocal range, including loudness, pitch, and sustained vocalization. Informal tasks and more formal screening tools are often used together to determine if further assessment is needed (including self-report questionnaires; Deary et al., 2003; Lee et al., 2004).

After a screening has occurred, there are several approaches to a more comprehensive assessment of a voice disorder. Assessment often begins with a referral to a voice disorders clinical team, and the team engages in observations to assess the quality of the patient's voice. Acoustic samples are collected to allow the team to assess articulation, phonation, speech rate, and overall vocal quality (including pitch, resonance, and loudness level); for this, a patient is asked to use their voice to sustain a vowel such as /a/ to reading sentences. An assessment of phonation includes an examination of vocal quality and any delay of voice onset as well as the ability to continually phonate while engaged in connected speech. The voice team might also examine the laryngeal area to detect any tension while phonating and when at rest.

An oral mechanism exam will be done to assess the structural components of the oral cavity. The team will examine structural differences or motor-based challenges that might impact the production of sound and the strength, speed, and range of motion of the oral musculature. Often, the assessment will involve observations of structures at rest and while talking to assess any asymmetry or unusual movements. Ultimately, the voice team will be listening for perceived differences in voice quality, such as the symptoms listed in Table 11–1.

Taking a case history is an important component of assessment because the patient can describe the onset of any atypical vocal characteristics as well as provide pertinent information regarding their medical history, including surgeries, chronic conditions, and medications that may have an impact on the voice. In addition, this is a good time for the team to get a sense of the patient's daily vocal habits, any previous voice therapy and the outcomes, and the patient's goals for assessment and intervention.

Self-assessment is frequently incorporated into a comprehensive assessment. This is done so that the team can determine the individual's perception of their own vocal quality, how they perceive their voice affects their self-image, and how their voice impacts their ability to communicate. Because vocal fatigue is often difficult to detect during a laryngeal exam, a self-assessment can be valuable to the team in understanding how an individual feels about their voice endurance, especially during times of physical exertion.

During a voice assessment, the respiratory system is assessed to examine breathing patterns, including abdominal, thoracic, and clavicular breathing, as well as how the individual coordinates their breath control with their phonation. Aerodynamic assessment using noninvasive procedures is completed to examine the airflow and pressure used during voice production. Acoustic assessment is implemented as an objective way to measure vocal loudness, pitch, and quality (Patel et al., 2018). In addition, a laryngoscopy may be done, which allows the visualization of the vocal folds and related airway structures. Laryngeal imaging is often used by physicians to measure the structure of the vocal mechanism through **videoendoscopy** and vocal fold vibration through **videostroboscopy**. Importantly, SLPs only diagnose functional differences in the voice, whereas otolaryngologists diagnose organic pathologies such as nodules and polyps.

See the **ASHA Vocal Tract Visualization and Imaging Practice Portal** for more information on clinical voice assessments.

An assessment of vocal resonance will usually be completed, including attention to **hypernasality**, **hyponasality**, and **cul-de-sac resonance** (i.e., sound resonates and is stuck in the throat or nose with no outlet for the sound, making it muffled-like speech). An assessment of stimulability for achieving normal resonance is also completed.

See the **ASHA Resonance Disorders Practice Portal** for more information on clinical voice assessments.

Both standardized and nonstandardized tools are part of the toolbox clinicians use to assess a voice disorder. **As part of the comprehensive voice assessment, these tools help examine body structure and function impairments**, other health conditions and medications that may affect the voice, and the impact of the voice on the individual's ability to fully participate and engage in interpersonal interactions and experience their desired quality of life.

See the **ASHA Assessment Tools, Techniques, and Data Sources Practice Portal** for more information on clinical voice assessments.

Explore and Find Out!

Roy, N., Barkmeier-Kraemer, J., Eadie, T., Sivasankar, M. P., Mehta, D., Paul, D., & Hillman, R. (2013). Evidence-based clinical voice assessment: A systematic review. *American Journal of Speech-Language Pathology, 22*(2), 212–226.

See ASHA's resource **"Person-Centered Focus on Function: Voice"** (PDF) for more information on assessment data.

When considering EILO, an SLP will likely consult with a laryngologist, particularly if the vocal changes in a child or youth are significant. For vocal nodules or polyps, the SLP is usually the first contact for assessment and intervention before any consideration of surgery and certainly following surgery if it is determined to be necessary.

As described previously, vocal quality can also be affected when psychological stressors lead to aphonia or dysphonia. SLPs may refer individuals suspected of having a psychogenic voice disorder to other appropriate professionals (e.g., psychologist and/or psychiatrist) for diagnosis and may collaborate in subsequent behavioral treatment.

Intervention for Voice Disorders

When intervening with individuals who exhibit a voice disorder, several basic principles guide the approach to intervention. First, the clinician educates the patient on vocal hygiene and practices that will support vocal health. Second, the clinician focuses on how to use an individual's strengths to help facilitate improvement in areas that are problematic for voice production. Third, it is valuable to increase the client's self-awareness of the quality of their voice and recognition of any tension that may exist in the laryngeal area. Fourth, the clinician's goals should foster the client's ability to fully engage in their environment through the acquisition of effective communication skills and vocal strategies. Finally, barriers to communication should be identified, and needed accommodations and training should be provided for those with voice disorders. Importantly, in different environmental settings (e.g., home, school, work, social gatherings), there are varying expectations for vocal use, so this needs to be a consideration in goal setting and intervention planning as well. Intervention for voice disorders requires a team approach, so multiple professions will be involved beyond the SLP. For example, when the clinician determines that the individual has a voice disorder that is not due to a structural difference or pathology, mental health counseling may be beneficial beyond the support provided by the SLP.

Clinicians often use questionnaires, counseling, and tasks that manipulate different aspects of the voice to help determine the factors influencing the voice disorder and the appropriate intervention path. Identifying the factors that may be contributing to a voice disorder is always a first step for clinicians. For example, we know that it is not good for our vocal mechanism to be consistently engaged in shouting or screaming, talking over loud noise, clearing our throat, coughing, or failing to hydrate sufficiently. So, the first step for any voice intervention is to reduce problematic vocal behaviors and teach the client to practice healthy vocal behavior (including drinking water and talking at a reasonable volume).

Part of voice therapy includes providing clients with strategies to increase their breath support, or breathing from their diaphragm, so they are not increasing the strain on their voice. Many strategies can be used to teach clients to decrease shoulder and neck tension as well as different ways to make sounds, such as like talking through a straw, humming, making lip trills, and so on. Intervention approaches often include both direct and indirect elements. A direct intervention approach changes an individual's vocal behavior by adjusting their phonatory, respiratory, and/or muscular function to increase healthy vocal production (Colton et al., 2011). An indirect approach changes the environment in which an individual's vocal function occurs through education on good vocal health and counseling that supports stress reduction and other issues impacting vocal health (Thomas & Stemple, 2007; Van Stan et al., 2015).

It may be necessary to treat voice disorders in children versus adults differently because of anatomical and structural differences that exist. For example, the size of the larynx and the vocal tract is not the same across the two populations; pediatric vocal folds are shorter and less layered than those of adolescents and adults (Braden, 2018). As a child grows and develops, pitch changes are also noted. It is important to keep these differences in mind when determining an appropriate therapeutic plan for children versus adults because adaptations may be needed to treat the same voice disorders (Braden, 2018). In the following sections, you will read about physiologic and symptomatic approaches to voice disorders as well as several direct and indirect intervention techniques for a variety of structural and functional voice disorders.

Physiologic and Symptomatic Techniques to Address Voice Disorders

Voice therapy that uses physiologic techniques is directed at modifying the vocal mechanism by focusing on balancing the respiratory, phonatory, and resonance systems. Examples of physiologic techniques include conversation training therapy, expiratory muscle strength training, Lee Silverman Voice Treatment (LSVT), Phonation Resistance Training Exercises (PhoRTE), and resonant voice therapy.

Symptomatic techniques for voice therapy, on the other hand, are designed to modify atypical vocal components using various facilitating strategies (Boone et al., 2010). Symptoms that are typically addressed include inappropriately low or high pitch, voicing that is too loud or soft, breathy phonation, and glottal attacks. Techniques to address these symptoms include, but are not limited to, amplification, auditory masking, biofeedback, relaxation, and inhalation phonation. Descriptions of these selected physiological and symptomatic strategies used in voice therapy are provided in Table 11–2.

See the **ASHA Voice Evidence Map** for more information on pertinent scientific evidence, expert opinion, and client/caregiver perspective on various voice therapy techniques.

Intervention for Laryngeal Cancer

For individuals who are in the advanced stages of cancer involving tumors in the larynx, an intervention option might be a total laryngectomy (or surgical removal of the larynx). Such a change to the physical structure of the vocal mechanism leads to a disruption of air moving through the upper and lower airways, leading to an alternative breathing pathway via a **tracheostomy**. Other functions that may be affected by the removal of the larynx could be smell, taste, the ability to talk, and the ability to swallow (St. Peter et al., 2022), ultimately impacting an individual's quality of life and emotional well-being (Perry et al., 2015). Notably, those who have had a family member with head and neck cancer leading to a total laryngectomy are also deeply impacted, which could have an impact on the patient's outcomes (Jeong et al., 2015). See Figure 11–2 for a visual that displays the larynx prior to and following a laryngectomy.

See the **ASHA Head and Neck Cancer Practice Portal**, which highlights intervention to support alaryngeal speech, for more information.

TABLE 11–2. Selected Examples of Physiologic and Symptomatic Voice Therapy Techniques

Technique	Description	Physiologic or Symptomatic
Conversation training therapy (Gartner-Schmidt et al., 2016; Gillespie et al., 2019)	Focuses on voice awareness and production while engaging in conversational speech. SLP reinforces, imitates, and models appropriate phonation with an emphasis on producing clear speech, prosody, pauses, rapport building, etc.	Physiologic
Expiratory muscle strength training (EMST) (Pitts et al., 2009)	Increases breathing strength during sound production through specific exercises over time; uses an external device that blocks airflow to achieve desired exhalation.	Physiologic
Lee Silverman Voice Treatment (LSVT) (Ramig et al., 1994, 2018)	Intensive intervention designed for those with Parkinson disease to increase sound production and breathing function; patients learn to produce and monitor their loudness level when speaking, including increased breath support, laryngeal muscle movement, articulation, and facial expression; uses visual biofeedback to show the effort needed to increase loudness.	Physiologic
Phonation Resistance Training Exercises (PhoRTE) (Ziegler et al., 2014; Ziegler & Hapner, 2013)	Adapted from LSVT involving four key exercises: sustained loud production of /a/, loud ascending and descending pitch glides producing /a/, using a loud and high-pitched voice during phrase production, and using a loud and low-pitched voice during phrase production; less intense than LSVT and effective for the aging voice.	Physiologic
Resonant voice therapy (Stemple et al., 2010)	Builds resonant voice production from attending to oral sensations in the alveolar ridge and lips to practicing easy phonation moving from gestures to conversation; goal is to find a strong voice with the least effort on the vocal folds and incorporates humming.	Physiologic
Amplification	Microphones are used to increase vocal loudness for weak voices and especially when speaking to large groups; helps prevent vocal hyperfunction that occurs when there is sustained vocal use at an increased volume.	Symptomatic
Auditory masking (Brumm & Zollinger, 2011)	Individuals read aloud while wearing headphones with noise to mask the sound of their voice; with this noise, vocal volume often increases; this behavior can be recorded and reviewed later to make comparisons during intervention.	Symptomatic
Biofeedback	Individual learns to control physiologic functions with feedback from an external device that monitors the body's internal state to provide reliable and real-time feedback about any changes in the individual's vocal productions.	Symptomatic

continues

TABLE 11–2. *continued*

Technique	Description	Physiologic or Symptomatic
Relaxation	Uses relaxation exercises to decrease body and laryngeal tension so that effortful phonation is also reduced; exercises start slow with muscles tensing and then relaxing in different muscle areas; visualization of calm and peaceful locations is encouraged, and deep breathing occurs.	Symptomatic
Inhalation phonation	Helps facilitate vocal vibration when engaged in ventricular fold phonation, aphonia, and/or dysphonia; uses a high-pitched voice on inhalation; with voicing on inhalation, the real vocal cords are stretched, adducted, and vibrate to make sound.	Symptomatic

Source: Adapted from ASHA Voice Disorders Practice Portal (https://www.asha.org/practice-portal/clinical-topics/voice-disorders).

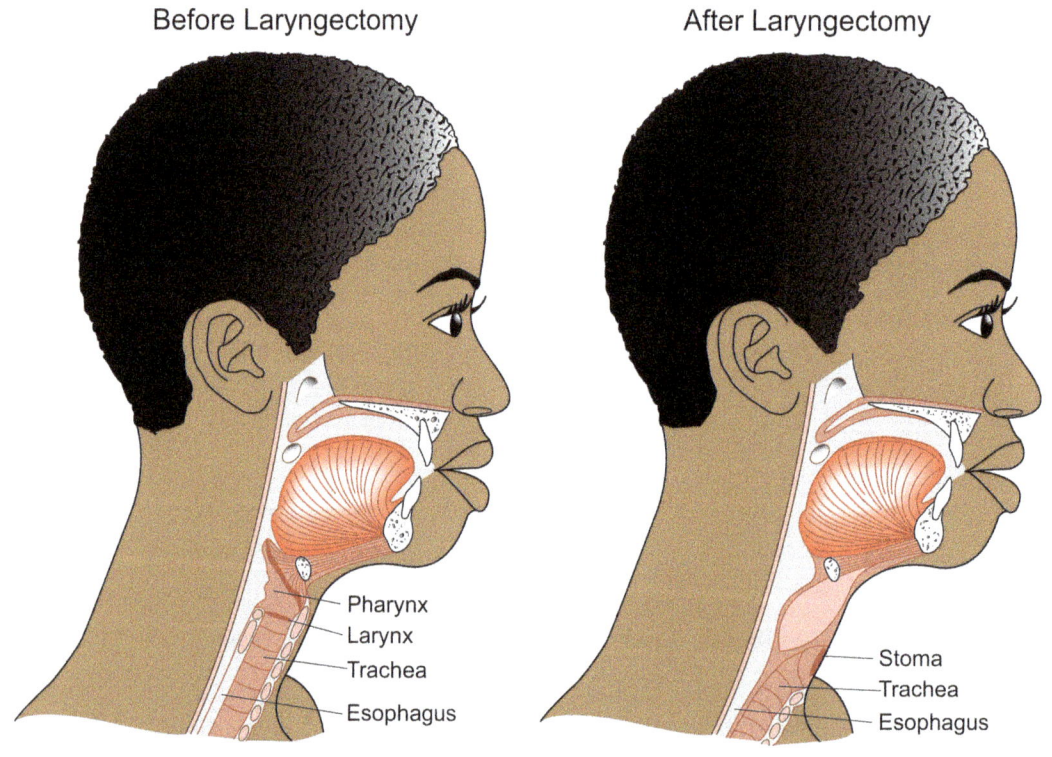

FIGURE 11–2. Total laryngectomy.

Intervention for Exercise-Induced Laryngeal Obstruction

Although pharmacological and psychological interventions, as well as treatments with airway devices, have been used for those with EILO, therapy provided by an SLP seems to be the most promising approach (Fujiki et al., 2023; Halevi-Katz et al., 2021; Mahoney et al., 2022; Schonman et al., 2022). Generally, the

SLP educates the individual on EILO, specifically the use of "lower thoracic breathing patterns, identification of triggers, teaching rescue techniques to address dyspnea symptoms, and practicing application of these techniques" (Fujiki et al., 2023, p. 1518). After three or more intervention sessions, symptoms can usually be managed (Fujiki et al., 2022). In fact, Fujiki et al. (2023) found that speech therapy for EILO led to clients being able to engage in more physical activity and exercise and lessen their use of inhalers.

Intervention for Vocal Cord Paralysis

When an individual demonstrates a paralysis of one of their **vocal cords** (also known as vocal folds), there are several strategies that might be initiated. First, the clinician engages in some education about how the vocal mechanism works. For children, the use of pictures, puppets, or other manipulatives to show the parts of the larynx and vocal folds is effective. Second, managing breath control is important, usually through shoulder and neck exercises, and production of nonnasal versus nasal sounds is used to increase awareness of nasal airflow (Barson et al., 2023). Children can be given visual or tactile cues to remind them to bring their breath from their diaphragm. A third strategy might be to change pitch and have the child glide through different pitches when making sounds (Barson et al., 2023). Finally, the clinician might add phrases to be produced with nasal sounds to relax muscles and facilitate a natural resonance when speaking in sentences.

Intervention to Support Gender-Affirming Voice Production

Gender-affirming voice therapy is an important area of study because gender-diverse individuals and those undergoing gender transition require special care to address any vocal concerns. Using a qualitative study approach, Holmberg and colleagues (2023) examined the goals and motivations of clients when undergoing gender-affirming voice intervention and found that person-centered intervention is crucial to the success of the intervention. Moreover, it is also important to outline the motivating factors that the individual has identified for changing their voice, along with addressing the likely challenges with making any desired changes. Holmberg et al. recommended that having this discussion prior to initiating intervention is key to ensuring that expectations are understood and practical barriers can be addressed. Notably, when one's biological sex at birth differs from their gender identity, they may experience the stress associated with this dissonance as well as how to navigate their desire to change their voice. This mismatch with gender identity and desired voice is part of what you may have heard as **gender dysphoria** (Coleman et al., 2022). Importantly, however, there are interventions that span from behavioral to drug-related to surgical approaches that can help an individual achieve their desired vocal changes (Coleman et al., 2022). Different approaches can also be used depending on whether the individual is male or female at birth. For an individual who was born a male and wishes to have a more feminine voice, intervention would likely involve voice training because the use of a female hormone such as estrogen has little impact on the voice (Mészáros et al., 2005). In contrast, a female at birth who desires a more masculine voice might be on a testosterone hormone regiment that lowers the pitch, although this may be insufficient in meeting all the individual's vocal needs (Azul, 2015, 2016; Nygren et al., 2016; Ziegler et al., 2018). Without meeting all the vocal needs of the individual seeking gender-affirming vocal care, vocal fatigue might result, and other voice problems might occur (Azul et al., 2017; Nygren et al., 2016). In addition, access to vocal care for gender diverse and transgender individuals often varies in terms of availability of expert SLPs in this area (Coleman et al., 2022; Holmberg et al., 2023)

A client's confidence and satisfaction with therapy must be part of the therapeutic process for it to be successful (Holmberg et al., 2023), especially when the client faces barriers to the changes being made (van Leer, 2021). It is valuable, then, for SLPs to work with their clients to identify possible barriers to achieving their goals so that strategies can be employed to facilitate self-efficacy (Dacakis et al., 2022).

See the **ASHA Gender Affirming Voice and Communication Practice Portal** for more information.

Intervention for Vocal Fatigue

Interestingly, online voice therapy using an **expiratory pressure device** (a small handheld device typically used to move mucous out of the lungs) in combination with voice rehabilitation training and phonatory exercises has been shown to effectively treat vocal fatigue (Acevedo et al., 2023). In this study, patient and provider satisfaction were also strong.

Why Is This Topic Important?

Understanding our voice and how we use it has implications for both monitoring unexpected changes and identifying ways to protect our voice so that we can fully participate in our daily activities and maintain an expected level of quality of life. Attending to our voice and changes in vocal quality (e.g., hoarseness, pitch, aphonia) may reveal structural or functional challenges that could be addressed with careful assessment and quality intervention. Vocal changes may suggest a pathology such as laryngeal cancer or growths on the vocal folds that can be addressed through surgery or behavioral interventions. It is important, therefore, to monitor your own vocal use or misuse, educate yourself on ways to protect your voice, and attend to vocal changes so that referrals for assessment can be made and intervention can be implemented as needed.

Application to a Child

James is a 10-year-old boy with Down syndrome. He is sociable and speaks using short sentences that are usually intelligible if the listener understands the context. Although he has an intellectual disability, he understands questions and can engage in a back-and-forth conversation. His voice, however, is characterized by low pitch, monotone, and variable loudness with a hoarse and breathy quality. James' SLP is working on James' vocabulary development and expanding his language structure, but the quality of his voice is interfering with his ability to be heard and understood, especially in noisy environments. The SLP decided it was time to address his voice disorder. She was trained in the LSVT LOUD protocol and learned that this protocol might have value in addressing the voice concerns of those with Down syndrome because the treatment includes motor learning (Ramig et al., 2018), and motor speech difficulties are common in this population. Although LSVT has typically been used to address voice disorders in individuals with Parkinson disease and cerebral palsy; more recently it has been applied to children with Down syndrome (Boliek et al., 2022). The primary aim of LSVT LOUD is for children to achieve a normal loudness level with adequate voice quality following the model of the clinician (Boliek et al., 2022). The intervention the SLP delivered included intensive 1-hour sessions on consecutive days for 4 weeks, and it was decided to revisit James' progress within 1 month. The parents supported James in this intervention because there were homework and generalization tasks following each intervention session. Each session comprised two parts. First, the SLP had James produce continuous vowels within a specific pitch range using 10 phrases familiar to him. Second, James moved from producing sounds in words to practicing conversational speech using simple language that James knew and understood. He learned to repeat sounds that his SLP modeled for him. He was provided with daily feedback regarding his vocal loudness and vocal quality. James made positive gains in his vocal loudness, and the quality of his voice improved, which made his speech more intelligible and improved his quality of life.

Because speech-language intervention for children with Down syndrome typically focuses on vocabulary development and increased use of connected and functional speech, do you think it was appropriate for the SLP to focus on James' voice quality? Why or why not? The SLP indicated that James made gains in his voice production. What do you think she did to assess the changes in his voice quality? Would it be important to assess others' perceptions of James' vocal change? If so, who would you ask?

Application to an Adolescent or Adult

 Jennifer is a 19-year-old college student who is studying to become an SLP. One of her instructors noticed that Jennifer frequently clears her throat in class and seems to have a hoarse vocal quality with frequent pitch breaks. After listening to her voice for 3 weeks, he talked with Jennifer after class and mentioned his concern. She dismissed his concern saying she just had a cold and a cough. He let it go, but after another 2 weeks, he met with her after class and expressed his continued concern. He noted that he had not seen any changes in her voice and was worried that her throat-clearing and hoarseness were persistent and might indicate a voice disorder. Jennifer was surprised because she generally liked the sound of her voice, and it did not seem to bother anyone else. Also, although she would lose her voice for a week at a time when she was a cheerleader in high school, her voice would always return in time for the next game.

Jennifer's teacher mentioned that the college had a faculty member who was a voice expert and that she would be willing to listen to Jennifer's voice and complete a voice assessment. Jennifer agreed and participated in a comprehensive voice assessment. The faculty voice expert interviewed Jennifer about her vocal history and found that she had been a cheerleader since seventh grade and had frequently lost her voice but would always get it back in time for the next game. Jennifer was asked to identify how she uses her voice. For example, does she go to concerts or places where the music is loud, or the noise level might cause her to strain her voice? Jennifer identified several situations in which she goes out dancing with her friends and attends her sorority's socials at which there are many other college students. She also mentioned that she intended to try out to be a member of the cheer team for her college's sports teams. In addition, Jennifer was asked how she stayed hydrated (and was she doing so with water), if she cleared her throat a lot, and if she felt like something was in her throat. She mentioned that she frequently cleared her throat, that she did not drink alcohol but usually drank soda and probably could drink more water, and that she sometimes had a sensation that there was something stuck in her throat. The voice assessment also included recording Jennifer's voice when she was phonating sounds, words, and sentences, as well as when reading a short passage. In addition, an otolaryngologist performed an indirect laryngoscopy in which he used a mirror to look down her pharynx to see the vocal folds when Jennifer phonated "ah." He also initiated videostroboscopy to visualize vocal fold vibration. He discovered bilateral vocal nodules.

Jennifer's voice was generally hoarse, low-pitched, and breathy because the vocal folds were thicker than normal due to the formation of the nodules. For this reason, air was being released during phonation because the vocal folds could not fully adduct. The SLP recommended immediate vocal rest and voice therapy because she believed that with intervention the nodules could be eliminated without a need for surgery. There was one complication to the plan the SLP put forward: Jennifer was planning on trying out for the cheer team at the university. The SLP counseled her that this would be a problem and that she needed to reconsider her plans, knowing that continued vocal misuse could permanently damage her vocal cords. Therapy began with both indirect and direct methods, including education about the vocal mechanism and ways to limit the stress on the vocal cords; learning to use diaphragmatic breathing when speaking loudly; and phonating with easy onset starting with vowels and moving to words, phrases, sentences, and conversation. Jennifer monitored her throat clearing and hydration and kept track of her vocal use. Within 8 weeks, Jennifer's nodules were gone. She felt she had a better handle on how to use her voice and was still contemplating trying out for the cheer team. She was reminded, however, of the short- and long-term consequences of vocal misuse.

What other assessment tools or strategies might you use to provide a comprehensive assessment and history of Jennifer's voice disorder? Did the clinician select appropriate strategies for addressing Jennifer's vocal nodules? How would you respond to Jennifer's desire to try out for the college cheer team? Who might help Jennifer monitor her vocal use so that she is careful to limit her involvement in loud and noisy environments or situations, reduce her throat clearing, and remember to hydrate?

Chapter Summary

Voice disorders can affect people of all ages and impact an individual's quality of life by reducing their vocal output and making it difficult for them to be understood. There are structural voice disorders that involve a change in the vocal mechanism, as well as functional voice disorders that result from no physical change in the vocal mechanism but insufficient use of the vocal mechanism. Assessment with a collaborative team across disciplines is crucial to assessing voice disorders, and technological advances make it easier to view the pharynx as well as the vocal folds to determine if a pathology exists. There are numerous interventions to address a voice disorder, ranging from education on vocal hygiene to surgery. The type of intervention selected to address a particular voice disorder is highly dependent on the specific condition, the patient's preferences and motivation, and access to a comprehensive assessment of the vocal mechanism and high-quality intervention with experienced voice clinicians. Often, a combination of direct and indirect intervention methods is used with ongoing monitoring of vocal use and the health status of the vocal mechanism.

Chapter Review Questions

1. What is the difference between structural and functional voice disorders?
2. What happens to the vocal mechanism when a person has a laryngectomy due to cancer or a traumatic accident?
3. What happens to the voice when you have vocal nodules? What is the reason for nodules developing on the vocal cords?
4. Describe the technology that is used to view the vocal mechanism and the movement of the vocal folds.
5. Explain the Lee Silverman Voice Therapy approach and the voice conditions for which it might be an appropriate intervention method.
6. What is exercise-induced laryngeal obstruction? When might it occur, who might it affect, and how might it be addressed for the person affected?
7. Give an example of an organic versus a neurogenic voice disorder?
8. What is voice dysphoria?
9. How might you approach gender-affirming therapy for an adolescent or young adult going through gender transition?
10. Who might experience vocal fatigue? What are the symptoms, and how might it be addressed?

Learning Activities

1. Listen to the voices of your peers and identify their level of loudness, their pitch level, and the quality of their voice. What do you notice? Are you hearing anyone with a hoarse, breathy voice quality? Did you notice anyone who frequently clears their throat or coughs even though they do not have a cold? Do you have a friend who often loses their voice? Why might you be hearing these differences in your peers' voice quality?
2. A friend of yours is gender diverse and is going through their transition. Your friend does not like the voice they currently have, and they want to change the quality of their voice, including their pitch and resonance. Who would you recommend they see as part of their treatment plan and why?
3. You have been engaged in a lot of exercise, an activity you enjoy, but lately you are feeling out of breath and intermittently losing your voice? Do you suspect EILO? Why or why not?

Suggested Reading

Adriaansen, A., Meerschman, I., van Lierde, K., & D'haeseleer, E. (2022). Effects of voice therapy in children with vocal fold nodules: A systematic review. *International Journal of Language & Communication Disorders, 57*(6), 1160–1193.

This systematic review found support for both direct and indirect voice therapy when treating children with vocal nodules. The level of evidence was determined as adequate, with improvements noted in both objective and subjective measures, showing positive outcomes for perceptual changes noted following voice therapy. The preferred treatment for children with vocal nodules is voice therapy, especially with the recurrence of nodules if a surgical approach is taken, because no effort will have been made to reduce the vocal abuse that was the primary cause of the nodules. Often, voice therapy for children includes both direct and indirect approaches. Further research of treatment effectiveness is needed.

Al-Kadi, M., Alfawaz, M. A., & Alotaibi, F. (2022). Impact of voice therapy on pediatric patients with dysphonia and vocal nodules: A systematic review. *Cureus, 14*(4), Article e24433.

Results of this review indicated the positive impact of direct, indirect, and combined intervention on pre- and post-test outcomes for children with vocal nodules and resulting dysphonia. Because of weak methodological designs, relatively small sample sizes, and the differences in targeted outcomes and interventions across the research reviewed, it was unclear if one intervention was more efficacious than the others.

Gelfer, M. P., & Tice, R. M. (2013). Perceptual and acoustic outcomes of voice therapy for male-to-female transgender individuals immediately after therapy and 15 months later. *Journal of Voice, 27*(3), 335–347.

The authors examined whether speech therapy for male-to-female (MtF) transgender individuals alters perceptions of other people about what gender the individual identifies as. There are different fundamental frequencies at which cis-gendered males and cis-gendered females speak. The differences in fundamental frequencies can be changed and maintained over time with speech therapy.

To investigate whether speech therapy can successfully change which gender is perceived when a MtF individual is speaking, the authors examined three groups of people. One group consisted of 5 MtF transgender participants who had been living as female for an average of 2 years and 2 months and had never undergone speech therapy before. A second group was a control group consisting of 5 cis-gendered males and 5 cis-gendered females who were matched to the transgender participants. The final group was the listener group, which consisted of 52 listeners and two subgroups. The first listener subgroup had no prior knowledge of or experience with communication and speech disorders. This group listened to transgender voices at the pretest and immediate post-test as well as to both the male and female controls. The second subgroup of listeners also had no prior experience in communication or speech disorders. This group listened to the transgender individuals at pretest and at long-term post-test as well as the male and female controls. The listener group listened to both transgender and cis-gender individuals repeating recordings of sounds, sentences, and short paragraphs before treatment, immediately after treatment, and 15 months after treatment.

The MtF individuals received 8 weeks of voice therapy, with sessions occurring twice a week for 60 minutes each session. This therapy included practice for the target pitch for participants and moved on to practice phrases focusing on intonation, pitch, and quality of speech. Full sentences were then targeted focusing on the same targets as for the phrases. Finally, multisentence production was elicited via role-playing, open-ended questions, and picture descriptions.

The pretreatment recording assessments showed that individuals were perceived as male 98.1% of the time. The immediate post-test recording assessments showed that on average, individuals were perceived as male 49.2% of the time and female (the voice they were working toward) 50.8% of the time. The long-term post-treatment recording assessment showed that individuals were perceived as male 66.9% of the time and female 33.1% of the time. However, the authors note that these percentages fluctuated depending on the individual.

The ratings for perceived masculinity and femininity were also compared pretest and post-test. For both the immediate- and long-term post-test, there was a marked decline in masculinity ratings and an increase in femininity ratings. Overall, this study shows that treatments can improve and show maintenance for perceived femininity and identification as a female voice. However, the number of participants and the time the participants had been living as female limit the study's generalizability.

Haines, J., Smith, J. A., Wingfield-Digby, J., King, J., Yorke, J., & Fowler, S. J. (2022). Systematic review of the effectiveness of non-pharmacological interventions used to treat adults with inducible laryngeal obstruction. *BMJ Open Respiratory Research, 9*(1), Article e001199.

The results of this article suggest that nonpharmacological voice interventions (muscle training, diaphragmatic breathing, education, etc.) decrease the symptoms of voice disorders and health care utilization by 59.5% in adults with inducible laryngeal obstruction. Because of the different interventions and outcomes examined, additional research is needed to investigate nonpharmacological treatment.

Leyns, C., Papeleu, T., Tomassen, P., T'Sjoen, G., & D'haeseleer, E. (2021). Effects of speech therapy for transgender women: A systematic review. *International Journal of Transgender Health, 22*(4), 360–380.

This review found positive outcomes for pitch, resonance, and voice perception following intervention for transgender women. Research quality, however, was limited, as was the number of published studies examining this area. More research is needed to assess the effectiveness of voice therapy for this population.

Morton, M. E., & Sandage, M. J. (2022). Sex and race reporting and representation in noncancerous voice clinical trials: A meta-analysis of National Institutes of Health–registered research between 1988 and 2021. *Journal of Speech-Language-Hearing Research, 65*(7), 2594–2607.

The authors examined the clinical trials registered with the National Institutes of Health/U.S. National Library of Medicine between January 1988 and September 2021 to determine the percentage of trials reporting demographics such as sex, race, and ethnicity. They reviewed 46 research studies and found more female subjects in the trials but no difference in sex. Only two trials described race and ethnicity, with Black and Hispanic participants participating in only one trial each. The authors conclude that clinical voice trials not related to cancer show disparities in representation across race and ethnicities, highlighting the need for more rigorous recruitment strategies for participants.

Additional Resources

- American Speech-Language-Hearing Association, "Code of Ethics"
  https://www.asha.org/policy/et2016-00342
- American Speech-Language-Hearing Association, "Consumer Resource Related to Voice Disorders"
  https://www.asha.org/public/speech/disorders/voice
- American Speech-Language-Hearing Association, "Gender-Affirming Voice and Communication Change for Transgender and Gender-Diverse People"
  https://www.asha.org/public/speech/disorders/voice-and-communication-change-for-transgender-people
- American Speech-Language-Hearing Association, "Multicultural Issues in the Treatment of Voice Disorders"
  https://pubs.asha.org/doi/10.1044/cds7.2.1
- American Speech-Language-Hearing Association, "Preferred Practice Patterns for the Profession of Speech-Language Pathology"
  https://www.asha.org/policy/pp2004-00191
- American Speech-Language-Hearing Association, Resonance Disorders Practice Portal
  https://www.asha.org/practice-portal/clinical-topics/resonance-disorders
- American Speech-Language-Hearing Association, "Scope of Practice in Speech-Language Pathology"
  https://www.asha.org/policy/sp2016-00343
- American Speech-Language-Hearing Association, "Supporting and Working With Transgender and Gender-Diverse Individuals"
  https://www.asha.org/practice/multicultural/supporting-and-working-with-transgender-and-gender-diverse-individuals
- American Speech-Language-Hearing Association, "The Role of the Speech-Language Pathologist, the Teacher of Singing, and the Speaking Voice Trainer in Voice Habilitation"
  https://www.asha.org/policy/tr2005-00147
- American Speech-Language-Hearing Association, Voice and Communication Services for Transgender and Gender Diverse Populations Practice Portal
  https://www.asha.org/practice-portal/professional-issues/gender-affirming-voice-and-communication
- Dysphonia International (formerly the National Spasmodic Dysphonia Association)
  https://dysphonia.org
- National Center for Voice and Speech
  https://ncvs.org

References

Acevedo, K., Guzman, M., Ortega, A., Aguirre, C., Diaz, S., Escudero, J., & Quezada, C. (2023). Remote voice therapy with an oscillatory positive expiratory pressure device in subjects with vocal fatigue: A randomized controlled trial. *Journal Speech, Language, and Hearing Research, 66*, 4801–4811.

American Speech-Language-Hearing Association. (2016). *Code of ethics.* https://www.asha.org/policy/et2016-00342

American Speech-Language-Hearing Association. (2023). *Voice disorders.* http://www.asha.org/Practice-Portal/Clinical-Topics/Voice-Disorders

Aronson, A. E., & Bless, D. M. (2009). *Clinical voice disorders* (4th ed.). Thieme.

Azul, D. (2015). Transmasculine people's vocal situations: A critical review of gender-related discourses and empirical data. *International Journal of Language & Communication Disorders, 50*(1), 31–47.

Azul, D. (2016). Gender-related aspects of transmasculine people's vocal situations: Insights from a qualitative content analysis of interview transcripts. *International Journal of Language Communication Disorders, 51*(6), 672–684.

Azul, D., Nygren, U., Södersten, M., & Neuschaefer-Rube, C. (2017). Transmasculine people's voice function: A review of the currently available evidence. *Journal of Voice, 31*(2), 261.e9–261.e23.

Bainbridge, K. E., Roy, N., Losonczy, K. G., Hoffman, H. J., & Cohen, S. M. (2017). Voice disorders and associated risk markers among young adults in the United States. *The Laryngoscope, 127*(9), 2093–2099.

Barson, P., Carroll, L., & Zur, K.B. (2023). Pediatric unilateral vocal fold paralysis. *Perspectives of the ASHA Special Interest Groups, 8,* 1345–1349.

Bhattacharyya, N. (2014). The prevalence of voice problems among adults in the United States. *The Laryngoscope, 124*(10), 2359–2362.

Boliek, C. A., Halpern, A., Hernandez, K., Fox, C. M., & Ramig, L. (2022). Intensive voice treatment (Lee Silverman Voice Treatment [LSVT LOUD]) for children with Down syndrome: Phase I outcomes. *Journal of Speech, Language, and Hearing Research, 65,* 1228–1262.

Boone, D. R., McFarlane, S. C., Von Berg, S. L., & Zraick, R. I. (2010). *The voice and voice therapy.* Allyn & Bacon.

Braden, M. (2018). Advances in pediatric voice therapy. *Perspectives of the ASHA Special Interest Groups, 3*(3), 68–76.

Brumm, H., & Zollinger, S. A. (2011). The evolution of the Lombard effect: 100 years of psychoacoustic research. *Behaviour, 148*(11–13), 1173–1198.

Byeon, H. (2019). The risk factors related to voice disorder in teachers: A systematic review and meta-analysis. *International Journal of Environmental Research and Public Health, 16*(19), Article 3675.

Christensen, P. M., Thomsen, S. F., Rasmussen, N., & Backer, V. (2011). Exercise-induced laryngeal obstructions: Prevalence and symptoms in the general public. *European Archives of Oto-Rhino-Laryngology, 268*(9), 1313–1319.

Coleman, E., Radix, A. E., Bouman, W. P., Brown, G. R., de Vries, A. L. C., Deutsch, M. B., . . . Arcelus, J. (2022). Standards of care for the health of transgender and gender diverse people, version 8. *International Journal of Transgender Health, 23*(Suppl. 1), S1–S259.

Colton, R. H., Casper, J. K., & Leonard, R. (2011). *Understanding voice problems: A physiological perspective for diagnosis and treatment* (4th ed.). Lippincott Williams & Wilkins.

Dacakis, G., Erasmus, J., Nygren, U., Oates, J., Quinn, S., & Södersten, M. (2022, May 2). Development and initial psychometric evaluation of the Self-Efficacy Scale for Voice Modification in Trans Women. *Journal of Voice,* S0892-1997(22)00078-9.

de Araújo Pernambuco, L., Espelt, A., Balata, P. M. M., & de Lima, K. C. (2014). Prevalence of voice disorders in the elderly: A systematic review of population-based studies. *European Archives of Oto-Rhino-Laryngology, 272*(10), 2601–2609.

Deary, I. J., Wilson, J. A., Carding, P. N., & MacKenzie, K. (2003). VoiSS: A patient-derived Voice Symptom Scale. *Journal of Psychosomatic Research, 54*(5), 483–489.

Desjardins, M., Halstead, L., Cooke, M., & Bonilha, H. S. (2017). A systematic review of voice therapy: What "effectiveness" really implies. *Journal of Voice, 31*(3), 392.e13–392.e32.

DeYoung, C. G. (2015). Cybernetic big five theory. *Journal of Research in Personality, 56*, 33–58.

Ersson, K., Mallmin, E., Malinovschi, A., Norlander, K., Johansson, H., & Nordang, L. (2020). Prevalence of exercise-induced bronchoconstriction and laryngeal obstruction in adolescent athletes. *Pediatric Pulmonology, 55*(12), 3509–3516.

Etter, N. M., Stemple, J. C., & Howell, D. M. (2013). Defining the lived experience of older adults with voice disorders. *Journal of Voice, 27*(1), 61–67.

Fujiki, R. B., Fujiki, A. E., & Thibeault, S. (2022). Factors impacting therapy duration in children and adolescents with paradoxical vocal fold movement (PVFM). *International Journal of Pediatric Otorhinolaryngology, 158*, Article 111182.

Fujiki, R. B., Olson-Greb, B., Braden, M., & Thibeault, S.L. (2023). Therapy outcomes for teenage athletes with exercise-induced laryngeal obstruction. *American Journal of Speech-Language Pathology, 32*, 1517–1531.

Fujiki, R. B., & Thibeault, S.L. (2023). Examining therapy duration in adults with voice disorders. *American Journal of Speech-Language Pathology, 32*, 1665–1678.

Gartner-Schmidt, J., Gherson, S., Hapner, E., Roth, D., Schneider, S., & Gillespie, A. (2016). The development of conversation training therapy: A concept paper. *Journal of Voice, 30*(5), 563–573.

Gillespie, A., Yabes, J., Rosen, C. A., & Gartner-Schmidt, J. (2019). Efficacy of conversation training therapy for patients with benign vocal fold lesions and muscle tension dysphonia compared to historical matched control patients. *Journal of Speech, Language, and Hearing Research, 62*(11), 4062–4079.

Gois, A. C. B., Pernambuco, L. D. A., & de Lima, K. C. (2018). Factors associated with voice disorders among the elderly: A systematic review. *Brazilian Journal of Otorhinolaryngology, 84*(4), 506–513.

Gregory, N. D., Chandran, S., Lurie, D., & Sataloff, R. T. (2012). Voice disorders in the elderly. *Journal of Voice, 26*(2), 254–258.

Guglani, L., Atkinson, S., Hosanagar, A., & Guglani, L. (2014). A systematic review of psychological interventions for adult and pediatric patients with vocal cord dysfunction. *Frontiers in Pediatrics, 2*, Article 82.

Haines, J., Smith, J. A., Wingfield-Digby, J., King, J., Yorke, J., & Fowler, S. J. (2022). Systematic review of the effectiveness of non-pharmacological interventions used to treat adults with inducible laryngeal obstruction. *BMJ Open Respiratory Research, 9*(1), Article e001199.

Halevi-Katz, D., Sella, O., Golan, H., Banai, K., Van Swearingen, J., Krisciunas, G. P., & Abbott, K. V. (2021). Buteyko breathing technique for exertion-induced paradoxical vocal fold motion (EI-PVFM). *Journal of Voice, 35*(1), 40–51.

Halvorsen, T., Walsted, E. S., Bucca, C., Bush, A., Cantarella, G., Friedrich, G., . . . Heimdal, J.-H. (2017). Inducible laryngeal obstruction: An official joint European Respiratory Society and European Laryngological Society statement. *European Respiratory Journal, 50*(3), Article 1602221.

Hoffman, H. J., Li, C.-M., Losonczy, K., Chiu, M. S., Lucas, J. B., & St. Louis, K. O. (2014). Voice, speech, and language disorders in the U.S. population: The 2012 National Health Interview Survey (NHIS) (Abstract No. 648). In *Abstracts of the 47th annual meeting of the Society for Epidemiologic Research, Seattle, WA* (p. 156). Annual Society for Epidemiologic Research.

Holmberg, J., Linander, I., Sodersten, M., & Karisson, F. (2023). Exploring motives and perceived barriers for voice modification: The views of transgender and gender-diverse voice clients. *Journal of Speech-Language-Hearing Research, 66*, 2246–2259.

Hseu, A., Nohamin, A., Kosuke, K., Woodnorth, G., & Nuss, R. (2018). Voice abnormalities and laryngeal pathology in preterm children. *Annals of Otology, Rhinology & Laryngology, 127*(8), 508–513.

Hunter, E. J., Cantor-Cutiva, L. C., van Leer, E., Van Mersbergen, M., Nanjundeswaran, C. D., Bottalico, P., & Whitling, S. (2020). Toward a consensus description of vocal effort, vocal load, vocal loading, and vocal fatigue. *Journal of Speech, Language, and Hearing Research, 63*(2), 509–532.

Jeong, A., Shin, D. W., Kim, S. Y., Yang, H. K., Shin, J. Y., Park, K., . . . Park, J. H. (2015). The effects on caregivers of cancer patients' needs and family hardiness. *PsychoOncology, 25*(1), 84–90.

Johansson, H., Norlander, K., Berglund, L., Janson, C., Malinovschi, A., Nordvall, L., . . . Emtner, M. (2015). Prevalence of exercise-induced bronchoconstriction and exercise-induced laryngeal obstruction in a general adolescent population. *Thorax, 70*(1), 57–63.

Johnson, C. M., Anderson, D. C., & Brigger, M. T. (2020). Pediatric dysphonia: A cross-sectional survey of subspecialty and primary care clinics. *Journal of Voice, 34*(2), 301.e1–301.e5.

Lee, L., Stemple, J. C., Glaze, L., & Kelchner, L. N. (2004). Quick screen for voice and supplementary documents for identifying pediatric voice disorders. *Language, Speech, and Hearing Services in Schools, 35*(4), 308–319.

Leyns, C., Papeleu, T., Tomassen, P., T'Sjoen, G., & D'haeseleer, E. (2021). Effects of speech therapy for transgender women: A systematic review. *International Journal of Transgender Health, 22*(4), 360–380.

Lin, K. J. Y., Chan, R. W., Wu, C.-H., & Liu, S. C. H. (2023). A vocal hygiene program for mitigating the effects of occupational vocal demand in primary school teachers. *Journal of Speech, Language, and Hearing Research, 66*, 1525–1540.

Mahoney, J., Hew, M., Vertigan, A., & Oates, J. (2022). Treatment effectiveness for vocal cord dysfunction in adults and adolescents: A systematic review. *Clinical & Experimental Allergy, 52*(3), 387–404.

Marmor, S., Horvath, K., Lim, K. O., & Misono, S. (2016). Voice problems and depression among adults in the United States. *The Laryngoscope, 126*(8), 1859–1864.

Martinez, C. C., & Cassol, M. (2015). Measurement of voice quality, anxiety, and depression symptoms after speech therapy. *Journal of Voice, 29*(4), 446–449.

Martins, R. H. G., do Amaral, H. A., Tavares, E. L. M., Martins, M. G., Gonçalves, T. M., & Dias, N. H. (2015). Voice disorders: Etiology and diagnosis. *Journal of Voice, 30*(6), 761.e1–761.e9.

Martins, R. H. G., Pereira, E. R., Hidalgo, C. B., & Tavares, E. L. M. (2014). Paradoxical vocal fold motion: A tutorial on a complex disorder and the speech-language pathologist's role. *American Journal of Speech-Language Pathology, 10*(2), 111–125.

Mayne, G. V., & Namazi, M. (2023). Social determinants of health: Implications for voice disorders and their treatment. *American Journal of Speech-Language Pathology, 32*, 1050–1064.

Meerschman, I., Lierde, K. V., Ketels, J., Coppieters, C., Claeys, S., & D'haeseleer, E. (2019). Effect of three semi-occluded vocal tract therapy programmes on the phonation of patients with dysphonia: Lip trill, water-resistance therapy and straw phonation. *International Journal of Language & Communication Disorders, 54*(1), 50–61.

Mészáros, K., Csokonai Vitéz, L., Szabolcs, I., Góth, M., Kovács, L., Görömbei, Z., & Hacki, T. (2005). Efficacy of conservative voice treatment in male-to-female transsexuals. *Folia Phoniatrica et Logopaedica, 57*(2), 111–118.

Morris, M. A., Meier, S. K., Griffin, J. M., Branda, M. E., & Phelan, S. M. (2016). Prevalence and etiologies of adult communication disabilities in the United States: Results of the 2012 National Health Interview Survey. *Disability and Health Journal, 9*(1),140–144.

Murry, T., & Milstein, C. F. (2016). Laryngeal movement disorders and their management. *Perspectives of the ASHA Special Interest Groups, 1*(3), 75–82.

Nanjundeswaran, C., Jacobson, B. H., Gartner-Schmidt, J., & Verdolini Abbott K. (2015). Vocal Fatigue Index (VFI): Development and validation. *Journal of Voice, 29*(4), 433–440.

Nascimento, T., & Tenenbaum, G. (2013). The psychological experience of athletes with vocal cord dysfunction. *Journal of Clinical Sport Psychology, 7*(2), 146–160.

Nygren, U., Nordenskjöld, A., Arver, S., & Södersten, M. (2016). Effects on voice fundamental frequency and satisfaction with voice in trans men during testosterone treatment—A longitudinal study. *Journal of Voice, 30*(6), 766.e23–766.e34.

Patel, R. R., Awan, S. N., Barkmeier-Kraemer, J., Courey, M., Deliyski, D., Eadie, T., . . . Hillman, R. (2018). Recommended protocols for instrumental assessment of voice: American Speech-Language-Hearing Association Expert Panel to Develop a Protocol for Instrumental Assessment of Vocal Function. *American Journal of Speech-Language Pathology, 27*(3), 887–905.

Patel, R. R., Venediktov, R., Schooling, T., & Wang, B. (2015). Evidence-based systematic review: Effects of speech-language pathology treatment for individuals with paradoxical vocal fold motion. *American Journal of Speech-Language Pathology, 24*(3), 566–584.

Perry, A., Casey, E., & Cotton, S. (2015). Quality of life after total laryngectomy: Functioning, psychological well-being and self-efficacy. *International Journal of Language & Communication Disorders, 50*(4), 467–475.

Pestana, P. M., Vaz-Freitas, S., & Manso, M. C. (2017). Prevalence of voice disorders in singers: Systematic review and meta-analysis. *Journal of Voice, 31*(6), 722–727.

Pitts, T., Bolser, D., Rosenbek, J., Troche, M., Okun, M. S., & Sapienza, C. (2009). Impact of expiratory muscle strength training on voluntary cough and swallow function in Parkinson disease. *Chest, 135*(5), 1301–1308.

Rahbar, R., Rouillon, I., Roger, G., Lin, A., Nuss, R. C., Denoyelle, F., . . . Garabedian, E. (2006). The presentation and management of laryngeal cleft: A 10-year experience. *Archives of Otolaryngology—Head & Neck Surgery, 132*(12), 1335–1341.

Ramig, L. O., Bonitati, C., Lemke, J., & Horii, Y. (1994). Voice treatment for patients with Parkinson disease: Development of an approach and preliminary efficacy data. *Journal of Medical Speech-Language Pathology, 2*, 191–209.

Ramig, L. O., Halpern, A., Spielman, J., Fox, C., & Freeman, K. (2018). Speech treatment in Parkinson's disease: Randomized controlled trial (RCT). *Movement Disorders, 33*(11), 1777–1791.

Roy, N., Kim, J., Courey, M., & Cohen, S. M. (2016). Voice disorders in the elderly: A national database study. *The Laryngoscope, 126*(2), 421–428.

Rundell, K. W., & Spiering, B. A. (2003). Inspiratory stridor in elite athletes. *Chest, 123*(2), 468–474.

Sapienza, C., & Ruddy, B. H. (2009). *Voice disorders*. Plural Publishing.

Schindler, A., Mozzanica, F., Maruzzi, P., Atac, M., De Cristofaro, V., & Ottaviani, F. (2013). Multidimensional assessment of vocal changes in benign vocal fold lesions after voice therapy. *Auris Nasus Larynx, 40*(3), 291–297.

Schonman, I., Mudd, P. A., Wiet, G. J., Ryan, M. A., Ongkasuwan, J., Prager, J., . . . Bauman, N. M. (2022). Multi-institutional study of patient-reported outcomes of paradoxical vocal fold motion. *The Laryngoscope, 133*(4), 970–976.

Smith, B., Milstein, C., Rolfes, B., & Anne, S. (2017). Paradoxical vocal fold motion (PVFM) in pediatric otolaryngology. *American Journal of Otolaryngology, 38*(2), 230–232.

Stemple, J. C., Glaze, L. E., & Klaben, B. G. (2010). *Clinical voice pathology: Theory and management* (4th ed.). Plural Publishing.

St. Peter, M., Ward, C., Nancy, N., & Sykes, K. J. (2022). Quality of life in caregivers, spouses, and partners of total laryngectomees: A scoping review. *Journal of Speech, Language, and Hearing Research, 65*, 1426–1434.

Tang, S. S., & Thibeault, S. L. (2017). Timing of voice therapy: A primary investigation of voice outcomes for surgical benign vocal fold lesion patients. *Journal of Voice, 31*(1), 129.e1–129.e7.

Thomas, L. B., & Stemple, J. C. (2007). Voice therapy: Does science support the art? *Communicative Disorders Review, 1*, 49–77.

Tibbetts, K. M., Dominguez, L., & Simpson, C. B. (2018). Impact of perioperative voice therapy on outcomes in the surgical management of vocal fold cysts. *Journal of Voice, 32*(3), 347–351.

Traister, R. S., Fajt, M. L., & Petrov, A. A. (2016). The morbidity and cost of vocal cord dysfunction misdiagnosed as asthma. *Allergy & Asthma Proceedings, 37*(2), e25–e31.

Vance, D., Heyd, C., Pier, M., Alnouri, G., & Sataloff, R. T. (2021). Paradoxical vocal fold movement: A retrospective analysis. *Journal of Voice, 35*(6), 927–929.

Van Leer, E. (2021). Enhancing adherence to voice therapy via social cognitive strategies. *Seminars in Speech and Language, 42*(1), 19–31.

Van Stan, J. H., Roy, N., Awan, S., Stemple, J. C., & Hillman, R. E. (2015). A taxonomy of voice therapy. *American Journal of Speech-Language Pathology, 24*(2), 101–125.

Verdolini, K., & Li, N. Y. K. (2019). Resonant voice therapy. In J. C. Stemple & L. B. Thomas (Eds.), *Voice therapy: Clinical studies* (3rd ed., pp. 132–140). Plural Publishing.

Welch, B., & Helou, L. B. (2022). Measuring communicative congruence and communicative dysphoria in a sample of individuals without voice disorders. *Journal of Speech-Language-Hearing Research, 65*(9), 3420–3437.

Welham, N. V., & Maclagan, M. A. (2003) Vocal fatigue: Current knowledge and future directions. *Journal of Voice, 17*(1), 21–30.

Wilson, J. J., Theis, S. M., & Wilson, E. M. (2009). Evaluation and management of vocal cord dysfunction in the athlete. *Current Sports Medicine Reports, 8*(2), 65–70.

Yi, J. S., Davis, A. C., Pietsch, K., Walsh, J. M., Scriven, K. A., Mock, J., & Ryan, M. A. (2021). Demographic differences in clinical presentation of pediatric paradoxical vocal fold motion (PVFM). *Journal of Voice, 9*, S0892-1997(21)00295-2.

Zalvan, C., Yuen, E., Geliebter, J., & Tiwari, R. (2021). A trigger reduction approach to treatment of paradoxical vocal fold motion disorder in the pediatric population. *Journal of Voice, 35*(2), 323.e9–323.e15.

Ziegler, A., Henke, T., Wiedrick, J., & Helou, L. B. (2018). Effectiveness of testosterone therapy for masculinizing voice in transgender patients: A meta-analytic review. *International Journal of Transgenderism, 19*, 25–45.

Ziegler, A., Verdolini Abbott, K., Johns, M., Klein, A., & Hapner, E. R. (2014). Preliminary data on two voice therapy interventions in the treatment of presbyphonia. *The Laryngoscope, 124*(8), 1869–1876.

Chapter 12

Feeding and Swallowing Disorders

With Dorothy Yang

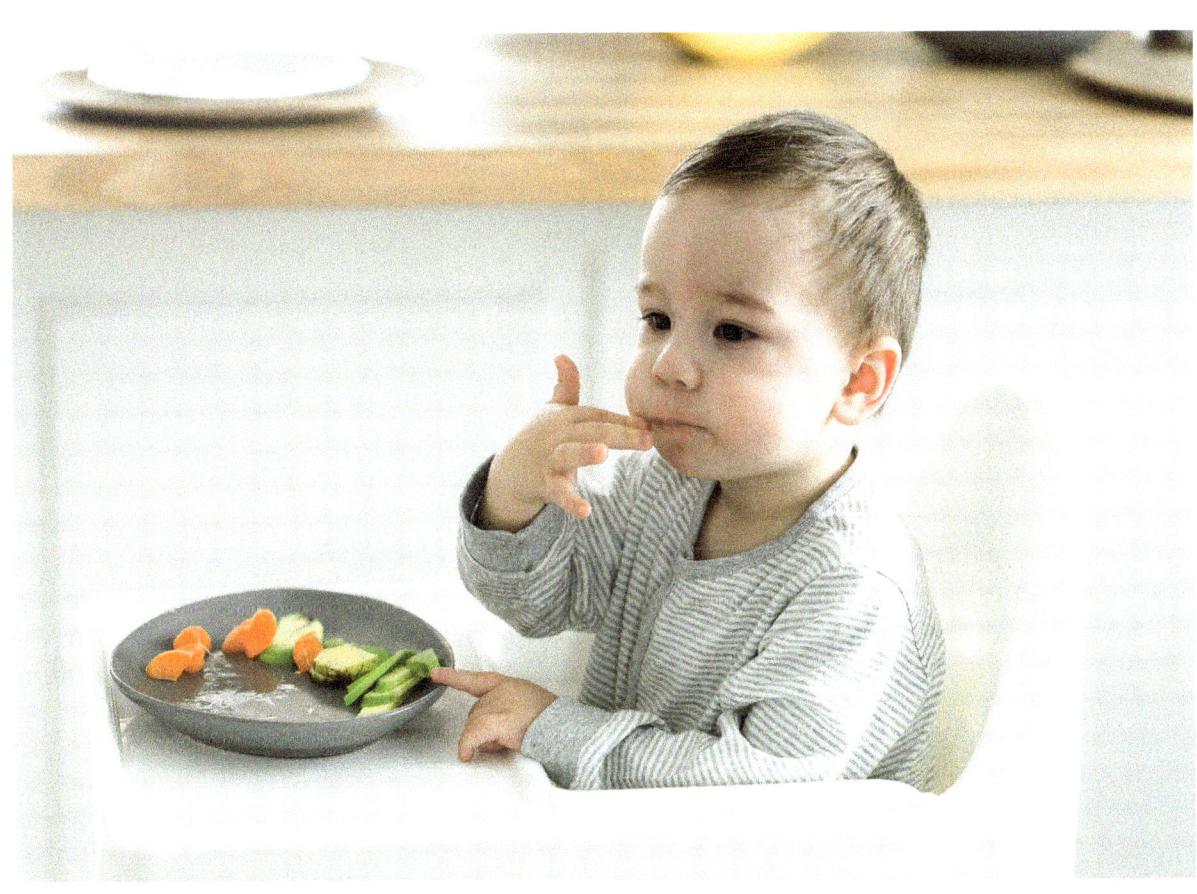

Learning Objectives

After reading this chapter, you will be able to:

- Describe the phases of a normal swallow and identify what challenges might be present at each phase of the swallow in a person with dysphagia.
- Describe the characteristics of dysphagia in children and adults.
- Identify appropriate methods for assessing dysphagia in pediatric and adult populations.
- Identify intervention approaches to support feeding and swallowing in children and adults with dysphagia as well as ways to support their caregivers.

Key Terms

amyotrophic lateral sclerosis
aspiration
bedside swallow evaluation
bolus
celiac disease
cleft lip/palate
clinical swallow evaluation
deglutition
dysphagia
edentulous
eosinophilic esophagitis
epiglottis
epistaxis
facial nerve
feeding
feeding disorder
fiberoptic endoscopic evaluation of swallowing (FEES)
gastroesophageal reflux disease (GERD)
hiatal hernia
hyoid bone
hypoglossal nerve
intraoral pressure
laryngospasm
mastication
modified barium swallow study (MBS)
nasal regurgitation
negative reinforcement
odynophagia
operant conditioning
penetration
peristalsis
positive reinforcement
postural changes
self-feeding
silent aspiration
swallowing
swallowing disorder
swallowing efficiency
swallowing maneuvers
syncope
trigeminal nerve
upper esophageal sphincter (UES)
vagus nerve
valleculae
videofluoroscopic swallowing study (VFSS)

Introduction

Have you ever eaten or drank something and when you swallowed, the food (or drink) "went down the wrong tube"? When this occurred, you were probably quick to recognize that something somewhere went awry during your swallow. The act of eating and swallowing is usually so seamless and automatic that we barely even think about it—that is, until something goes wrong. In this chapter, we describe the various phases that are associated with swallowing: the preoral, oral/oral preparatory, oral, pharyngeal, and esophageal phases in individuals who have normal swallowing function and in individuals who present with disordered swallowing (or **dysphagia**). We then discuss what a swallowing disorder might look like in children and adults who have various conditions. Assessment of swallowing disorders is key to understanding what phase(s) of the swallow is affected, which will be necessary for implementing appropriate intervention. Appropriate assessment and intervention of swallowing disorders in pediatric and adult populations are crucial because feeding is how our bodies get many of the nutrients that are necessary for healthy development and functioning. We describe several intervention strategies and techniques that speech-language pathologists (SLPs) use when managing dysphagia cases, as well as how families can be incorporated into intervention practices.

What We Know About This Topic

Before we discuss disorders associated with feeding and swallowing, it is essential to understand how a normal swallow works. Like other areas of speech-language pathology and audiology, we need to know what something is supposed to look like before we can identify it as disordered and requiring intervention. For this reason, let's dive into healthy feeding and swallowing processes. But first, let's define some key terms. **Feeding** refers to the process of eating food, and a **feeding disorder** occurs when an individual (usually an infant or child) has trouble eating foods based on textures or even dislike of certain food groups or types. **Swallowing** (also referred to as **deglutition**) refers to the act of transporting food from the oral cavity to the stomach, and a **swallowing disorder** (or dysphagia) often occurs when there are physical/anatomical (or psychological) concerns that impact a person's ability to successfully complete the swallow cycle. The swallow cycle consists of four phases—the preoral phase, the oral preparatory/oral phase, the pharyngeal phase, and the esophageal phase (Figure 12–1)—which are discussed in the following sections. Breaking up the swallow process into phases can be a helpful way for students to conceptualize what is happening in the body. At the same time, we note that these phases are not as distinct

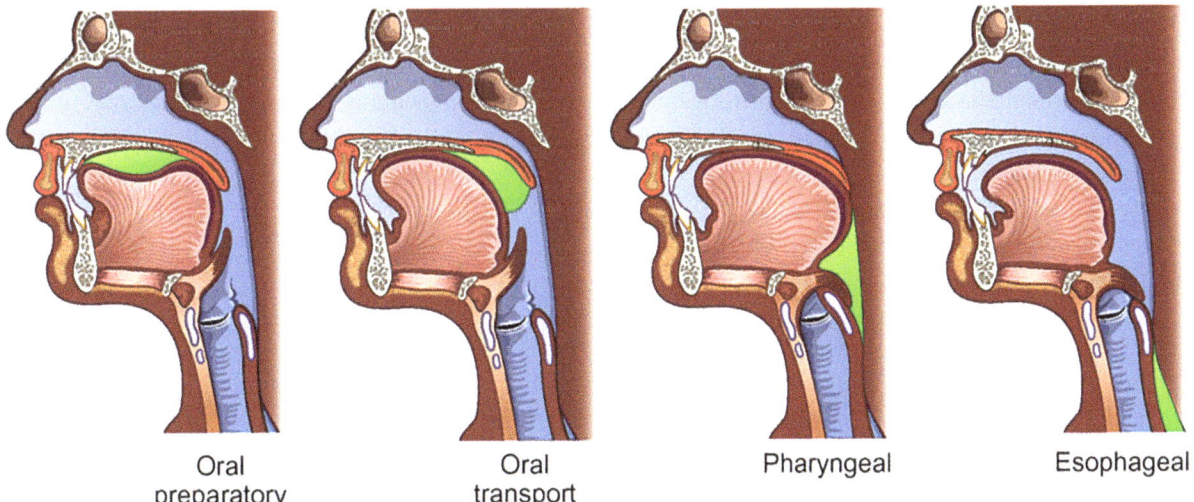

FIGURE 12–1. Phases of the swallow. *Source:* Ento Key (http://entokey.com/swallowing-2).

as we make them out to be. When you swallow, you may notice that it is in fact a continuous and (usually) seamless process; the phases are functionally interconnected to achieve this continuity. In the following sections, we also highlight how dysphagia can occur at any point. Note, however, that swallowing can deviate from what is considered "normal" in healthy individuals who do not present with dysphagia, and this is influenced by a variety of factors. Imagine taking a bite of something only to realize that the bite you took was too big. This will certainly affect how you manage that bite of food without corresponding to a disordered swallow. In addition, older adults may experience changes in their swallow function that are associated with healthy aging and may not rise to the level of a diagnosed swallowing disorder.

Preoral Phase

The preoral phase of swallowing occurs before food even touches your lips. Have you ever smelled something cooking and noticed that suddenly you were hungry? Or were presented with a dish that was visually unappealing and lost your appetite? It turns out that our senses (particularly our visual and olfactory senses) are associated with both feeding and swallowing (Ebihara et al., 2006; Sanders et al., 1992). Other external factors at the preoral phase include a person's cognition and executive functioning skills, such as attention and impulsivity.

Although the preoral phase is not typically associated with disordered swallowing, there are a few considerations to keep in mind. Oral movements do in fact occur during the preoral phase of swallowing, as the oral structures anticipate the arrival of food or drink. If these anticipatory movements are impaired or disrupted, this may lead to challenges at later stages of the swallow. In addition, sensory factors are key in the preoral phase. If an individual does not have access to visual or auditory cues associated with feeding, or has attention difficulties, they may be less likely to engage in the feeding process altogether. Moreover, having food aversions may impact an individual's desire and motivation to eat.

Oral Preparatory/Oral Phase

Normal

During the oral preparatory phase, food or drink enters the mouth and we begin to chew. During **mastication** (i.e., chewing), saliva is mixed with the food or drink to create a **bolus**. Once the bolus is formed, the oral phase of swallowing begins. In this phase, the bolus makes its way from the front of the mouth to the back of the tongue in preparation for the next phase of the swallow cycle: the pharyngeal phase. During the oral preparatory/oral phase, the bolus is contained in the mouth by the tongue, cheeks, lips, and soft palate.

Disordered

Because several anatomical structures are involved in the oral preparatory/oral phase, there are many potential causes of dysphagia at this early stage. Drooling and food spillage can occur if the person does not have adequate lip closure, challenges with chewing can result from weak muscles or tooth concerns, and reduced saliva production can hinder the construction of the bolus. Moreover, weak muscles can also interfere with moving the bolus from the front of the mouth to the back of the tongue for preparation of the pharyngeal phase.

12 ◆ Feeding and Swallowing Disorders

Pharyngeal Phase

Normal

After the bolus has been adequately prepared and moved toward the back of the tongue, the pharyngeal phase of the swallow can happen. The primary job in this phase is to keep the bolus out of undesirable places, such as the nasal cavity and the larynx, so that it can go where it needs to go: the pharynx. To allow this to happen, the soft palate (i.e., the velum) raises to close off the nasal cavity. For the bolus to make its way into the pharynx, enough pressure must be created by the movement of the tongue to the pharyngeal wall (i.e., **intraoral pressure**). As all of this is occurring, the larynx is moved upward by the **hyoid bone**, which causes the **epiglottis** to lower over the vocal folds and protect the airway. The bolus then moves through the pharynx into the esophagus.

Disordered

When problems are present in the pharyngeal phase of the swallow, this can result in serious complications. If the velum does not sufficiently close off the nasal cavity, liquid or solid bolus can be expelled from the nose (i.e., **nasal regurgitation**). In addition, if the larynx does not raise quickly enough and the epiglottis does not fully cover the airway, penetration and aspiration can occur. **Penetration** occurs when the bolus enters the top of the airway, above the vocal folds. Have you ever taken a sip of water and coughed because "it went down the wrong tube"? If so, that is penetration. Figure 12–2 shows an example of penetration. **Aspiration** occurs when the bolus enters the lower part of the airway, below the vocal

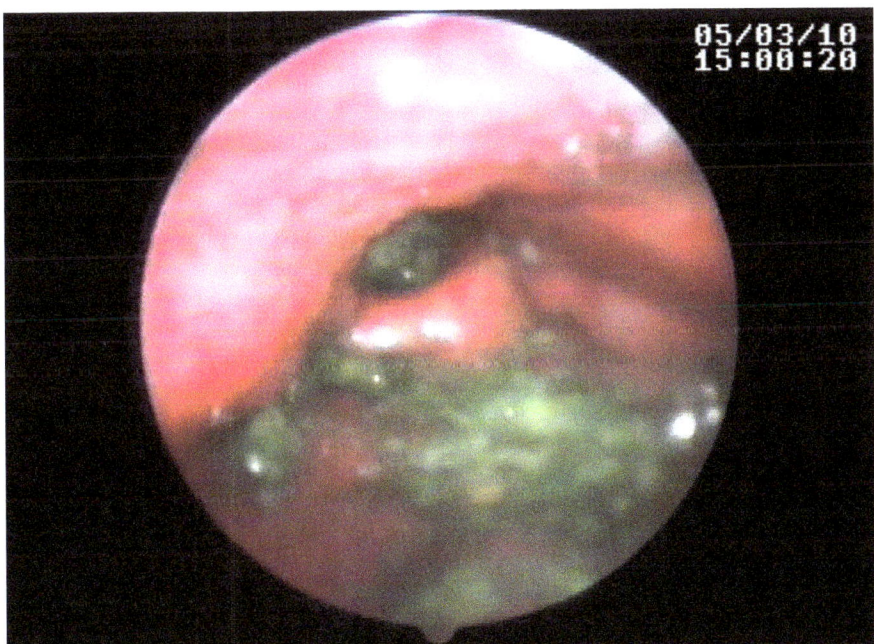

FIGURE 12–2. A portion of the bolus is shown at the vocal folds before the patient expels it. *Source: From Clinical Management of Swallowing Disorders, Sixth Edition* (in press) by Murry, T., Chan, K., & Walsh. E. H. Copyright © 2026 Plural Publishing, Inc. All rights reserved.

folds and into the larynx (and potentially the lungs). Aspiration is often considered a primary marker of dysphagia, but remember that this is not the only symptom associated with a disordered swallow.

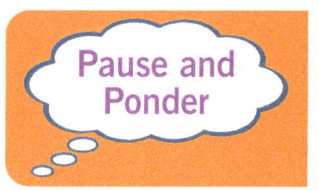 **Pause and Ponder** Consider how challenges other than aspiration (at any phase of the swallow) can lead to malnutrition and reduced quality of life in patients.

Esophageal Phase

Normal

After the bolus has been propelled from the pharynx into the esophagus, the muscles of the esophagus contract, which causes the bolus to move into the stomach. This contraction is referred to a **peristalsis**.

Disordered

If peristaltic contractions do not occur or are weak, the bolus might not be fully transported into the stomach and remain on the linings of the esophageal walls. If food does not make its way into the stomach, a person may experience nutritional deficits and, potentially, infections.

Characteristics of Dysphagia

Feeding and swallowing disorders occur in both children and adults for different reasons, and the causes are many. In infants, the processes involved in feeding and swallowing tend to be intricately linked (Lefton-Grief, 2008), and so when we think about pediatric dysphagia, we tend to lump together disorders of feeding and swallowing. In adults, however, we primarily focus on disorders of swallowing (i.e., dysphagia). In the following sections, we discuss some of the primary conditions associated with dysphagia in children and adult populations.

Pediatric Dysphagia

In the United States, approximately 1 in 23 to 1 in 37 children ages birth to 5 years are diagnosed with dysphagia (Kovacic et al., 2021), and for children who have co-occurring conditions, feeding disorders are more common. Children who have various health conditions can be diagnosed with pediatric dysphagia, including those with cognitive/developmental or neurological conditions, structural abnormalities, certain infections associated with the immune system, and those who were born prematurely.

Infants who are born with damage to their central nervous system, such as those with cerebral palsy, may have feeding or swallowing challenges that result from abnormal muscle tone or muscle movements. Hypo- or hyperactive movement of muscles in the torso can directly impact the structures that are associated with oral and pharyngeal phases of swallowing (Benfer et al., 2013; Malandraki et al., 2022). Not only can the structures involved in swallowing be impacted by a child's muscle tone and coordination but these structures can also be abnormal at birth. Consider a child who has **cleft lip/palate**. A child who has a cleft lip may have challenges in the oral preparatory phase of swallowing, when lip closure is necessary. A child born with a cleft lip and cleft palate may experience more serious complications during the pharyngeal phase of swallowing. That is, their soft palate may not adequately seal off the nasal cavity, which could result in food being expelled from the nose. In addition, for infants who are breastfeeding or drinking from a bottle, the inability to seal off the nasal cavity can severely impact their ability to intake food because they are unable to create the negative intraoral pressure required for sucking. Children who are born with other congenital conditions experience different structural abnormalities that can impact the swallowing mechanism. These include syndromes associated with smaller jaws and retracted tongues (which can obscure the airway) and heart defects (which impact feeding endurance).

Finally, children who are born prematurely may not have adequately developed structures or muscle coordination necessary for feeding. They may have difficulty coordinating the movements required for the pattern of feeding/breathing. In addition, infants and children who are born preterm and considered medically fragile may have respiratory challenges that preclude oral feeding. Because of this, they may receive intervention to support their breathing, which may pose safety challenges for oral food intake (for a review, see Rice & Lefton-Greif, 2022).

Children who are diagnosed with cognitive or developmental conditions such as intellectual disability or autism may present with motor difficulties that impact their ability to independently eat food without the use of adapted equipment (e.g., specialized feeding utensils, plates, cups). In addition, these children may prefer to eat foods that are restricted in texture, color, or food group (e.g., only eating orange foods or food that is puréed). These factors may contribute to negative behaviors associated with mealtime, which is a primary concern of caregivers because the frequency of mealtimes is high and it can be particularly stressful when they do not go as planned (Piazza, 2008).

Adult Dysphagia

Although children can and do have dysphagia, it is more common to see adult patients who have conditions that are associated with an impaired swallow. Many acquired conditions are associated with both primary and secondary complications for swallowing. Primary complications with swallowing occur as a direct result of the disorder, such as tongue weakness. Secondary complications are not directly associated with the swallow mechanism but, rather, occur because of something else. For example, perhaps a patient does not experience any structural or anatomical difficulties, but their condition is associated with fatigue that results in a disinterest in eating and reduced oral intake. The most common disorders associated with dysphagia can be classified as neurological or structural in origin.

Neurological Etiologies

Neurological conditions associated with dysphagia include cerebrovascular accident (i.e., stroke), traumatic brain injury, degenerative conditions (e.g., **Parkinson's disease**, **amyotrophic lateral sclerosis**, **Huntington's disease**), and tumors on the brain. Because these conditions are a result of neurological damage, and swallowing requires a complex integration of neural regions, there are multiple pathways to dysfunction following a neurological disorder (Daniels & Huckabee, 2014). How a person's swallow is affected will depend on which part of the brain is implicated and the ensuing neural damage. This means that two people who have a stroke can present with very different dysphagias. However, individuals who have a neurogenic dysphagia will have impairments at the oral, pharyngeal, and esophageal stages that are often the result of muscle weakness, paralysis, and/or incoordination. Table 12–1 lists common symptoms associated with each stage of swallowing for individuals who have a neurogenic condition.

In addition to the physiological complications associated with dysphagia in individuals with neurogenic conditions, behavioral difficulties can also contribute to disruptions in feeding and swallowing. A person who sustains a traumatic brain injury or who develops dementia (see Chapter 9) may present with cognitive challenges that impact attention and memory. These individuals may forget to eat altogether or not have the sustained attention to focus on the task of consuming food.

Structural Etiologies

Structural etiologies associated with dysphagia include congenital abnormalities (e.g., cleft lip/palate, as discussed in the section on pediatric dysphagia), trauma (accidental and medical), infections, and head and neck cancer. As implied, dysphagia results from anatomical factors associated with one or more of the structures involved in deglutition. As you might guess, any resulting dysphagia will depend on which components of the swallow were impacted and to what extent. The most common structural cause of dysphagia is treatment associated with head and neck cancer. When a person receives a diagnosis of head and neck cancer, they may undergo surgery to remove the tumor or cancer cells. Sometimes this means removing part of a person's muscle or bone. Surgery for head and neck cancer may involve removal of all or part of the lips, tongue, jaw, hard or soft palate, hyoid bone, larynx, epiglottis, vocal folds, and so on. Sometimes it is even necessary to surgically remove the entire pharynx, larynx, or esophagus. When these structures are implicated, challenges with swallowing ensue.

Aside from surgical treatment for head and neck cancer, a person may undergo radiation or chemotherapy. Although radiation therapy may allow swallowing structures to remain intact, side effects can include dry mouth and reduced saliva production, damage to soft tissue, and swelling of laryngeal tissue, all of which can lead to dysphagia. Figure 12–3 shows a photograph of a larynx that has received radiation therapy for laryngeal cancer. Despite these side effects, radiation therapy has been found to be associated with higher levels of quality of life in patients with head and neck cancer compared to surgical intervention (Terrell et al., 1998).

TABLE 12–1. Common Symptoms Associated With Each Phase of the Swallow

Phase of Swallow	Common Symptoms
Oral	Drooling
	Pocketing of food in the cheeks
	Difficulty with chewing
	Difficulty moving the bolus in the oral cavity
Pharyngeal	Delayed swallow trigger
	Nasal regurgitation
	Penetration
	Aspiration
Esophageal	**Odynophagia** (i.e., pain with swallowing)

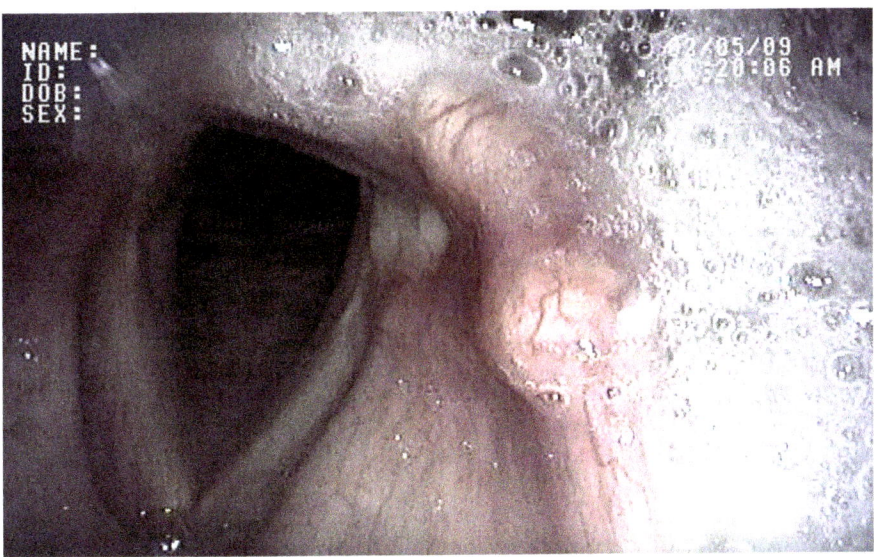

FIGURE 12–3. The larynx following radiation therapy (XRT) for laryngeal cancer. *Source:* From *Clinical Management of Swallowing Disorders, Fifth Edition* (pp. 1–350) by Murry, T., Carrau, R. L., & Chan, K. Copyright © 2022 Plural Publishing, Inc. All rights reserved.

In addition to treatments for head and neck cancer, trauma to the oral, pharyngeal, or esophageal structures can also result in temporary or permanent dysphagia. Trauma is defined loosely here, as it includes accidental incidents (e.g., a vehicle accident or gunshot wound) or more purposeful (and often necessary) medical causes, such as surgery to position a breathing or tracheostomy tube. Another common structural cause of dysphagia is acidic substances in the stomach refluxing into the esophagus, pharynx, or larynx. Although this can, and often does, happen in healthy individuals, when acid reflux becomes chronic and contributes to heartburn or other pain, the person may be experiencing **gastroesophageal reflux disease (GERD)**.

Impact of the Disorder Across the Lifespan

The reason for a dysphagia diagnosis may be associated with other challenges related to a person's speech, language, hearing, and/or cognition. For example, children and adults who have structural differences in the oral cavity will also likely have compromised articulation and intelligibility. In addition, those who have a swallowing disorder resulting from a neurogenic condition may also have neurological damage that affects their language, cognition, and/or hearing.

Of course, having a swallowing disorder will not only impact how a person swallows their food and drink but also result in secondary and sometimes tertiary consequences. Perhaps less obvious are the social, emotional, and cultural repercussions of dysphagia. Eating and drinking are not merely acts that we engage in to fuel our bodies. Although consumption of food and beverages is necessary for our survival, eating and drinking are highly social activities. Think about the past week: How many times did you eat or drink as a part of a social function? When we meet new friends, potential romantic partners, or old colleagues, what activity is usually proposed? Grabbing coffee, lunch, or dinner. Children and adults who have dysphagia may feel self-conscious about sharing a meal with someone, even if that person is familiar with and understanding of their challenges. Similarly, if a person's swallow is affected in such a way that they require a feeding tube, the act of grabbing a drink or meal with someone as a social event might feel awkward or uncomfortable. In addition, eating and swallowing have been reported to lead to increased levels of fatigue in older adults with dysphagia (Brates et al., 2022). A person who relies on others to help them eat may feel frustrated that they cannot care for themself. Perhaps not surprisingly, dysphagia can co-occur with depression. As such, individuals who feel depressed may not consume enough food, may feel too tired to eat, and may even experience tightness in their throat which can lead to pain with swallowing.

Dysphagia has a negative impact not only on the person with the disorder but also on the person's caregivers. Caregivers and family members of adults with dysphagia report increased levels of caregiver burden and decreased levels of quality of life associated with changes in family roles and daily routines/interactions, increased social isolation because of reduced outside social engagements, and fear and anxiety associated with the health and safety of their loved one (for a review of caregiver burden, see Shune et al., 2022). Moreover, the health of the caregiver in turn plays a role in the health of the person with dysphagia. That is, evidence suggests that poor caregiver mental health results in an increased risk of the person with dysphagia dying (Lwi et al., 2017).

Parents of children with swallowing disorders are also faced with a complicated task. When an infant presents with feeding or swallowing challenges, they are at risk for further developmental and nutritional deficits. What has the potential to make this even more complicated is the role that early feeding has on parent–child attachment. Because bonding between a caregiver and their child tends to occur during mealtimes (Cormack et al., 2020), a feeding or swallowing disorder has the potential to impede bonding, resulting in increased stress for both the parent and the child during mealtimes and other routine events (Cohen & Dilfer, 2022). Moreover, parents have reported that feeding challenges are a contributing factor to their children's reduced social participation and overall quality of life (Simione et al., 2020).

Cross-Cultural Information

The act of eating and sharing meals with others is a highly social activity that is also culturally rooted. Various cultures have traditions and rules associated with food, and these can extend outside of mealtimes (e.g., religious practices). When, where, how, and what food is consumed may be linked to a person's cultural identity, and these preferences may be at odds with the health risks and intervention procedures associated with dysphagia management (Kenny, 2015). That is, whereas from the perspective of the SLP, increased quality of life for the patient might be associated with a safe swallow, a patient may place higher value on maintaining the relationship with their culture through food. As culturally responsive clinicians, SLPs must consider the role that food plays in a person's culture, as well as the person's/family's beliefs and preferences regarding feeding tubes and end-of-life care, if necessary (Riquelme, 2007). Patients and families should be asked about their understanding of and perspective toward their swallowing disorder, as well as more specific information about food preferences and mealtime experiences using open-ended, non-leading questions (Hall & Johnson, 2020). Shared decision making between the healthcare team and the patient/family is a valuable way to ensure that all perspectives are considered to support an individual's quality of life (Kenny, 2015).

Assessment

Assessment Considerations for Adult Populations

Swallow Screening

The 3-ounce water test, or Yale Swallow Protocol, is a screening tool that can be used to identify individuals who are at risk for aspiration. The use of this screening measure is not restricted to SLPs but, rather, can be given by any medical professional, such as registered nurses and physicians, who are trained to recognize the signs and symptoms of aspiration (e.g., coughing, throat clearing, wet/gurgly vocal quality). In the 3-ounce water test, the client/patient is instructed to drink 3 ounces of water without stopping until the water is finished. The client/patient is considered to have passed the screening if they are able to drink the entire amount of water without stopping and without demonstrating any overt signs and symptoms of swallowing difficulty during the task, immediately after the task, and 1 minute after completing the task. If, however, they are unable to meet all of these criteria, they fail the screening and are referred to speech-language pathology for further evaluation. In most cases, once speech-language pathology is consulted, an SLP will proceed with a clinical swallow evaluation as a first step to evaluating the patient's swallow function.

Clinical Swallow Evaluation

The **clinical swallow evaluation** (CSE), also referred to as the **bedside swallow evaluation**, allows the SLP to determine if an individual/patient presents with signs and symptoms of dysphagia within the context of other variables, such as mealtime performance, feeding posture/positioning, and environmental conditions (American Speech-Language-Hearing Association [ASHA], n.d.-a). To conduct a thorough CSE, the SLP should begin by collecting a thorough case history, which includes a review of the patient's medical chart, patient and/or family interview, and a self-assessment of swallowing ability usually presented in the form of a questionnaire (e.g., Eating Assessment Tool [EAT-10], Swallowing Quality of Life [SWAL-QOL] questionnaire). Following the case history, the SLP should proceed to examine the structural and functional integrity of the oral mechanism (e.g., jaw, lips, tongue) and the cranial nerves (e.g., **trigeminal**, **facial**, **vagus**, **hypoglossal**) that innervate it, assess cognitive status as it impacts swallowing and swallow safety, and administer PO (i.e., Latin for *per os*, meaning "by mouth") trials of different liquid (e.g., thin liquids or thickened liquids if indicated) and solid consistencies (e.g., purée, soft solids, hard solids).

In the CSE, the SLP looks for signs and symptoms of dysphagia during the administration of PO trials, including, but not limited to, reduced lip seal or closure (resulting in material spilling out between the lips); prolonged chewing/mastication; throat clearing and/or coughing before, during, or after the swallow; and wet/gurgly vocal quality after the swallow (which may indicate that material has entered the airway). The SLP also uses information from the CSE to identify factors that increase a patient's risk of aspiration and possible strategies that may help decrease that risk. It is important to recognize that the CSE is a non-instrumental swallowing assessment, meaning that it does not provide the examiner with direct visualization of the laryngeal, pharyngeal, and esophageal structures and their physiology during swallowing. As such, SLPs must use the CSE with caution, understanding that it is limited in its ability to accurately determine the presence or absence of "**silent aspiration**" (i.e., when swallowed material enters the airway but no behavioral response, such as a cough or throat clear, is elicited due to decreased sensation in the upper respiratory tract). Therefore, the SLP must carefully consider and weigh all information obtained from the CSE to determine whether further evaluation via an instrumental swallowing assessment is warranted and appropriate for a given patient.

Videofluoroscopic Swallowing Study

The **videofluoroscopic swallowing study (VFSS)**, also called the **modified barium swallow study (MBS)**, is a type of instrumental swallowing assessment that provides SLPs with a direct view of the oral, pharyngeal, and esophageal phases of swallowing. In VFSS, liquids and solids of various consistencies are mixed with barium, a contrast material, so that the SLP can visualize the bolus on an x-ray and follow its path as it travels down from the mouth to the stomach during a swallow in real time (Logemann, 1986). As such, VFSS is a valuable tool that SLPs can use to evaluate the safety and efficiency of a patient's swallow. The term **swallowing safety** refers to whether swallowed material enters the airway (i.e., whether material is penetrated and/or aspirated), and the term **swallowing efficiency** refers to the amount of residual material left behind in the oral and/or pharyngeal cavities after the swallow. In a normal swallow, swallowing should be safe, meaning that material should not enter the airway, and it should be highly efficient, meaning that no material should remain in the pharynx after the swallow. However, in individuals with dysphagia, these aspects of swallowing are compromised. VFSS thus allows the SLP to determine the presence, extent, and timing of penetration and/or aspiration (i.e., before, during, and/or after the swallow), the presence and extent of any residue remaining in the pharynx after the swallow, and the underlying anatomical and/or physiological impairments that are contributing to these problems. Furthermore, the SLP can use VFSS to confirm whether certain compensatory strategies (e.g., posture/positional, dietary texture modifications) are effective in reducing the impact of the anatomical and physiological deficits on swallowing (Martin-Harris et al., 2000).

As with any assessment tool, VFSS is not without its advantages and limitations. As previously discussed, one of the major advantages of VFSS is that it provides direct, moment-by-moment visualization of swallowing anatomy and physiology for all phases of swallowing. Although VFSS is considered a noninvasive, relatively low-risk procedure, it still involves radiation exposure because this method uses x-ray; however, many facilities have adopted general safety guidelines to ensure that patient exposure to radiation is kept to a minimum (e.g., less than 3–5 minutes; Leonard & Kendall, 2019). Even still, the SLP must be strategic in their approach to obtaining the information necessary to develop an appropriate treatment plan within a limited time frame because VFSS only provides a quick snapshot in time of the patient's swallowing ability and may not be representative of how a patient swallows over the course of an entire meal. In addition, the SLP must be sensitive to the quantity of material (which is mixed with barium) that a patient may aspirate and must recognize when it is appropriate to defer trialing a given texture or perhaps end the examination. Patients with cognitive and/or behavioral limitations that limit their ability to follow instructions and cooperate in the examination, patients who are unable to tolerate or may be allergic to barium, patients who are unable to achieve optimal positioning, and/or patients who are too ill to be brought to the radiology suite (e.g., those who are in the intensive care unit) may not be good candidates for this procedure.

Flexible Endoscopic Evaluation of Swallowing

Another type of instrumental swallowing assessment available to SLPs is flexible endoscopy evaluation of swallowing, also known as **fiberoptic endoscopic evaluation of swallowing (FEES)**. In FEES, a flexible endoscope with a light source and camera attached to the end of the scope is inserted into the nose and passed through the nasal cavity to visualize the larynx and pharynx below (Figure 12–4). Similar to VFSS, liquids and solids of different consistencies are administered to the patient during a FEES exam, allowing for direct visualization of the bolus as it passes through the pharynx (Langmore et al., 1988). Furthermore, FEES shares similarities with VFSS in that it also provides SLPs with information about the safety and efficiency of the patient's swallow, such as the presence, extent, and timing of penetration and/or aspiration (i.e., before, during, and/or after the swallow) and the presence and extent of any residue remaining in the pharynx after the swallow. Once these problems are identified, the SLP can develop an appropriate treatment plan that targets and aims to remediate the underlying swallowing impairment(s). Compensatory strategies can also be trialed during a FEES examination to confirm whether they are appropriate for use.

FEES offers several unique advantages over VFSS. First, it allows for direct observation of any anatomical deviations in the larynx if suspected. Second, if there is a strong concern for aspiration, FEES

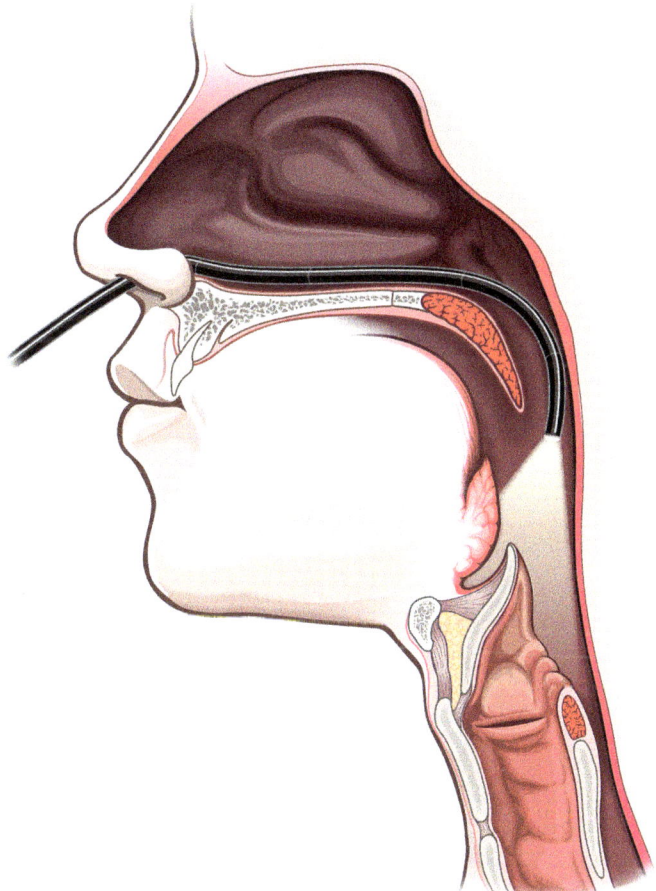

FIGURE 12–4. Drawing from lateral view showing proper placement of scope prior to feeding the patient. Note the scope is above the epiglottis. *Source:* From *Clinical Management of Swallowing Disorders, Sixth Edition* (in press) by Murry, T., Chan, K., & Walsh, E. H. Copyright © 2026 Plural Publishing, Inc. All rights reserved.

can be used to initially evaluate how well a patient manages their own secretions prior to the administration of any PO trials. Third, there is no radiation exposure with FEES and therefore no time limitations, and solids and liquids can be given without barium or other contrast material. This is particularly helpful when trying to determine how a patient swallows across an entire meal or if frequent retesting of the patient's swallow function is warranted. FEES can also be easily implemented in therapy as a biofeedback tool to increase patients' awareness of their own swallow function and to teach patients how to correctly execute compensatory strategies. Fourth, FEES may be a good alternative for patients who are unable to be transported to radiology for VFSS, as FEES equipment is much more portable. Patients with mobility and/or postural deficits or who wear external devices that obstruct a clear view on VFSS are also good candidates for FEES. Finally, FEES is a more accessible method compared to VFSS because it is less costly overall.

In terms of limitations, one cannot directly visualize the oral and esophageal phases of swallowing with FEES; only the pharyngeal phase can be observed. However, some aspects of the pharyngeal phase are more difficult to analyze with FEES compared to VFSS (e.g., the extent of posterior pharyngeal wall constriction, laryngeal elevation, upper esophageal segment opening). Patients who are unable to follow instructions and cooperate in the examination, unable to tolerate the procedure due to discomfort or a hyperactive gag reflex, have experienced recent nasal trauma or have increased susceptibility to **epistaxis** (i.e., nose bleeding), and have a history of **laryngospasm** (i.e., spasming of the vocal folds) or **syncope** (i.e., fainting) may not be good candidates for this procedure.

Both VFSS and FEES are considered the clinical gold standards of swallowing assessment. It is important to remember that one method is not superior to the other; instead, the two techniques are complementary to each other and provide valuable insight into a patient's swallow function. What determines the selection of one method over another (or perhaps deciding to do both) will depend on the diagnostic information that is needed, the weighing of each method's advantages and disadvantages, and careful consideration of the needs and abilities of the patient.

Assessment Considerations for Pediatric Populations

Like the assessment processes discussed throughout this book, the assessment of pediatric dysphagia follows a multidisciplinary approach. Although an interprofessional approach to assessment is important for all populations treated by an SLP, children with feeding and swallowing disorders are a special population that requires a particularly high level of collaboration across disciplines to ensure safety and healthy physical development. The assessment team is often composed of an SLP, occupational therapist, pediatrician, dietitian, and psychologist, each with expertise in the various aspects associated with feeding and swallowing. To conduct an assessment, the team collects a medical history, performs an interview with the caregiver/family, observes the child during a feeding activity, and collects data from caregiver–informant questionnaires. As always, it is important to gather insight into the family's concerns with their child's feeding as well as what the family hopes to achieve through assessment and intervention.

In addition to the assessment components, the SLP examines the child's physical and anatomical structures that are necessary for safe and efficient feeding. This can be done merely by watching the child eat or by using instrumentation to observe swallowing behaviors. Instrumentation methods discussed in the section on assessment considerations for adults can be modified for use with pediatric populations. One popular instrumentation method for use with this population is the VFSS, which can provide information about the physical characteristics of a child's swallow at the different phases of swallowing, including (but not limited to) total pharyngeal transit time, bolus clearance ratio, and opening of the pharyngeal esophageal segment, which separates the pharynx from the esophagus. VFSS has been validated as an appropriate instrumentation method for bottle-fed infants (ages 0–9 months) and children (up to age 21 years; Miles et al., 2022).

Treatment

Treatment Considerations for Adult Populations

Recall that during a VFSS or FEES, SLPs often trial compensatory strategies with patients to determine if the strategies can be used to mitigate the swallowing symptoms (e.g., laryngeal penetration, aspiration, pharyngeal residue) and improve swallowing safety and efficiency during PO intake. As such, SLPs are often engaging in the treatment process as early as when they evaluate a patient. Keep in mind that compensatory strategies only help manage the symptoms; if the goal is to rehabilitate specific physiological aspects of the swallowing mechanism (identified only through an instrumental swallowing evaluation) with the purpose of reducing the severity of the physiological deficit, then the SLP may also recommend techniques such as swallowing exercises to the patient.

Compensatory Strategies

Compensatory strategies are often used to change bolus flow and/or the dimensions of the vocal tract to reduce the swallowing symptoms that a patient may be experiencing. These include behavioral strategies, postural changes, and swallowing maneuvers.

Behavioral strategies are perhaps the easiest compensatory strategies to implement. They include, but are not limited to, using a liquid wash, producing a double or multiple swallows, changing bolus size, and modifying dietary textures. A patient may use a liquid wash after swallowing a solid bolus for the purpose of "washing away" or clearing any residue that may be present in the oral and/or pharyngeal cavities after the swallow. A double or multiple swallows may also be used for this purpose. For some patients, a smaller bolus size may be beneficial in decreasing the amount of oral and/or pharyngeal residue after the swallow or laryngeal penetration and/or aspiration; in contrast, other patients may benefit from a larger bolus size (e.g., patients with sensory issues who depend on the weight of the bolus to swallow safely and effectively). Finally, swallowing safety and efficiency may be improved simply by changing the viscosity or texture of solids and liquids. For a description of the various viscosities and textures of liquids and solids, see the International Dysphagia Diet Standardisation Initiative (IDDSI) framework (IDDSI, 2024).

The most common **postural changes** are the chin tuck, neck extension, head rotation (to the left or right), and head tilt (to the left or right). In the chin tuck, a patient is instructed to bring their chin down to their chest prior to swallowing a bolus. In this posture, the base of the tongue and the epiglottis are positioned closer to the posterior pharyngeal wall, which may help protect the airway during swallowing for some patients.

The neck extension posture uses gravity to move the bolus in an anterior-to-posterior direction in the oral cavity for delivery to the pharynx. This posture is particularly helpful for patients who are unable to move their tongue or have limited movement of the tongue, perhaps because of neurological damage, or those who have had part or all of their tongue removed likely due to oral cancer. In addition, patients must demonstrate good ability to protect their airway when using this strategy because this posture can increase aspiration risk if there are also problems with the pharyngeal phase of swallowing.

To perform the head rotation posture, patients are instructed to turn their head to the left or right and look over their shoulder prior to swallowing a bolus. This posture changes the dimensions of the vocal tract, thereby changing the pressures generated in the vocal tract during swallowing. As such, some patients may benefit from using this posture to help reduce or clear residue in the pharynx. Furthermore, if a patient exhibits any unilateral (i.e., one-sided) pharyngeal or laryngeal weakness, having them turn their head to the weak side helps redirect the flow of the bolus to the stronger side. This may also help improve airway protection and/or reduce residue collected in the pharynx.

Finally, to perform the head tilt posture, patients are instructed to tilt their head (or upper body if they have good trunk control) to the left or the right. Patients who present with unilateral oral or pharyngeal weakness are most likely to benefit from this posture because this posture uses gravity to redirect the flow of the bolus to the stronger side.

The next group of compensatory strategies are **swallowing maneuvers**, which aim to bring certain involuntary aspects of the swallow under the patient's voluntary control. The most common swallowing maneuvers are the supraglottic swallow, the super-supraglottic swallow, the effortful swallow, and the Mendelsohn maneuver. These are described next.

Patients who have difficulties protecting their airway when swallowing may be good candidates for the supraglottic swallow or the super-supraglottic swallow. The supraglottic swallow is a technique that requires the patient to breathe in, hold their breath, place the bolus in their oral cavity, swallow while still holding their breath, and then produce an immediate cough after they swallow prior to breathing normally again. By holding their breath before and during the swallow, patients voluntarily close their true vocal folds, preventing material from passing below the vocal folds and entering the trachea. The cough at the end ensures that any material remaining in the larynx above the vocal folds after the swallow is quickly ejected and cleared from the airway. The super-supraglottic swallow shares similarities with the supraglottic swallow, with one additional component: bearing down throughout the breath hold. With this added component of bearing down, a patient may be able to achieve even greater airway protection by closing their false (i.e., ventricular) vocal folds in addition to their true vocal folds.

In the effortful swallow maneuver, a patient is instructed to "swallow hard," squeezing tightly all the muscles that they use for swallowing. Performing this maneuver may assist with anterior-to-posterior bolus propulsion in the oral cavity. In addition, this maneuver generates greater pressure in the pharynx, which may help reduce or clear residue in the pharynx (Lazarus et al., 2002).

The final swallowing maneuver is the Mendelsohn maneuver, which can be difficult to perform. It is important, therefore, that the SLP trains a patient to execute this maneuver accurately prior to implementing it during PO intake. The SLP will often begin by encouraging the patient to perform several dry swallows and feel how their larynx elevates during the swallows. Once the patient confirms that they can feel their larynx elevating during a swallow, the SLP then instructs the patient to swallow again; however, instead of allowing the larynx to return to its resting state, the patient is to hold up their larynx in an elevated position for several seconds. Passing the bolus from the pharynx into the esophagus through a structure called the **upper esophageal sphincter (UES)** depends on effective laryngeal elevation. Thus, as a compensatory strategy, the Mendelsohn maneuver may be helpful for patients who have difficulties with UES opening.

It is important to emphasize that if any of the previously discussed compensatory strategies are to be adopted, the SLP must ensure that these strategies are successful in increasing swallowing safety and efficiency based on the results of a comprehensive and thorough clinical assessment. In some cases, this may require an instrumental swallowing evaluation to confirm that the recommended strategies are appropriate.

Swallowing Exercises

Swallowing exercises should be considered one of the aims of therapy to remediate or improve the underlying physiological deficits of the swallowing mechanism. These exercises often involve improving the strength, timing, range of motion, and/or coordination of the various structures involved in swallowing and include oral motor exercises, the Masako, the Shaker, chin tuck against resistance (CTAR), expiratory muscle strength training (EMST), the effortful swallow, and the Mendelsohn maneuver, which are described next. As is true of any exercise regimen, the frequency, intensity, and duration of the swallowing exercise(s) prescribed must be appropriate if long-term change is desired.

Oral motor exercises are often used to strengthen and improve control of structures involved in swallowing, such as the lips, tongue, jaw, and larynx. There are many variations of these exercises, such as pushing the weakened structure (e.g., lips, tongue, jaw) against resistance, mimicking chewing or sucking behaviors, producing a yawn, coughing, and completing phonation tasks that increase vocal fold closure.

The Masako, or tongue hold maneuver, works to improve contraction of the posterior pharyngeal wall, which is important for propelling the bolus effectively and efficiently through the pharynx into the esophagus (Fujiu & Logemann, 1996). To perform the Masako, patients are instructed to stick out their tongue and hold it gently between their teeth (or gumline for patients who are *edentulous* or have no teeth). Then they are told to swallow their saliva hard while remaining in this position.

The purpose of the Shaker or head lift exercise is to improve passage of the bolus from the pharynx to the esophagus by increasing UES opening (Shaker et al., 1997). Because UES opening is largely dependent on laryngeal elevation, this exercise works to strengthen the muscles that elevate the larynx. In this exercise, patients are positioned flat on their back in a supine position and then instructed to raise their head and look down at their feet without lifting their shoulders. This exercise can be done as either an isometric or isotonic exercise. The isometric form of the Shaker requires the patient to keep their head raised for 1 minute, rest for 1 minute, and then repeat the cycle two more times; for the isotonic form, the patient completes 20 to 30 consecutive head lifts without holding, followed by a 1-minute rest period, and then repeats the cycle two more times. It is important to note that the Shaker is a difficult and fatiguing exercise; if a patient is unable to perform the exercise accurately or is susceptible to fatigue, then CTAR may be a better alternative. Like the Shaker, CTAR also helps improve UES opening by targeting the muscles of laryngeal elevation (Yoon et al., 2013). In CTAR, patients are seated in an upright position with a small rubber ball placed underneath their chin to squeeze down on as they tuck their chin. For the isometric version of CTAR, the patient uses their chin to compress the ball against their chest without interruption for 1 minute, rests for 1 minute, and then repeats the cycle two more times. The isotonic version of the exercise involves completion of 20 to 30 consecutive squeezes followed by a 1-minute rest period and then two more repetitions of this cycle.

In EMST, patients are instructed to blow quickly and forcefully through a special respiratory device that contains an adjustable one-way valve which varies the resistance provided to expiratory airflow.

As such, patients must generate sufficient expiratory pressure to overcome the resistance of the valve and successfully pass air through the device. As the name suggests, EMST helps strengthen expiratory muscles, and research has shown that a broad range of benefits can be obtained with use of the device, such as improvements in breathing, voice, cough, and swallowing (Kim & Sapienza, 2005).

The effortful swallow and the Mendelsohn maneuver, both of which were described previously as compensatory strategies, can also be incorporated into a swallowing exercise program. When used as an exercise, the effortful swallow has been shown to improve laryngeal elevation, UES opening, airway protection, and muscular contraction of oral and pharyngeal structures such as the tongue and posterior pharyngeal wall. Use of the Mendelsohn maneuver as an exercise has also resulted in improvements in laryngeal elevation, UES opening, and airway protection.

Intervention for swallowing disorders often involves a combination of compensatory strategies to manage the symptoms of the dysphagia and rehabilitative approaches to directly target the underlying physiologic impairments of the swallowing mechanism. When developing a treatment plan, SLPs must consider multiple factors to maximize quality of life, including the nutrition and hydration needs of the patient, burden of oral intake, and potential to rehabilitate swallow function. As such, intervention must be highly individualized to meet the goals of each patient and their caregivers across unique settings and situations.

Treatment Considerations for Pediatric Populations

As described previously, some infants who present with pediatric dysphagia were born prematurely and are medically fragile. This means that SLPs are often tasked with a complex job—making sure that the infant or child can breathe and obtain the adequate nutrients necessary for survival. Furthermore, SLPs are vital players in determining when pediatric patients are ready to safely begin oral feeding. Remember that feeding and breathing are highly linked, and we run the risk of food or liquid entering the lungs (i.e., aspiration) if breathing and swallowing are not coordinated. For patients who require ventilation support, we must consider several factors with regard to introducing food orally, including the child's birth, medical, and feeding history; current nutrient levels; and indicators that they are ready to orally intake food (e.g., alertness, sucking abilities). Instrumental and clinical examinations may also inform this decision (Rice & Lefton-Grief, 2022). A review of the evidence suggests that the practice of oral feeding can be done safely when pediatric patients undergo ventilation intervention (Rice & Lefton-Grief, 2022).

An interprofessional team that often includes an SLP, dietician, occupational therapist, psychologist, and the child's caregiver is paramount to the successful treatment of children with feeding disorders (Desai et al., 2022). Goals for feeding tend to center around three broad areas: teaching skills for self-feeding, using behavioral and/or sensorimotor interventions to increase the types of foods that are tolerated, and improving oral–motor skills that are required for safe feeding (Howe & Wang, 2013). Furthermore, parent interventions are also vital to supporting feeding in children because feeding usually involves both the child and the caregiver. It is not surprising, then, that the evidence suggests that feeding and swallowing outcomes in children are improved when a combination of intervention strategies is used. Several interventions are associated with improvements in feeding and swallowing in children, including those targeting nutritional intake, behavioral factors associated with eating, and sensory approaches to feeding, with observed outcomes in infants' mealtime behaviors and weight, as well as caregiver stress.

Several approaches can be taken to target the various physiological components of feeding and swallowing, including preparatory behaviors, acquisition of feeding skills, and environmental supports for feeding. Preparatory approaches focus on behaviors that are associated with feeding but do not involve the actual act of feeding or swallowing. These include activities such as nonnutritive sucking, oral desensitization, and mother–child skin-to-skin contact (which is important for breastfeeding). Techniques to support the acquisition of feeding skills include oral stimulation, olfactory stimulation, and tactile stimulation of the tongue. Finally, environmental approaches to pediatric dysphagia intervention include positioning techniques of the neck and upper body as well as the use of adaptive feeding equipment. For a review of the outcomes associated with each of these interventions, see Howe and Wang (2013).

Behavioral interventions for feeding are based on the principles of **operant conditioning** (i.e., a behavioral modification strategy in which behaviors are shaped based on rewards and punishments). **Positive reinforcement** is a technique in which the child's behaviors are praised or celebrated. The idea is that the child begins to associate the behavior with a positive outcome. For example, imagine that you are trying to expand the types of food tolerated by a child who only eats orange foods. You offer the child a small piece of a different-colored food (perhaps a yellow banana), and they take a small bite. Positively reinforcing the behavior of trying a new type of food might look like verbally praising the child (e.g., "You did it! You ate the banana! I'm so proud of you!") or even offering the child something that they like as a reward (e.g., a toy, song, tablet) for trying the new food. **Negative reinforcement**, on the other hand, involves the removal of an aversive stimuli when a specific behavior is performed. Here, the idea is that the child learns that they can avoid situations or tasks that they do not like by engaging in certain other desired behaviors. For example, when the goal of therapy is for a child to feed themselves (i.e., **self-feeding**), it is necessary to wean the child from being fed by their caregiver. To do this, the caregiver or clinician might teach the child that they can be finished with mealtime (the aversive stimuli) sooner if they feed themselves compared to if the caregiver feeds them (Haney et al., 2023). This might look like offering the child the following option: "You can take five more bites if I feed you or one more bite if you feed yourself." Other behavioral modification techniques include extinction, shaping, and physical guidance (for a review of these techniques, see Hong & Wang, 2012). Behavioral interventions are associated with a variety of improvements in feeding skills as well as decreased caregiver stress.

Parent-directed intervention and educational practices are also common approaches to supporting feeding in children with pediatric dysphagia, and in fact, evidence suggests that parents prefer family-centered approaches to feeding therapy (Simione et al., 2020). These approaches include providing education about the purpose of the selected intervention techniques, incorporating parents into the intervention sessions, modeling intervention strategies, and coaching parents to use these approaches with their children during mealtimes (Silverman, 2015). Not only do parent-directed interventions lead to positive outcomes regarding children's feeding behaviors, they also lead to improvements in parent–child interactions (Howe & Wang, 2013).

Although many of the interventions discussed so far target infants and young children with dysphagia, we must also consider older, school-aged children who present with this diagnosis. Children engage in eating several times throughout the school day, including breakfast, snack, and lunch. For those who have dysphagia, it is the responsibility of the school-based SLP to provide dysphagia therapy and safe eating practices throughout the school day. Many of the interventions described so far are appropriate for school-aged children with dysphagia, and it is important that the school-based SLP be up to date on best practices for safe feeding and swallowing. In addition, it is the responsibility of the school-based SLP to collaborate with the child's school and medical teams to ensure that the school team is informed about the child's dietary restrictions and modifications for safe eating practices (West, 2024).

Why Is This Topic Important?

Our ability to swallow contributes significantly to our overall quality of life and well-being. Consider how your life would be impacted if you were not able to eat or drink. How would you meet your basic nutritional and hydration needs for survival? For many individuals, eating and drinking are more than just a requirement needed to live; they are a pleasurable and sociable activity. Think about all the activities that you engage in on a regular basis that involve food and drink. How would your participation in these activities change if you were unable to swallow? For example, consider a meal that you had over the weekend. What were you doing while you were partaking in that meal? Were you at a restaurant with friends? Were you by yourself in front of the television watching Netflix? What was your emotional state? Were you happy? Tired? Perhaps sad? As you can imagine, for individuals with dysphagia, the presence of a swallowing problem can (and often does) lead to significant and adverse life changes.

According to ASHA (n.d.-b), the overall objective of an SLP should be to "optimize individuals' ability to communicate and swallow, thereby improving quality of life." As discussed in this chapter, there are many physical, social, and emotional ramifications of dysphagia, including malnutrition and dehydration, pulmonary compromise such as aspiration pneumonia, reduced interest in eating and drinking, isolation as it relates to PO intake, and embarrassment. In addition, individuals with dysphagia are not the only ones negatively affected by the swallowing impairment; often, their caregivers experience significant physical, emotional, social, and/or financial stress in providing dysphagia care. As the preferred providers of dysphagia services, SLPs are in a unique position to help individuals with dysphagia and their families. Working closely with other disciplines within the interdisciplinary medical team (e.g., otolaryngology, gastroenterology), SLPs work to assess, diagnose, and treat swallowing disorders (ASHA, n.d.-b). Throughout the assessment and treatment process, SLPs must carefully consider the impact of various clinical decisions on quality of life and determine if the outcomes align with the patient's and/or their family's goals.

Finally, recall the *International Classification of Functioning, Disability, and Health* (ICF) model (World Health Organization, 2001) from Chapter 2. Let's apply the ICF framework to an older adult, Gertrude, with dysphagia (Figure 12–5). To get a better sense of how Gertrude's disability interacts with various environmental and personal factors to support or hinder her participation in activities throughout her day, let's look at a completed ICF diagram. Here, we want to know about Gertrude's ability to participate in a commonly occurring activity for her: sharing a meal with her adult children. We consider the factors that are both supportive of and barriers to her participation in this activity. Several factors contribute to Gertrude's ability to share a meal with her adult children. Gertrude primarily presents with dysphagia at the oral and pharyngeal phases. She has difficulty with foods of mixed textures, such as chicken and rice soup, particularly with holding the liquid bolus in her oral cavity while she chews the chicken and rice. The liquid either escapes through her lips or enters her airway (body function and structures). This is especially the case when she eats with others because she enjoys chatting around the dinner table. Modifying the meal that is served at these family dinners to include single-textured food helps Gertrude to be able to be a part of the conversation at the dinner table, as does providing education to Gertrude and her children about the importance of waiting until she has finished swallowing her food to speak. Environmental factors that may impact her participation in this activity include the types of foods available at any given meal and how her adult children encourage her to participate in conversation (e.g., waiting until she has finished chewing and swallowing to ask her a question). Moreover, personal factors can impact Gertrude's ability to safely share a meal with her children, including her ability to remember to chew and swallow before talking and her focused attention to chewing and swallowing.

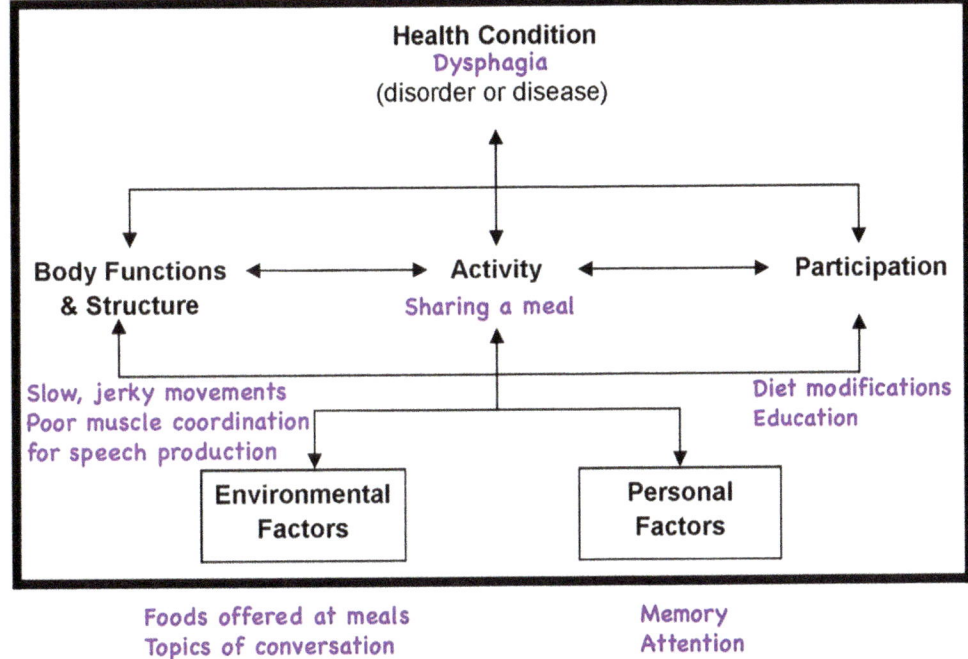

FIGURE 12–5. ICF model example. *Source:* Adapted from the World Health Organization (2021).

Application to a Child

 Ramon is a 14-year-old boy who was diagnosed with autism when he was aged 30 months. At that time, he spoke using delayed echolalia, repeating the last word someone had said to him. For example, if Mom asked, "Do you want milk?" Ramon would respond with "milk." He also would only speak in two-word utterances when his body was in motion, despite being able to say longer utterances when his body was still. At the same time, Ramon easily labeled nouns and was able to read. As a toddler, he was provided with a low-tech augmentative and alternative communication device to support his communication, and by age 3 years, Ramon began developing more generative language.

As a child, Ramon exhibited left-sided weakness in his whole body, including his limbs and his face. Although this left-sided weakness did not impact his ability to walk, he presented with an asymmetrical smile, and he had difficulty forming sounds and chewing food. At approximately age 3 or 4 years, Ramon would stuff his mouth with food and swallow it without chewing. At that time, he was eating mainly pureed and soft foods (e.g., applesauce, mashed vegetables). Ramon was not choking, and his parents were unaware that he had swallowing difficulties. At age 8 years, Ramon attended a summer camp for children interested in wilderness exploration. In the evenings, within 10 minutes of laying down for bed, Ramon would begin coughing and vomiting. At approximately this same time, Ramon began choking on his foods. These eating challenges halted Ramon's growth and led to significant weight loss. His parents and medical team were concerned. There was speculation that Ramon had either eosinophilic esophagitis (an immune disease in the esophagus resulting from a buildup of white blood cells) or celiac disease (an autoimmune disorder that causes damage to the small intestine when the individual consumes foods containing gluten). To determine if Ramon had eosinophilic esophagitis, the otolaryngologist (ear, nose, and throat doctor) performed an upper endoscopy, in which she inserted an endoscope through Ramon's mouth and down his esophagus to identify any inflammation. No inflammation was identified, so the medical team decided to conduct an MBS. The MBS revealed that Ramon's esophagus and stomach were both unremarkable (i.e., normal). Further inspection revealed that he did not have a hiatal hernia (in which part of the stomach pushes into an opening in the diaphragm and into the chest) and that his stomach emptied well. In addition, Ramon's blood tests were negative for celiac disease. After all this testing and no answers, Ramon's parents were confused, frustrated, and concerned for their child's health and safety. To help ensure that he was getting at least some nutrients, his parents continued to feed him at home. At school, Ramon was unable to eat in the cafeteria with the rest of his third-grade class. As a result, he ate in the special education classroom with his 1:1 aide, who sometimes struggled to get him to eat any food at all. Lunchtime often carried over into recess time, and there were many days that Ramon missed out on playing with his classmates on the playground. Because eating was a priority for Ramon's health, his aide kept data throughout the day on what Ramon ate, when he ate, and how much he ate. This feeding log went back and forth between home and school so that Ramon's team could monitor his eating patterns. After many months of taking data, it was difficult to determine any patterns, and adults were still feeding Ramon even though he was now 9 years old. Although they were still feeding him soft foods, they also introduced some harder finger foods (e.g., small pieces of fruit, diced chicken). With no answers from any medical tests and no patterns in her son's food data log, Ramon's mother began to believe that he had become dependent on others feeding him, a form of learned helplessness. To remedy this, she began resisting helping Ramon eat at mealtimes, giving him the opportunity to feed himself. Without his mother feeding him, Ramon simply sat at the dinner table, either completely engrossed in telling his family about his favorite Minecraft game or expressing discomfort (e.g., "my stomach hurts"). After trying this for a week, Ramon's parents rescinded their belief that Ramon's behavior was a form of learned helplessness and sought additional help. At age 10 years, Ramon was sent for a feeding evaluation at his local hospital.

The SLP at the hospital gathered a comprehensive case history from Ramon's parents, which included a long list of foods that he ate, foods that he avoided, and foods that he choked on or vomited. She then conducted a CSE, during which she collected data on Ramon's ability to feed himself independently and his feeding skills when he was being fed. She trialed different food textures and consistencies and noticed that when Ramon fed himself, he would stuff his mouth full of food before initiating a swallow. This was true for all foods she trialed, regardless of texture and consistency. Aside from stuffing his mouth with food, when Ramon consumed foods that were smooth in texture, he presented with a normal swallow. However, when given foods that had a mixed texture (e.g., cereal in milk, yogurt with fruit pieces), the SLP noted that Ramon did not seem to know what to do orally. Again, he continued to stuff his mouth with the food until he felt that his mouth was full and then chewed the food just enough to be able to swallow. This often resulted in choking. Because of this, the SLP noted that Ramon presented with the swallow skills of a 12- to 18-month-old. In addition to choking, the SLP noticed that Ramon presented with postural challenges (inability to maintain upright position when feeding), which seemed to impact his endurance, stability, and positioning when eating. She also noted that he demonstrated deficits in fine motor abilities, which impacted his ability to hold and use eating utensils. Many of his oral motor challenges were related to the sensory abilities required to find and manage food in his mouth and tolerate changes in texture.

When he fed himself, he tended to take excessively large bites of food, which he had difficulty chewing, and it was difficult to determine where he was positioning the food in his mouth. He exhibited a munching chewing pattern and had to stop chewing and swallow some of the bolus before continuing to chew the food he had stuffed into his mouth. Because his mouth was stuffed, food was pocketing under his lips and in his cheeks, and he had to use a hard swallow pattern to create enough force to clear the food (although it took three or four swallows for every mouthful of food). When he was given more appropriate bite sizes, the SLP noticed that he was positioning the food under his tongue and used appropriate tongue lateralization, although he still had decreased strength and endurance for eating. Presenting Ramon with food that he found visually unappealing would elicit a gag reflex. Additional challenges that the SLP noted were that Ramon was unaware that he had food on his hand or face, he was unable to answer questions while he was chewing, and he had difficulty discriminating between tastes (e.g., sweet vs. sour). As a result of this clinical evaluation, Ramon was diagnosed with oral dysphagia and a feeding disturbance.

Based on the CSE, the SLP recommended that Ramon receive feeding therapy for his dysphagia. The SLP recognized the importance of incorporating Ramon's family into the therapy and considered the family's priorities for intervention. The primary goals for intervention were to have Ramon eat 100% independently while maintaining a healthy weight. The SLP collaborated with the family to construct a plan to scaffold Ramon's feeding abilities. At each mealtime, the goal was for Ramon to eat 25% of his food on his own, 50% of the food together (e.g., Mom would cut the food and load his fork), and 25% of the food by being fed directly. Over time, Ramon increased the percentage of time that he was eating independently and decreased the amount of time that he required being fed. Ramon and his family followed this intervention plan for 2 years, at which time Ramon was eating 100% of his food independently and maintaining a healthy weight.

Now, at age 14 years, Ramon prefers foods that are consistent in texture. For example, when given a sandwich, he will deconstruct it and eat each component separately (although he does eat grilled cheese sandwiches in the typical fashion). In addition, although he does eat tacos, he prefers to have others feed him the tacos (a food of mixed textures). Because the goals that the family had identified at the beginning of the intervention have been met (Ramon is eating independently and maintaining a healthy weight), his family has decided to put a pause on the feeding intervention for now. Although Ramon still presents with challenges in this area, other areas of development are a greater priority currently, including social communication skills, advocacy, and developing independence.

Application to an Adolescent or Adult

 Thomas Jones is a 59-year-old male who underwent anterior cervical discectomy and fusion (i.e., a surgical procedure to remove a herniated or degenerative disk in the neck) to cervical spinal segments C4 through C7 approximately 4 years ago. At his most recent doctor's appointment, Thomas informed his primary care physician that he had been experiencing persistent problems with his swallowing since his surgery, reducing his desire to eat. He told his primary care physician that he eats only one meal per day, which has caused him to lose weight unintentionally. In response to this, Thomas' primary care physician placed a referral to speech-language pathology so that Thomas' swallowing could be further evaluated. Thomas was promptly scheduled for an outpatient VFSS at his local hospital.

The SLP began her assessment by collecting a thorough case history. Thomas endorsed long-term difficulties swallowing since his spinal surgery. Although his chronic dysphagia had remained stable, it had lessened his interest in eating, resulting in a 145-pound weight loss during the past 4 years. He reported experiencing the following swallowing symptoms daily: occasional coughing or "choking" on thin liquids; feeling of obstruction in his throat and/or chest; heartburn/indigestion; and GERD, for which he regularly took medication. He also informed the SLP that he had difficulty taking his pills because they often felt like they got "stuck" in his throat; as such, he crushed his pills to increase the ease of swallowing his medication. To prevent coughing or "choking" on thin liquids, Thomas would drink thin liquids at a slower rate, and to reduce the feeling of obstruction in his throat and/or chest, he would chew his food thoroughly until it became "mush" and would often produce multiple swallows for each bite that he took.

After interviewing Thomas, the SLP completed an oral mechanism examination. Overall, results were unremarkable, and no significant anatomical abnormalities or motor impairments were noted. The SLP then began the VFSS, instructing Thomas to take sips of thin liquids via a cup as well as bites of purée, mixed textures/soft solids, and hard solids. All of these textures contained barium so that the SLP could examine Thomas' ability to swallow these different textures in real time on x-ray. Regarding the oral phase of swallowing, the SLP did not notice anything abnormal. Thomas was able to achieve a tight lip seal, maintain good control of the bolus, and transport the bolus quickly in an anterior-to-posterior direction. Although mastication was slightly prolonged, it remained functional and was not attributable to an oral deficit (recall that Thomas informed the SLP that he chews his food for a long time to reduce possible feelings of obstruction in his throat and/or chest when swallowing solids). In addition, no residue remained in the oral cavity after the swallow, suggesting that Thomas' oral musculature was operating within functional limits.

When assessing Thomas' pharyngeal phase, the SLP noted that Thomas presented with incomplete epiglottic inversion, reduced laryngeal elevation and excursion, and reduced laryngeal closure (i.e., airway protection). These deficits negatively impacted both swallowing safety and efficiency. In terms of swallowing safety, the SLP noted consistent laryngeal penetration above the vocal folds during the swallow with thin liquids. Regarding swallowing efficiency, the SLP observed mild residue in the **valleculae** with all consistencies following the initial swallow. Then the SLP trialed several compensatory strategies during the examination to determine if any were successful in mitigating the laryngeal penetration observed with thin liquids during the swallow and/or reducing the residue in the valleculae from all consistencies after the swallow. Of the strategies trialed, a left turn was most effective in reducing the symptoms of Thomas' swallowing deficits. Not only did it eliminate the laryngeal penetration of thin liquids during the swallow but also it cleared the residue in the valleculae for all consistencies.

Results of the esophageal screening revealed esophageal retention with retrograde bolus flow below the upper esophageal segment (i.e., the muscle segment that separates the pharynx from the esophagus), particularly for solids (such an observation may be indicative of reflux). Passage of solids from the esophagus into the stomach was slow but eventually cleared.

The SLP reviewed the results of the VFSS and shared her recommendations with Thomas after completing the exam. She informed Thomas that based on the findings of his VFSS, he would likely be able to continue tolerating a regular diet but should use a left head turn to help mitigate some of his swallowing symptoms and increase swallowing safety and efficiency during PO intake. She also informed him that using a left head turn when eating/drinking was only a temporary fix to his problem. She explained that if he wanted to produce long-term change and improve the overall functioning of his swallowing mechanism, he would need to engage in swallowing exercises targeting the deficits identified on his VFSS (i.e., incomplete epiglottic inversion, reduced laryngeal elevation and excursion, and reduced laryngeal closure) to help rehabilitate his swallow. Thomas was amenable to the SLP's recommendations, and a swallowing exercise program was initiated that included the effortful swallow and Mendelsohn maneuver.

To address the findings from the esophageal screening, the SLP provided Thomas with education on dietary and lifestyle modifications that he could incorporate into his daily life to minimize the effects of GERD. The SLP also referred Thomas back to his primary care physician to discuss next steps and to determine if he needed additional esophageal workup by gastroenterology.

Chapter Summary

Whereas feeding involves eating food, swallowing involves the transport of food from the mouth to the stomach and is comprised of the following interconnected phases: preoral, oral preparatory/oral, pharyngeal, and esophageal. Dysphagia, or a swallowing disorder, occurs when a person has an impairment in one or more of the phases of swallowing. Children may present with pediatric dysphagia because of a neurological condition or structural abnormalities that impact muscle tone and coordination. Premature birth can also affect feeding and swallowing development. In adults, dysphagia is often associated with neurological conditions or structural abnormalities, such as head and neck cancer. Dysphagia not only directly impacts a person's feeding and swallowing abilities but also can play a role in the social, emotional, and cultural aspects of their lives and lead to depression, social isolation, and increased caregiver burden. Culturally sensitive and family-/client-centered approaches in dysphagia management must be taken into consideration throughout the assessment and intervention processes.

Assessment of dysphagia includes an interprofessional approach that often involves an SLP, medical doctor, dietitian, and other health care professionals. In adult populations, assessment involves various methods, including a screening and a CSE. During the CSE, the SLP gathers a case history, examines the patient's oral structures and functions, and conducts feeding/swallowing trials with different consistencies of solids and liquids. In addition, instrumental assessments can be used to provide direct visualization of swallowing anatomy and physiology, allowing SLPs to assess swallowing safety and efficiency. In pediatric populations, assessment involves gathering a medical history, observing feeding activities, and using instrumentation methods to assess physical characteristics of swallowing. These assessments aim to ensure safe and efficient feeding for children with feeding and swallowing disorders.

Intervention for adults with dysphagia includes compensatory strategies and swallowing exercises. Compensatory strategies include behavioral techniques, postural adjustments (which change bolus flow by altering the dimensions of the vocal tract), and swallowing maneuvers (which bring involuntary aspects of the swallow under voluntary control). Whereas compensatory strategies aim to manage symptoms, swallowing exercises work to strengthen various swallowing muscles and improve swallow function by targeting physiological deficits directly. Interventions for pediatric populations involve a multidisciplinary team approach to dysphagia, including various interventions aimed at addressing feeding skills, behavioral factors associated with feeding, sensory processing, and environmental supports. Parent-directed interventions and educational practices are crucial for children with dysphagia, leading to positive outcomes in feeding behaviors and parent–child interactions. In addition, school-based SLPs play a vital role in providing dysphagia therapy and ensuring safe eating practices for school-aged children with dysphagia, collaborating with school and medical teams to accommodate dietary restrictions and modifications.

Chapter Review Questions

1. Describe the phases of a normal swallow.
2. What is a common symptom of dysphagia in the oral phase? Pharyngeal? Esophageal?
3. Name two neurological conditions associated with dysphagia in adults.
4. What are some structural abnormalities that can lead to dysphagia in children?
5. What are some social and emotional consequences of dysphagia for both individuals and their caregivers?
6. Explain the difference between penetration and aspiration during swallowing.
7. How can cultural preferences influence dysphagia management?
8. How is a swallow screening different from a clinical swallow evaluation?
9. Describe the advantages and disadvantages of the clinical swallow evaluation, videofluoroscopic swallow study, and flexible endoscopic evaluation of swallowing.
10. How are compensatory strategies different from swallowing exercises?
11. Describe the various types of compensatory strategies, how they work, and when they might be used.
12. Describe the various types of swallowing exercises and explain what each does to improve swallow function.

Learning Activities

1. Two types of thickened liquids that SLPs may recommend to patients are mildly (nectar) thick liquids and moderately (honey) thick liquids. Examples of items that have a mildly thick liquid consistency include fruit nectars, milkshakes, cream-based soups, and tomato juice. Examples of items that have a moderately thick liquid consistency include honey and molasses. Now imagine if you had dysphagia and someone told you that the only way you could drink liquids safely is if you thickened them. How would this news make you feel? Would you accept this as a long-term solution to your swallowing problem? Why or why not?

2. Pick one of your favorite foods to eat and pay attention to what you are doing as you are eating it. What did you eat? Describe what you did with the food as it was in your mouth and throat. Consider the following questions to help guide your response: (a) If your food required chewing, how long did it take? (b) What was your tongue doing throughout the entire eating process? (c) How many swallows did it take for you to get the food down? (d) Did you still have food in your mouth after your first swallow? If so, what did you do? (e) Did anything go wrong as you were eating? If so, what happened and what did you do to try to fix the problem?

3. It is the SLP's role to provide a recommendation for dietary textures after completing a swallowing evaluation. What impact do you think an SLP's recommendations could have on a patient and their quality of life? To help guide your response, consider a patient who was given a diet recommendation of mildly thick liquids with soft and bite-sized solids or a patient who was given a diet recommendation of thin liquids with pureed solids (for descriptions and characteristics of the different liquid and solid consistencies that SLPs can recommend to patients, see the IDDSI framework [IDDSI, 2024]).

Suggested Reading

Desai, H., Lauridson, S., Nhuyen, M., Ornelas, E., & Schomberg, J. (2022). Feeding skill and behavior changes in children with complex feeding disorders following therapy in an intensive multidisciplinary feeding program. *Perspectives of the ASHA Special Interest Groups, 7*, 1155–1165.

This study examined the effects of a multidisciplinary feeding intervention program on the oral feeding skills and mealtime behaviors of children with complex cases of pediatric dysphagia. Participants were 34 children between the ages of 13 months and 6½ years and caregivers who were responsible for feeding. The intervention program consisted of direct child intervention and caregiver training implemented by a multidisciplinary team of several professionals: gastroenterologist, nurse practitioner, registered dietitian, SLP, occupational therapist, psychologist, and clinical social worker. Intervention approaches focused on a range of techniques, including behavioral modification, oral motor skills, sensory processing strategies, food selection, and specific caregiver training and education.

    Results of this study indicate that an individualized, multidisciplinary approach to pediatric dysphagia supports feeding overall. Of note, this intervention approach demonstrated a significant reduction in frequency of inappropriate mealtime behaviors, including throwing food, eating only small amounts of food, and avoiding eating altogether. Children also demonstrated improvements in oral motor and sensory skills, including a reduction in pocketing food in the cheeks, spitting food out instead of chewing it, and accepting a variety of food textures. This study highlights the value of a multidisciplinary approach, including caregiver education and training, to the treatment of children with complex cases of dysphagia.

Haney, S., Ibañez, V., Kirkwood, C., & Piazza, C. (2023). An evaluation of negative reinforcement to increase self-feeding and self-drinking for children with feeding disorders. *Journal of Applied Behavior Analysis, 56*(4), 757–776.

This study examined self-feeding behaviors in six children with pediatric feeding disorders. The researchers were interested in examining caregiver and child feeding behaviors after caregiver training, as well as the effect of negative reinforcement on self-feeding and self-drinking. All children in the study were between the ages of 3 and 8 years; had diagnoses of autism, Down syndrome, or DiGeorge syndrome (except for one participant who had received a liver and small bowel transplant and had vitamin D deficiency); and were deemed by an SLP and pediatrician/gastroenterologist to safely intake food orally. None of the children engaged in self-feeding independently and consistently. Whereas some of the children would self-feed only for preferred food items, others had never self-fed. For this study, each child was accompanied by at least one caregiver who underwent training in a behavioral intervention to facilitate self-feeding. Once the caregivers were trained using the behavioral strategies, the researchers collected data on the children's acceptance of food and inappropriate mealtime behaviors during self-fed and caregiver-fed conditions.

During a second part of the study, researchers were specifically interested in the effects of negative reinforcement on the development of children's self-feeding and self-drinking. In the control conditions, children were given the chance to self-feed but were not required to for the duration of the mealtime. In the treatment condition (referred to as the mealtime termination condition), children had the power to end the mealtime session early by engaging in self-feeding. Researchers found that using negative reinforcement resulted in increased self-feeding behaviors and that children were motivated to self-feed during this intervention. Although this study examined oral intake of small amounts of foods, the authors propose that this is a promising intervention technique for children who do not self-feed and recommend that future research examine greater portions of foods, such as full meals.

Rangira, D., Najeeb, H., Shune, S. E., & Namasivayam-MacDonald, A. (2022). Understanding burden in caregivers of adults with dysphagia: A systematic review. *American Journal of Speech-Language Pathology, 31*(1), 486–501.

The term *caregiver burden* is often used to describe the impact of caregiving on a caregiver's emotional well-being, physical health, social life, and/or financial situation over time. In this article, the authors detail a systematic review and meta-analysis investigating dysphagia-related caregiver burden in caregivers of adults with dysphagia. Only literature meeting the authors' inclusion criteria for this systematic review and meta-analysis were evaluated. All literature included in the analyses examined caregiver burden through interviews, questionnaires, and/or surveys, but the caregivers interviewed and/or surveyed varied across patient populations (e.g., head and neck cancer, stroke, neurodegenerative diseases). Different sources of caregiver burden were identified for each of the unique medical diagnoses leading to dysphagia, with some similarities shared across diagnoses, including changes in meal preparation, disruption in lifestyle, effects on social life, degree of support, decisions regarding non-oral feeding methods such as feeding tubes, and fear of aspiration.

This study demonstrated that caregiver burden is prevalent among caregivers of adults with dysphagia and does not appear to be influenced by other factors, such as caregiver age, caregiver–care recipient relationship, and patient population. In fact, the meta-analysis described in this article revealed that 71% of caregivers reported some degree of burden in caring for an adult with dysphagia and managing their swallowing impairments. Given this information, clinicians should consider how to best support caregivers within their approach to dysphagia management. The authors conclude with some recommendations that can be readily adopted in practice to help reduce caregiver burden.

Sura, L., Madhavan, A., Carnaby, G., & Crary, M. A. (2012). Dysphagia in the elderly: Management and nutritional considerations. *Clinical Interventions in Aging, 7,* 287–298.

Elderly adults are at particular risk for dysphagia given that they experience age-related changes to the swallowing mechanism and have increased susceptibility to age-related diseases such as stroke and dementia. This article specifically discusses dysphagia as it occurs in three elderly populations: (a) those with dementia, (b) those who have suffered from stroke, and (c) those dwelling in the community. There is strong evidence that dysphagia can compromise nutritional status and pulmonary health in each group, increasing an individual's risk of becoming malnourished and acquiring a lung infection such as pneumonia. In addition, this article provides a general overview of approaches to swallowing intervention, including compensatory strategies and swallow rehabilitation techniques, and discusses how these approaches can decrease the risk of malnutrition and pneumonia in the elderly with dysphagia.

References

American Speech-Language-Hearing Association. (n.d.-a). *Adult dysphagia.* Retrieved February 15, 2024, from https://www.asha.org/practice-portal/clinical-topics/adult-dysphagia

American Speech-Language-Hearing Association. (n.d.-b). *Scope of practice in speech-language pathology.* Retrieved February 15, 2024, from https://www.asha.org/policy/sp2016-00343

Bratcs, D., Harel, D., & Molfcntcr, S. (2022). Perception of swallowing-related fatigue among older adults. *Journal of Speech, Language, and Hearing Research, 65,* 2801–2814.

Cohen, S., & Dilfer, K. (2022). Pediatric feeding disorder in early intervention: Expanding access, improving outcomes, and prioritizing responsive feeding. *Perspectives of the ASHA Special Interest Groups, 7,* 829–840.

Daniels, S., & Huckabee, M. (2014). *Dysphagia following stroke* (2nd ed.). Plural Publishing.

Desai, H., Lauridson, S., Nhuyen, M., Ornelas, E., & Schomberg, J. (2022). Feeding skill and behavior changes in children with complex feeding disorders following therapy in an intensive multidisciplinary feeding program. *Perspectives of the ASHA Special Interest Groups, 7,* 1155–1165.

Ebihara, T., Ebihara, S., Maruyama, M., Kobayashi, M., Itou, A., Arai, H., & Sasaki, H. (2006). A randomized trial of olfactory stimulation using black pepper oil in older people with swallowing dysfunction. *Journal of the American Geriatrics Society, 54*(9), 1401–1406.

Fujiu, M., & Logemann, J. A. (1996). Effect of a tongue-holding maneuver on posterior pharyngeal wall movement during deglutition. *American Journal of Speech-Language Pathology, 5*, 25–30.

Hall, K., & Johnson, L. (2020). The three CCCs of dysphagia management: Culturally competent care. *Perspectives of the ASHA Special Interest Groups, 5*, 1000–1005.

Haney, S., Ibañez, V., Kirkwood, C., & Piazza, C. (2023). An evaluation of negative reinforcement to increase self-feeding and self-drinking for children with feeding disorders. *Journal of Applied Behavior Analysis, 56*(4), 757–776.

Howe, T.-H., & Wang, T.-N. (2013). Systematic review of interventions used in or relevant to occupational therapy for children with feeding difficulties ages birth–5 years. *American Journal of Occupational Therapy, 67*, 405–412.

International Dysphagia Diet Standardisation Initiative. (2024). *The IDDSI framework*. https://iddsi.org/Framework

Kenny, B. (2015). Food culture, preferences and ethics in dysphagia management. *Bioethics, 29*(9), 1467–8519.

Kim, J., & Sapienza, C. M. (2005). Implications of expiratory muscle strength training for rehabilitation of the elderly: Tutorial. *Journal of Rehabilitation Research & Development, 42*(4), 211–224.

Kovacic, K., Rein, L., Szabo, A., Kommareddy, S., Bhagavatula, P., & Goday, P. (2021). Pediatric feeding disorder: A prevalence study. *Journal of Pediatrics, 228*, 126–131.

Langmore, S. E., Schatz, K., & Olsen, N. (1988). Fiberoptic endoscopic examination of swallowing safety: A new procedure. *Dysphagia, 2*(4), 216–219.

Lazarus, C., Logemann, J. A., Song, C. W., Rademaker, A. W., & Kahrilas, P. J. (2002). Effects of voluntary maneuvers on tongue base function for swallowing. *Folia Phoniatrica et Logopaedica, 54*(4), 171–176.

Lefton-Grief, M. (2008). Pediatric dysphagia. *Physical Medicine and Rehabilitation Clinics of North America, 19*(4), 837–851.

Leonard, R., & Kendall, K. (2023). *Dysphagia assessment and treatment planning: A team approach*. Plural Publishing.

Logemann, J. A. (1986). *Manual for the videofluorographic study of swallowing*. Little, Brown.

Lwi, S., Ford, B., Casey, J., Miller, B., & Levenson, R. (2017). Poor caregiver mental health predicts mortality with neurodegenerative disease. *Proceedings of the National Academy of Sciences of the United States of America, 114*(28), 7319–7324.

Malandraki, G., Mitchell, S., Hahn Arkenberg, R., Brown, B., Craig, B., Burdo-Hartman, W., . . . Goffman, L. (2022). Swallowing and motor speech skills in unilateral cerebral palsy: Novel findings from a preliminary cross-sectional study. *Journal of Speech, Language, and Hearing Research, 65*, 3300–3315.

Martin-Harris, B., Logemann, J. A., McMahon, S., Schleicher, M., & Sandidge, J. (2000). Clinical utility of the modified barium swallow. *Dysphagia, 15*(3), 136–141.

Miles, A., Dharmarathna, I., Fuller, L., Jardine, M., & Allen, J. (2022). Developing a protocol for quantitative analysis of liquid swallowing in children. *American Journal of Speech-Language Pathology, 31*, 1244–1263.

Piazza, C. (2008). Feeding disorders and behavior: What have we learned? *Developmental Disabilities Research Review, 14*(2), 174–181.

Rice, J., & Lefton-Grief, M. (2022). Treatment of pediatric patients with high-flow nasal cannula and considerations for oral feeding: A review of the literature. *Perspectives of the ASHA Special Interest Groups, 7*, 543–552.

Riquelme, L. (2007). The role of cultural competence in providing services to persons with dysphagia. *Topics in Geriatric Rehabilitation, 23*(3), 228–239.

Sanders, H., Hoffman, S., & Lund, C. (1992). Feeding strategy for dependent eaters. *Journal of the American Dietetic Association, 92*(11), 1389–1390.

Shune, S., Linville, D., & Namasivayam-MacDonald, A. (2022). Integrating family-centered care into chronic dysphagia management: A tutorial. *Perspectives of the ASHA Special Interest Groups, 7*, 795–806.

Silverman, A. (2015). Behavioral management of feeding disorders in childhood. *Annals of Nutrition & Metabolism, 66*(5), 33–42.

Simione, M., Dartley, A., Cooper-Vince, C., Martin, V., Hartnick, C., Taveras, E., & Fiechtner, L. (2020). Family-centered outcomes that matter most to parents: A pediatric feeding disorders qualitative study. *Journal of Pediatric Gastroenterology and Nutrition, 71*(2), 270–275.

Terrell, J., Fisher, S., & Wolf, G. (1998). Long-term quality of life after treatment of laryngeal cancer: The Veterans Affairs Laryngeal Cancer Study Group. *Archives of Otolaryngology, Head and Neck Surgery, 124*, 964–971.

West, K. (2024). Treating pediatric feeding disorders and dysphagia: Evidence-based interventions for school-based clinicians. *Language, Speech, and Hearing Services in Schools, 55*(2), 444–457.

World Health Organization. (2001). *International classification of functioning, disability and health*.

Yoon, W. L., Khoo, J. K., & Liow, S. J. (2013). Chin tuck against resistance (CTAR): New method for enhancing suprahyoid muscle activity using a shaker-type exercise. *Dysphagia, 29*(2), 243–248.

Chapter 13

Hearing Disorders and Their Impact on Communication

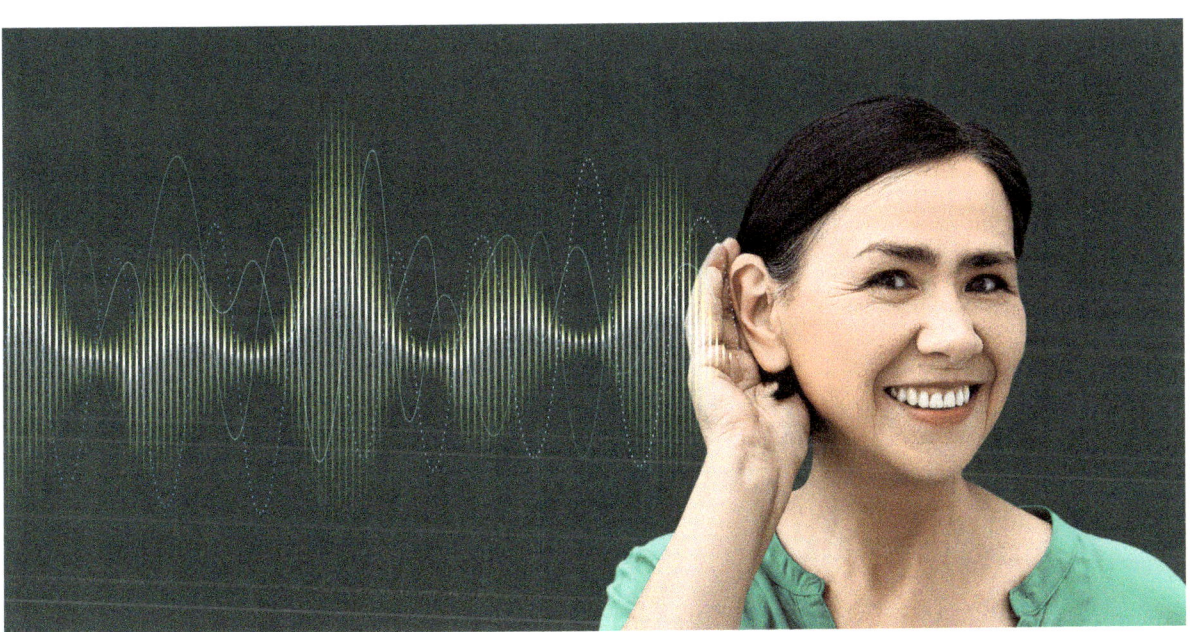

Learning Objectives

After reading this chapter, you will be able to:

- Explain the types of hearing loss experienced across the lifespan.
- Describe the tools used to assess hearing.
- Identify approaches to addressing the needs of those who are deaf and hard of hearing.
- Describe social–cultural differences in identification.
- Explain the disparities in access to hearing testing and management.

Key Terms

acoustic immittance testing	malleus
acoustic or auditory nerve	masking
acoustic reflex testing	mastoid process
air conduction	Ménière's disease
atresia	nasopharynx
audiogram	organ of Corti
auditory brainstem response (ABR) test	ossicular chain
auditory evoked potential	otitis media
auditory neuropathy	otitis media with effusion
autoimmune inner ear disease	otoacoustic emissions (OAEs)
basilar membrane	otoscopy
bilateral hearing loss	oval window
bone conduction	Pendred syndrome
bone oscillator	pinna
cerumen	presbycusis
CHARGE syndrome	pseudohypacusis
cholesteatoma	retrocochlear pathology
cochlea	semicircular canals
cochlear synaptopathy	signal-to-noise ratio
conditioned play audiometry	sound pressure level (SPL)
decibel (dB)	stapes
enlarged vestibular aqueduct syndrome	temporal bone
eustachian tube	tinnitus
external auditory meatus	tympanic membrane
frequency	tympanometry
hair cells	unilateral hearing loss
hearing or auditory threshold	Usher syndrome
hertz (Hz)	vestibulocochlear nerve
incus	Waardenburg syndrome
intensity	

Introduction

Have you ever had an ear infection or flown on a plane and your ears were plugged, which resulted in difficulty hearing and discriminating sounds and words? Auditory input is incredibly important to our understanding of oral language. The ability to hear sounds, words, and conversation helps us understand language and engage in conversation. When a child or adult has a hearing loss, they miss out on the sounds crucial to understanding and using oral language.

In the United States, more than 37 million adults (15%) aged 18 years or older identify that they have difficulty hearing (Blackwell et al., 2014). Worldwide, more than 432 million adults have a hearing loss that is greater than 40 **decibels (dB)**, which can be disabling. A decibel is a unit of measurement for **sound**

pressure level (SPL). Prevalence data suggest that 7.6% of adults aged 15 years or older have a hearing loss, and this prevalence is greater for males (8.5%) than females (6.7%; World Health Organization [WHO], 2018). Prevalence rates seem to be increasing, and predictions suggest that by 2050, one in four people are likely to have some level of hearing loss, with 10% of those exhibiting a disabling hearing loss (WHO, 2021a, 2021b).

Approximately 3 of every 1,000 U.S. children are born with a hearing loss impacting one or both ears (Centers for Disease Control and Prevention [CDC], 2010). Notably, 60% of childhood hearing loss could be prevented (American Speech-Language-Hearing Association [ASHA], 2016) because it is often associated with infections such as mumps, measles, and rubella as well as birth complications or ototoxic medication used by mothers. Almost 10% of the world's population with hearing loss are children in low- and middle-income countries (Prelock & Hutchins, 2018). Childhood hearing loss could be decreased with immunizations, improved prenatal and postnatal care, and avoidance of drugs during pregnancy that have a toxic impact on the hearing mechanism.

To address early identification of hearing loss, nearly 98% of U.S.-born infants are screened immediately after birth as part of universal newborn hearing screening (CDC, 2021. Approximately 3 newborns in 1,000 births have a congenital hearing loss, and this prevalence increases into the school years, with 19.5% of adolescents (ages 12–19 years) diagnosed with **unilateral** or bilateral hearing loss (Kingsbury et al., 2022; Shargorodsky, Curhan, Curhan, et al., 2010). Even with this proactive approach to newborn hearing screening, some mild or progressive hearing losses may not be identified. Furthermore, nearly 40% of children with hearing loss have other conditions impacting their day-to-day functioning (Gallaudet Research Institute, 2011). For example, **otitis media** is a common ear infection experienced by children that can have an intermittent impact on their hearing and learning. Thus, providing hearing screening, assessment, and support on an ongoing basis is crucial to a child's ability to engage in daily communication and fully participate in their community because childhood hearing loss can have long-term impacts on educational achievement and social engagement (Idstad & Engdahl, 2019).

For adults between the ages of 20 and 69 years, the prevalence of hearing loss was reduced slightly from 16% (or 28 million people) in the 1999 to 2004 period to 14% (27.7 million) in the 2011 and 2012 period; adults older than age 60 years experience the greatest losses, with men being affected twice as often as women (Hoffman et al., 2017). Notably, non-Hispanic Black adults have the lowest prevalence of hearing loss and non-Hispanic White adults have the highest prevalence of hearing loss compared to all other racial and ethnic groups (Hoffman et al., 2017). The type of hearing loss also varies, with 18% of adults exhibiting a hearing loss in both ears from 5 or more years of work-related noise exposure compared to 5.5% with no reported work-related noise exposure (Hoffman et al., 2017). Approximately 30 million people (13%) in the United States older than age 12 years have **bilateral hearing loss**. Approximately 2% of these cases occur in adults aged 45 to 54 years, increasing to 8.5% for those aged 55 to 64 years, 50% for those aged 65 to 74 years, and 75% for those older than age 75 years (Lin et al., 2011).

Hearing loss is the third most common chronic condition in the United States (Masterson et al., 2016, and 16.5% of adults identify having trouble hearing without the use of listening devices (including hearing aids; National Center for Health Statistics, 2018). As might be expected, hearing difficulties increase with age; 6.1% of adults aged 18 to 44 years report trouble hearing, increasing to 47.2% of adults aged 75 years or older (Villarroel et al., 2019). By age 80 years or older, 81.4% of adults report some level of hearing loss (Sharma et al., 2020).

Tinnitus, the conscious awareness of a noise (usually a ringing or buzzing sound) when there is no actual sound (De Ridder et al., 2021; Kikidis et al., 2021), occurs in approximately 10% to 15% of adults (McCormack et al., 2016; Shargorodsky, Curhan, & Farwell, 2010). A primary risk for tinnitus is exposure to loud noise, and it can occur with or without hearing loss (Baracca et al., 2011). Chronic tinnitus impacts an individual's quality of life specifically in the areas of emotional well-being, hearing, sleep, and cognitive deficits such as executive control of attention (Khan & Husain, 2020). This may lead to more effortful listening and understanding of speech (Degeest et al., 2022).

Adults with hearing loss do benefit from using hearing aids, but only approximately 30% of individuals older than age 70 years and 16% of people between the ages of 20 and 69 years wear them. Figure 13–1 shows the percentage of adults with hearing loss who wear hearing aids. The higher the percentage of use, the better the outcomes.

This chapter briefly describes the development of hearing, the anatomy of the auditory system, and the most common hearing impairments, as well as approaches to assessing hearing. Intervention strategies are discussed, and opportunities to apply your knowledge through case studies are provided.

What We Know About This Topic

Anatomy of the Hearing Mechanism

Several structures contribute to our ability to hear, including the eighth cranial nerve (auditory and vestibular) and auditory areas of the brain (Prelock & Hutchins, 2018). Figure 13–2 depicts the structure of the outer, middle, and inner ear. The **pinna** or **auricle**, what you see as the outer ear, supports sound

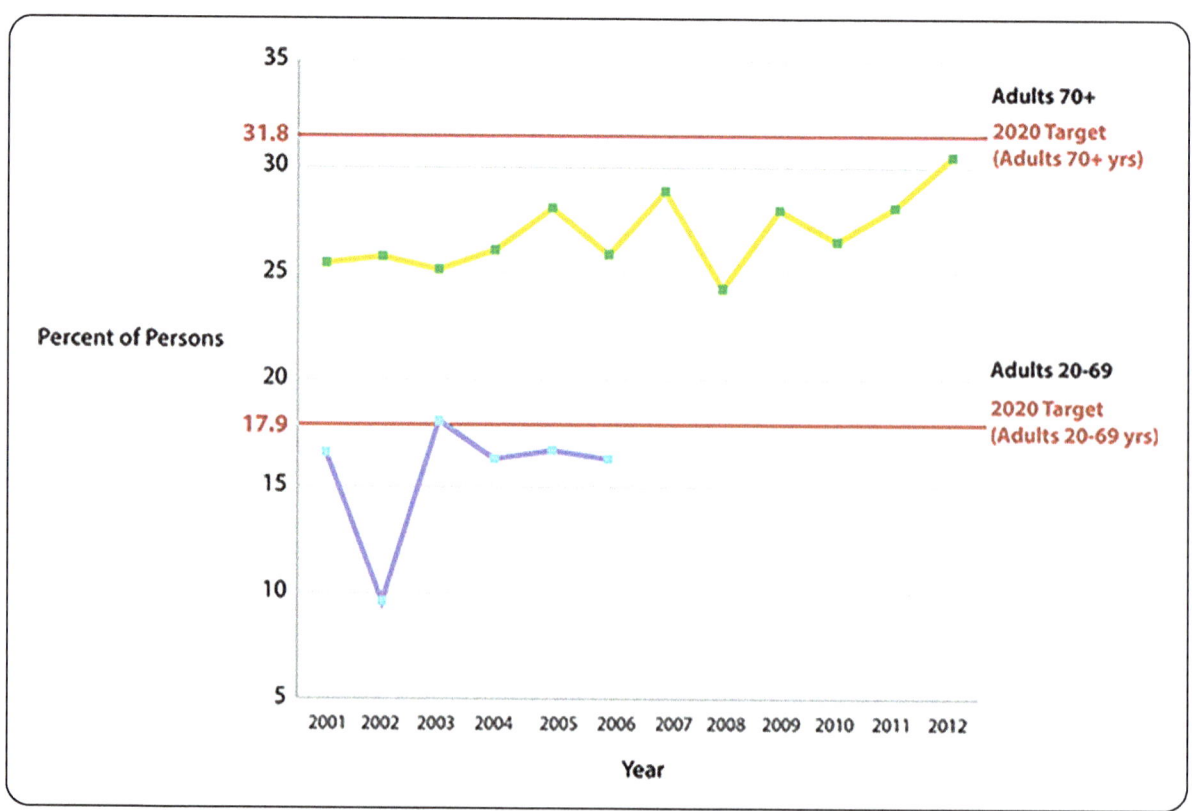

FIGURE 13–1. Percentage of persons with hearing loss who have used hearing aids. *Source:* https://www.nidcd.nih.gov/health/statistics/use-hearing-aids-adults-hearing-loss Retrieved February 16, 2024.

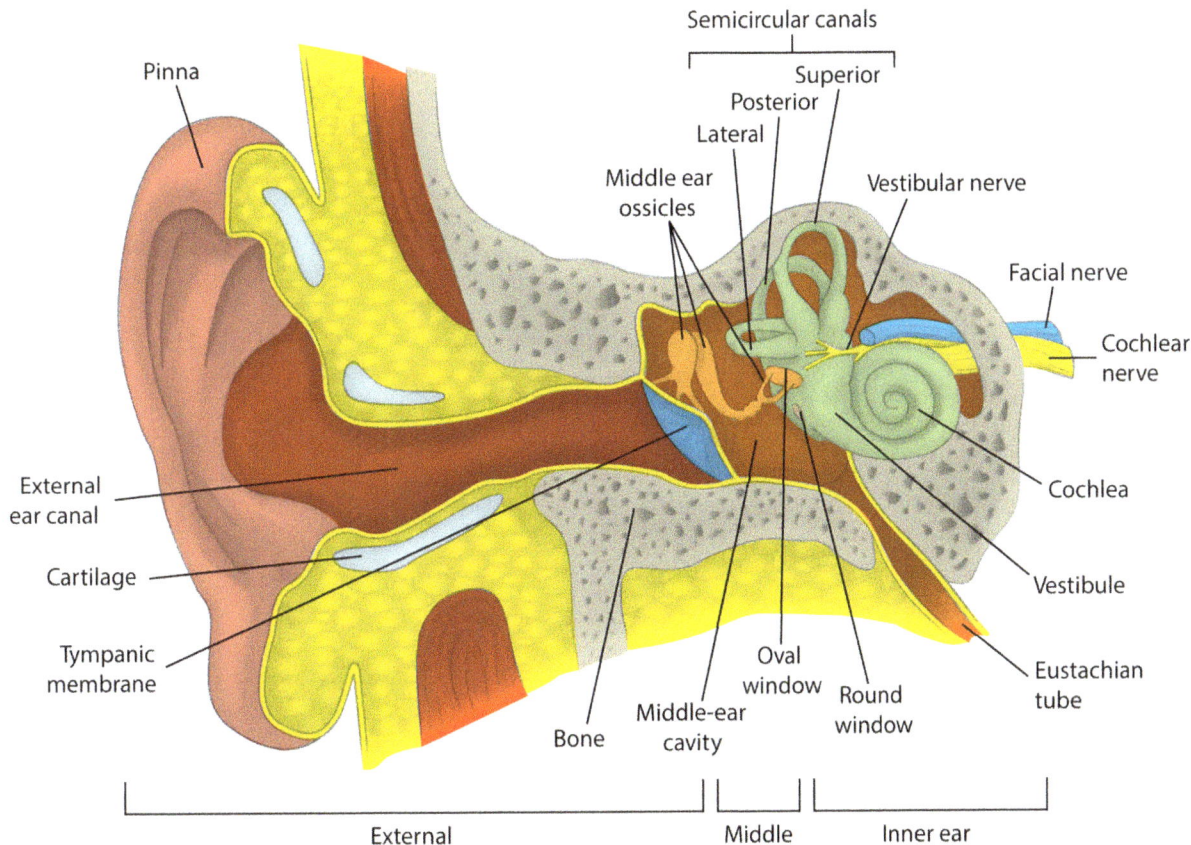

FIGURE 13–2. Anatomy of the ear. *Source:* From *Clinical Audiology: An Introduction, Third Edition* (pp. 1–575) by Brad A. Stach and Virginia Ramachandran. Copyright © 2022 Plural Publishing, Inc. All rights reserved.

localization as well as produces cerumen and protects the eardrum. The external ear canal (also known as the **external auditory meatus**) has wax (also known as **cerumen**) that traps debris from entering the middle ear. The middle ear is full of air and is composed of the eardrum (i.e., the **tympanic membrane**, which separates the middle and outer ear), the ossicular chain, and the **eustachian tube**. Sudden pressure changes can damage and even rupture the eardrum, and although it usually heals on its own, the initial damage can cause scarred tissue and decrease the membrane's mobility.

The three small bones in the middle ear (i.e., the ossicular chain) are the **malleus**, **incus**, and **stapes**. The first of the bones is the largest and looks like a hammer; it is attached to the eardrum so that vibrations move from the eardrum to the malleus, which is attached to the second bone (the incus). The incus is attached to the stapes, which fits into the **oval window**—a small opening into the inner ear (Hegde, 2010; Prelock & Hutchins, 2018). All three bones in this ossicular chain are sound transmitters. The auditory tube, also called the eustachian tube, is connected to the middle ear and the **nasopharynx** (opening to the nasal passage), and its job is to maintain equal air pressure within and outside the middle ear. The eustachian tube also creates a pathway for eliminating any debris or fluid from the middle ear. Figure 13–3 shows a clear depiction of the bones of the middle ear.

The inner ear is a complex structure in the auditory mechanism that is composed of the oval window and interconnecting tunnels (labyrinths) filled with fluid that are in the **temporal bone**. There are two

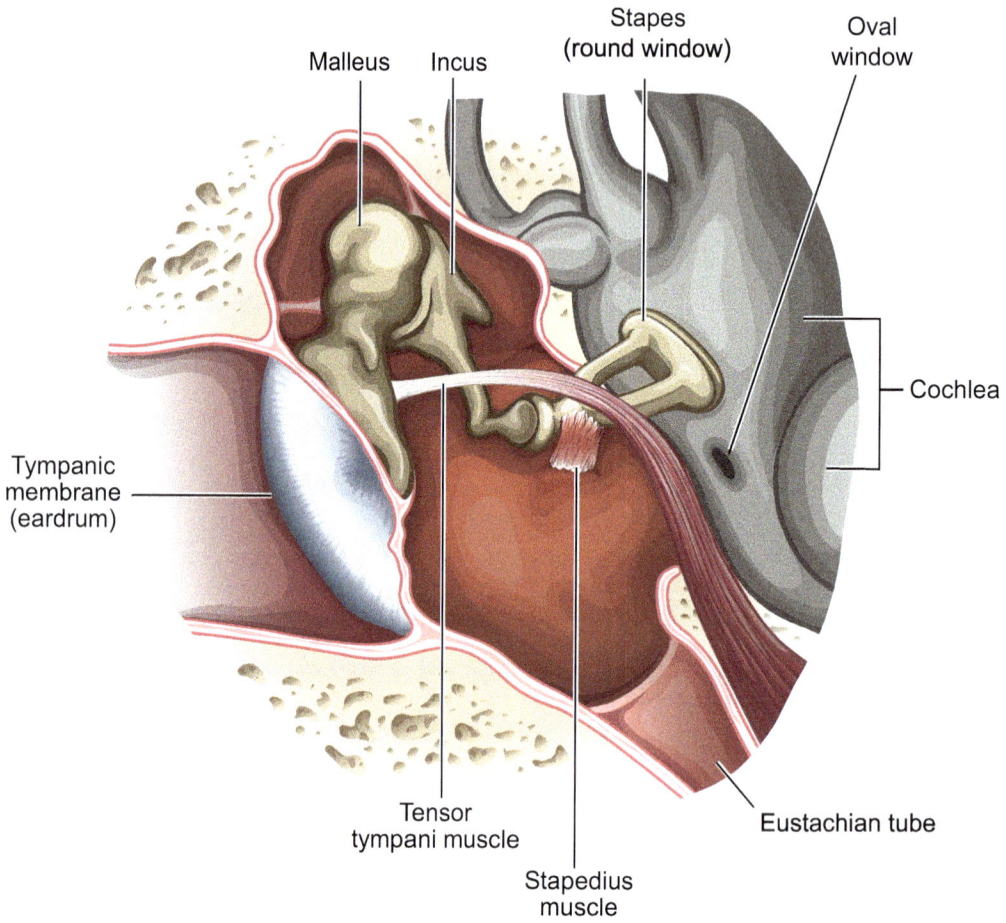

FIGURE 13–3. Illustration (anterior view) of key structures in the middle ear interfacing with the cochlea. *Source:* Adapted from *Foundations of Speech and Hearing: Anatomy and Physiology, Second Edition* (pp 1–348) by Hoit, J. D., Weismer, G., & Story, B. Copyright © 2022 Plural Publishing, Inc. Modified with permission.

inner ear structures, the vestibular system and the cochlea, that have unrelated functions. The three **semicircular canals** of the vestibular system affect movement, balance, and body position. For hearing, the cochlea has a critical role and is in fact the most important structure for hearing. It is a snail-shaped, fluid-filled coiled tunnel containing the basilar membrane and the **organ of Corti** with thousands of **hair cells** that respond to sound. The final component of the inner ear is the **auditory nerve**, also known as cranial nerve VIII, with two branches: a vestibular branch and an acoustic branch connecting the cochlear hair cells supporting sound transmission. The **acoustic nerve**, composed of a bundle of neurons, transmits sound impulses from the cochlea to the brain (Hegde, Prelock & Hutchins, 2018). Figure 13–4 provides a representation of the cochlea and semicircular canals.

Normal Hearing Development

The development of the auditory system begins as a 20-week-old fetus responds to sounds as evidenced by an increased heart rate (Hegde, 2010). Early on, infants will blink their eyes when they hear sound, or

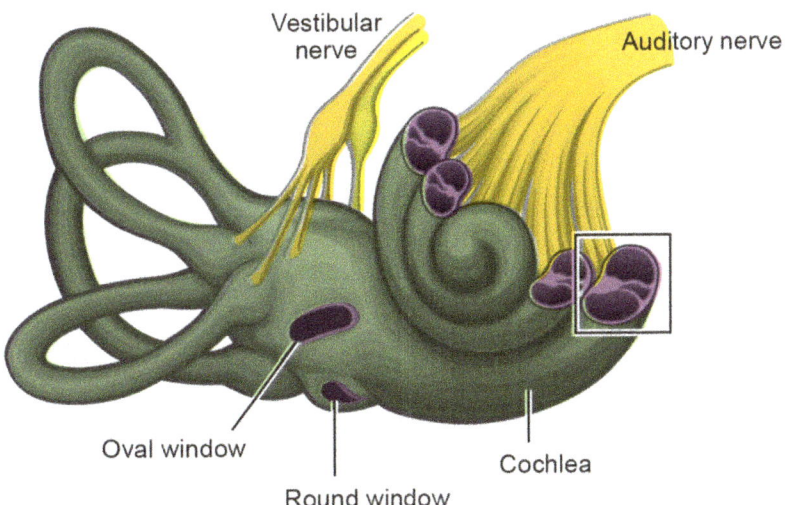

FIGURE 13–4. Cochlea and semicircular canals. The cross-section through the cochlear spiral shows the three chambers of the membranous labyrinth. *Source:* From *Neuroscience Fundamentals for Communication Sciences and Disorders, Second Edition* (pp. 1–802) by Andreatta, R. D. Copyright © 2024 Plural Publishing, Inc. All rights reserved.

they will move an arm or leg suddenly as a startle response to sound (Prelock & Hutchins, 2018). By the time they are 3 months old, infants respond to the voice of their mothers, and between 3 and 4 months of age they turn their head toward sounds. This localization to sound continues to improve as infants age to 6 or 7 months.

When an individual hears normally, sound is conducted through either air conduction or bone conduction. If it is conducted through **air conduction**, sound moves through the air and hits the eardrum, where it gets sent to the middle ear. Within the middle ear are three bones that make up the **ossicular chain**, and sound in the middle ear causes movement of fluid in the inner ear, which results in vibrations on the **basilar membrane** of the **cochlea** (Prelock & Hutchins, 2018). Cochlear hair cells are connected to the acoustic nerve so vibrations that occur cause sound to move to the brain. If, however, sound is conducted through **bone conduction**, it moves through vibrations to the skull and three middle ear bones (instead of being sent to the eardrum) and causes inner ear fluid movement and then ultimately acoustic nerve stimulation (Hegde, 2010; Prelock & Hutchins, 2018).

The loudness or volume of a sound is a result of the level of sound pressure. The higher the sound pressure level, the louder the sound. The decibel, developed by Alexander Graham Bell, is the physical measurement of sound pressure. The pitch of a sound or our perception of how high or low a sound is produced has a physical measurement in **hertz** (Hz; named after the German physicist Heinrich Rudolf Hertz) and is described as the **frequency** or the number of vibrations that occur per second (e.g., 30 Hz indicates 30 vibrations per second). Slow vibrations would lead to a sound that you could barely hear, whereas fast vibrations would lead to higher pitches. Humans can hear between 20 and 20,000 Hz, depending on the amplitude of the sound. Figure 13–5 shows where speech sounds typically fall on an audiogram (a graph representing what we hear), which is often referred to as the speech banana.

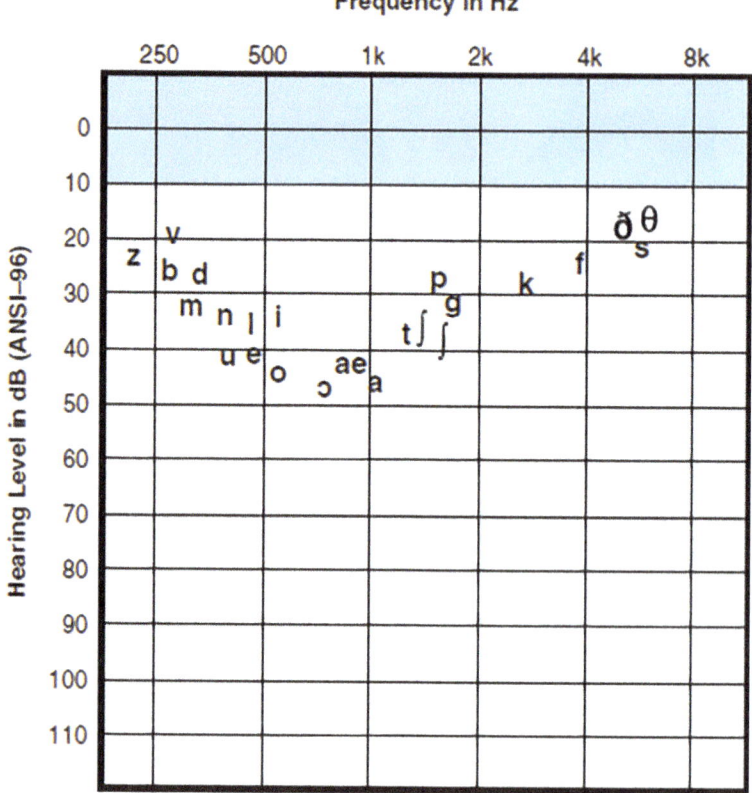

FIGURE 13–5. Representation of the sounds of human speech on an audiogram. *Source:* From *Foundations of Aural Rehabilitation: Children, Adults, and Their Family Members, Sixth Edition* (pp. 1–567) by Nancy Tye-Murray. Copyright © 2024 Plural Publishing, Inc. All rights reserved.

You might be wondering what sounds we can hear daily and if there are sounds that are too loud and can be harmful to our ears. For you to hear any sound, it must be above a certain level or what is called the **auditory or hearing threshold**. Humans have a hearing threshold level of approximately 0 dB, and when sounds are above this threshold, they are audible (Occupational Safety and Health Administration, 2024). Hearing damage can occur if people are exposed to greater than 85 dB SPL on a regular basis. Above 110 dB SPL, sounds become uncomfortable (our threshold for discomfort), and 130 dB SPL seems to be our threshold for painful sound. Notably, adult hearing often becomes less efficient because of the natural aging process as well as years of noise exposure. Figure 13–6 shows a chart of familiar sounds and the approximate decibels at which you would hear those sounds. For example, quiet conversation might be approximately 40 dB SPL, whereas normal conversation occurs at approximately 60 dB SPL, and traffic noise is approximately 80 dB SPL. Louder noises such as music at a concert would be approximately 120 dB SPL, and the engine of a jet might be approximately 140 dB SPL. When you are exposed to sounds that are louder than 130 dB SPL, this can be problematic and cause acute hearing loss. Notably, a temporary threshold shift might be experienced for those with noise-induced hearing loss that persists for 4 hours without permanent loss because of very loud music exposure above 100 dB SPL (Kramer et al., 2006; Le Prell et al., 2012, 2016). In fact, you may have heard about occupational hearing conservation

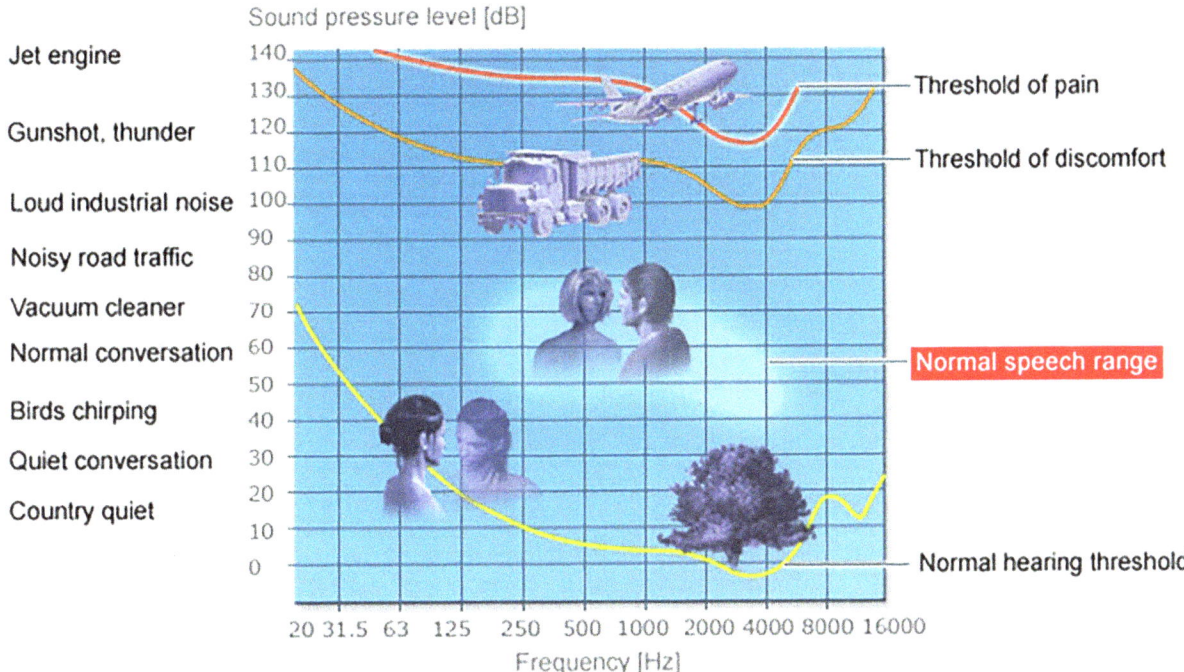

FIGURE 13–6. Sound pressure levels for environmental sounds and noises you might hear. *Source:* National Library of Medicine.

programs that require industry workers to wear ear plugs or headphones to protect their hearing when working in conditions with exposure to noise at these high sound levels.

What Does Hearing Impairment Look Like?

As described previously, hearing loss is often associated with aging, but it can impact a person at any age. Hearing loss can be mild to profound, and it can have varying effects on communication, including how an individual understands language and the way in which they express themself. Table 13–1 summarizes the typical degrees of hearing loss. It includes a unit for **intensity** (i.e., perceptual correlate being loudness), as measured in decibels, as well as the ranges for normal hearing and hearing loss. Someone who is described as hard of hearing will likely have hearing that still works for them but not as effectively as it did in the past. Notably, hearing loss can be present at birth or develop after an illness or with aging, and it can be temporary or permanent.

Some common symptoms that characterize hearing loss are the avoidance of social situations, asking to have things repeated, difficulty discriminating speech in noise or on the telephone, and describing others' speech as mumbling (National Institute on Aging, n.d.). You might also see an individual turning the television or radio volume up too high, exhibiting fatigue after periods of listening, and speaking too softly or loudly.

A person can have a conductive hearing loss, a sensorineural hearing loss, or both. In addition, some individuals exhibit auditory neuropathy or an auditory processing disorder. Table 13–2 describes these types of hearing disorders and identifies the typical causes reported for these hearing impairments. Conductive hearing losses are usually due to difficulty conducting sound through the ear canal, the eardrum, or the middle ear. There are several causes that would explain a conductive hearing loss, such

TABLE 13–1. Degree and Range of Hearing Loss

Degree of Hearing Loss	Hearing Loss Range (dB HL)
Normal	−10 to 15
Slight	16 to 25
Mild	26 to 40
Moderate	41 to 55
Moderately severe	56 to 70
Severe	71 to 90
Profound	91+

Note: A classification system by the National Institutes of Health, National Library of Medicine (retrieved February 17, 2024, from https://www.ncbi.nlm.nih.gov/books/NBK390300) shows slightly different ranges: normal hearing (up to 20 dB HL), mild hearing loss (20–40 dB HL), moderate hearing loss (41–60 dB HL), severe hearing loss (61–80 dB HL), and profound hearing loss (81+ dB HL). In either classification system, a hearing loss of greater than 40 dB HL would be considered a hearing impairment. HL, hearing loss.

Source: ASHA (https://www.asha.org/practice-portal/clinical-topics/hearing-loss).

as a malformation in the auditory mechanism, fluid in the middle ear, impacted wax or the presence of a foreign body, infection in the ear canal or the middle ear, perforated eardrum or limited function of the eustachian tube, limited vibrations of the middle ear bones, or a benign tumor or head trauma.

A sensorineural hearing loss is the result of a dysfunction of the cochlea or the **vestibulocochlear (auditory) nerve** (cranial nerve VIII). Damage to the cochlear hair cells prevents the brain from receiving sound impulses. Sensorineural hearing loss can be caused by ototoxic drugs taken early in the gestational period, infections (bacterial, viral, or parasitic), and ongoing noise exposure. The most common conditions responsible for sensorineural hearing loss include meningitis and maternal rubella, birth defects, or an acoustic neuroma. Other conditions include **autoimmune inner ear disease** (immune system attacks the inner ear); **enlarged vestibular aqueduct syndrome** (inner ear malformation causing both hearing loss and vestibular problems); **Ménière disease** (inner ear disease causing vertigo, tinnitus, and fluctuating hearing loss); head trauma affecting the inner ear; vascular deficits (vertebrobasilar insufficiency and sickle cell anemia); **presbycusis** (hearing loss related to aging); and genetic causes that are syndrome related (**CHARGE syndrome**, **Pendred syndrome**, and **Waardenburg syndrome**) or not syndrome related, such as a genetic mutation (ASHA, n.d.-a [children]; n.d.-b [adults]).

A **mixed hearing loss** means there has been damage to the outer and/or middle ear pathways and the inner ear's sensory hair cells. Any combination of conditions described for conductive and sensorineural hearing loss can account for a mixed hearing loss.

Hearing Loss in Children

The first 3 years of life have often been described as a critical period for brain development and learning, during which children's brains make millions of neural connections (Leadsom et al., 2013). At age 16 weeks, auditory information is available to the fetus, which contributes to an infant's ability to discriminate their native from nonnative speech early after birth (Graven & Browne, 2008; Moon et al., 2013).

TABLE 13–2. Types and Descriptions of Hearing Disorders and Likely Conditions Responsible for the Specific Hearing Disorders

Type of Hearing Disorder	Description and Cause	Examples of Conditions
Conductive hearing loss	Reduced movement of sound to the middle or inner ear caused by anything that blocks the external ear canal, such as foreign bodies. There could also be structural difference in the ear canal, the tympanic membrane, or the ossicular chain, usually the result of a birth defect or disease.	• Aural atresia: Causes the external ear canal to be closed off. • Stenosis: When the external ear canal is extremely narrow. • External otitis: Infection resulting in the swelling of the ear canal tissues; often seen in swimmers. • Bony growths or tumors: Structure that blocks the ear canal. • Otitis media: A middle ear infection associated with upper respiratory infections. • Cholesteatoma: Skin growth in the middle ear behind the tympanic membrane usually a result of middle ear infections and poor functioning of the eustachian tube.
Sensorineural hearing loss	Damage to the cochlear hair cells or the acoustic nerve which keeps the brain from receiving sound impulses. Can be caused by ototoxic drugs taken during gestation week 6 or 7, infections, and/or ongoing noise exposure that damages the cochlear hair cells.	• Meningitis and maternal rubella: Infections that attack the inner ear. • Birth defects: Impact on the development of the acoustic nerve and/or the cochlea. • Acoustic neuroma(s): Rare noncancerous, slow-growing tumor(s) that interferes with the conduction of sound through the acoustic nerve because the tumor forms along the branches of the acoustic nerve.
Mixed hearing loss	Both the middle and inner ear function poorly.	• Any of the conditions described above or combination of conditions.
Auditory processing disorders	Affects the ability to segment and sequence sounds, particularly when auditory input is distorted as in a noisy environment.	• Lesions are not present in children but auditory processing disorder can be.
Auditory neuropathy	Normal or near normal cochlear hair cell function but there is no acoustic nerve response, usually the result of a mitochondrial genetic condition.	• Mitochondrial encephalopathy, lactate acidosis, and stroke-like episodes (MELAS): A progressive deterioration of the nervous system leading to impairment and dementia in adolescence and early adulthood.

continues

TABLE 13–2. *continued*

Type of Hearing Disorder	Description and Cause	Examples of Conditions
Auditory neuropathy		• Maternally inherited diabetes and deafness (MIDD): Usually results in hearing loss in the high pitch range. • Myoclonic epilepsy with ragged red fibers (MERRF): Multisystem mitochondrial syndrome with sensorineural hearing loss, dementia, progressive myoclonus or twitch/jerking of muscles, seizures, etc. • Progressive external ophthalmoplegia (PEO): Weakness of eye muscles occurring between ages 18 and 40 years that can include sensorineural hearing loss and neuropathy.

Source: Adapted from Prelock and Hutchins (2018).

If a child has a congenital hearing loss, however, they have reduced access to auditory information in utero as well as in the first months of life before their hearing loss is detected and amplification is provided (Rudge et al., 2022). Without this auditory system development early on, children who are deaf and hard of hearing (DHH) have difficulty establishing their expressive vocabulary in the same way as children who do not have a hearing loss. With early intervention, however, growth in vocabulary development can be realized. In fact, Rudge and colleagues (2022) found that children who are DHH and who receive more intervention hours prior to their third birthday will have greater outcomes for vocabulary development.

Otitis media and cholesteatoma are the most frequent causes of conductive loss in children. As described previously, otitis media is a middle ear infection that commonly occurs during the first 2 years of life. Nearly 95% of all children are impacted at least once, and children often have recurrent otitis media (Prelock & Hutchins, 2018). Frequent occurrences of otitis media may impact the development of a child's speech and language because ear infections tend to occur during that critical language period. Children who are particularly impacted by otitis media include those with Down syndrome and cleft palate (Hegde, 2010).

Cholesteatoma is rare and can be congenital, but it is most often the result of a chronic ear infection leading to an abnormal collection of skin cells inside the ear. This collection of skin cells can damage ear structures, especially if untreated, which ultimately impacts balance and the ability to hear. Interestingly, although typically caused by an ear infection, cholesteatoma can also lead to an ear infection with discharge from the ear. Other conditions causing conductive hearing loss include aural **atresia** (lack of a fully developed ear canal), stenosis (a narrowing of the ear canal), external otitis (swelling of ear canal often seen in swimmers), and bony growths that block the ear canal.

An auditory processing disorder is described as a condition affecting a child's academic performance because of difficulty with sound localization and direction following. Notably, however, this is a controversial research and clinical area, and many suggest this may just be another way to explain language processing difficulties. If a child has **auditory neuropathy**, they will likely exhibit adequate cochlear hair cell function but poor acoustic nerve function. That is, the problem lies not with the detection of the acoustic signal but, rather, with transmitting the sound to the brain. This can lead to problems hearing in noise and poor speech perception (Rance et al., 1999; Starr et al., 1996). Auditory neuropathy occurs in more than 13% of children with severe to profound hearing loss (Sanyebhaa et al., 2009), and in 40% of these children, there is a genetic basis for the neuropathy (Clarin, 2015), most often a mitochondrial genetic condition and other genetic syndromes (Manchaiah et al., 2011). Interestingly, children with auditory neuropathy can benefit from cochlear implantation, although more research is needed (Jafari et al., 2023).

Hearing loss in children affects speech and language functioning, social interactions, and academic success. For example, children with hearing loss may not learn words as quickly as those without hearing loss and may have greater difficulty hearing soft or unvoiced sounds (e.g., s, t, k), comprehending what they hear, hearing word endings that have meaning (e.g., plurals, past tense, possessives), and producing more complex sentences (ASHA, n.d.-a [children]). Academic challenges are also likely for children with hearing loss, especially in reading and math, and connecting with hearing peers presents its own difficulties. Therefore, it is important to provide speech and language support, assistive listening devices in the classroom, and education for the child, their family, and their peers about hearing loss.

Nearly 15% of 6- to 19-year-olds in the United States are identified as deaf or hard of hearing in at least one ear and are at increased risk for not developing adequate receptive and expressive language and may lag academically (ASHA, n.d.-a [children]; CDC, 2020). Children who are DHH often struggle with the production of complex syntax and vocabulary knowledge compared to hearing peers (Lund, 2016; Werfel et al., 2021). Use of mental state verbs (i.e., words that represent more abstract thinking which are not easily observed, such as *wonder, think, remember*) seems to be a particularly challenging area that is influenced by age, syntactic knowledge, and exposure to mental state terms (Choi & Jeong, 2023; Pluta et al., 2023; Yu et al., 2021). Mental state verb use is also important for literacy and academic success. Vachio and colleagues (2023) investigated the diversity and frequency of mental state verb use in preschool children with hearing loss compared to those without hearing loss. They found that children who were DHH used fewer mental state verbs than those who were not DHH, and there were no demonstrable differences between children who had cochlear implants (CIs) and those who used hearing aids.

The narratives of young school-age children who are hard of hearing are significantly different than those of hearing children, and this is particularly true for narrative retell (Walker et al., 2023). Although hearing loss cannot explain pragmatic difficulties during social communication opportunities, certainly the limited language access that often accompanies hearing loss from infancy on may impact a child's ability to make sense of complex social–pragmatic contexts (Crowe & Dammeyer, 2021; Matthews & Kelly, 2022; Mood et al., 2020; Paul et al., 2020). Typically, issues of language use have been less of a focus in children with hearing loss, and intervention usually emphasizes basic speech and language abilities (Goberis et al., 2012). Tuohimaa and colleagues (2023) assessed the pragmatic abilities of 86 preschool children with bilateral hearing aids, bilateral CIs, and normal hearing, and they found that children with bilateral hearing aids and CIs were at risk for challenges in pragmatic language understanding and use even with early identification and amplification/implantation. This highlights the importance of ongoing assessment of pragmatic skills and availability of interventions to support social–pragmatic abilities.

Farquharson and colleagues (2022) examined the interconnections among speech sound production, hearing experience, and literacy in children who were hard of hearing. They found that hearing experience and speech sound production were, in fact, relevant for literacy development. Academic and linguistic achievement is also compromised in this population, particularly for those with severe hearing loss and other co-occurring conditions that may impact cognitive function (Cupples et al., 2018). Additional educational support, such as access to teachers of the deaf, speech-language pathologists (SLPs), smaller classrooms, interpreters, preferential seating, and technology, is often needed to facilitate students' potential (e.g., National Association of State Directors of Special Education, 2019).

Notably, however, Epstein and colleagues (2022) found that from 2012 to 2018, children who were deaf or hard of hearing spent more time in general education than special education, and most were high school graduates with a low dropout rate similar to those without hearing loss. The importance and impact of positive educational supports in the general education classroom appear to be facilitative of educational achievement for this population.

Hearing Loss in Adults

Hearing loss in adults that was present at birth or in early childhood usually has a genetic cause. Common genetic syndromes that are associated with hearing loss include CHARGE syndrome and Usher syndrome. Genetic inheritance that is not syndrome specific usually is the result of an autosomal dominant hearing loss or X-linked hearing loss (Sheffield & Smith, 2019).

Excessive noise exposure is a common and preventable cause of hearing loss in young and middle-aged adults, and occupational noise exposure is the most common cause of hearing loss worldwide (Carroll et al., 2017; Chen et al., 2020; Lie et al., 2017). Recreational noise exposure places individuals at risk for developing hearing challenges, and long-term exposure can lead to permanent hearing loss with an impact on quality of life (Tordrup et al., 2022). Notably, the recreational habits of teens and young adults, such as going to nightclubs, concerts, sporting events, movie theaters, and the ongoing noise exposure while listening to music through smartphones and iPods place them at great risk for noise-induced hearing loss (Armitage et al., 2020; Elmazoska et al., 2023).

Almost 50% of Americans who are aged 75 years or older have hearing loss (Villarroel et al., 2019), and some have both hearing and cognitive losses that affect their quality of life (Pichora-Fuller et al., 2013). Presbycusis, hearing loss related to age, affects a significant percentage of the older population and is usually the result of multiple factors, including environmental exposure, an aging cochlea, a familial or genetic predisposition for hearing loss, or other medical conditions (Bowl & Dawson, 2019). Notably, age-related hearing loss leads to increased rates of depression, social isolation, loneliness, and cognitive decline (Gopinath et al., 2016; Lawrence et al., 2020; Lin et al., 2013; Loughrey et al., 2018; Mick et al., 2014, 2018; Thomson et al., 2017).

Another condition, cochlear synaptopathy, commonly described as hidden hearing loss, is usually undetectable using standard pure tone testing and suggests damage to the neuronal connections between the cochlear and the vestibulocochlear nerve (Barbee et al., 2018). Typically, this condition is the result of aging, noise exposure, or ototoxic drugs and leads to difficulty comprehending what is being said, particularly in a noisy environment (Kohrman et al., 2020).

What Do We Do to Address This Communication Challenge?

A comprehensive, patient-centered approach to hearing assessment is important to understanding an individual's hearing difficulties and needs. To assess hearing, an audiologist gathers information for several different reasons, including the following (ASHA, n.d.-a [children]; n.d.-b [adults]):

- To determine how the auditory system is working in both ears
- To identify the type of hearing loss
- To measure hearing across frequencies
- To establish a hearing baseline for comparison in future assessments
- To provide information specific to each ear, which is important to determine amplification needs
- To assess the effect of hearing loss on quality of life
- To initiate hearing education and support for the patient and the family

Hearing Assessment

A hearing assessment typically includes taking a case history; making a medical referral if the findings indicate this is needed; and having the patient complete a self-assessment of their hearing, including identifying their specific needs and the impact on communication. To make an accurate diagnosis, the audiologist considers both the assessment approach they use and the findings of their audiological assessment in the context of the individual's developmental and medical history (including family history of hearing loss).

For example, a case history may provide information about different disabilities the individual has that may require some alteration in the approach to assessment. Questions usually consider general health, history of ear infections, use of medication, previous hearing testing, pain or discharge from the ears, any history of falls, balance problems or dizziness, or the presence of tinnitus (ASHA, n.d.-b [adults]). Questions might also ask about when difficulty hearing first occurred, whether the onset was sudden or gradual, if one ear is more affected than the other, if there are certain situations in which hearing seems to be more difficult than others (e.g., noisy environment), if the person has been exposed to loud noises, whether communication difficulties are occurring (e.g., missing what people are saying), and if the person has used hearing aids or assistive hearing devices in the past.

See the **ASHA Cultural Responsiveness Practice Portal** for information on gathering a case history.

Medical referrals might occur because deformity of the ear is noted in the assessment, pain or dizziness are reported, or there has been a sudden and rapid decline in hearing. A cognitive screen is included so that audiologists can observe and experience a patient's cognitive changes during the assessment or during ongoing hearing visits (Shen et al., 2016; Souza, 2018). In addition, several specific audiological assessments are completed, which are explained in the sections that follow.

Specific Audiological Assessment Procedures

Otoscopy (i.e., an inspection of the outer ear and ear canal) occurs before any hearing testing to ensure there are no foreign objects or materials in the ear canal, the ear canal is free of wax, and there is no active pathological condition present. **Acoustic immittance testing** is conducted to assess the middle ear, including the function of the eardrum and the reflexes of the surrounding muscles. If hearing loss is present, this testing helps identify where a lesion might exist. Acoustic immittance testing involves **tympanometry** and **acoustic reflex testing**. Middle ear function is measured through tympanometry, in which a probe is placed in the ear canal generating a pure tone so that the response of the eardrum (i.e., tympanic membrane) to the sound can be assessed. Results are graphed onto a tympanogram. Response to the sound, known as middle ear compliance, is also graphed on the tympanogram. Ultimately, the audiologist is looking for middle ear compliance that occurs when the pressure in the middle ear is aligned with the pressure in the ear canal. As you might expect, different middle ear pathologies (otitis media, perforated ear drum, etc.) would have distinctive tympanograms. Figures 13–7 and 13–8 show examples of a tympanogram representing normal and abnormal middle ear function, respectively.

When we hear a sound, a small reflex occurs in the middle ear. One assessment of hearing loss includes **acoustic reflex testing**, which measures how loud a sound must be for the reflex in the middle ear to occur. When there is a conductive hearing pathology, acoustic reflexes will either not occur because the pathology limits the immittance changes at the probe tip or will be elevated because the stimulus reaching the cochlea is reduced. In the case of a sensorineural hearing loss and pathology, hearing sensitivity determines the acoustic reflex thresholds. If an individual has a **retrocochlear pathology** (i.e., a condition that impacts the vestibulocochlear nerve or other components of the central auditory system), acoustic reflexes are absent or above what would be expected when a person has a sensorineural hearing loss (ASHA, n.d.-b [adults]).

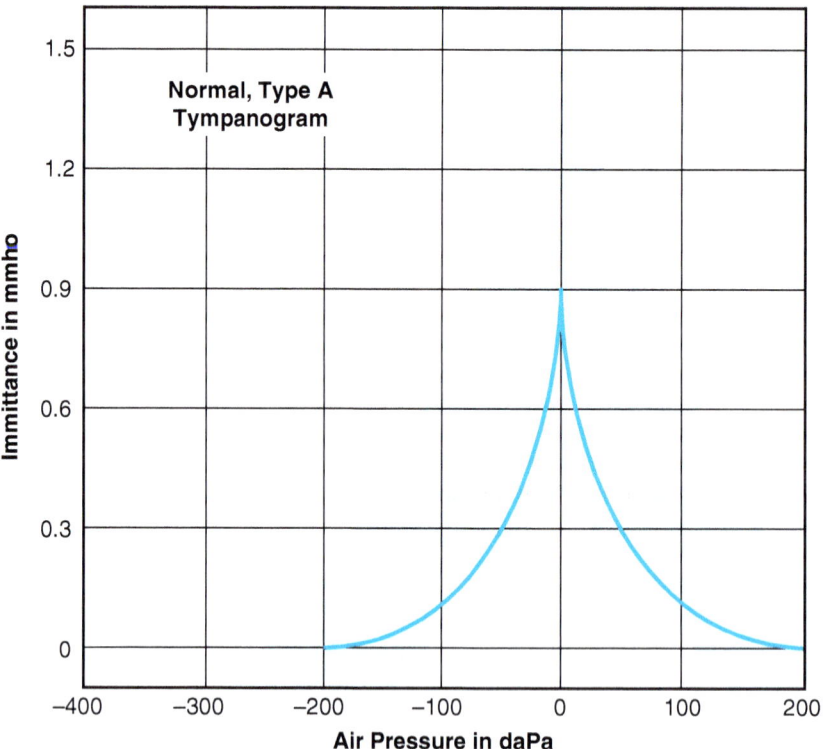

FIGURE 13–7. A tympanogram representing normal middle ear function. *Source:* From *Clinical Audiology: An Introduction, Third Edition* (pp. 1–575) by Stach, B. A., & Ramachandran, V. Copyright © 2022 Plural Publishing, Inc. All rights reserved.

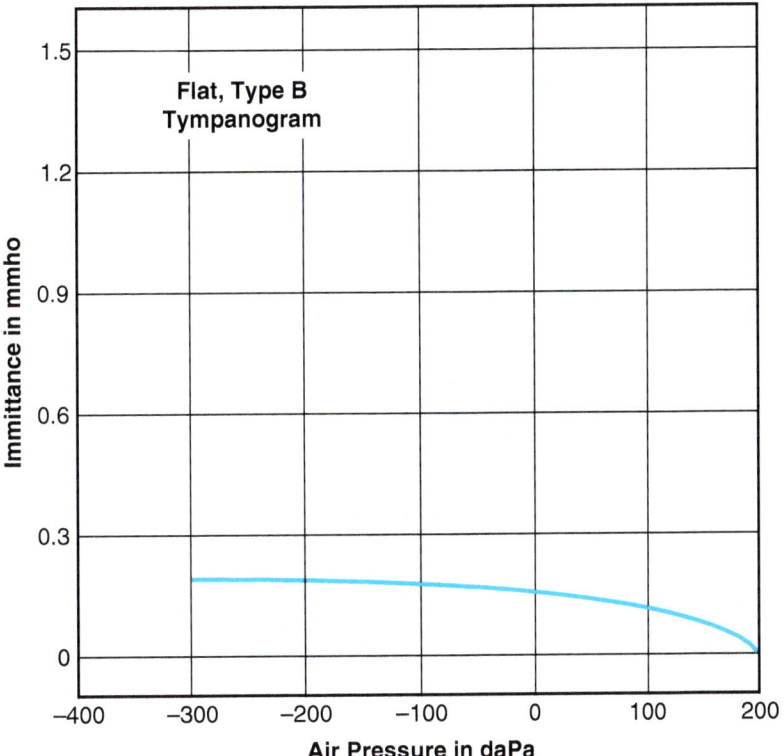

FIGURE 13–8. A tympanogram representing abnormal middle ear function. *Source:* From *Clinical Audiology: An Introduction, Third Edition* (pp. 1–575) by Stach, B. A., & Ramachandran, V. Copyright © 2022 Plural Publishing, Inc. All rights reserved.

Whereas acoustic reflex testing provides information about the middle ear, otoacoustic emissions (OAE) testing offers information about the function of the inner ear and cochlea. OAE testing involves generating a sound from the cochlear in response to an auditory stimulation. Individuals with normal hearing will generate OAEs; however, those with hearing loss will likely not produce any OAEs. OAE measurements examine cochlear function and help with differential diagnoses (ASHA, n.d.-b [adults]).

Another type of audiological assessment that measures hearing sensitivity is pure-tone audiometry testing. Results of the testing are visualized on an audiogram, noting the frequency of the sound (pitch) on the horizontal axis and the loudness of the sound (intensity) on the vertical axis. Testing can be done using air or bone conduction measures. Figure 13–9 shows an audiogram with air and bone conduction testing. Pure-tone air conduction testing uses earphones to deliver a pure tone to each ear. Pure-tone thresholds are assessed at the lowest loudness level in decibels at which a pure tone at a given frequency is responded to 50% of the time. Hearing thresholds are usually assessed between 250 and 8000 Hz. A standard frequency order is usually delivered to ensure consistency and limit omissions (American National Standards Institute [ANSI], 2018). Sometimes testing involves frequencies between 9000 and 20,000 Hz if there is a concern with ultra-high-frequency loss and particularly if the individual has been exposed to ototoxic chemicals or significant noise (Hunter et al., 2020; Valiente et al., 2016). Notably, air conduction pure-tone audiometry can be compromised if there is crossover of the signal (i.e., when a

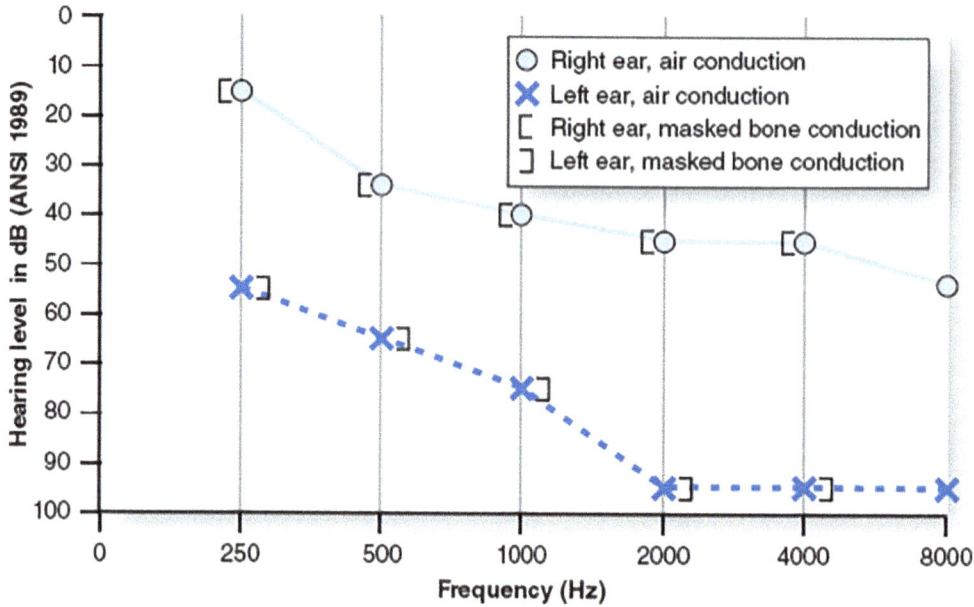

FIGURE 13–9. Visual of an audiogram representing air and bone conduction testing. *Source:* From *Foundations of Aural Rehabilitation: Children, Adults, and Their Family Members, Sixth Edition* (pp. 1–567) by Tye-Murray, N. Copyright © 2024 Plural Publishing, Inc. All rights reserved.

signal presented to one ear is perceived by the other ear). **Masking** noise can be presented to the non-test ear to address this problem.

For pure-tone **bone conduction audiometry,** vibrations of the skull are used as testing stimuli in which **bone oscillators** create vibrations directly that stimulate the cochlea, bypassing any outer and middle ear problems. A bone conduction vibrator is placed on the **mastoid process** and the test ear is not covered. Masking can be used for the ear not being tested. Thresholds are usually assessed from 500 to 4000 Hz.

Speech audiometry testing focuses on the detection or awareness of speech thresholds, speech and word recognition testing, and speech-in-noise (SIN) testing. Speech audiometry is used to assess speech perception, hearing sensitivity, and potential site of lesion (ASHA, n.d.-b [adults]). A speech detection threshold is the minimum hearing level at which an individual can detect speech, usually running speech or familiar words, at least 50% of the time without having to identify what is being said. In contrast, a speech reception threshold is the minimum hearing level at which a person can recognize and repeat back the speech heard, usually presented as two-syllable words (i.e., spondees), 50% of the time (Stach & Ramachandran, 2021). Speech thresholds can support the results of a pure-tone audiogram, and if there are discrepancies among the results, it may be an indication of **pseudohypacusis** (i.e., false hearing loss) or the influence of other variables, such as misunderstanding instructions.

Word recognition testing includes the use of phonetically balanced monosyllabic words from a variety of available word lists. Words are presented using either live or recorded voice, and scores on this test are determined by calculating the percentage of correctly identified words. For individual who are English language learners or non-English speakers, a bilingual audiologist provides the assessment of the services or an interpreter or translator is used.

See the **ASHA Collaborating With Interpreters, Transliterators, and Translators Practice Portal** for information.

SIN testing is done to address the often-reported difficulty of understanding what is being said by a communication partner when there is background noise. This type of testing provides hearing information in the context of real-world experiences. The audiologist considers the speech stimulus, the type of noise, and the signal to noise ratio when implementing SIN testing.

Auditory brainstem response (ABR) testing is used to identify hearing loss and estimate hearing thresholds when other testing is not possible or it is extremely difficult to obtain accurate results because of other disabilities or conditions. ABR testing is also used for differential diagnosis of cochlear hearing loss. It involves placing electrodes on the skin in specific areas and then delivering sound stimuli in the form of clicks or tone bursts through insert earphones (ASHA, n.d.-a [children]). **Auditory evoked potentials** (evoked responses to auditory stimuli) coming from the vestibulocochlear nerve/cranial nerve VIII and auditory brainstem are shown on a waveform consisting of five to seven identifiable peaks that represent the neural function of the auditory pathways. Measurement abnormalities may be indicative of pathology.

Importantly, audiologic assessment accuracy relies on calibrated equipment and maintaining appropriate hearing specifications for the testing equipment and environments used. Equipment for hearing assessment must function properly, and testing must be held in an environment that will ensure accurate and reliable testing results (ANSI, 2012, 2018a, 2018b).

Hearing Assessment in Children

In the diagnosis of hearing loss, it is important to both assess and meet the individual needs of families and the children affected so they can make informed decisions about the next steps for treatment. Important considerations for families and children include whether hearing aids will be used and what communication approach (e.g., verbal speech, sign language) will be emphasized (Hyde et al., 2010; Okubo et al., 2008). These decisions are usually made under stress with little time to think through all the options (Quittner et al., 2010) because families often want to get their child into early intervention as soon as possible and early intervention should begin no later than age 3 to 6 months (Joint Committee on Infant Hearing, 2019).

In children, a hearing concern should lead to an immediate referral to an audiologist. The audiologist works with the child and family to implement a comprehensive assessment. Most often, the child will be assessed using pure-tone audiometry, speech audiometry, and acoustic immittance testing, as previously described. To address the status of the inner ear without the need for a specific behavioral response from the child, otoacoustic emissions are used to determine the functioning of the cochlea's outer hair cells, and electrophysiological audiometry measures such as ABR are used to detect the brain's response to sound, including signals from the cochlea, acoustic nerve, and auditory centers of the brain.

Hearing assessment for infants and young children is critical because of the potential impact of hearing loss on language acquisition. Although traditional audiometry may not be effective for young children, behavioral observation audiometry can be used. This approach to hearing assessment can be used for children from birth to 6 months of age and considers the reflexive response of young children to sound through noisemakers and calling the infant's name. For older infants, sound localization is often used, in which the audiologist watches for the child to turn their head in the direction of a sound stimuli. Between ages 6 and 30 months, some infants and toddlers can be conditioned to wear headphones and respond to pure tones delivered through the headphones, but they usually require **conditioned play audiometry**. In this context, a child learns to place a block in a container each time a sound is heard (Prelock & Hutchins, 2018).

There is also a need for assessment that can better describe the language profiles of children with hearing loss, specifically to profile complex syntax because this continues to be an area of vulnerability for school-age children with hearing loss (Klieve et al., 2023). In addition, Nickbakht and colleagues (2022) identified informational support (e.g., nature and type of hearing loss), professional support (e.g., roles of different professionals), peer support (e.g., parent support groups), skills and knowledge (e.g., ways to communicate with their child), financial support (e.g., available funding to help meet the child's needs), and methods of information provision (phone, e-mail, in person, etc.) that can help families of children with hearing loss transition to early intervention.

Treatment Planning, Management, and Options for Individuals With Hearing Loss

Once an assessment is complete, the audiologist reviews the assessment results with the family and the individual with the identified hearing loss and identifies areas of hearing needs. Priority intervention goals are jointly defined with the family, and a plan for services is put in place that may include amplification, aural rehabilitation, assistive technology systems, counseling regarding the hearing loss, and identification of other professionals who may be appropriate intervention supports. For example, SLPs may be identified as having a critical role in the implementation of the intervention plan. SLPs typically know how to maintain a hearing aid or assistive hearing device and use them appropriately in academic and job situations. As a member of the interprofessional team serving the needs of an individual with a hearing loss and their family, the SLP helps educate the public and other professionals on the potential communication needs of the individual with a hearing loss, provides hearing screenings, offers culturally and linguistically appropriate speech and language evaluations, and implements aural rehabilitation plans. An aural rehabilitation plan usually involves counseling, education for the individual and the family about the hearing loss and what it means for participation in daily activities, sensory management, and perceptual training (Boothroyd, 2007). When a hearing loss is the result of a medical condition, a referral is usually made to a physician because symptoms often suggest the presence of some type of physical trauma, a tumor, or an infection.

⊘ www

See the **ASHA Aural Rehabilitation for Adults Practice Portal** for information.

Intervention Options for Adults

Several options are available for addressing the needs of adults with hearing loss. Auditory rehabilitation (AR) includes four primary elements: (a) the use of hearing aids, CIs, or other listening devices;

(b) instruction on device use; (c) auditory training or lipreading; and (d) counseling to address the impact of hearing loss on quality of life (Boothroyd, 2007, 2017). However, there are a variety of practice patterns and professional perspectives on implementing AR for adults, which suggests a greater need for closer examination as to why such variability exists and what barriers must be addressed so a standard of care can be achieved (Ray et al., 2022).

See the **ASHA Hearing Loss (Adults) Evidence Map** for more information on models of service delivery.

For example, an amplification care plan for an individual with a hearing loss may involve a sensory device such as a hearing aid or a CI along with the instruction on how to use the device and counseling on what to expect. Figure 13–10 provides a visual of a CI.

See the **ASHA Cochlear Implants Practice Portal** and the **ASHA Hearing Aids for Adults Practice Portal** for more information.

Audiological rehabilitation is important for adults with CIs, where an electrode is placed on the skull behind the ear to stimulate the acoustic nerve and facilitate the brain's ability to process sound, bypassing the damaged inner ear (Tye-Murray, 2020). Those with CIs usually undergo auditory training to ensure that they fully benefit from their CIs and can adequately engage with other communication partners (Moberly et al., 2016). Typically, this training emphasizes performing auditory tasks, managing hearing challenges, increasing speech perception, and refining auditory skills (Henshaw & Ferguson, 2013). For adult CI users, some factors that will impact hearing outcomes are the age at which the CIs were

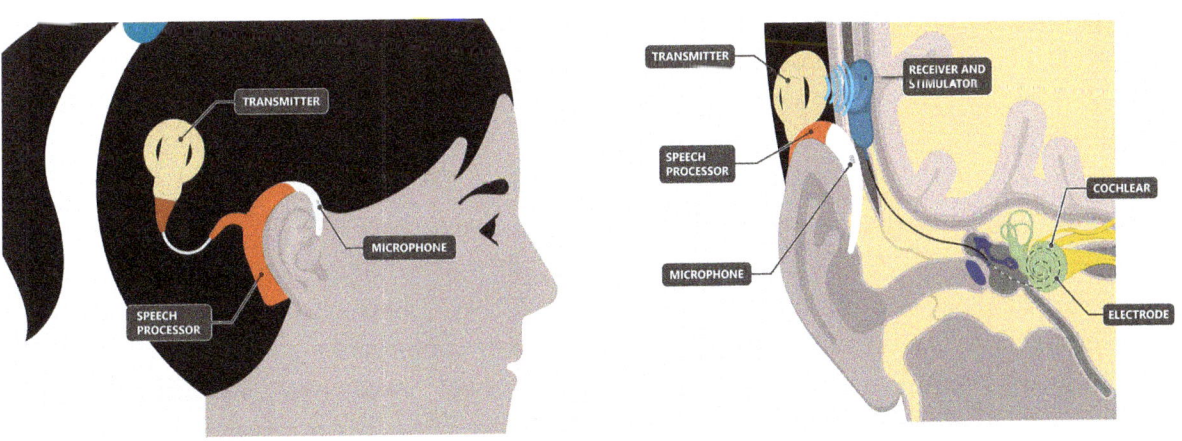

FIGURE 13–10. Internal and external components of a typical cochlear implant. *Source:* From *Foundations of Aural Rehabilitation: Children, Adults, and Their Family Members, Sixth Edition* (pp. 1–567) by Tye-Murray, N. Copyright © 2024 Plural Publishing, Inc. All rights reserved.

implanted, how long they have been deaf, and if they have any residual hearing (Philpott et al., 2023). It is important, then, if positive and less variable outcomes are to be achieved, that an individualized rehabilitation approach is implemented for adult CI users (Philpott et al., 2023).

Intervention might also include the use of hearing assistive technologies systems (HATS) to increase hearing in particular listening situations. The following are examples (taken from ASHA, n.d.-b [adults]):

- Alerting device: The use of lights or vibrations to signal that a sound (e.g., phone, smoke alarm, timer) has occurred.
- Frequency modulation system: Radio waves are used to move sound from its source to a receiver that is worn by an individual.
- Induction loop system: Hardwire loops that are located under floors or around the walls to convert sound to magnetic forces; hearing aids and CIs can then convert the magnetic force back to sound.
- Infrared system: Sound is sent via infrared waves to a listener's receiver.
- Personal amplification system: Uses streamers such as Bluetooth or a digital application to amplify sound.
- Telephone amplifier: Increases the volume of speech heard when speaking on the phone.
- Television assistive device and/or accessories: Increases television volume using wireless streaming or a loop system.
- Text telephone (TTD or TTY): Typed messages are sent and received via telephone lines.
- Voice carryover telephone: A person with hearing loss is connected to a local relay service.

Counseling and education comprise another intervention strategy that is frequently used for those with a hearing loss. The audiologist and/or SLP offer information to the individual and the family that is provided in clear, plain language so that it is easily understood. Usually, the nature of the hearing loss and how it might impact the individual's quality of life are explained. Social and vocational implications are described. Compensatory strategies to minimize the impact of hearing loss are discussed, and ways to self-manage are provided. Often, handouts are provided that clarify how to use and maintain listening devices and what to expect in terms of ability to hear and understand speech.

See "Audiology Patient Education Handouts" on the ASHA website for resources to use with patients.

One example of an education program for those with hearing loss and cognitive communication difficulties was developed by Postman and colleagues (2022), who investigated disparities in hearing and cognitive health for an older African American population. They examined the effects of an established group intervention, cognitive stimulation therapy, along with comprehensive audiology services. This evidence-based program was adapted to a group of low-income older African American adults integrating audiological services and education about hearing health. During weekly group sessions, discussions were held about ways to foster social interaction and cognition, and education about comprehensive audiological services was provided. The participants reported increased knowledge of their cognitive and hearing needs, leading to the use of audiological services.

To address the challenges associated with tinnitus, sound therapy is used to refocus attention by having the individual listen to external sounds (Sheppard et al., 2020). This approach is seldom recommended, however, because it currently lacks a strong evidence base for those with persistent tinnitus, although it is considered an option to provide some sense of relief (Jin et al., 2021; Tyler et al., 2020). To test the impact of sound therapy on the functional and emotional impact of tinnitus, Jin and colleagues (2022) evaluated sound therapy duration to determine whether a longer period of daily sound therapy would facilitate some level of relief. They found that extended sound therapy each day led to greater impact on perceived tinnitus level and the patient's emotional response.

The impact of hearing aids, when used in conjunction with counseling, to address tinnitus is unclear. Wang and colleagues (2023) examined the difference between hearing aids plus education counseling and educational counseling alone to determine what approach to intervention was most effective. After studying 72 adults with tinnitus, they found inadequate evidence that hearing aids plus counseling versus counseling alone was more effective, indicating more research is needed for addressing the needs of those experiencing tinnitus.

There are notable differences reported in health care access and use for individuals with and without hearing loss. This raises red flags for adults who are deaf or hard of hearing and have a higher occurrence of chronic health conditions that require health care management (Gonzalez et al., 2023). Clearly, health care providers must carefully consider options for communication when working with DHH populations to ensure better health care outcomes.

See **"Reaching Consumers"** on the American Academy of Audiology website for resources to use with patients.

Intervention Options for Children

There are a handful of intervention options for children with hearing loss, including amplification in the form of hearing aids or CIs, assistive listening devices, language intervention, and parent training. In addition, children with hearing loss watch the movement of a speaker's articulators, which allows them to speech- or lipread so they can better understand spoken language. Like adults with hearing loss, children who are deaf or hard of hearing employ assistive listening devices to use the telephone and watch television. To support learning in the classroom, frequency modulation (FM) systems are used to provide amplified access to classroom instruction. An FM system requires the teacher to talk into a microphone that is directly transmitted to a child's hearing aid.

Many children with a bilateral, severe to profound hearing loss may be unlikely to benefit from amplification using hearing aids, so CIs have become the standard of care (Beer et al., 2014; Sarant & Garrard, 2014). When using a CI, as described previously, an electrode is placed on the skull behind the ear and is used to stimulate the acoustic nerve and facilitate the brain's ability to process sound, bypassing the damaged inner ear (O'Donoghue et al., 2000). A CI does not restore hearing, but earlier implantation increases a child's ability to understand and produce language with the support of speech and language intervention. In addition, the language acquisition of children with CIs is better than that of those without an implant (Prelock & Hutchins, 2018), although delays in both speech and language skills and literacy skills may persist (Montgomery et al., 2010; Nittrouer et al., 2012). For example, Hasnain and colleagues (2023) investigated verbal fluency in children and adolescents with early cochlear implantation and found that compared to their peers without hearing loss, CI users demonstrated deficits in their ability to fluently retrieve semantic and phonological information for words from their working memory.

Currently, the recommended age for cochlear implantation is 9 months or older for those with profound bilateral sensorineural hearing loss (SNHL; U.S. Food and Drug Administration). However, research suggests earlier implantation and activation can improve outcomes for spoken language. Culbertson and colleagues (2022) examined young children's ability to acquire auditory information considering age as an influencing factor and tried to discern if CI prior to 9 months led to demonstrable change in auditory skills compared to those with later CI activation. They found that compared to children who were implanted between 9 and 24 months, those who were implanted prior to 9 months had more auditory skills that approximated those of hearing children. Culbertson and colleagues also found greater auditory skills at age 4 years for earlier implanted CI users and recommended that consideration be given to earlier CI activation for children with bilateral congenital SNHL. In fact, congenitally deaf children with bilateral CIs that are activated before their first birthday can develop language skills appropriate for their age by the time they are school age and attending formal educational programs (Ilig et al., 2023).

Children with a hearing loss in the mild to severe range are at risk for literacy challenges often related to their less well-developed phonological systems, vocabulary, and morphosyntactic understanding (Camarata et al., 2018; Herman et al., 2019; Tomblin et al., 2020; Walker et al., 2020). With inconsistent speech sound input, it is predictable that sound production would be impacted in children who are hard of hearing, even for those who have access to hearing aids and early intervention (Ambrose et al., 2014; Asad et al., 2018; Walker et al., 2015). Professionals can lessen the impact for children who are deaf or hard of hearing by initiating a habilitation plan that emphasizes function and the child's full participation. The audiologist has responsibility for hearing loss assessment, hearing aid fittings and use, and child and family counseling. The SLP supports the child's speech and language and socialization as well as their voice and prosody. The deaf educator provides education on the use of American Sign Language (ASL) and offers academic support.

Behavior problems are an area of risk for deaf or hard of hearing children; however, these children may not have similar access to intervention as their hearing peers, and nearly half have persistent behavioral problems (including those who receive early intervention that focuses primarily on hearing health care and speech-language therapy; Fellinger et al., 2012; Sessa & Sutherland, 2013; Theunissen et al., 2014). In the absence of behavioral intervention, challenging behaviors are likely to be seen in adolescence and beyond, often accompanied by anxiety and depression (Lavigne et al., 2009). Persistent behavioral problems may also increase the stress levels of families and impact their overall functioning (Reinke et al., 2012).

Studts and colleagues (2022) investigated a behaviorally based parent training intervention called the Family Check-Up for Children Who Are Deaf and Hard of Hearing (FCU-DHH) for young deaf and hard of hearing children. The intervention used a focused assessment approach and motivational interviewing in which parents engaged in mindful parenting using proactive monitoring. Parents also provided structured feedback to their children using positive behavior support, setting healthy limits, and building family relationships that capitalized on strengths and defining areas for positive change (Dishon et al., 2008; Stormshak & Dishon, 2009; Studts et al., 2022). Intervention was provided via home visits, with the initial sessions emphasizing building a relationship with the family and identifying their primary concerns and strengths. Parenting skills were assessed using both questionnaires and review of videotaped parent–child interactions followed by a discussion with the family regarding the assessment findings, parent motivation, and possible options for skill development. If families identified skills training as a priority for them, then several strategies were provided, including "visual aids, videotaped interactions, role play, coaching, in vivo practice, and homework" (Studts et al., 2022, p. 1169). Studts and colleagues adapted the training for parents of young children who are DHH in several ways, including the following:

- Use of a parent of a child who is DHH as a peer coach
- Provision of examples of role play and targeted homework suggestions
- Identification of resources that help improve parent–child interaction, increase knowledge regarding child development, and offer advocacy strategies to address the family's individual needs

Six, 1-hour intervention sessions were provided by the same peer coach via online technology within a 6- to 12-week period. The researchers also examined the feasibility and acceptability of the adapted intervention and found that it has promise for addressing the behavioral challenges that are often reported for children who are DHH.

Ambrose and colleagues (2023) investigated the effectiveness of Caregivers Optimizing Achievement of Children With Hearing Loss (COACH), an intervention incorporating interaction strategies delivered in the natural environment to support language development. Their findings indicated that although parents can be taught to use the natural language interaction strategies through the COACH model with some variability, children learned the targeted language and families were happy with the intervention. Ultimately, parent training will be critical to a child's success in learning to communicate and engage socially with others.

Cultural and Linguistic Considerations

Many children who are deaf or hard of hearing are exposed to more than one language in their homes and are multilingual learners (Crowe, 2018). As such, clinicians must consider in what language they are offering language support. Data indicate that 82% of children who are DHH use English, 18% use Spanish, 13% use ASL, and 5% use other languages (Benitez-Barrera et al., 2023; Office of Research Support and International Affairs, 2014). Being a culturally competent clinician requires professionals to support families in determining the language they would like to speak with their child in their home (Moeller et al., 2013). Unfortunately, Spanish-speaking caregivers of children who are DHH are often told to focus on the development of English language with sign language support. This is discouraging because it suggests that there may be a limited number of children who are DHH who actually speak their home language (Steinberg et al., 2003), which ultimately impacts the family dynamic. Interestingly, the beliefs of families regarding oral bilingualism "might impact language practices and ultimately child language proficiency" (Ronderos et al., 2022, p. 225; see also Hwang et al., 2022). Benitez-Barrera and colleagues (2023) examined professional recommendations regarding oral bilingualism and found that less than one-fourth of parents were encouraged to offer a bilingual option for their child. Most parents were given recommendations that violated best practice guidelines, suggesting training remains a priority to build cultural competence in the profession.

When their child is diagnosed with hearing loss in the first year of life, parents are faced with many decisions regarding their child's communication. Roughly 90% of children who are born DHH are born to hearing parents. Thus, caregivers must learn about the various means of communication available to their young child so they can make an informed decision (Reynolds et al., 2023). The decision is often complicated by the ongoing debate regarding the use of sign versus spoken language or the use of total communication (Hall et al., 2019). To add to this, complexities associated with myriad sociocultural factors must be considered in this decision (Lucas, 2014). Jones and Roberts (2023) investigated the advice parents receive and what they consider in their decision-making process regarding communication. They found that a parent's greatest priority is making sure they consider how their decision will impact their child's future, including their ability to take advantage of opportunities available to them.

Why Is This Topic Important?

Approximately 3 newborns in 1,000 births have a congenital hearing loss, and this prevalence increases into the school years, with 19.5% of adolescents (aged 12–19 years) diagnosed with unilateral or bilateral hearing loss (Kingsbury et al., 2022; Shargorodsky, Curhan et al., 2010). Importantly, childhood hearing loss can have long-term impacts on educational achievement and social engagement (Idstad & Engdahl, 2019).

Hearing is crucial to language acquisition, sound production, and comprehension. Hearing assessment, follow-up, and intervention are key to the academic, occupational, and community success of an individual who is deaf or hard of hearing. Because a congenital hearing loss will likely have a greater impact across the lifespan, early assessment and intervention are critical, and options for managing the hearing loss must be provided so that a child and their family can determine if amplification or a CI is possible. Furthermore, children who acquire language before losing their hearing will fare better than those who do not, and the degree of hearing loss will certainly be an important consideration for language development. Although deaf children may learn to communicate using ASL, approximately 95% have hearing parents who are less fluent in sign, which limits their children's access to language and socialization (Prelock & Hutchins, 2018).

Universal newborn hearing screening programs in the United States were first implemented in the 2000s, and hearing screening currently is done with 98.5% of newborns (CDC, 2020); international screening rates are consistent with these data (Mackey et al., 2021). Early Hearing Detection and Intervention (EHDI) programs are important for screening infants by age 1 month, confirming hearing loss by age 3 months, and enrolling infants in early intervention no later than age 6 months (Joint Committee on Infant Hearing, 2019). This is crucial because evidence indicates the value of early intervention for supporting language and cognition (Butcher et al., 2019; Ching et al., 2013; Moeller, 2000; Yoshinaga-Itano et al., 2021).

Not moving through the EHDI system puts children at risk for poor outcomes (Yoshinaga-Itano et al., 2017). Kingsbury and colleagues (2022) reviewed the evidence for hearing health care barriers in children who are deaf and hard of hearing. They found that SLPs and audiologists have a responsibility to ensure culturally responsive hearing health care. In addition, SLPs and audiologists are important advocates for policy change so that hearing follow-up is implemented in rural communities, families are informed about insurance coverage and financial support, and there is a qualified workforce to address hearing health care needs in culturally and linguistically diverse communities (Kingsbury et al., 2022).

For adolescents and young adults, repeated exposure to noise can damage the hearing mechanism. For this reason, education about hearing protection and the impact of noise exposure is important for this population to avoid hearing loss that can have far-reaching impacts on quality of life. For aging adults, hearing loss can lead to increased isolation and depression, so recognizing the loss and providing options for amplification are important. In addition, when there is a sudden loss in hearing, it may be indicative of a pathology that requires immediate attention. Thus, attending to our hearing is also attending to our physical health, our mental health, and our overall well-being.

Application to a Child

Christopher is a 6-year-old boy in first grade who has had a history of chronic otitis media. Because of this, his hearing has fluctuated, and his mother has noticed some frustration in school, especially related to literacy, including sounding out words as the first graders are learning to read. Christopher's mother has had his hearing tested, and it is generally within normal limits, but the audiologist recognizes that his hearing could fluctuate during a repeat occurrence of his otitis media. The pediatric ear, nose, and throat (ENT) doctor is considering placing myringotomy or tympanostomy tubes (ear tubes) in his ears. The tubes are tiny, hollow, and inserted into the eardrum. This allows air to flow into the middle ear and is often needed for children who have repeated ear infections. Ear tubes can also help drain the fluid that collects in the ear after an infection clears up (**otitis media with effusion**). Most tubes are designed to naturally exit the tympanic membrane between ages 4 and 18 months.

Christopher loves to swim, and his parents are worried that placing tubes in his ears will impact his ability to continue to do so. The ENT doctor explains that ear tube placement is a minimally invasive surgical procedure. The family is also told that Christopher can continue to swim if he does not dive deep under water. In addition, he can also use earplugs when he swims if he feels any pressure or discomfort. Furthermore, the doctor explains that hearing will likely improve and mild speech delays or difficulty hearing specific speech sounds may dissipate.

In the meantime, the SLP in Christopher's school has been consulting with his teacher and has recommended strategies to help Christopher understand the teacher's instructions and the lessons she is focused on related to sound–letter correspondence and early word learning. She suggested that Christopher be given priority seating in the classroom, away from noisy areas (e.g., the door and windows) and close to where most of the classroom instruction occurs. The SLP also provided an assistive listening device so that the teacher could wear a microphone that directs her voice to a small amplifier on Christopher's desk.

As you consider Christopher's case and what you have learned about hearing so far, reflect on the following questions:

- What are the advantages and potential disadvantages of placing ear tubes in a child's ears?
- Are there other strategies the teacher and SLP should consider so that Christopher's speech and reading are not impacted during periods of chronic otitis media?
- How often should Christopher's hearing be tested?
- What signs of potential hearing difficulty might a teacher or parent look for in a child with chronic otitis media?

Application to an Adolescent or Adult

Billy is a 60-year-old male who is married and a practicing attorney. Following a situation in court in which he could barely hear a soft-spoken judge in the courtroom during a case he was litigating, he shared the experience with his wife. She reminded him that she had been complaining that he frequently does not answer her when she is talking to him, and when the radio or television is on, he seems to have even more difficulty hearing. She also shared with him that several times when they have been out with friends, he asked people to repeat what they said or asked his wife to tell him what they said. In fact, sometimes he misinterprets a question for a comment and ignores the question being asked of him. During this discussion with his wife, Billy agreed that it was time for him to receive an audiological evaluation.

Billy was initially seen at a university clinic and shared the difficulties he had been having hearing in his job, at home, and when out with friends. He also reported that his hearing had been a problem for a few years but that he just was not ready for the possibility of needing hearing aids at age 60 years. He described how much effort it took to hear and explained that he would avoid certain restaurants that were just too noisy. He also shared that he found himself extremely tired at the end of a workday because of the extra effort he expended to listen to clients and the dialogue that occurred in the courtroom. In addition, he did not enjoy going to the movie theater because the dialogue was sometimes difficult to understand, and when watching television, he had to turn the volume up to a level that was uncomfortable to others.

A case history did not reveal any familial or medical conditions that would explain his hearing loss, and no one in his family had a hearing loss. Billy did explain, however, that he was in the Marine Corps and had served in Vietnam. He was on fire support bases with artillery for 9 months, during which time he had significant exposure to noise.

Otoscopic inspection revealed large osteomas (or bony growths) in both ear canals. There was no significant cerumen in either ear. Pure-tone testing revealed excellent low-frequency hearing, with sloping to mild to moderate hearing loss in the higher frequencies. The right ear was slightly better than the left ear. Bone conduction thresholds revealed no significant air–bone gaps, consistent with a permanent sensorineural hearing loss. Word recognition scores were good at 84% in the left ear and 88% in the right ear. Billy was diagnosed with a bilateral sensorineural hearing loss and was fitted with bilateral in-the-ear-canal–style hearing aids.

After wearing his hearing aids for a brief time, Billy mentioned to his wife that he was hearing the birds outside and that he could hear much better in the courtroom. His wife found that he was asking to have things repeated much less and did not seem to be as tired at the end of the day as he had been before being fitted with hearing aids.

Billy had annual hearing evaluations, and 3 years after his hearing loss was diagnosed, he transitioned to newer, small behind-the-ear hearing aids that were programmed to address his specific hearing loss. Although no significant progression in his hearing loss was noted over the 3 years, he continues to have difficulty understanding conversational speech without his hearing aids because he is not hearing high-frequency sounds such as [s, f, th]. He reported to the audiologist that he does not function as well without his hearing aids.

As you consider Billy's case, reflect on what you have learned about hearing so far, and answer the following questions:

- How might Billy's quality of life have been impacted because of his hearing loss?
- What additional information would you want to know about Billy's hearing to make sure that all his hearing needs were being met?
- Why is it important for a person with a hearing loss to have their hearing tested on an annual basis?
- What recommendations would you make to his wife and friends to ensure that their conversations with him can be heard and understood?
- Are there other assisting hearing technologies you might recommend for Billy that might support other aspects of his life?

Chapter Summary

Hearing loss can impact an individual's hearing either partially or totally and can result from problems with the outer, middle, or inner ear or the auditory nerve. Hearing loss can affect one or both ears; can be present at birth or acquired; and can be sudden, progressive, or fluctuate over time. Hearing loss is usually diagnosed as a conductive, sensorineural, or mixed hearing loss, and the degree of hearing loss certainly impacts an individual's quality of life.

Making a hearing loss diagnosis, assessing the specific conditions of a hearing loss, and ultimately the management of hearing loss require an interdisciplinary team approach. SLPs often screen hearing, and audiologists complete a comprehensive assessment to describe the hearing loss and decide on possible amplification strategies. Otolaryngologists and primary care physicians provide medical consultation and support if the hearing loss is related to a specific medical condition. Educators of the deaf, SLPs, and other educational and health care providers support implementation of the intervention plan. Collaboration with the family and the individual with a hearing loss is crucial to the decision-making process and the management approach that best meets their needs (Grenness et al., 2014; Scarinci et al., 2013).

It is estimated that in the United States, 2 to 3 children are born with hearing loss per 1,000 births (National Institute on Deafness and Other Communication Disorders, 2024), with nearly 90% born to hearing parents who use only spoken language (Mitchell & Karchmer, 2004). Thus, language input may be inaccessible depending on the child's degree of hearing loss, their access to sign language, and the use of amplification (Campbell & Bergelson, 2022). Notably, there is strong evidence that sign language exposure early on is beneficial to children with hearing loss (e.g., Clark et al., 2016; Davidson et al., 2014; Hrastinski & Wilbur, 2016). It is important to note, too, that acquiring sign language does not interfere with the acquisition of spoken vocabulary and that often children exposed to ASL early on are likely to develop vocabulary in spoken English as well as ASL (Pontecorvo et al., 2023).

Some children will develop spoken language commensurate with their hearing peers (Geers et al., 2017), but for many, language deficits will persist (Luckner & Cooke, 2010; Moeller et al., 2007) and may impact academic achievement and specifically reading (Qi & Mitchell, 2012). In addition, there is performance variability in that gender and other disabilities (Ching et al., 2013; Yoshinaga-Itano et al., 2017), degree of hearing loss (Ching et al., 2013; de Diego-Lázaro et al., 2018; Yoshinaga-Itano et al., 2017), use of amplification (Walker et al., 2015), and early intervention (Yoshinaga-Itano et al., 2017, 2018) will impact outcomes. In fact, timely diagnosis and service access lead to developmentally appropriate language outcomes (Stika et al., 2015).

Campbell and Bergelson (2022) investigated the relationships among demographic and hearing characteristics and outcomes for vocabulary development in 100 DHH children in early intervention and found that age, amplification, and whether hearing loss was unilateral or bilateral influenced the variability in productive vocabulary. Ultimately, it is crucial to provide access to early intervention and language access to ensure learning success.

Furthermore, more than half of the cases of hearing loss in childhood are due to preventable causes (WHO, 2021b). Hearing loss has a significant impact on a child's ability to produce speech, develop language, and use an appropriate vocal tone and resonance. Challenges in the ability to hear create potential difficulties not only with talking but also with school and job success and access to positive social interactions. If you or someone you know is having difficulty hearing, getting tested is critical, especially for the youngest children. There are also guidelines for hearing loss assessment and diagnosis that can be useful to practicing clinicians (Alfred et al., 2014).

Chapter Review Questions

1. What is the ossicular chain, and what is its importance to hearing?
2. What are the components of the inner ear and their function?
3. How does sound travel from the outer ear to the brain?
4. What is the typical decibel level for conversation, and when is sound too low to hear versus so loud that it is uncomfortable or painful?
5. What types of hearing loss might an individual experience?
6. What are the typical causes of hearing loss in children versus adults?
7. How does a cochlear implant support the hearing of an individual considered deaf or hard of hearing?
8. What is the importance of hearing assessment for infants and those with acute or chronic otitis media?
9. What are the components of a comprehensive audiological assessment?
10. How effective are hearing aids in supporting a child's and/or adult's hearing, and why is the use of hearing aids important?

Learning Activities

1. Identify sources of noise exposure in your school, job, and/or community and determine where noise exposure has the potential to impact your hearing or that of the community members. What recommendations might you provide to your school, job, or community setting to conserve the hearing of its population beyond eliminating the noise?

2. Review the volume or intensity levels of the devices you use (iPods, iPhones), concerts you attend, sporting events, and clubs you go to, and describe those that are above the accepted threshold for potential impact to your hearing. If you have an Apple Watch, there is an app that can help you measure intensity levels. What steps can you and your friends take to protect your ears when using devices or attending social, sports, and music events where the sound level is beyond what is safe for your hearing?
3. Explore what clinics or agencies in your area perform hearing screenings. Have your hearing tested and ask the audiologist to explain the air and bone conduction testing they administered. Review your audiogram with the audiologist and ask if there are any situations that might make it more difficult for you to hear and understand speech.

Suggested Reading

Almufarrij, I., Dillon, H., & Munro, K. J. (2023). Do we need audiogram-based prescriptions? A systematic review. *International Journal of Audiology, 62*(6), 500–511.

Programming hearing aids usually involves using the individual's hearing thresholds on a hearing test. With technology, direct-to-consumer devices are available that are not typically developed from an individual's hearing thresholds. This systematic review examined the best ways to program an individual's hearing aids. Studies reviewed several fitting types: (a) using the individual's audiogram results, (b) comparative fitting in various settings, (c) having the patient choose preset responses, and (d) allowing self-fit adjustments. The findings suggest that hearing aid programing using the individual's audiogram improves outcomes relative to the comparative and client choice fitting approaches. Self-adjustment may lead to better outcomes than the audiogram approach when considering daily use. Limitations of the review include that there is little research in this area and study quality is reduced, indicating more research is needed.

Melo, I. M. M., Silva, A. R. X., Camargo, R., Cavalcanti, H. G., Ferrari, D. V., Taveira, K. V. M., & Balen, S. A. (2022). Accuracy of smartphone-based hearing screening tests: A systematic review. *CoDAS, 34*(3), Article e20200380.

This article describes hearing screening tools (i.e., uHear, Digit-in-Noise Test, HearTest, and HearScreen) that have adequate specificity and sensitivity for screening possible hearing difficulty. However, many methodological differences exist between the studies reviewed, limiting the ability to complete a full meta-analysis. Therefore, additional research is needed.

Rosenfeld, R. M., Tunkel, D. E., Schwartz, S. R., Anne, S., Bishop, C. E., Chelius, D. C., . . . Monjur, T. M. (2022). Clinical practice guideline: Tympanostomy tubes in children (update). *Otolaryngology—Head & Neck Surgery, 166*(1 Suppl.), S1–S55.

This guideline provides recommendations about which children (aged 6 months to 12 years) might be most appropriate for tympanostomy tubes. There are three primary recommendations. First, a hearing evaluation should be done if a child has otitis media that lasts for more than 3 months. Second, children with chronic otitis media who do not receive tympanostomy tubes should be periodically assessed until the fluid is gone or hearing loss is identified. Third, a determination should be made if the child is at risk for speech and language difficulties or learning concerns with recurrent otitis media.

Warner-Czyz, A. D., Roland, J. T., Jr., Thomas, D., Uhler, K., & Zombek, L. (2022). American Cochlear Implant Alliance Task Force guidelines for determining cochlear implant candidacy in children. *Ear and Hearing, 43*(2), 268–282.

Several recommendations provided in this guideline focus on screening, assessment, and intervention for children who are appropriate candidates for CIs. The following are some of the key recommendations:

- Hearing screening should be completed on all infants by age 1 month, and a more comprehensive audiological evaluation should be performed by 2 or 3 months if needed.
- Several criteria are considered in determining candidacy, including audiometric data such as speech recognition, benefit of hearing aids, and quality of life. In addition, parent and clinical feedback and responses to questionnaires regarding the child's auditory awareness, auditory responsiveness, and language progress are critical.
- A CI team should include physicians, SLPs, audiologists, teachers of the deaf, early interventionist specialists in deaf and hard of hearing children, psychologists, counselors, and social workers, as well as the child's family.
- When doing a history of hearing health, note should be made of hearing loss onset, use of hearing aids, and etiology of the hearing loss.
- A test battery is important so that appropriate care coordination can occur and support can be provided to the family in their decision making.
- An assessment of functional listening should also occur, including suprasegmental features (e.g., duration, intensity, pitch) as well as the ability to hear sound features to help identify consonants and vowels and ways in which hearing changes when at a distance or in noise.
- Objective measures should be used to verify hearing aid fittings. Subjective measures can be used to assess progress and determine whether the child should be referred for further evaluation.
- Frequent speech and language assessments should occur to determine whether a child is achieving the expected developmental milestones.
- Because children with hearing loss exhibit variable outcomes, nontraditional factors should also be considered in the assessment of speech and language.
- Fitting for amplification should be performed following a confirmed hearing loss within 1 month of identification, with intervention occurring within 3 to 6 months.

Additional Resources

- American Academy of Audiology
  https://www.audiology.org
- American Academy of Pediatrics (AAP)
  - AAP policy on reducing harm from excessive noise exposure
    https://publications.aap.org/aapnews/news/26437/New-AAP-policy-technical-report-offer-advice-on?autologincheck=redirected

- AAP policy on hearing assessment for infants, children, and adolescents
  https://www.aap.org/en/news-room/news-releases/aap/2023/american-academy-of-pediatrics-updates-guidance-on-assessing-hearing-in-infants-children-and-adolescents
- American Speech-Language-Hearing Association, "Autoimmune Inner Ear Disease"
  https://www.asha.org/articles/autoimmune-inner-ear-disease
- American Speech-Language-Hearing Association, Hearing-Related Topics: Terminology Guidance Practice Portal
  https://www.asha.org/practice-portal/hearing-related-topics-terminology-guidance
- American Speech-Language-Hearing Association, "Ototoxic Medications (Medication Effects)"
  https://www.asha.org/public/hearing/ototoxic-medications
- American Speech-Language-Hearing Association, "Person-Centered Care in Audiology"
  https://www.asha.org/aud/person-centered-care-in-audiology
- American Speech-Language-Hearing Association, "Self-Test for Hearing Loss"
  https://www.asha.org/public/hearing/self-test-for-hearing-loss
- Educational Audiology Association
  https://edaud.org
- Hearing Loss Association of America
  https://www.hearingloss.org
- Ida Institute
  https://idainstitute.com
- U.S. Department of Labor, Occupational Safety and Health Administration, standards on occupational noise exposure
  https://www.osha.gov/noise
- World Health Organization and International Telecommunication Union, standard on safe listening devices and systems
  https://iris.who.int/bitstream/handle/10665/280085/9789241515276-eng.pdf

References

Alfred, R. L., Arnos, K. S., Fox, M., Lin, J. W., Palmer, C. G., Pandya, A., . . . Yoshinaga-Itano, C. (2014). ACMG guideline for the clinical evaluation and etiologic diagnosis of hearing loss. *Genetics in Medicine, 16*(4), 347–355.

Ambrose, S. E., Appenzeller, M., & Kaiser, A. P. (2023). Teaching caregivers to implement the Caregivers Optimizing Achievement of Children with Hearing Loss (COACH) intervention. *American Journal of Speech-Language Pathology, 32*, 1131–1153.

Ambrose, S. E., Unflat Berry, L. M., Walker, E. A., Harrison, M., Oleson, J., & Moeller, M. P. (2014). Speech sound production in 2-year-olds who are hard of hearing. *American Journal of Speech-Language Pathology, 23*(2), 91–104.

American National Standards Institute. (2018). *Specification for audiometers* (Rev. ed.; (ANSI/ASA S3.6-2018). Acoustical Society of America.

American Speech-Language-Hearing Association. (n.d.-a). *Hearing loss (ages 5+)*. Retrieved February 17, 2024, from https://www.asha.org/practice-portal/clinical-topics/hearing-loss

American Speech-Language-Hearing Association (n.d.-b). *Hearing loss in adults*. Retrieved February 5, 2024 https://www.asha.org/practice-portal/clinical-topics/hearing-loss

American Speech-Language-Hearing Association. (2016, June). 60 percent of childhood hearing loss is preventable. *The ASHA Leader, 21*, 12.

Armitage, C. J., Loughran, M. T., & Munro, K. J. (2020). Epidemiology of the extent of recreational noise exposure and hearing protection use: Cross-sectional survey in a nationally representative UK adult population sample. *BMC Public Health, 20*(1), Article 1529.

Asad, A. N., Purdy, S. C., Ballard, E., Fairgray, L., & Bowen, C. (2018). Phonological processes in the speech of school-age children with hearing loss: Comparisons with children with normal hearing. *Journal of Communication Disorders, 74*, 10–22.

Baracca, G., Del Bo, L., & Ambrosetti, U. (2011). Tinnitus and hearing loss. In A. R. Møller, B. Langguth, D. De Ridder & T. Kleinjung (Eds.), *Textbook of tinnitus* (Vol. 1, pp. 285–290). Springer.

Barbee, C. M., James, J. A., Park, J. H., Smith, E. M., Johnson, C. E., Clifton, S., & Danhauer, J. L. (2018). Effectiveness of auditory measures for detecting hidden hearing loss and/or cochlear synaptopathy: A systematic review. *Seminars in Hearing, 39*(2), 172–209.

Beer, J., Kronenberger, W. G., Castellanos, I., Colson, B. G., Henning, S. C., & Pisoni, D. B. (2014). Executive functioning skills in preschool children with cochlear implants. *Journal of Speech, Language, and Hearing Research, 57*, 1521–1534.

Benitez-Barrera, C., Reiss, L., Majid, M., Chau, T., Wilson, J., Rico, E. F., . . . de Diego-Lazaro, B. (2023). Caregiver experiences with oral bilingualism in children who are deaf and hard of hearing in the United States: Impact on child language proficiency. *Language, Speech, and Hearing Services in Schools, 54*, 224–240.

Blackwell, D. L., Lucas, J. W., & Clarke, T. C. (2014, February). Summary health statistics for U.S. adults: National Health Interview Survey, 2012. *Vital Health Statistics Series 10: Data from the National Health Survey*, (260), 1–161.

Boothroyd, A. (2007). Adult aural rehabilitation: What is it and does it work? *Trends in Amplification, 11*(2), 63–71.

Boothroyd, A. (2017). Aural rehabilitation as comprehensive hearing health care. *Perspectives of the ASHA Special Interest Groups, 2*(7), 31–38.

Bowl, M. R., & Dawson, S. J. (2019). Age-related hearing loss. *Cold Spring Harbor Perspectives in Medicine, 9*(8), Article a033217.

Butcher, E., Dezateux, C., Cortina-Borja, M., & Knowles, R. L. (2019). Prevalence of permanent childhood hearing loss detected at the universal newborn hearing screen: Systematic review and meta-analysis. *PLoS ONE, 14*(7), Article e0219600.

Camarata, S., Werfel, K., Davis, T., Hornsby, B. W., & Bess, F. H. (2018). Language abilities, phonological awareness, reading skills, and subjective fatigue in school-age children with mild to moderate hearing loss. *Exceptional Children, 84*(4), 420–436.

Campbell, E., & Bergelson, E. (2022). Characterizing North Carolina's deaf and hard of hearing infants and toddlers: Predictors of vocabulary, diagnosis, and intervention. *Journal of Speech, Language, and Hearing Research, 65*, 1894–1905.

Carroll, Y. I., Eichwald, J., Scinicariello, F., Hoffman, H. J., Deitchman, S., Radke, M. S., . . . Breysse, P. (2017). Vital signs: Noise-induced hearing loss among adults—United States 2011–2012. *MMWR Morbidity and Mortality Weekly Report, 66*(5), 139–144.

Centers for Disease Control and Prevention. (2010). Identifying infants with hearing loss—United States, 1999–2007. *MMWR Morbidity and Mortality Weekly Report, 59*(8), 220–223.

Centers for Disease Control and Prevention. (2020). *Data and statistics about hearing loss in children.* https://www.cdc.gov/hearing-loss-children/data/?CDC_AAref_Val=https://www.cdc.gov/ncbddd/hearingloss/data.html

Centers for Disease Control and Prevention (2021). *National Center on Birth Defects and Developmental Disabilities 2021 Summary of hearing screening among total occurrent births.* https://www.cdc.gov/ncbddd/hearingloss/2021-data/02-screen.html

Chen, K. H., Su, S. B., & Chen, K. T. (2020). An overview of occupational noise-induced hearing loss among workers: Epidemiology, pathogenesis, and preventive measures. *Environmental Health and Preventive Medicine, 25*(1), 1–10.

Ching, T. Y. C., Dillon, H., Marnane, V., Hou, S., Day, J., Seeto, M., . . . Yeh, A. (2013). Outcomes of early- and late-identified children at 3 years of age: Findings from a prospective population-based study. *Ear and Hearing, 34*(5), 535–552.

Choi, Y. M., & Jeong, S. W. (2023). Theory of mind in children with cochlear implants: Comparison with age- and sex-matched children with normal hearing. *American Journal of Otolaryngology, 44*(2), Article 103693.

Clarin, G. (2015). Auditory nerve pathway. In *A resource guide to early hearing screening and intervention* [e-book]. National Center for Hearing Assessment and Management.

Clark, M. D., Hauser, P. C., Miller, P., Kargin, T., Rathmann, C., Guldenoglu, B., . . . Israel, E. (2016). The importance of early sign language acquisition for deaf readers. *Reading and Writing Quarterly, 32*(2), 127–151.

Crowe, K. (2018). Deaf and hard-of-hearing multilingual learners: Language acquisition in a multilingual world. In H. Knoors & M. Marschark (Eds.), *Evidence-based practice in deaf education* (pp. 59–79). Oxford University Press.

Crowe, K., & Dammeyer, J. (2021). A review of the conversational pragmatic skills of children with cochlear implants. *Journal of Deaf Studies and Deaf Education, 26*(2), 171–186.

Culbertson, S. R., Dillon, M. T., Richter, M. E., Brown, K. D., Anderson, M. R., Hancock, S. L., & Park, L. R. (2022). Younger age at cochlear implant activation results in improved auditory skill development for children with congenital deafness. *Journal of Speech, Language, and Hearing Research, 65,* 3539–3547.

Cupples, L., Ching, T. Y. C., Leigh, G., Martin, L., Gunnourie, M., Button, L., . . . Van Buynder, P. (2018). Language development in deaf or hard-of-hearing children with additional disabilities: Type matters! *Journal of Intellectual Disability Research, 62*(6), 532–543.

Davidson, K., Lillo-Martin, D., & Pichler, D. C. (2014). Spoken English language development among native signing children with cochlear implants. *Journal of Deaf Studies and Deaf Education, 19*(2), 238–250.

de Diego-Lázaro, B., Restrepo, M. A., Sedey, A. L., & Yoshinaga-Itano, C. (2018). Predictors of vocabulary outcomes in children who are deaf or hard of hearing from Spanish-speaking families. *Language, Speech, and Hearing Services in Schools, 50*(1), 113–125.

Degeest, S., Kestens, K., & Keppler, H. (2022). Investigation of the relation between tinnitus, cognition, and the amount of listening effort. *Journal of Speech, Language, and Hearing Research, 65,* 1988–2002.

De Ridder, D., Schlee, W., Vanneste, S., Londero, A., Weisz, N., Kleinjung, T., . . . Langguth, B. (2021). Tinnitus and tinnitus disorder: Theoretical and operational definitions (an international multidisciplinary proposal). In W. Schlee, B. Langguth, T. Kleinjung, S. Vanneste, & D. De Ridder (Eds.), *Progress in brain research* (pp. 1–25). Elsevier.

Elmazoska, I., Maki-Torkko, E., Granberg, S., & Widen, S. (2023). Associations between recreational noise exposure and hearing function in adolescents and young adults: A systematic review. *Journal of Speech, Language, and Hearing Research, 67*, 688–710.

Epstein, S., Christianson, E., Ou, H. C., Norton, S. J., Sie, K. C. Y., & Horn, D. L. (2022). Educational environments and secondary school outcomes among students who are D/deaf and hard of hearing in special education. *Language, Speech, and Hearing Services in Schools, 53*, 1161–1167.

Farquharson, K., Oleson, J., McCreery, R. W., & Walker, E. A. (2022). Auditory experience, speech sound production growth, and early literacy in children who are hard of hearing. *American Journal of Speech-Language Pathology, 31*, 2092–2107.

Gallaudet Research Institute. (2011, April). *Regional and national summary report of data from the 2009–10 Annual Survey of Deaf and Hard of Hearing Children and Youth.*

Geers, A. E., Mitchell, C. M., Warner-Czyz, A., Wang, N. Y., & Eisenberg, L. S. (2017). Early sign language exposure and cochlear implantation benefits. *Pediatrics, 140*(1), Article e20163489.

Goberis, D., Beams, D., Dalpes, M., Albrosch, A., Baca, R., & Yoshinaga-Itano, C. (2012). The missing link in language development of deaf and hard of hearing children: Pragmatic language development. *Seminars in Speech and Language, 33*(4), 297–309.

Gonzalez, V. C., Santiago, Z. Y., Jacobs, M., & Ellis, C. (2023). Disparities in health care utilization among deaf and hard of hearing adults. *Perspectives of the ASHA Special Interest Groups, 8*, 675–682.

Gopinath, B., McMahon, C. M., Burlutsky, G., & Mitchell, P. (2016). Hearing and vision impairment and the 5-year incidence of falls in older adults. *Age and Ageing, 45*(3), 409–414.

Graven, S. N., & Browne, J. V. (2008). Sensory development in the fetus, neonate, and infant: Introduction and overview. *Newborn and Infant Nursing Reviews, 8*(4), 169–172.

Grenness, C., Hickson, L., Laplante-Lévesque, A., & Davidson, B. (2014). Patient-centered care: A review for rehabilitative audiologists. *International Journal of Audiology, 53*(Suppl. 1), S60–S67.

Hall, M. L., Hall, W. C., & Caselli, N. K. (2019). Deaf children need language, not (just) speech. *First Language, 39*(4), 367–395.

Hasnain, F., Herran, R. M., Henning, S. C., Ditmars, A. M., Pisoni, D. B., Sehgal, S. T., & Kronenberger, W. G. (2023). Verbal fluency in prelingually deaf, early implanted children and adolescents with cochlear implants. *Journal of Speech, Language, and Hearing Research, 66*(4), 1394–1409.

Hegde, M. N. (2010). Audiology: Hearing and its disorders. In *Introduction to communicative disorders* (4th ed., pp. 487–529). Pro-Ed.

Henshaw, H., & Ferguson, M. A. (2013). Efficacy of individual computer-based auditory training for people with hearing loss: A systematic review of the evidence. *PLoS ONE, 8*(5), Article e62836.

Herman, R. E., Kyle, F., & Roy, P. (2019). Literacy and phonological skills in oral deaf children and hearing children with a history of dyslexia. *Reading Research Quarterly, 54*(4), 553–575.

Hoffman, H. J., Dobie, R. A., Losonczy, K. G., Themann, C. L., & Flamme, G. A. (2017). Declining prevalence of hearing loss in US adults aged 20 to 69 years. *JAMA Otolaryngology—Head & Neck Surgery, 143*(3), 274–285.

Hrastinski, I., & Wilbur, R. B. (2016). Academic achievement of deaf and hard-of-hearing students in an ASL/English bilingual program. *Journal of Deaf Studies and Deaf Education, 21*(2), 156–170.

Hunter, L. L., Monson, B. B., Moore, D. R., Dhar, S., Wright, B. A., Munro, K. J., . . . Siegel, J. H. (2020). Extended high frequency hearing and speech perception implications in adults and children. *Hearing Research, 397,* Article 107922.

Hwang, J. K., Mancilla-Martinez, J., Flores, I., & McClain, J. B. (2022). The relationship among home language use, parental beliefs, and Spanish-speaking children's vocabulary. *International Journal of Bilingual Education and Bilingualism, 25*(4), 1175–1193.

Hyde, M., Punch, R., & Komesaroff, L. (2010). Coming to a decision about cochlear implantation: Parents making choices for their deaf children. *Journal of Deaf Studies and Deaf Education, 15*(2), 162–178.

Idstad, M., & Engdahl, B. (2019). Childhood sensorineural hearing loss and educational attainment in adulthood: Results from the HUNT study. *Ear and Hearing, 40*(6), 1359–1367.

Ilig, A., Adams, D., Lesinski-Schiedat, A., Lenarz, T., & Kral, A. (2023). Variability in receptive language development following bilateral cochlear implantation. *Journal of Speech, Language, and Hearing Research, 67,* 618–632.

Jafari, Z., Fitzpatrick, E. M., Schramm, D., Rouillon, I., & Koravand, A. (2023). An umbrella review of cochlear implant outcomes in children with auditory neuropathy. *Journal of Speech, Language, and Hearing Research, 66,* 4160–4176.

Jin, I. K., Choi, S.-J., Ku, M., Sim, Y., & Lee, T. (2022). The impact of daily hours of sound therapy on tinnitus relief for people with chronic tinnitus: A randomized controlled study. *Journal of Speech, Language, and Hearing Research, 65,* 3079–3099.

Jin, I. K., Choi, S.-J., Yoo, J., Jeong, S., Heo, S., & Oh, H. (2021). Effects of tinnitus sound therapy determined using subjective measurements. *Journal of the American Academy of Audiology, 32*(4), 212–218.

Joint Committee on Infant Hearing. (2019). Year 2019 position statement: Principles and guidelines for early hearing detection and intervention programs. *Journal of Early Hearing Detection and Intervention, 4*(2), 1–44.

Jones, M. K., & Roberts, M. Y. (2023). Speech, sign, or both? Factors influencing caregivers' communication method decision making for deaf/hard of hearing children. *Journal of Speech, Language, and Hearing Research, 67,* 187–195.

Khan, R. A., & Husain, F. T. (2020). Tinnitus and cognition: Can load theory help us refine our understanding? *Laryngoscope Investigative Otolaryngology, 5*(6), 1197–1204.

Kikidis, D., Vassou, E., Schlee, W., Iliadou, E., Markatos, N., Triantafyllou, A., & Langguth, B. (2021). Methodological aspects of randomized controlled trials for tinnitus: A systematic review and how a decision support system could overcome barriers. *Journal of Clinical Medicine, 10*(8), Article 1737.

Kingsbury, S., Khvalabov, N., Stirn, J., Held, C., Fleckenstein, S. M., Hendrickson, K., & Walker, E. A. (2022). Barriers to equity in pediatric hearing health care: A review of the evidence. *Perspectives of the ASHA Special Interest Groups, 7,* 1060–1071.

Klieve, S., Eadie, P., Graham, L., & Leitao, S. (2023). Complex language use in children with hearing loss: A scoping review. *Journal of Speech, Language, and Hearing Research, 66,* 688–719.

Kohrman, D. C., Wan, G., Cassinotti, L., & Corfas, G. (2020). Hidden hearing loss: A disorder with multiple etiologies and mechanisms. *Cold Spring Harbor Perspectives in Medicine, 10*(1), Article a035493.

Kramer, S., Dreisbach, L., Lockwood, J., Baldwin, K., Kopke, R., Scranton, S., & O'Leary M. (2006). Efficacy of the antioxidant N-acetylcysteine (NAC) in protecting ears exposed to loud music. *Journal of the American Academy of Audiology, 17*(4), 265–278.

Lawrence, B. J., Jayakody, D. M. P., Bennett, R. J., Eikelboom, R. H., Gasson, N., & Friedland, P. L. (2020). Hearing loss and depression in older adults: A systematic review and meta-analysis. *The Gerontologist, 60*(3), e137–e154.

Leadsom, A., Field, F., Burstow, P., & Lucas, C. (2013). *1001 critical days: The importance of the conception to age two period.* https://www.nwcscnsenate.nhs.uk/files/8614/7325/1138/1001cd manifesto.pdf

Le Prell, C. G., Dell, S., Hensley, B., Hall, J. W., Campbell, K. C. M., Antonelli, P. J., . . . Guire, K. (2012). Digital music exposure reliably induces temporary threshold shift in normal-hearing human subjects. *Ear and Hearing, 33*(6), e44–e58.

Le Prell, C. G., Fulbright, A., Spankovich, C., Griffiths, S. K., Lobarinas, E., Campbell, K. C. M., . . . Miller, J. M. (2016). Dietary supplement comprised of β-carotene, vitamin C, vitamin E, and magnesium: Failure to prevent music-induced temporary threshold shift. *Audiology and Neurotology Extra, 6*(2), 20–39.

Lie, A., Engdahl, B., Hoffman, H. J., Li, C. M., & Tambs, K. (2017). Occupational noise exposure, hearing loss, and notched audiograms in the HUNT Nord-Trøndelag hearing loss study, 1996–1998. *The Laryngoscope, 127*(6), 1442–1450.

Lin, F. R., Niparko, J. K., & Ferrucci, L. (2011). Hearing loss prevalence in the United States. *Archives in Internal Medicine, 171*(20), 1851–1852.

Lin, F. R., Yaffe, K., Xia, J., Xue, Q., Harris, T. B., Purchase-Helzner, E., . . . Simonsick, E. M. (2013). Hearing loss and cognitive decline among older adults. *JAMA Internal Medicine, 173*(4), 293–299.

Loughrey, D. G., Kelly, M. E., Kelley, G. A., Brennan, S., & Lawlor, B. A. (2018). Association of age-related hearing loss with cognitive function, cognitive impairment, and dementia: A systematic review and meta-analysis. *JAMA Otolaryngology—Head & Neck Surgery, 144*(2), 115–126.

Lucas, C. (2014). *The sociolinguistics of the deaf community.* Elsevier.

Luckner, J. L., & Cooke, C. (2010). A summary of the vocabulary research with students who are deaf or hard of hearing. *American Annals of the Deaf, 155*(1), 38–67.

Lund, E. (2016). Vocabulary knowledge of children with cochlear implants: A meta-analysis. *Journal of Deaf Studies and Deaf Education, 21*(2), 107–121.

Mackey, A. R., Bussé, A. M. L., Hoeve, H. L. J., Goedegebure, A., Carr, G., Simonsz, H. J., & Uhlén, I. M., for the EUSCREEN Foundation. (2021). Assessment of hearing screening programmes across 47 countries or regions II: Coverage, referral, follow-up and detection rates from newborn hearing screening. *International Journal of Audiology, 60*(11), 831–840.

Manchaiah, V. K. C., Zhao, F., Danesh, A. A., & Duprey, R. (2011). The genetic basis of auditory neuropathy spectrum disorder (ANSD). *International Journal of Pediatric Otorhinolaryngology, 75*, 151–158.

Masterson, E., Bushnell, P., Themann, C., & Morta, T. (2016). Hearing impairment among noise-exposed workers—United States, 2003-2012. *Morbidity and Mortality Weekly Report, 65*(15), 389–394.

Matthews, D., & Kelly, C. (2022). Pragmatic development in deaf and hard of hearing children: A review. *Deafness & Education International, 24*(4), 296–313.

McCormack, A., Edmondson-Jones, M., Somerset, S., & Hall, D. (2016). A systematic review of the reporting of tinnitus prevalence and severity. *Hearing Research, 337,* 70–79.

Mick, P., Kawachi, I., & Lin, F. R. (2014). The association between hearing loss and social isolation in older adults. *Otolaryngology—Head & Neck Surgery, 150*(3), 378–384.

Mick, P., Parfyonov, M., Wittich, W., Phillips, N., & Kathleen Pichora-Fuller, M. (2018). Associations between sensory loss and social networks, participation, support, and loneliness: Analysis of the Canadian Longitudinal Study on Aging. *Canadian Family Physician, 64*(1), e33–e41.

Mitchell, R. E., & Karchmer, M. A. (2004). Chasing the mythical ten percent: Parental hearing status of deaf and hard of hearing students in the United States. *Sign Language Studies, 4*(2), 138–163.

Moberly, A. C., Bates, C., Harris, M. S., & Pisoni, D. B. (2016). The enigma of poor performance by adults with cochlear implants. *Otology & Neurotology, 37*(10), 1522–1528.

Moeller, M. P. (2000). Early intervention and language development in children who are deaf and hard of hearing. *Pediatrics, 106*(3), Article e43.

Moeller, M.P., Carr., G., Seaver, L., Stredler-Brown, A., & Holzinger, D. (2013). Best practices in family-centered early intervention for children who are deaf and hard of hearing: An international consensus statement. *Journal of Deaf Studies and Deaf Education, 18*(4), 429-445.

Moeller, M. P., Tomblin, J. B., Yoshinaga-Itano, C., Connor, C. M. D., & Jerger, S. (2007). Current state of knowledge: Language and literacy of children with hearing impairment. *Ear and Hearing, 28,* 740–753.

Montgomery, J. W., Magimairaj, B. M., & Finney, M. C. (2010). Working memory and specific language impairment: An update on the relation and perspectives on assessment and treatment. *American Journal of Speech-Language Pathology, 19,* 78–94.

Mood, D., Szarkowski, A., Brice, P. J., & Wiley, S. (2020). Relational factors in pragmatic skill development: Deaf and hard of hearing infants and toddlers. *Pediatrics, 146*(Suppl. 3), S246–S261.

Moon, C., Lagercrantz, H. K., & Kuhl, P. K. (2013). Language experienced in utero affects vowel perception after birth: A two-country study. *Acta Paediatrica, 102*(2), 156–160.

National Association of State Directors of Special Education. (2019). *Optimizing outcomes for students who are Deaf or hard of hearing: Educational service guidelines* (3rd ed.). http://www.nasdse.org/docs/nasdse-3rd-ed-7-11-2019-final.pdf

National Center for Health Statistics. (2018, August 27). *Crude percentages of hearing trouble for adults aged 18 and over, United States, 2015–2018.* Centers for Disease Control and Prevention. https://www.cdc.gov/nchs/nhis/ADULTS/www/index.htm

National Institute on Aging. (n.d.). *Hearing loss: A common problem for older adults.* Retrieved February 5, 2024, from https://www.nia.nih.gov/hearing-loss

National Institute on Deafness and Other Communication Disorders. (2024, March 4). *Quick statistics about hearing, balance, and dizziness.* Retrieved August 11, 2024, from https://www.nidcd.nih.gov/health/statistics/quick-statistics-hearing#1

Nickbakht, M., Meyer, C., Beswick, R., & Scarinci, N. (2022). Minimum data set for families of children with hearing loss: An eDelphi study. *Journal of Speech, Language, and Hearing Research, 65,* 1615–1629.

Nittrouer, S., Caldwell, A., & Holloman, C. (2012). Measuring what matters: Effectively predicting language and literacy in children with cochlear implants. *International Journal of Pediatric Otorhinolaryngology, 76,* 1148–1158.

Occupational Safety and Health Administration. (2024). *Occupational noise exposure.* Retrieved April 28, 2024, from https://www.osha.gov/noise

O'Donoghue, G. M., Nikolopoulos, T. P., & Archbold, S. M. (2000). Determinants of speech perception in children after cochlear implantation. *Lancet, 356,* 466–468.

Office of Research Support and International Affairs. (2014, October). *Regional and national summary report of data from the 2013–14 Annual Survey of Deaf and Hard of Hearing Children and Youth.* Gallaudet University.

Okubo, S., Takahashi, M., & Kai, I. (2008). How Japanese parents of deaf children arrive at decisions regarding pediatric cochlear implantation surgery: A qualitative study. *Social Science & Medicine, 66*(12), 2436–2447.

Philpott, N., Philips, B., Tromp, K., Kramer, S., Mylanus, E., & Huinck, W. (2023). Phoneme training for adult cochlear implant users: A review of the literature and study protocol. *Journal of Speech, Language, and Hearing Research, 66,* 5071–5086.

Pichora-Fuller, M. K., Dupuis, K., Reed, M., & Lemke, U. (2013). Helping older people with cognitive decline communicate: Hearing aids as part of a broader rehabilitation approach. *Seminars in Hearing, 34*(4), 308–330.

Pluta, A., Krysztofiak, M., Zgoda, M., Wysocka, J., Golec, K., Gajos, K., . . . Haman, M. (2023). Theory of mind and parental mental-state talk in children with CIs. *Journal of Deaf Studies and Deaf Education, 28*(3), 288–299.

Pontecorvo, E., Higgins, M., Mora, J., Lieberman, A. M., Pyers, J., & Caselli, N. K. (2023). Learning a sign language does not hinder acquisition of a spoken language. *Journal of Speech, Language, and Hearing Research, 66*(4), 1291–1308.

Postman, W. A., Fischer, M., Dalton, K., Leisure, K., Thompson, S., Sankey, L., & Watkins, H. (2022). Coupling hearing health with community-based group therapy for cognitive health in low-income African American elders. *Perspectives of the ASHA Special Interest Groups, 7,* 367–399.

Prelock, P. A., & Hutchins, T. L. (2018). *Clinical guide to assessment and treatment of communication disorders.* Springer.

Qi, S., & Mitchell, R. E. (2012). Large-scale academic achievement testing of deaf and hard-of-hearing students: Past, present, and future. *Journal of Deaf Studies and Deaf Education, 17*(1), 1–18.

Quittner, A. L., Barker, D. H., Cruz, I., Snell, C., Grimley, M. E., Botteri, M., & CDaCI Investigative Team. (2010). Parenting stress among parents of deaf and hearing children: Associations with language delays and behavior problems. *Parenting, Science and Practice, 10*(2), 136–155.

Rance, G., Beer, D., Cone-Wesson, B., & Shepherd, R. (1999). Clinical findings for a group of infants and young children with auditory neuropathy. *Ear and Hearing, 20,* 238–252.

Ray, C., Glade, R., & Culbertson, D. S. (2022). Cross-disciplinary practices and perspectives of auditory rehabilitation for adults with cochlear implants. *Perspectives of the ASHA Special Interest Groups, 7,* 1048–1059.

Reinke, W. M., Eddy, J. M., Dishion, T. J., & Reid, J. B. (2012). Joint trajectories of symptoms of disruptive behavior problems and depressive symptoms during early adolescence and adjustment problems during emerging adulthood. *Journal of Abnormal Child Psychology, 40*(7), 1123–1136.

Reynolds, G., Werfel, K. L., Vachio, M., & Lund, E. A. (2023). Early experiences of parents of children who are deaf or hard of hearing: Navigating through identification, intervention, and beyond. *Journal of Early Hearing Detection and Intervention, 8*(1), 56–68.

Ronderos, J., Castilla-Earls, A., & Marissa Ramos, G. (2022). Parental beliefs, language practices and language outcomes in Spanish–English bilingual children. *International Journal of Bilingual Education and Bilingualism, 25*(7), 2586–2607.

Rudge, A. M., Brooks, B. M., & Grantham, H. (2022). Expressive vocabulary growth rates of very young children who are deaf or hard of hearing: How much is enough? *Journal of Speech, Language, and Hearing Research, 65*, 1978–1987.

Sarant, J., & Garrard, P. (2014). Parenting stress in parents of children with cochlear implants: Relationships among parent stress, child language, and unilateral versus bilateral implants. *Journal of Deaf Studies and Deaf Education, 19*, 85–106.

Scarinci, N., Meyer, C., Ekberg, K., & Hickson, L. (2013). Using a family-centered care approach in audiologic rehabilitation for adults with hearing impairment. *Perspectives on Aural Rehabilitation and Its Instrumentation, 20*(3), 83–90.

Sessa, B., & Sutherland, H. (2013). Addressing mental health needs of deaf children and their families: The National Deaf Child and Adolescent Mental Health Service. *The Psychiatrist, 37*(5), 175–178.

Shargorodsky, J., Curhan, G. C., & Farwell, W. R. (2010). Prevalence and characteristics of tinnitus among US adults. *American Journal of Medicine, 123*(8), 711–718.

Shargorodsky, J., Curhan, S. G., Curhan, G. C., & Eavey, R. (2010). Change in prevalence of hearing loss in US adolescents. *JAMA, 304*(7), 772–778.

Sharma, R. K., Lalwani, A. K., & Golub, J. S. (2020). Prevalence and severity of hearing loss in the older old population. *JAMA Otolaryngology—Head & Neck Surgery, 146*(8), 762–763.

Sheffield, A. M., & Smith, R. J. (2019). The epidemiology of deafness. *Cold Spring Harbor Perspectives in Medicine, 9*(9), Article a033258.

Shen, J., Anderson, M. C., Arehart, K. H., & Souza, P. E. (2016). Using cognitive screening tests in audiology. *American Journal of Audiology, 25*(4), 319–331.

Sheppard, A., Stocking, C., Ralli, M., & Salvi, R. (2020). A review of auditory gain, low-level noise and sound therapy for tinnitus and hyperacusis. *International Journal of Audiology, 59*(1), 5–15.

Souza, P. E. (2018). Cognition and hearing aids: What should clinicians know? *Perspectives of the ASHA Special Interest Groups, 3*(6), 43–50.

Stach, B. A., & Ramachandran, V. (2021). *Clinical audiology: An introduction* (3rd ed.). Plural Publishing.

Starr, A., Picton, T., Hood, L. J., & Berlin, C. (1996). Auditory neuropathy. *Brain, 119*, 741–753.

Stika, C. J., Eisenberg, L. S., Johnson, K. C., Henning, S. C., Colson, B. G., Ganguly, D. H., & DesJardin, J. L. (2015). Developmental outcomes of early-identified children who are hard of hearing at 12 to 18 months of age. *Early Human Development, 91*(1), 47–55.

Stormshak, E. A., & Dishion, T. J. (2009). A school-based, family-centered intervention to prevent substance use: The family check-up. *American Journal of Drug and Alcohol Abuse, 35*(4), 227–232.

Studts, C. R., Jacobs, J. A., Bush, M. L., Lowman, J., Creel, L. M., & Westgate, P. M. (2022). Study protocol: Type 1 hybrid effectiveness-implementation trial of a behavioral parent training intervention for parents of young children who are deaf or hard of hearing. *American Journal of Speech-Language Pathology, 31*, 1163–1178.

Theunissen, S. C., Rieffe, C., Kouwenberg, M., De Raeve, L. J., Soede, W., Briaire, J. J., & Frijns, J. H. (2014). Behavioral problems in school-aged hearing-impaired children: The influence of sociodemographic, linguistic, and medical factors. *European Child and Adolescent Psychiatry, 23*(4), 187–196.

Thomson, R. S., Auduong, P., Miller, A. T., & Gurgel, R. K. (2017). Hearing loss as a risk factor for dementia: A systematic review. *Laryngoscope Investigative Otolaryngology, 2*(2), 69–79.

Tomblin, J. B., Oleson, J., Ambrose, S. E., Walker, E. A., McCreery, R. W., & Moeller, M. P. (2020). Aided hearing moderates the academic outcomes of children with mild to severe hearing loss. *Ear and Hearing, 41*(4), 775–789.

Tordrup, D., Smith, R., Kamenov, K., Bertram, M. Y., Green, N., Chadha, S., & WHO HEAR Group. (2022). Global return on investment and cost-effectiveness of WHO's HEAR interventions for hearing loss: A modelling study. *Lancet Global Health, 10*(1), E52–E62.

Tuohimaa, K., Loukusa, S., Lopponen, H., Valimaa, T., & Kunnari, S. (2023). Development of social–pragmatic understanding in children with congenital hearing loss and typical hearing between the ages of 4 and 6 years. *Journal of Speech, Language, and Hearing Research, 66*, 2502–2520.

Tye-Murray, N. (2020). *Foundations of aural rehabilitation: Children, adults, and their family members* (5th ed.). Plural Publishing.

Tyler, R. S., Perreau, A., Powers, T., Watts, A., Owen, R., Ji, H., & Mancini, P. C. (2020). Tinnitus sound therapy trial shows effectiveness for those with tinnitus. *Journal of the American Academy of Audiology, 31*(1), 6–16.

Vachio, M., Lund, E., & Werfel, K. L. (2023). An analysis of mental state verb and complex syntax use in children who are deaf and hard of hearing. *Language, Speech, and Hearing Services in Schools, 54*, 1282–1294.

Valiente, A. R., Fidalgo, A. R., Villarreal, I. M., & Berrocal, J. R. G. (2016). Extended high-frequency audiometry (9000–20000 Hz): Usefulness in audiological diagnosis. *Acta Otorrinolaringologica, 67*(1), 40–44.

Villarroel, M. A. B. D., Blackwell, D. L., & Jen, A. (2019). *Tables of summary health statistics for U.S. adults: 2018 National Health Interview Survey.* National Center for Health Statistics. https://ftp.cdc.gov/pub/Health_Statistics/NCHS/NHIS/SHS/2018_SHS_Table_A-6.pdf

Walker, E. A., Harrison, M., Baumann, R., Moeller, M. P., Sorensen, E., Oleson, J. J., & McCreery, R. W. (2023). Story generation and narrative retells in children who are hard of hearing and hearing children. *Journal of Speech, Language, and Hearing Research, 66*, 3550–3573.

Walker, E. A., Holte, L., McCreery, R. W., Spratford, M., Page, T., & Moeller, M. P. (2015). The influence of hearing aid use on outcomes of children with mild hearing loss. *Journal of Speech, Language, and Hearing Research, 58*(5), 1611–1625.

Walker, E. A., Sapp, C., Dallapiazza, M., Spratford, M., McCreery, R. W., & Oleson, J. J. (2020). Language and reading outcomes in fourth-grade children with mild hearing loss compared to age-matched hearing peers. *Language, Speech, and Hearing Services in Schools, 51*(1), 17–28.

Wang, X., Guo, L., Tian, R., Fei, Y., Ji, J., Diao, C., . . . Zheng, Y. (2023). Hearing aids combined with educational counseling versus educational counseling alone for tinnitus treatment in patients with hearing loss: A longitudinal follow-up study. *Journal of Speech, Language, and Hearing Research, 66*, 2490–2502.

Werfel, K. L., Reynolds, G., Hudgins, S., Castaldo, M., & Lund, E. A. (2021). The production of complex syntax in spontaneous language by 4-year-old children with hearing loss. *American Journal of Speech-Language Pathology, 30*(2), 609–621.

World Health Organization. (2018). *WHO global estimates on prevalence of hearing loss* [PowerPoint slides]. https://www.who.int/deafness/Global-estimates-on-prevalence-of-hearing-loss-Jul2018.pptx?ua=1

World Health Organization. (2021a, March 2). *WHO: 1 in 4 people projected to have hearing problems by 2050* [News release]. https://www.who.int/news/item/02-03-2021-who-1-in-4-people-projected-to-have-hearing-problems-by-2050

World Health Organization. (2021b, April 1). *Deafness and hearing loss* [Fact sheet]. https://www.who.int/news-room/fact-sheets/detail/deafness-and-hearing-loss

Yoshinaga-Itano, C., Mason, C. A., Wiggin, M., Grosse, S. D., Gaffney, M., & Gilley, P. M. (2021). Reading proficiency trends following newborn hearing screening implementation. *Pediatrics, 148*(4), Article e2020048702.

Yoshinaga-Itano, C., Sedey, A. L., Wiggin, M., & Chung, W. (2017). Early hearing detection and vocabulary of children with hearing loss. *Pediatrics, 140*(2), Article e20162964.

Yoshinaga-Itano, C., Sedey, A. L., Wiggin, M., & Mason, C. A. (2018). Language outcomes improved through early hearing detection and earlier cochlear implantation. *Otology and Neurotology, 39*(10), 1256–1263.

Yu, C. L., Stanzione, C. M., Wellman, H. M., & Lederberg, A. R. (2021). Theory-of-mind development in young deaf children with early hearing provisions. *Psychological Science, 32*(1), 109–119.

Chapter 14

Augmentative and Alternative Communication

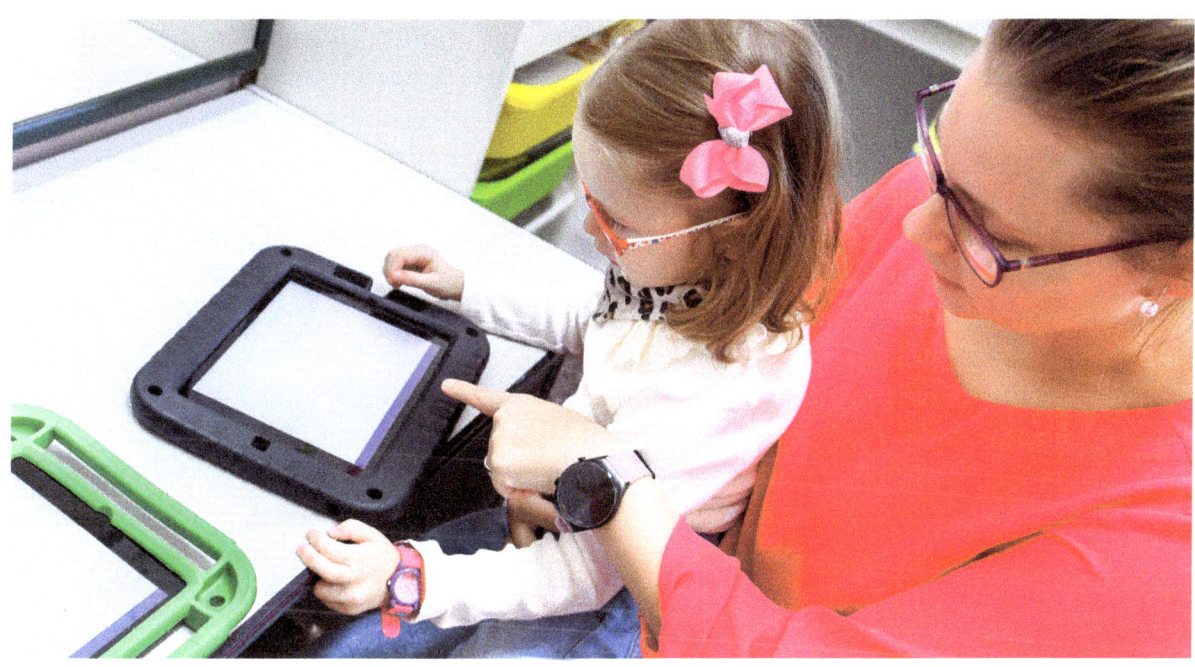

Learning Objectives

After reading this chapter, you will be able to:

- Describe the different methods of augmentative and alternative communication (AAC), including aided and unaided systems; no-, low-, and high-tech systems; and direct selection versus scanning.
- Compare and contrast intervention techniques for children with developmental conditions compared to adults with acquired communication disorders.
- Argue against the four main myths associated with AAC.

Key Terms

AAC abandonment
access barriers
aided AAC
aided language stimulation
augmentative and alternative communication
communication partner training
core vocabulary
fringe vocabulary

high-tech systems
modeling
no-tech systems
opportunity barriers
spontaneous novel utterance generation (SNUG)
unaided AAC
visual scene display

Introduction

Unlike many of the chapters in this book, this chapter does not describe a specific condition but, rather, seeks to offer information regarding communication that may be applicable to individuals with various communication disorders. The focus of this chapter is on augmentative and alternative communication (AAC). According to the American Speech-Language-Hearing Association (n.d.), **augmentative and alternative communication** is any form of communication that supplements or replaces verbal speech. AAC is used by children and adults who may be unable to use verbal speech at all, who may use verbal speech in some settings but not others, or who use verbal speech but may be unintelligible to their listeners. AAC is important because it allows individuals with complex communication needs (CCNs) the opportunity to participate in activities that without communication would be extremely difficult. Although not an exhaustive list, AAC may be used by individuals with developmental conditions, such as autism, Down syndrome, apraxia of speech, cerebral palsy, and Angelman syndrome, as well as by people with acquired communication disorders, including those who have experienced a stroke, traumatic brain injury (TBI), or a degenerative condition such as dementia or amyotrophic lateral sclerosis (ALS). As you read this chapter, keep in mind that AAC is not a tool, nor is it technology; AAC is communication that is accessed through a mode other than verbal speech (and often this is a technological mode).

Characteristics of AAC

As previously mentioned, AAC is any form of communication other than verbal speech that allows individuals with CCNs to participate in everyday activities. AAC includes unaided and aided means of communication. **Unaided AAC** refers to any mode of communication that a person uses that does *not* rely on an external tool, and includes facial expressions, gestures, and pointing. **Aided AAC**, on the other hand, refers to augmentative systems used for communication that are external to the speaker, including picture boards, electronic communication devices, and typing. Although this chapter focuses primarily on aided AAC, we highlight the importance of unaided communication throughout.

Another important distinction in the AAC world is that of no-tech/low-tech versus high-tech systems. No-tech and low-tech options do not rely heavily, if at all, on technology. These include communication books, picture boards, spelling by pointing to letters, and so on. High-tech systems rely on the use of technology and include apps that are commercially available on personal tablets and computer devices specifically designed for communication. It is important to note that no-, low-, and high-tech AAC tools can be accessed by the AAC user by directly selecting the message by touching it, using a laser pointer, through eye gaze, or even by scanning through and selecting messages through blinking or small muscle movements.

Unaided AAC

When we first think about AAC and supporting individuals who are complex communicators, we might not immediately think of unaided AAC or communication modalities that do not rely on external methods. Unaided AAC includes using gestures, eye gaze, body language, and facial expressions to communicate, all of which are considered nonverbal communication. We all use nonverbal communication (and thus unaided AAC) daily, so much so that nonverbal communication is present in most, if not all, of our communication encounters, especially those that happen face-to-face (Burgoon et al., 2021). Individuals with CCNs who have little or no verbal speech also communicate through nonverbal communication. This can occur on its own or in conjunction with aided AAC. It is particularly important to note that how a person uses unaided AAC to communicate will vary by culture. The meanings associated with nonverbal communicative acts (e.g., gestures, eye gaze) are not universal; each culture has its own set of rules for the meaning behind specific nonverbal behaviors.

Although unaided AAC is vital to communicating with others, it is often limiting in that it is insufficient to meet the broad range of communicative needs that we have as humans. For individuals with CCNs, this is where aided AAC comes in.

Aided AAC

When a person's verbal speech and use of unaided AAC are not enough to meet their communication needs, external modes of communication (aided AAC) can be used. Aided AAC is often thought about in terms of the symbols that are used to communicate. These include objects, photographs, line drawings, and the written alphabet. The type of symbols that are used depends on several factors, including the AAC user's physical, sensory, and literacy skills (Hall et al., 2023). A thorough assessment of the AAC user's strengths and challenges will be necessary to determine which aided system(s) is most appropriate to meet the individual's communication needs.

No-Tech/Low-Tech AAC

There are many options to consider when selecting an aided AAC system, ranging from no-tech/low-tech to high-tech. **No-tech systems** (also referred to as low-tech or lite-tech) do not require any technology, and therefore do not have a voice output. No-tech AAC systems include picture boards, alphabet boards, language boards, and communication books, all of which offer a way for individuals to access communication in various environments. Figure 14–1 presents an example of no-tech AAC. These boards or symbols can be placed throughout the individual's environment, can be easily transported with the individual across settings, and can be duplicated and updated relatively easily. No-tech systems can be used

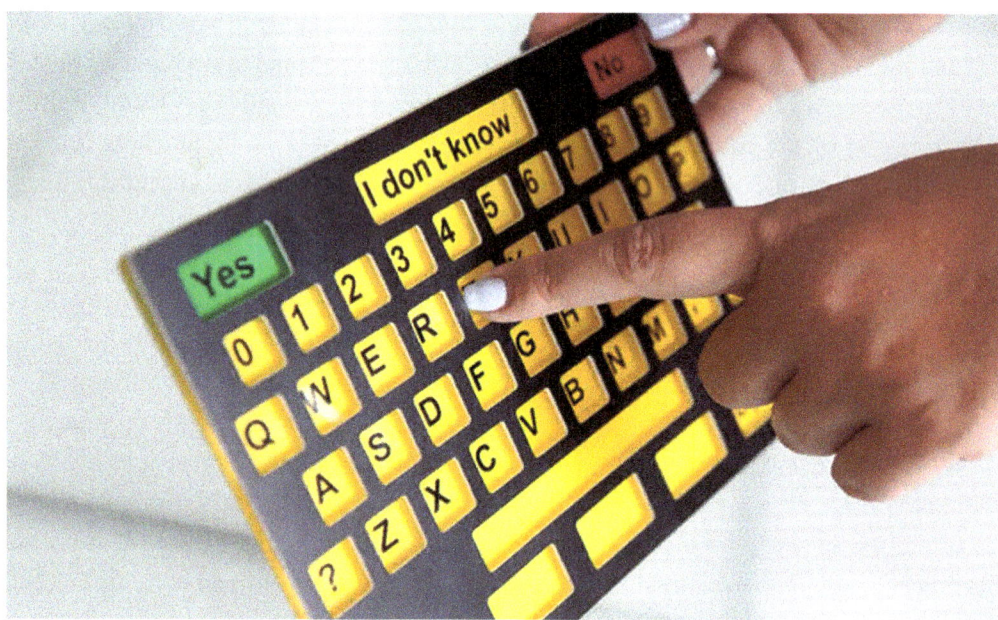

FIGURE 14–1. No-tech alphabet board. *Source:* CandLE (https://candleaac.com/low-techresources).

alone or in conjunction with high-tech AAC systems to provide more comprehensive and robust access to language. Pages from a person's high-tech AAC system can be printed and used as no-tech boards. This is particularly useful in places where using technology is prohibited or ill-advised (e.g., in the pool or at the water table). Premade downloadable no-tech communication boards are offered by various companies, including Saltillo and AssistiveWare.

Saltillo

AssistiveWare

High-Tech AAC

High-tech systems come in the form of computers or tablets and are sometimes called speech-generating devices because a key feature of these systems is that they have voice output (either a digitized voice or from a voice bank). Figure 14–2 shows some examples of high-tech AAC. High-tech devices allow for a more robust vocabulary than no-tech systems. This is because they are equipped with software that supports multiple vocabulary sets. In addition, the software often has various voice output settings and languages, as well as the ability to connect to e-mail and text messaging so that messages can be sent digitally. A robust vocabulary makes high-tech AAC stand out from no-tech AAC because it is with a robust vocabulary that individuals can communicate a range of messages, have access to all parts of speech, and generate infinite grammatical utterances. This allows AAC users to communicate using **spontaneous novel utterance generation** (**SNUG**; Hill, 2014), supporting participation in all communication

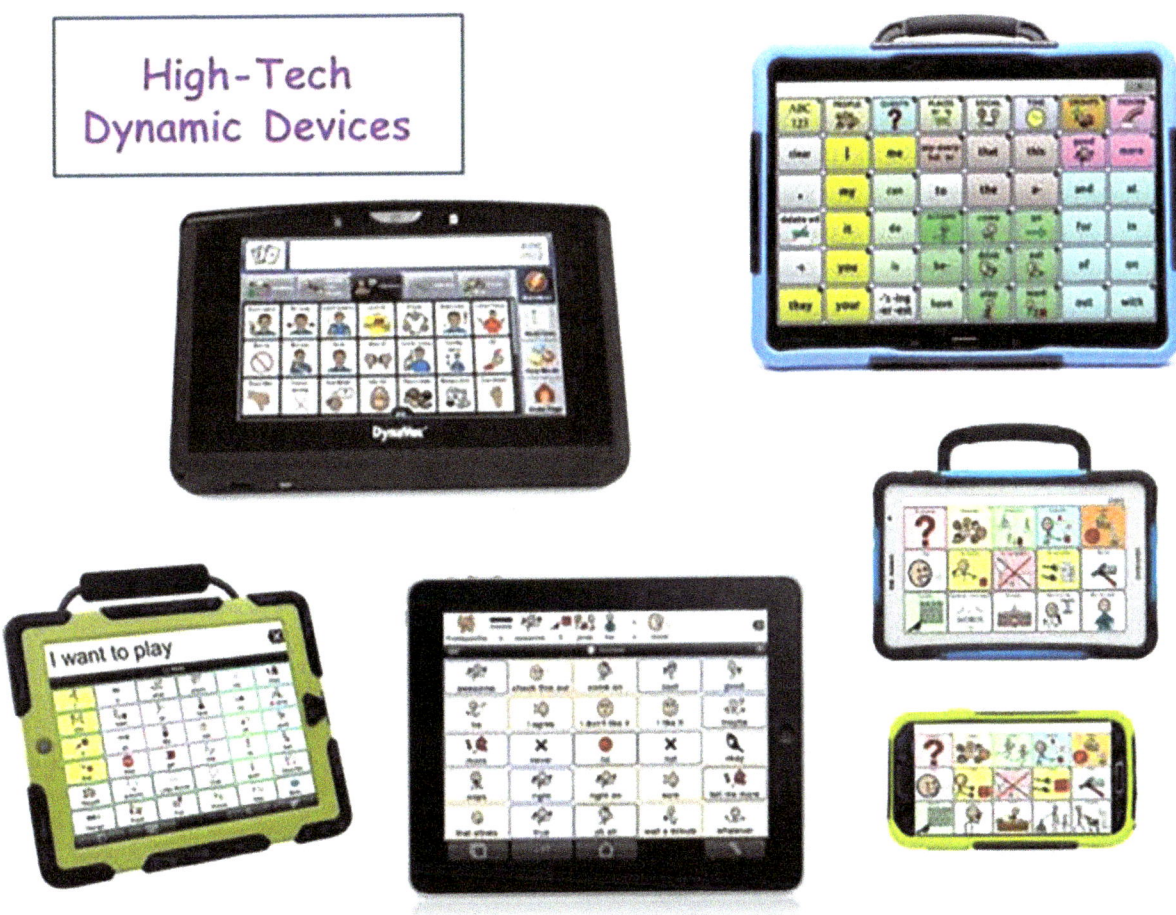

FIGURE 14–2. High-tech AAC. *Source:* The Autism Helper (https://theautismhelper.com/what-is-aac).

activities. Because high-tech systems are designed to support a robust vocabulary, they are well suited to support a range of communicative functions.

Access

Whether the person uses no-tech or high-tech AAC, another important consideration is how they access their system. There are two main access methods for AAC: direct selection and scanning. As implied, with direct selection, the AAC user can select their message directly by touching the symbol with their finger, hand, or even toe. Direct selection methods also include eye-gaze technologies in which the individual with CCN fixates their eyes on a symbol for a specific amount of time to select it.

When an individual does not have the ability to physically select a message, another mode of access is through scanning. Scanning (also known as indirect selection) involves the AAC technology scanning through a set of symbols and the AAC user selecting the symbol they want to say (e.g., by activating a switch, blinking) when the symbol is highlighted (Figure 14–3). Scanning can also be done using a communication partner instead of an electronic device. Here, the communication partner verbally scans through a set of letters or words and the communication partner indicates which letter/word they want the communication partner to stop at (again by blinking or gesturing, etc.).

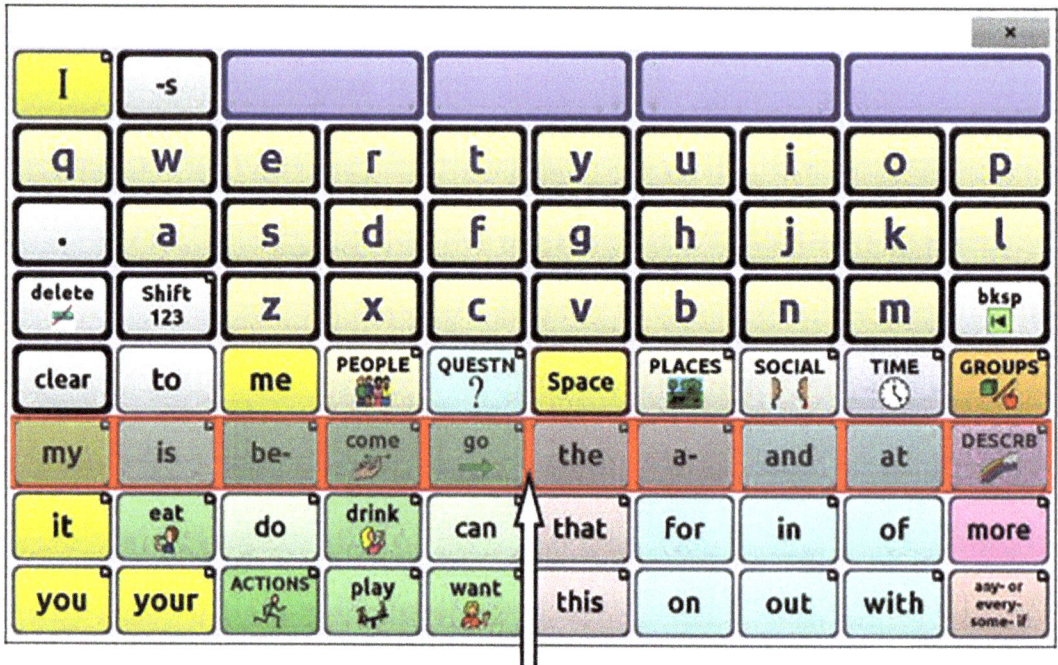

Row highlighted

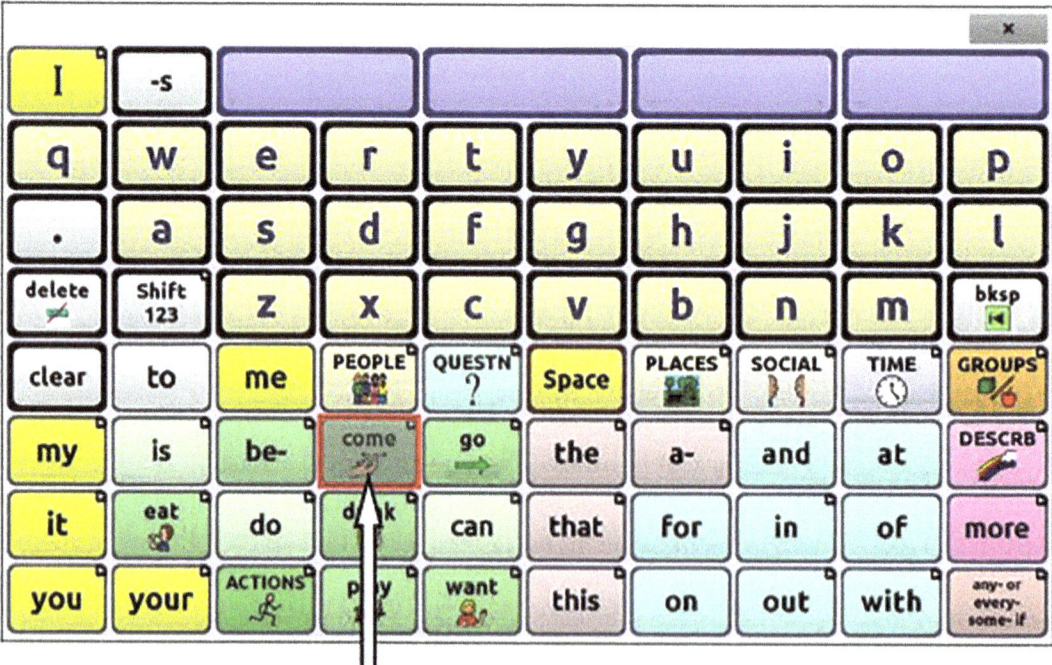

Button highlighted

FIGURE 14–3. Scanning selection method. *Source:* Saltillo (https://saltillo.com/support/article/scanning-patterns).

Symbols and Vocabulary

One of the main factors to consider when selecting an AAC system is what symbols and vocabulary will be used to communicate the speaker's messages. Symbols usually include alphabet-, word-, and picture-based systems. If the individual has already developed or is learning literacy skills, having an alphabet-based symbol system incorporated into their AAC will be important. Many AAC systems have a combination of alphabet, word, phrase, and picture symbols.

In addition to the type of symbols, the type of vocabulary the person will have access to must also be considered. When an AAC system includes word- and/or picture-based symbols, there are two main types of vocabulary words: core and fringe. **Core vocabulary** refers to high-frequency words that are used across people and settings and serve various grammatical purposes. Core words are a small class of words that make up roughly 80% of the words we speak and include pronouns (e.g., I, you, he, she, it), verbs (e.g., want, like, see, eat), prepositions (e.g., in, on, over), and articles (e.g., a, the). A defining feature of core words is that they can be used for various purposes and combined with other core words and fringe vocabulary to generate numerous phrases and sentences. **Fringe vocabulary**, on the other hand, refers primarily to nouns that are specific to certain contexts (e.g., ball, bubbles, goldfish, cookie, cat, dog). These vocabulary words are less frequently occurring in our everyday communication and are important for talking about specific events or activities. Fringe words are most useful when they are combined with core words. Table 14–1 lists the "first 40" core vocabulary words.

Importance of AAC

We communicate for so many reasons. On a daily basis, we communicate to get our needs met, ask questions and gain information, share information, tell stories, empathize, refuse or refute, plan, tell jokes or deceive, self-regulate, persuade, and so much more. Having a wide range of communicative functions allows us to engage meaningfully with other people, participate in daily activities, and contribute to

TABLE 14–1. Dynamic Learning Maps Core Vocabulary "First 40"

1.	I	like	not	want
2.	help	it	more	different
3.	who	she	you	he
4.	where	up	on	in
5.	me	make	get	look
6.	what	need	are	is
7.	some	put	all	this
8.	don't	that	go	do
9.	when	finished	can	here
10.	open	turn	stop	over

Source: Dynamic Learning Maps.

society. We do not just communicate verbally with others; we also communicate through writing. We write papers to support our arguments, we e-mail others to schedule appointments, we text friends to keep in touch, and we post on social media to share ideas with larger audiences. These communicative experiences are a form of self-expression that help shape our identities and contribute to our sense of self. And this is the reason why AAC (and a properly selected one at that) is so important to individuals with CCNs. AAC provides those with CCNs the opportunity to engage with the world in ways that are fundamental to the development of oneself. So, let's talk about who can benefit from AAC.

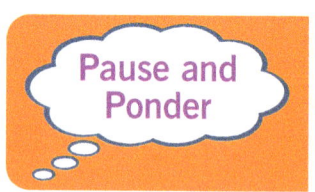 Think about the reasons that you communicate every day. Write them down. What did you come up with?

AAC Users

Augmentative and alternative communication is useful for anyone. There are no specific conditions or criteria that a person must meet to be eligible to use AAC. Although we often think of people who are nonspeaking as being the beneficiaries of aided communication, it is also the case that those who speak can use AAC. For example, perhaps a person has some verbal speech or can verbally communicate in some settings or with some people but has challenges doing so in other settings. This person is a candidate for AAC. Perhaps a person has verbal speech and primarily relies on echolalia to communicate with others. This person is a candidate for AAC. Perhaps the person has verbal speech and can verbally communicate early in the day when their energy level is optimal but begins to become fatigued as the day goes on or the verbal demands increase. This person is also a candidate for AAC. The point here is that there are no set rules to follow or boxes to check with regard to deciding who can benefit from AAC. However, because AAC is useful for those with CCNs, some groups of people rely on AAC more than others. These include children and adults with either developmental or acquired conditions. Some common developmental conditions that are associated with the use of AAC include autism, Down syndrome, childhood apraxia of speech, and cerebral palsy. AAC assessment and intervention will look different in these populations compared to those with acquired conditions because AAC is the primary mode through which they are *learning* language (more on this in a later section). Adults who have an acquired communication disorder, such as aphasia, dysarthria, or apraxia of speech, most often have already learned language and verbally communicated before their injury or disease, and thus AAC assessment and intervention will focus more on rehabilitation or maintenance of language structures.

AAC Assessment

One of the first and most important components of AAC assessment is that it is not a one-person job. Although SLPs are professionals who focus on language and communication (and thus are key players in an AAC assessment), there are other aspects of AAC that are important to consider when conducting an assessment of this kind. Consider the myriad skills that must go into using an AAC system. Yes, we must focus on language (both receptive and expressive), but we also need to think about motor skills (both fine and gross motor), visual and auditory functioning, and literacy skills. Therefore, the assessment team for an AAC evaluation must be interdisciplinary, bringing in perspectives and expertise from various professions. These teams should include the SLP, AAC specialist (if the SLP is not one), physical therapist, occupational therapist, vision and hearing specialists, general or special education teacher as necessary (and appropriate), and, as always, the client and their caregiver(s).

As with any evaluation, a necessary first step is to interview the client and/or their caregivers. Doing so will give the team valuable information not only about the person's present communication abilities but also about their strengths, values, and goals. Designing an intervention plan without understanding a person's values and goals will very likely result in abandonment of the AAC system and reduced or missed communicative opportunities. The interview part of the evaluation includes gathering information about how the client currently communicates—verbally, using signs, or through gestures or objects—and for what purposes—to requests, refuse, share information, or for social purposes. Conducting a semistructured interview with the client/caregivers can give the team valuable information to consider when implementing AAC. Consider why gaining an understanding of the client's goals and values would be an integral part of the assessment.

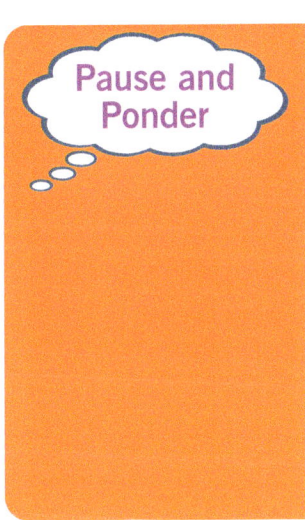

Questions that are important to ask during a semistructured interview include the following:

- How does the client currently communicate? With whom?
- What does the client usually communicate about? (functions)
- If there is a communication breakdown/miscommunication, how do they attempt to solve it?
- What are the client's strengths/challenges around communication?
- What does the client like/is interested in? What motivates them?
- What goals and values does the client have? What goals and values do caregivers have?

From here, the SLP can evaluate the client's receptive and expressive language skills. Standardized assessment tools can be used to assess language; however, observing the client in numerous settings and with various communication partners will be of utmost value because it will provide the team with a comprehensive picture of the client's language abilities in real-world settings. It is also important to gather information about the client's abilities from multiple people who know the individual well, including caregivers, spouses, teachers, siblings, and so on. Obtaining information from several sources allows the SLP to form a comprehensive understanding of how the client participates and engages in activities throughout their day.

AAC assessment often includes evaluation of the client's literacy skills, gross and fine motor abilities, as well as vision and hearing. These parts of the assessment will be completed by other members of the interdisciplinary team, including special educators, physical and occupational therapists, as well as vision and hearing specialists. Results from these components of the evaluation will help determine the most appropriate access features to consider when selecting an AAC system.

Once information about the client's abilities has been gathered, it is time to get to the actual AAC part of the evaluation—matching the client with the most appropriate tools to communicate. By this point in the assessment, the SLP has likely determined whether the client will rely solely on AAC or will use it to supplement existing verbal speech, and if a no-tech or high-tech system will be most appropriate. If it is determined that a high-tech device is most appropriate, ensuring that the system is equipped with a robust vocabulary will support SNUG and lead to a greater number of communicative functions. In any case, it is important that the client try multiple systems over a period of time and in various settings before one is selected. This helps the team decide which system will be the most successful and have the least risk of abandonment.

AAC Intervention

After completing the AAC assessment and matching the client with the most appropriate system, the SLP can start using the AAC system to support the person's language and communication goals. As previously mentioned, this will look different depending on whether the client has a developmental or acquired communication disorder. Although there are certainly myriad factors to consider, for the purpose of this book, we break AAC intervention down into two categories: supporting language and communication in (a) individuals with developmental conditions and (b) individuals with acquired conditions. Regardless of the type of communication disorder the person has, successful AAC intervention has three main components. Successful AAC intervention for any client (a) aligns with their current communication abilities and needs, (b) is set up to meet their future communication abilities and needs, and (c) focuses on communication in real-world settings (Light & Mcnaughton, 2015). For these reasons, a comprehensive AAC assessment is necessary to ensure that the intervention will be as effective as possible. In addition, the overall goal of AAC intervention is to support participation and communication in various contexts for all. For some, AAC intervention will serve to support and supplement verbal speech by increasing intelligibility, as may be the case with someone who has apraxia of speech and is highly unintelligible. For others, AAC will be the primary verbal means by which a person communicates because verbal speech is not sufficient.

AAC Intervention for Developmental Conditions

Using AAC with individuals with developmental conditions means that AAC is supporting language acquisition—that is supporting the development of language. This is important because these individuals will need the same instruction in language as their non-AAC user peers who are developing spoken language. And this is why a system with a robust vocabulary is key. Imagine teaching the domains of language—phonology, semantics, syntax, morphology, and pragmatics—using only a handful of selected nouns. If it sounds impossible, that's because it is. Language instruction involves the integration of all domains and functions of language, and language is complex! To teach language, AAC systems need to have robust vocabularies that include both core and fringe vocabulary.

One of the key strategies to teach language to AAC users involves others modeling language input on the AAC system. This is called **modeling** (also referred to as **aided language stimulation**). Modeling occurs when the communication partner uses AAC (paired with verbal speech) to talk with the person with a CCN. This approach to teaching language is precisely how non-AAC users learn language—adults providing rich language environments by modeling vocabulary, grammatical structures, and language organization. Modeling is most appropriate when it is done at a level that is slightly higher than the individual's current language output (within their zone of proximal development; Vygotsky, 1978). For example, if someone with a CCN is just learning language and AAC, the communication partner would model one-word utterances. If the AAC user frequently uses one-word utterances, the communication partner would model using two-word utterances (and so on). In addition, modeling does not mean finding every single word on the device that you are verbally saying. For example, if you are talking to a child who uses AAC and verbally say, "I like to watch movies," you might only model one or two of those words on the AAC device (e.g., "I" or "LIKE" or "I LIKE"). The words you choose to model will depend on the focus of your treatment session and what vocabulary you are targeting. An important component of modeling is that it should be done *without expecting* the AAC user to communicate in return (i.e., *modeling without expectation*). And modeling takes time. Think about language development in young children. From the moment a child is born, adults are constantly modeling language, and it is not until children are roughly 1 year old that we expect them to say their first words. We then wait another year or so before we expect children to combine words. And this is at a rate of children hearing around 125,000 words per week (Sennott et al., 2016). That's a lot of modeling language! The same principles are true for AAC users. We cannot expect language output with AAC if we are not modeling it extensively over time, in various settings, and using all communicative functions of language.

AAC Intervention for Acquired Conditions

For individuals who have an acquired communication disorder (including ALS, TBI, a motor speech disorder, or dementia), it is highly likely that they had mastery over their expressive language prior to the onset of their communication disorder. This means that intervention will likely not focus on language acquisition but, rather, on explicit instruction of the system for the AAC user as well as their primary caregivers. Providing ongoing training to communication partners is crucial to the success of AAC intervention (Beukelman et al., 2007) because caregivers and communication partners are likely to change over time. For individuals who have a progressive motor disorder without cognitive deficits, such as ALS, setting the person up with a high-tech eye-tracking AAC system early on in their disease will likely be important for continued communicative success as their motor skills deteriorate over time. For many adults who rely on literacy skills, such as those with ALS and TBI, word prediction technology can allow for increased effectiveness and efficiency of communication. For individuals whose condition results in a severe language impairment, such as various aphasias (i.e., loss of language following damage to portions of the brain responsible for language), a variety of low- and high-tech systems, such as personalized communication books, written word messages, and picture-based speech generative devices, can be used to support communication; however, acceptance of these systems by those with aphasia and their family members has historically been low (Beukelman et al., 2007). **Visual scene displays**, which are contextualized photographs with embedded messages or text, may be one strategy for those with aphasia to share stories and engage in meaningful communication (Beukelman et al., 2007; Light et al., 2019). Figure 14–4 provides an example of a visual scene display used with an adult.

An important feature of AAC intervention for both those with developmental conditions and those with acquired conditions is communication partner training (Kent-Walsh et al., 2015). **Communication partner training** involves teaching those who frequently communicate with the AAC user how to use the system, what to expect from the AAC user, and how to model language. Primary communication partners often include parents, caregivers, teachers, and siblings. This teaching strategy is crucial because the AAC user spends most of their day *without* the SLP. It is not enough to simply teach others the ins

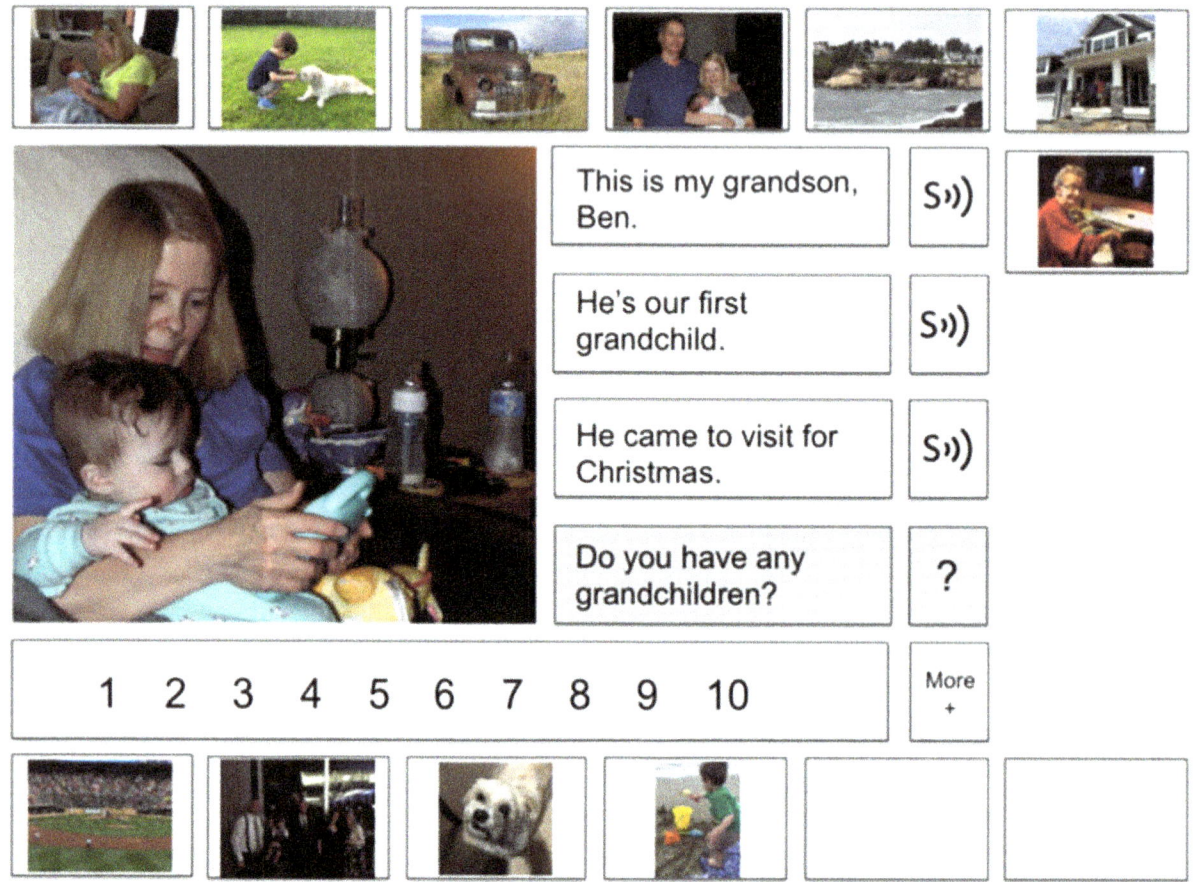

FIGURE 14–4. Visual scene display for an adult. *Source:* Janice Light, Krista M. Wilkinson, Amber Thiessen, David R. Beukelman, & Susan Koch Fager (2019): Designing effective AAC displays for individuals with developmental or acquired disabilities: State of the science and future research directions, *Augmentative and Alternative Communication, 35*(1), 42–55. https://doi.org/10.1080/07434618.2018.1558283

and outs of the AAC system and how it operates; communication partner training involves teaching how to use the system to support language in real time during actual communication activities (Kent-Walsh & Mcnaughton, 2005; Marra & Micco, 2019). Training others how to communicate with AAC users supports communication across people and environments (Kent-Walsh et al., 2015), reduces the likelihood that AAC will be abandoned or discontinued, and provides opportunities for more meaningful communication interactions.

Considerations for AAC

As we hope you are aware by now, AAC is important for so many reasons. It allows those who cannot fully rely on verbal speech to participate in so many aspects of life. In this section, we discuss a variety of factors that must be considered to ensure that AAC is successful. Here, we discuss AAC abandonment, multimodal communication, bilingual AAC users, and myths surrounding the use of AAC.

AAC Abandonment

Now that we have discussed what AAC is, as well as how to assess and provide intervention to AAC users, let's talk about factors that can make or break the use of AAC. **AAC abandonment**, or the discontinuation/rejection of AAC, occurs frequently despite AAC being an important tool for supporting individuals with complex communication needs (Johnson et al., 2006). Communication partner education and training are key factors in reducing the likelihood of AAC abandonment. Families and caregivers have reported myriad reasons that they reject AAC for their loved ones, including the additional work required of families to implement the AAC system into their daily routines, the individual not using the system in a way that feels like meaningful communication, caregivers themselves not being satisfied with the system, a perceived lack of knowledge of and support from the SLP, as well as lack of communication with the caregivers on the part of the SLP (Moorcroft et al., 2019a, 2021). Other factors that play a role in AAC abandonment are barriers that come with using AAC. These include opportunity barriers and access barriers (Beukelman & Light, 2020), which can also be thought of as environmental and personal barriers, respectively (Moorcroft et al., 2019b). **Opportunity barriers** include ways in which the environment limits the person's ability to participate in communicative activities using AAC. Examples include negative attitudes about AAC users' abilities, communication partners having inadequate knowledge or skills to communicate with AAC users, and policies and practices that prohibit use of technology in certain settings or transfer of AAC devices across environments over time (Beukelman & Light, 2020; Moorcroft et al., 2019b). **Access barriers**, on the other hand, result from challenges that are directly related to the AAC user, whether that be their own limitations in communicating using the system or their ability to physically access the system as intended. Examples include lack of motivation to communicate using a given system, being unable to physically access the system because of motor or vision challenges, and discrepancies between the language spoken at home and at school and ensuring that language and culture are reflected on the AAC device (Beukelman & Light, 2020; Moorcroft et al., 2019b).

Evidence suggests that just as there are barriers that can lead to AAC abandonment, there are also facilitators that can support the maintenance of AAC use. That is, environmental and personal factors can also facilitate and promote the use of AAC. Examples of environmental facilitators include communication partners being knowledgeable and skilled in the use of AAC (often through communication partner training), collaboration between stakeholders implementing AAC intervention, and societal awareness of AAC (Beukelman & Light, 2020; Moorcroft et al., 2019b). Examples of personal factors that facilitate AAC use include the client being motivated to use the AAC system, having the appropriate access method to support effective and efficient communication, and having a system that aligns with the person's cultural values (Beukelman & Light, 2020; Moorcroft et al., 2019b).

Multimodal Communication

Because several personal factors that facilitate AAC use have to do with the system itself, selecting the most appropriate AAC systems, and making sure they are accessible, is key. One way to increase the accessibility and utility of AAC is through multimodal communication. This means teaching AAC users to communicate in a variety of ways and honoring all forms of their communication. Sometimes a person with a CCN will rely on high-tech AAC systems to communicate, and other times that same person will communicate using a low-tech communication board, writing, or gestures. Teaching AAC users to communicate using numerous methods will allow them access to communication that is efficient and effective given the circumstance (Sigafoos & Drawsgow, 2001). This should not come as a surprise because most people frequently engage in multimodal communication. For example, a person can simply nod their head to indicate "yes" without verbally speaking the word, gesture toward an object out of reach to request it without verbally asking for it, and give a "thumbs up" to communicate affirmation.

Bilingual AAC Users

Much of the research and information regarding AAC use have centered around monolingual speakers despite the growing number of bilingual individuals who have speech and/or language impairments (Soto & Yu, 2014). Assessment, customization, and intervention for AAC with monolingual speakers require an interprofessional approach in which each team member has a unique skill set related to language development, access, technology, and so on. SLPs who have specific knowledge in bilingualism are practiced in skills pertaining to assessment and intervention to support language development across languages, as well as how to engage with and support families from various cultural and linguistic backgrounds (Soto & Yu, 2021). This means that to address AAC needs in bilingual language learners, SLPs must understand the various components of AAC assessment, intervention, and personalization, as well as have a solid understanding of bilingual and multilingual language development and impairment.

Bilingual individuals often switch between the language they use at home, school, and in the community, and they indicate the importance of being able to communicate across these settings (Tönsing et al., 2019). As such, it is critical that AAC intervention focus on both (or all) languages, not just the language spoken with the SLP (King et al., 2021), so that individuals can be better understood by those around them as well as feel a sense of belonging in their communities (Tönsing et al., 2019). Evidence suggests that English–Spanish-speaking bilingual children with and without language disorders can differentiate between the different visual layouts of Spanish versus English vocabulary on two separate AAC devices (King et al., 2021); however, the children in this study did not rely on AAC to communicate. AAC users who speak more than one language may also switch between communication modalities. That is, they may use high-tech AAC with voice output in one language while using verbal speech or sign in a second language (King & Soto, 2022).

One important consideration for bilingual AAC systems (as with monolingual AAC systems) is the selection of the most appropriate vocabulary. Because languages do not have the same core vocabulary words (Mngomezulu et al., 2019; Shin & Hill, 2016), using translations of English core vocabulary for bilingual AAC users is not linguistically or culturally appropriate. Core vocabulary lists have been researched and developed for various languages, including, but not limited to, Hebrew (Savaldi-Harussi & Uziel, 2023), Korean (Shin & Hill, 2016), Mandarin (Liu & Sloane, 2006), Spanish (Soto & Cooper, 2021), Yolnu (Amery et al., 2022), and Zulu (Mngomezulu et al., 2019). Despite the growing interest in bilingual AAC access, more research is necessary to better understand the way that bilingual speakers can have the best possible access to AAC in various modalities across their language environments.

Myths of AAC

By now, it should be apparent how important AAC is for individuals who cannot rely on verbal speech to communicate fully. Unfortunately, there are some common misconceptions about the value and utility of AAC. Although these claims are unsubstantiated, and a large body of research has debunked these myths, it is important to call attention to them so that we can continue to spread awareness around AAC (Jensen et al., 2023).

Myth 1

One of the main myths surrounding AAC is that children who are taught to use AAC will not develop verbal language. The belief is that when children rely on an external tool to access language, they will not develop language in the same ways as their speaking peers. Decades of research shows that AAC in fact promotes expressive and receptive language development, even in early childhood (Lal, 2010; Romski et al., 2015; Rose et al., 2020). Research also suggests that AAC positively impacts social behavior (Lal, 2010) and literacy skills, including letter–sound correspondence, phonemic awareness, and word reading (for a review, see Machalicek et al., 2010). To ensure that children who use AAC have access to evidence-based reading instruction, it is essential to understand their baseline literacy skills (e.g., print awareness) early on in childhood (Collins et al., 2023).

Myth 2

A similar myth regarding AAC use is that children will not be motivated to use verbal speech if they become accustomed to using an AAC system. To dispel this belief, research shows that using AAC can promote the development of verbal speech production for some children (Millar et al., 2006; Romski et al., 2015; White et al., 2021).

Myth 3

A third myth associated with AAC is that young children are too young and thus not ready to use it. This myth is not valid because young children develop communication skills as they are exposed to language input in their environment. Verbally speaking children develop verbal language through exposure, and this exposure happens as soon as the child is born. Moreover, a body of research supports the use of unaided AAC (e.g., gestures, sign) with infants and toddlers, and the existing evidence is promising for the use of aided AAC with this population (for a review, see Branson & Demchak, 2009).

Myth 4

Another main myth associated with AAC is that individuals require certain cognitive prerequisite skills to use AAC, such as understanding cause and effect, receptive language, and use of eye contact. In fact, the opposite has been shown to be true. That is, these skills can develop in conjunction with the development of communication through AAC use (Holyfield et al., 2019; Kangas & Lloyd, 1998; Romski & Sevcik, 1998).

Application to a Child

Jacob Finnley (pseudonym) is a 7-year-old male in first grade. Jacob is White and lives in a two-parent household with two older siblings in which the only language spoken is English. Jacob attends a public elementary school in the United States. At birth, Jacob was diagnosed with Down syndrome. Jacob enjoys playing outside with friends, dancing, and playing with his Bert and Ernie dolls.

Jacob began receiving speech-language therapy at age 2 years. Early intervention at this time was focused on the production of speech sounds at the sound level and following simple one-step directions. At age 3 years, in his first year of preschool, speech and language services focused on receptive language, particularly identifying nouns (e.g., animals, toys, food), colors, and shapes, as well as following one-step directions. At this time, Jacob was also given access to a choice board to request preferred activities and foods. In his second year of preschool (age 4 years), Jacob began seeing a new SLP who continued to work on the aforementioned goals and also introduced a no-tech communication system. In his third year of preschool (age 5 years), Jacob transitioned from using solely a no-tech AAC system to using a high-tech speech-generating device on an iPad. Jacob currently attends a first-grade general education class with 30 minutes per week of pullout occupational therapy, 30 minutes per day of speech-language therapy, and 30 minutes per day of academic support.

Jacob was recently referred for an AAC evaluation. The results presented here summarize his language, motor, cognitive, literacy, and visual/auditory skills, along with information gathered from his parents and teachers.

Jacob's receptive language and vocabulary are significantly below average. He can follow simple one-step directions in structured settings and identify basic shapes, colors, and nouns. In addition to his below average receptive language skills, Jacob's current expressive speech and language skills are severely impaired. He can vocalize the following sounds: /b/, /p/, /w/, /t/, /d/, /m/, /n/, /æ/, /ɛ/, /i/, /ɪ/, /o/, /u/, /ə/, /ɑ/, and /ʌ/. Jacob can also vocalize the following words: /mɑ/, /bɑ/, /dæ/, /dædæ/, /mɑmɑ/, and /bʌbʌ/. His expressive language also consists of shaking and nodding of his head, vocalizing, and using refusal gestures and facial expressions to indicate "no" and "yes." He also has a few approximations of manual signs (e.g., touches pointer fingers together to indicate "more") and initiates interactions with familiar people by grabbing their hands. He can request preferred items (nouns and people) on his AAC device at the one-word level but demonstrates inconsistent use of the device for other communicative functions and longer utterances.

Jacob demonstrates relatively good gross motor skills; he is ambulatory and demonstrates functional use of his upper and lower extremities. He can carry items up to 5 pounds in weight and carry a backpack on his back or bag across his shoulder. Although Jacob demonstrates below average fine motor abilities and has difficulty holding a writing utensil, he has demonstrated the ability to point to and distinguish between pictures as small as ¼ inch.

Cognitive testing was challenging to complete due to Jacob's limited expressive language and poor receptive language abilities. Jacob's reading and writing skills are significantly below grade level. He is unable to read any sight words. Jacob's visual abilities are within normal limits. He presents with a mild sensorineural bilateral hearing loss.

Jacob's parents report that they understand his communication 50% of the time because they know their son well and are accustomed to his likes and wants. They also report that they want Jacob to use verbal speech as his primary mode of communication. Although they have recently become more open to him using AAC, they were hesitant to use it in the past. One of the family's primary goals for Jacob is for him to learn to read.

Jacob's teachers report that Jacob has difficulty expressing his needs, wants, and ideas in class and that he often attempts to share his ideas with peers and teachers without much success. His limited expressive language skills impact his ability to participate in both academic and social classroom activities. He often resorts to communicating through behaviors that are disruptive to other students' learning, which has begun to increase since the classroom demands have increased. This results in Jacob spending more time in the resource room than in the general education environment. His teachers report that Jacob often becomes frustrated when his teachers and friends do not understand what he is trying to communicate.

To support Jacob's communication and participation in everyday activities, the most effective AAC intervention technique is modeling. As part of the intervention, the SLP teaches Jacob's family and school team about the value of AAC, the myths associated with AAC, and how modeling language using an AAC device is invaluable to support Jacob's language development. Because the SLP does not have much time to connect with Jacob's family during the school day, she sends home videos of her and Jacob using AAC in therapy sessions and highlights what words she is focusing on for modeling each week. Because Jacob is currently using his AAC device at the one-word level inconsistently, the SLP begins by modeling one- and two-word utterances on the AAC device without expecting Jacob to use the device. Intervention is primarily play-based using toys, games, and activities that Jacob enjoys. Jacob's Bert and Ernie dolls are often incorporated into the sessions because Jacob is highly motivated to play with these dolls. During these sessions, the SLP uses the device to model various communicative functions during play, including requesting (e.g., "I WANT to play with Bert"), commenting (e.g., "I LIKE Ernie's shirt"), rejecting (e.g., "I DON'T THINK that Bernie likes his soup"), and for social purposes (e.g., "Bert is saying HI to Ernie and to you!"). In addition, because Jacob is in first grade and one of his family's primary goals for him is to learn to read, the SLP incorporates reading books into her instruction. When reading books, she models certain target words on the AAC device. For example, when reading *Brown Bear, Brown Bear, What Do You See?* with Jacob, the SLP models the words "YOU SEE" and "I SEE." Because the book is repetitive, this provides various models of these phrases. From there, the SLP continues modeling the word "SEE" in the intervention session, commenting on what she sees in the classroom, and so on.

Application to an Adult

Callum Dristol (pseudonym) is a 51-year-old White male who lives in a single-family home with his wife, Leslie, and twin teenage daughters. Callum speaks English as his first language and French as his second language, as he was born in a French-speaking province of Canada. Although Callum currently lives in the northern United States, his parents and siblings reside in Canada. Soon after his 51st birthday, Callum was diagnosed with ALS and was given 2 years to live. Prior to his diagnosis, Callum was a pediatrician at the local hospital and was in charge of the local running club.

Prior to his diagnosis of ALS, Callum had no speech or language concerns. A few months after receiving the ALS diagnosis, Callum started noticing changes in his voice and speech and decided to undergo a speech evaluation. During the evaluation, Callum noted that he had more articulatory imprecision and his rate of speech was slower than usual, although these changes went unnoticed by others. In addition, Callum noted that he became fatigued by the end of the day, and during these times speaking felt tiring and cumbersome. Ultimately, Callum's symptoms aligned with a mixed flaccid/spastic dysarthria.

Given his diagnosis of ALS, Callum was referred for an AAC evaluation. During this evaluation, the SLP interviewed Callum and his wife to gather a more complete picture of Callum's communication environments (e.g., home, community) and needs (e.g., with whom he communicates, in what capacity). The SLP also gathered information about Callum's current motor skills, sensory capabilities (i.e., vision and hearing), and his familiarity with technology. Because ALS is a degenerative disease that affects muscle movements, the SLP assessed Callum's current motor skills to determine which type of AAC system would be most useful for Callum now and in the future. The SLP examined Callum's eye movements (i.e., his ability to move his eyes up, down, side to side, and diagonally); the movement of his arms, hands, legs, feet, and head; his sensory abilities (i.e., hearing, vision, and residual voice); and his cognition. Eye movements were assessed to determine if Callum was a candidate for eye-tracking technology. Limb and head movement were assessed to determine if Callum was a candidate for AAC devices that rely on scanning and are thus switch operated. Moreover, residual voice was assessed as an option for voice banking. Finally, cognition was assessed to provide information on whether Callum would be able to operate an AAC device, as well as understand the purpose of and how to use the device.

Results of the assessment revealed that Callum has functional movements of his eyes, a desire to record his residual voice and transfer these recordings to a high-tech AAC system, and the cognitive skills to understand the purpose of communicating with an eye-tracking AAC device. In addition to ordering the eye-tracking AAC device and beginning the process of recording and storing Callum's voice, the SLP also provided Callum with a no-tech communication board to use during times when he no longer has functional use of his voice and his high-tech device is unavailable or needs updating/fixing. The no-tech communication board consists of phrases that are deemed important to Callum as determined by Callum and his family (e.g., "I need help," "please readjust my head," "yes," "no").

Intervention for Callum primarily consists of teaching him and his family how to use his AAC systems (eye gaze and communication board) while he is in the early stages of his disease progression. Integrating his AAC into his daily life early on is an important step to ensuring that Callum will have a meaningful way to communicate when he can no longer use his voice to speak. To decrease the likelihood of AAC abandonment, the SLP conducts periodic check-ins to see how the device is being used in Callum's home. Moreover, these check-ins also serve to monitor Callum's physical and cognitive skills as his ALS progresses to ensure that his AAC matches his capabilities. For example, if Callum loses range of motion in his eye movements and is no longer able to use his high-tech eye-tracking device, the SLP will need to adjust his communication system based on his intact functions. This may mean using a no-tech communication system that relies purely on yes/no questions such as "Are you in pain?" "Do you need your head adjusted?" and "Are you feeling anxious?"

Chapter Summary

This chapter focuses on AAC, which is any form of communication that supplements or replaces verbal speech. A wide range of individuals use ACC, including both adults and children who may have no verbal speech, only use verbal speech in certain settings, and whose verbal speech may be unintelligible to their listeners. AAC allows individuals with CCNs to participate in activities that would be difficult without communication. It is important to remember that AAC is communication—it is just accessed through a mode other than verbal speech.

There are different types of AAC, which can best be categorized into two main groups: aided and unaided. Unaided AAC refers to any mode of communication that a person uses which does not rely on an external tool. Unaided AAC consists of nonverbal communication, which varies by culture based on the set of rules that culture has for the meaning behind specific nonverbal behaviors. Aided AAC comprises systems that are used for communication that are external to the speaker. Important subgroups of aided AAC include no-tech/low-tech and high-tech systems. No-tech and low-tech options have either very little or no technology involved. High-tech systems rely heavily on the use of technology and often include apps that are commercially available on personal tablets and computers designed for communication. AAC systems can be accessed by the user through directly selecting the message by touching it, using a laser pointer, through eye gaze, or even by scanning through and selecting messages by blinking or using small muscle movements. No-tech systems are often used in conjunction with high-tech systems to create more comprehensive and robust access to language, especially in environments in which technology cannot be used. High-tech devices allow for a stronger vocabulary than no-tech devices because they are equipped with software that supports multiple vocabulary sets; have various voice output settings and languages; and can be connected to e-mail and text messaging, allowing for messages to be sent digitally. Although there are advantages and disadvantages to both no-tech/low-tech and high-tech systems, the most appropriate choice will depend on the individual and their specific needs.

We use communication for a wide variety of reasons. Our communicative experiences are a form of self-expression that help shape our identities and contribute to our sense of self. This highlights the reason why a properly selected AAC is so important for individuals with CCNs. AAC assessment teams need to be interdisciplinary so that different perspectives and expertise can be brought from various professions. The first step in the evaluation is to conduct an interview, thus allowing the team to gain valuable information about the person's current communication abilities, strengths, values, and goals. Ensuring that an intervention plan is focused on the client's goals will minimize abandonment of the AAC system. AAC assessment will often also include observations of the client in different communication settings, evaluation of the client's literacy skills and gross and fine motor abilities, and vision and hearing testing. It is important to have the client try multiple systems in different settings to ensure a good fit and ultimately provide the best results.

AAC intervention is used to support language and communication in individuals with developmental conditions and individuals with acquired conditions. Individuals with developmental conditions use AAC to support language development and benefit from a system that includes both core and fringe vocabulary. For individuals with acquired conditions, intervention will likely focus more on explicit instruction of the system for the client and their caregiver. Communication partner training is important whether the individual has a developmental or acquired condition because the partner will be with them more than will the SLP. Proper communication partner training can help avoid AAC abandonment.

The use of multimodal communication can increase accessibility and utility of AAC. Having the AAC user be able to communicate using numerous methods will allow them to communicate more effectively and efficiently because they can change how they communicate depending on the circumstance.

AAC is heavily centered around monolingual speakers, but it is important for SLPs to understand bilingual and multilingual language development and impairment. Bilinguals often switch between languages depending on the setting they are in or who they are talking to, which is why AAC intervention for bilinguals must focus on all languages spoken by the individual. It is important to note that just as with monolingual AAC systems, bilingual AAC systems must be equipped with the most appropriate vocabulary to support language use across settings. More research is needed regarding AAC systems for bilingual users.

Chapter Review Questions

1. What is AAC and who can use it?
2. What are the two main types of AAC and how do they differ from each other?
3. Why might it be beneficial to use the different levels of technology systems in conjunction with each other?
4. How do you determine what level of technology is appropriate for the AAC user?
5. Why is it important to ensure that an individual with CCN receives a properly selected AAC device?
6. Is AAC limited to those who are nonspeaking? Why or why not?
7. Name some common developmental conditions that are associated with AAC use.
8. Who is involved in AAC assessment?
9. This chapter discusses the importance of conducting an interview as the first step in the evaluation process. Why? What do you think might be some consequences to not doing this?
10. What is core vocabulary? Fringe vocabulary? Why is it important for AAC systems to have both?
11. List three reasons why an individual might abandon their AAC system.
12. What are opportunity barriers? Access barriers?
13. What are the three main components to successful AAC intervention for any client?
14. Discuss why using modeling is important in teaching language to AAC users and why modeling without expectation should be implemented.
15. The focus for AAC users with developmental conditions is language learning. What is the focus for AAC users with acquired conditions?
16. Why is the communication partner's role important in the AAC user's success?
17. What are some examples of facilitators that can support the maintenance of AAC use?
18. Multimodal communication is discussed as a valuable way to increase the accessibility and utility of AAC. Why is this the case?
19. Why is it important for AAC devices to support all languages spoken by the individual?
20. Why is it not appropriate to use translations of English core vocabulary for bilingual AAC users?

Learning Activities

1. Observe an individual without a communication disorder. Take notes on the messages that they are communicating. Note which functions they use to communicate (to request, reject, share information, get information, entertain, etc.).

2. Choose a video, film, or piece of literature to watch/read that tells the story of a person using AAC. Write a 3- or 4-page paper describing the AAC used, including the following:
   a. Brief synopsis of the film and character, including the disability represented.
   b. Information about the type of AAC used.
   c. The advantages and disadvantages of the AAC modality.
   d. The main communicative function(s) the device was used for.
   e. What other AAC methods could be appropriate for this person? And why?

3. When we model with AAC, we do not model every word that we verbally speak. For the following sentences, indicate which words you would choose to model if your client spoke in one-word utterances, two-word utterances, or three-word utterances:
   a. I want more cookies.
   b. I like your jacket.
   c. Do you want to make a cake?

4. Select a children's book. Highlight the core and fringe vocabulary words on each page. Then, with this list of core and fringe vocabulary words, see how many utterances you can come up with by combing them in generative ways.

5. Select a photo that has personal meaning to you (e.g., a photo of your birthday party or your last family vacation). Design a visual scene display using this photo. What sentences would you create to tell the story associated with this picture?

6. Create a handout/visual on debunking AAC myths and how to prevent AAC abandonment. Make sure your information is accessible to your target audience. Present your handout to the class. Create your handout for one or more of the following populations:
   a. Parents of children: Preschool, elementary, and middle/high school
   b. Teachers of children: Preschool, elementary, and middle/high school
   c. Client who is in college/young adult
   d. Client who is an older adult
   e. Caregiver/spouse of a young adult
   f. Caregiver/spouse of an older adult

Suggested Reading

Fäldt, A., Fabian, H., Thunberg, G., & Lucas, S. (2020). "All of a sudden we noticed a difference at home too": Parents' perception of a parent-focused early communication and AAC intervention for toddlers. *Augmentative and Alternative Communication, 36*(3), 143–154.

This article describes ComAlong Toddler, an intervention course aimed to support parents' understanding of and experiences with using AAC with their toddlers. This intervention was composed of individual and group sessions in which the course leader (SLP, psychologist, or special educator) taught parents about how AAC could be used with their own children who were between the ages of 1 and 3 years. During the sessions, parents were also provided with tools that could be used when interacting with their child outside of the sessions. This study describes parents' perception of the ComAlong Toddler intervention, as well as the communicative interactions between the caregiver and the child. After partaking in this intervention, parents described the strategies as being useful in understanding the communication abilities of their child, as well as how to best interact with their child (and even other siblings who were not AAC users). Parents also indicated that after the training, their children were more engaged and interactive with their caregivers. It was also noted that the modeling and instruction provided by the SLP was important to integrating the intervention into their daily lives.

Meinzen-Derr, J., Sheldon, R., Altaye, M., Lane, L., Mays, L., & Wiley, S. (2021). A technology-assisted language intervention for children who are deaf or hard of hearing: A randomized clinical trial. *Pediatrics, 147*(2), Article e2020025734.

This study examined a technology-assisted language intervention (TALI) compared to treatment as usual (TAU) for individuals with mild or greater bilateral hearing loss, aged 3 to 12 years. The authors examined syntax (as measured by mean length of utterances in morphemes [MLU_m] and mean turn length [MTL] in words), semantics (as determined by the number of different words [NDW] in 50 consecutive and complete utterances), and receptive and expressive language scores. Language samples were taken at baseline, 12 weeks, and 24 weeks.

Children in the TAU group received 24 weeks of weekly hour-long therapy sessions targeting language and communication skills without the use of AAC. The goal for each child varied but included discrimination of sounds and phonemes; segmentation of words; and understanding words, phrases, and sentences in context. Children in the TALI group received 24 weeks of therapy (a combination of SLP-directed therapy and self-guided at-home intervention) targeting language and communication, but with the use of AAC as a language-teaching tool. The AAC provided visual support for abstract concepts and gave voice to the selections a child made, thus providing a consistent model for verbalization of target words and concepts. The device was used to help the child create longer and more complex sentences. Children in the TALI group showed greater progress with MLU_m, MTL, and NDW scores, as well as receptive and expressive language, than the TAU group. This suggests that the use of AAC in conjunction with speech-language therapy led to faster improvements than speech-language therapy without the use of AAC. This was consistent with previous studies examining how AAC aid supports language development in other populations.

Morin, K., Ganz, J., Gregori, E. M., Foster, M., Gerow, S., Genç-Tosunn, D., & Hong, E. (2018). A systematic quality review of high-tech AAC interventions as an evidence-based practice. *Augmentative and Alternative Communication, 34*(2), 104–117.

This article is a systematic review that evaluates 17 studies that have used high-tech AAC to teach social communication skills to individuals with complex communication needs who had autism or intellectual disability. The 17 articles that were evaluated had different study designs (i.e., multiple probe, multiple baseline, and alternative treatment designs), which are useful in determining if an intervention is evidence-based. The results of this systematic review suggest that using high-tech AAC to support communication development in individuals with autism and/or intellectual disability in natural contexts is evidence-based; however, this review did not consider which communicative functions high-tech AAC was supporting. More research is needed to conclusively support the evidence base of using AAC to support a variety of communicative functions.

References

American Speech-Language-Hearing Association. (n.d.). *Augmentative and alternative communication (AAC)*. https://www.asha.org/public/speech/disorders/aac

Amery, R., Wunungmurra, P., Bukulatjpi, G., Baker, R., Gumbula, F., Barker, R., . . . Lowell, A. (2022). Augmentative and alternative communication for Aboriginal Australians: Developing core vocabulary for Yolnu speakers. *Augmentative and Alternative Communication, 38*(4), 209–220.

Beukelman, D., Fager, S., Ball, L., & Dietz, A. (2007). AAC for adults with acquired neurological conditions: A review. *Augmentative and Alternative Communication, 23*(3), 230–242.

Beukelman D., & Light, J. (2020). *Augmentative & alternative communication: Supporting children and adults with complex communication needs* (5th ed.). Brookes.

Branson, D., & Demchak, M. (2009). The use of augmentative and alternative communication methods with infants and toddlers with disabilities: A research review. *Augmentative and Alternative Communication, 25*(4), 274–286.

Burgoon, J., Manusov, V., & Guerrer, L. (2021). *Nonverbal communication*. Taylor & Francis.

Collins, S., Barton-Hulsey, A., Timm-Fulkerson, C., & Therrien, M. (2023). AAC & literacy: A scoping review of print knowledge measures for students who use aided augmentative and alternative communication. *Journal of Developmental and Physical Disabilities.* https://doi.org/10.1007/s10882-023-09934-4

Hall, N., Juengling-Sudkamp, J., Gutmann, M., & Cohn, E. (2023). *Fundamentals of AAC: A case-based approach to enhancing communication.* Plural Publishing.

Hill, K. (2014). *Achieving success in AAC: Assessment and intervention*. https://aacinstitute.org/wp-content/uploads/2014/12/Achieving-Success-In-AAC.pdf

Holyfield, C., Caron, J., & Light, J. (2019). Programming AAC just-in-time for beginning communicators: The process. *Augmentative and Alternative Communication, 35*, 309–318.

Jensen, E., Douglas, S., & Gerde, H. (2023). Dispelling myths surrounding AAC use for children: Recommendations for professionals. *Inclusive Practices, 2*(1), 30–36.

Johnson, J., Inglebret, E., Jones, C., & Ray, J. (2006). Perspectives of speech language pathologists regarding success versus abandonment of AAC. *Augmentative and Alternative Communication, 22*, 85–99.

Kangas, K., & Lloyd, L. (1998). Early cognitive skills as prerequisites to augmentative and alternative communication use: What are we waiting for? *Augmentative and Alternative Communication, 4*, 211–221.

Kent-Walsh, J., & Mcnaughton, D. (2005). Communication partner instruction in AAC: Present practices and future directions. *Augmentative and Alternative Communication, 21*(3), 195–204.

Kent-Walsh, J., Murza, K., Malani, M., & Binger, C. (2015). Effects of communication partner instruction on the communication of individuals using AAC: A meta-analysis. *Augmentative and Alternative Communication, 31*(4), 271–284.

King, M., Romski, M., & Sevcik, R. (2021). Language differentiation using augmentative and alternative communication: An investigation of Spanish–English bilingual children with and without language impairments. *American Journal of Speech-Language Pathology, 30*(1), 89–104.

King, M., & Soto, G. (2022). Code-switching using aided AAC: Toward an integrated theoretical framework. *Augmentative and Alternative Communication, 38*(1), 67–76.

Lal, R. (2010). Effect of alternative and augmentative communication on language and social behavior of children with autism. *Educational Research and Reviews, 5*(3), 119–125.

Light, J., & Mcnaughton, D. (2015). Designing AAC research and intervention to improve outcomes for individuals with complex communication needs. *Augmentative and Alternative Communication, 31*, 85–96.

Light, J., Wilkinson, K., Thiessen, A., Beukelman, D., & Fager, S. (2019). Designing effective AAC displays for individuals with developmental or acquired disabilities: State of the science and future research directions. *Augmentative and Alternative Communication, 35*(1), 42–55.

Liu, C., & Sloane, Z. (2006). Developing a core vocabulary for a Mandarin Chinese AAC system using word frequency data. *International Journal of Computer Processing of Oriental Language, 19*(4), 285–300.

Machalicek, W., Sanford, A., Lang, R., Rispoli, M., Molfenter, N., & Mbeseha, M. (2010). Literacy interventions for students with physical and developmental disabilities who use aided AAC devices: A systematic review. *Journal of Developmental and Physical Disabilities, 22*, 219–240.

Marra, L., & Micco, K. (2019). Communication partner training to increase interactive communication using augmentative and alternative communication: A case study. *Perspectives of the ASHA Special Interest Groups, 4*, 584–592.

Millar, D., Light, J., & Schlosser, R. (2006). The impact of augmentative and alternative communication intervention on the speech production of individuals with developmental disabilities: A research review. *Journal of Speech, Language, and Hearing Research, 49*(2), 248–264.

Mngomezulu, J., Tönsing, K., Dada, S., & Bokaba, N. (2019). Determining a Zulu core vocabulary for children who use augmentative and alternative communication. *Augmentative and Alternative Communication, 35*(4), 274–284.

Moorcroft, A., Scarinci, N., & Meyer, C. (2019a). Speech pathologist perspectives on the acceptance versus rejection or abandonment of AAC systems for children with complex communication needs. *Augmentative and Alternative Communication, 35*(3), 193–204.

Moorcroft, A., Scarinci, N., & Meyer, C. (2019b). A systematic review of the barriers and facilitators to the provision and use of low-tech and unaided AAC systems for people with complex communication needs and their families. *Disability and Rehabilitation: Assistive Technology, 14*(7), 710–731.

Moorcroft, A., Scarinci, N., & Meyer, C. (2021). "I've had a love–hate, I mean mostly hate relationship with these PODD books": Parent perceptions of how they and their child contributed to AAC rejection and abandonment. *Disability and Rehabilitation: Assistive Technology, 16*(1), 72–82.

Romski, M., & Sevcik, R. (1998). Augmentative and alternative communication systems: Considerations for individuals with severe intellectual disabilities. *Augmentative and Alternative Communication, 4*(2), 83–93.

Romski, M., Sevcik, R., Barton-Husley, A., & Whitmore, A. (2015). Early intervention and AAC: What a difference 30 years makes. *Augmentative and Alternative Communication, 31*(3), 181–202.

Rose, V., Paynter, J., Vivanti, G., Keen, D., & Trembath, D. (2020). Predictors of expressive language change for children with autism spectrum disorder receiving AAC-infused comprehensive instruction. *Journal of Autism and Developmental Disorders, 50,* 278–291.

Savaldi-Harussi, G., & Uziel, S. (2023). Frequency of word usage by Hebrew preschoolers: Implications for AAC core vocabulary. *Augmentative and Alternative Communication, 39*(2), 123–134.

Sennott, S., Light, J., & Mcnaughton, D. (2016). AAC modeling intervention research review. *Research and Practice for Persons with Severe Disabilities, 41*(2), 101–115.

Shin, S., & Hill, K. (2016). Korean word frequency and commonality study for augmentative and alternative communication. *International Journal of Language & Communication Disorders, 51*(4), 415–429.

Sigafoos, J., & Drawsgow, E. (2001). Conditional use of aided and unaided AAC: A review and clinical case demonstration. *Focus on Autism and Other Developmental Disabilities, 16*(3), 152–161.

Soto, G., & Cooper, B. (2021). An early Spanish vocabulary for children who use AAC: Developmental and linguistic considerations. *Augmentative and Alternative Communication, 37*(1), 64–74.

Soto, G., & Yu, B. (2014). Considerations for the provision of services to bilingual children who use augmentative and alternative communication. *Augmentative and Alternative Communication, 30*(1), 83–92.

Tönsing, K., van Nieker, K., Schlünz, G., & Wilken, I. (2019). Multilingualism and augmentative and alternative communication in South Africa—Exploring the views of persons with complex communication needs. *African Journal of Disabilities, 8,* 1–13.

Vygotsky, L. (1978). *Mind in society.* MIT Press.

White, E., Ayers, K., Snyder, S., Cagliani, R., & Ledford, J. (2021). Augmentative and alternative communication and speech production for individuals with autism: A systematic review. *Journal of Autism and Developmental Disorders, 51,* 4199–4212.

Chapter 15

Understanding Research and Evidence-Based Practice

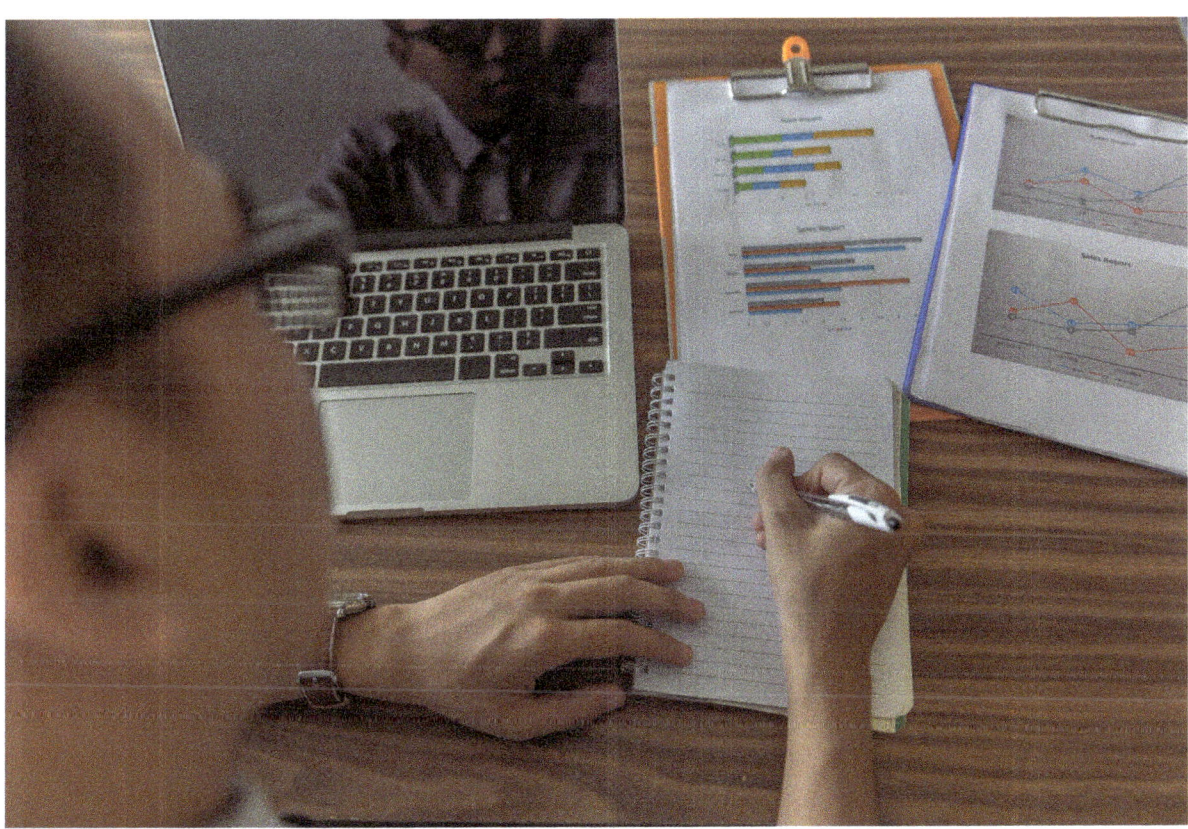

Learning Objectives

After reading this chapter, you will be able to:

- Describe the difference between experimental and nonexperimental research.
- Describe advantages and disadvantages of various types of research.
- Explain the importance of study limitations.
- Describe the three legs of the evidence-based practice triangle and give examples of each.

Key Terms

- between-subjects design
- case–control design
- case study
- clinical expertise
- cohort design
- confounding variable
- correlation
- covert observation
- dependent variable
- descriptive research
- empirical research
- evidence-based practice
- experimental research
- external evidence
- fidelity
- hypothesis
- independent variable
- internal evidence
- literature review
- meta-analysis
- negative correlation
- nonempirical research
- nonexperimental research
- observational study
- overt observation
- peer-reviewed
- phenomenology
- positive correlation
- qualitative data
- quantitative data
- quasi-experimental research
- randomized clinical trial
- randomized controlled trial
- research question
- semistructured interview
- study limitation
- survey study
- systematic review
- within-subjects design

Introduction

Fill in the blank: "Research is _____." What word(s) did you choose? After years of teaching research methods and evidence-based practice to undergraduate and graduate students studying health care professions, we have found that students often describe research as "boring," "laborious," "time-consuming," "tedious," "not for me," and "only important for people who want to get their PhD." But every so often, students will fill in the blank with words such as "important," "necessary," "exciting," and "useful for clinicians." Although the former descriptors might be true, it is this latter perspective about research that we hope will gain traction among students at all levels and in all health care professions.

Often in many curricula, research courses are the ones that students take not because they necessarily want to but because they are courses needed to fulfill a degree requirement. The disdain for these courses may come from preconceived notions about research methodology being stale and unexciting or from previous experiences reading dense research articles without understanding how to read and interpret them. In addition, the general stance has been that research is its own entity that lives *over there* and is separate from the workings of everyday life. This viewpoint could not be further from the truth because research is everywhere! We are researchers and consumers of research every day, whether we like it or not. We are researchers when we search for a major that will fit our skills and interests, when we are deciding where we want to live and who we want to be in a relationship with, when we decide which brand of cat food is best, and when we decide to switch from Android to iPhone (or vice versa). We are consumers of research when we watch the news, scroll through Instagram, watch TED Talks, and read the latest book on becoming a better partner or investing in Bitcoin.

In this chapter, we discuss the various types of research that you may encounter as a student or professional in communication sciences and disorders. We talk about the advantages and disadvantages of the different types of methodologies and how to use this information to inform how we interpret and share research findings. Finally, we discuss the value of understanding research as it pertains to the field of communication sciences and how we can stay informed and up to date in our clinical practices.

Types of Research

One of the reasons why students often get tripped up about research is because there are so many different types of research, and they each tell us something different. Without a fundamental understanding of the methods involved in each, and an understanding of the advantages and disadvantages of specific methods, the concept of research can be overwhelming. In this section, we offer brief descriptions of the different types of research (although certainly not all of them) that are often used in communication sciences and disorders and describe some of the strengths and limitations of each methodology. We then offer tips on how the information from each type of research can be useful to clinical practice. A more in-depth description of the types of research can be found in various research textbooks, including *Understanding Research and Evidence-Based Practice in Communication Disorders: A Primer for Students and Practitioners* by William Haynes and Carole Johnson (2009) and the fourth edition of *Research in Communication Sciences and Disorders: Methods for Systematic Inquiry* by Lauren Nelson and Jaimie Gilbert (2021).

To begin, let's distinguish empirical research from nonempirical research. **Empirical research** is what typically comes to mind when we think about "research" and occurs when an individual or group of researchers collects new data. This can be done through observation or more structured measures such as collecting language samples, conducting surveys, gathering information through rating scales or questionnaires, or directly measuring a behavior or skill through a testing protocol. The information or data gathered can then be analyzed and interpreted. Empirical research is required when researchers have new questions that they want answered pertaining to a specific research topic. Empirical research can be broken down into two main types of data collection or data observation: quantitative and qualitative (discussed later). The purpose of **nonempirical research**, on the other hand, is not to gather new information but, rather, to make use of data that has already been collected, analyzed, and interpreted. This includes summarizing information in the form of a literature review, analyzing existing findings to address a specific clinical question through a **systematic review** or **meta-analysis**, or explaining and summarizing complex phenomena through a **literature review**. Nonempirical research is particularly important for teaching us about topics that have already been studied, often at length.

Regardless of whether the research is empirical or nonempirical, all studies should have an aim or a purpose. The purpose of the study is usually to address an identifiable problem in the field. Once a researcher has an identifiable problem, they can set out to address it. From there, the researcher may pose a research question, offer a hypothesis, or both. A **hypothesis**, which is usually informed by some sort of existing research or knowledge, is a prediction about the outcome of a study or the relationship between the variables under study. Although also often informed by any extant literature, a **research question** is a specific question that the researchers are aiming to answer. Note that when investigators ask a research question, they are not offering a prediction about what they will find. When conducting research, the purpose and hypothesis/research questions of a study guide the research so that it can be conducted and interpreted in a systematic way. It also allows readers of the research to determine if the study that was conducted is applicable to their clinical interests. Note that whereas some authors specifically state the purpose of their study in their research article, others are less explicit and leave it up to the reader to infer the aim of the study based on the identified problem and research question or hypothesis.

Consider the following paragraph from Walker and Chung (2022). Identify the problem, the purpose of the study, and the hypothesis or research question.

> To our knowledge, few case studies have specifically investigated whether and how AAC [augmentative and alternative communication] systems are implemented to address different communication functions within natural environments, such as school-based settings. This information is critical given the growing prevalence of individuals relying on AAC (Light et al., 2019) and the limited information on AAC use in classrooms. Identifying the ways in which AAC is used within schools and the limitations that exist within the environment can further expand the resources available for those who benefit from AAC. Such findings may also inform future research in developing support strategies that promote effective communication methods and access to communication rights (e.g., Brady et al., 2016) for individuals with severe disabilities, along with practices to inform the provision of communication supports among practitioners in school-based settings. Therefore, this case study specifically addressed the following research question: How are AAC systems implemented within an elementary school setting among students with severe disabilities who have complex communication needs that necessitate the use of AAC? (p. 169)

Before we dive into discussing the differences between quantitative and qualitative data observation, let's make sure that we understand some terms that are important for understanding all kinds of research that we will be talking about. Let's begin with variables. You may have heard the term "variable" before and even used it in your causal talk, but understanding how we use the term "variable" in research is key to understanding what is being studied, how it is being studied, and how research can be translated into clinical practice. Although you will be exposed to other variables as you advance your research career, the two main types of variables to understand are independent and dependent variables (Figure 15–1). An **independent variable** is essentially *the thing that the researchers want to study* that does not depend on any other variable. This could be a specific intervention, a manipulation of a construct, or simply the difference between two (or more) groups. For example, if I want to study the impact that spending time with cats has on mild depression in adults, I might design a study in which I have two groups of adults

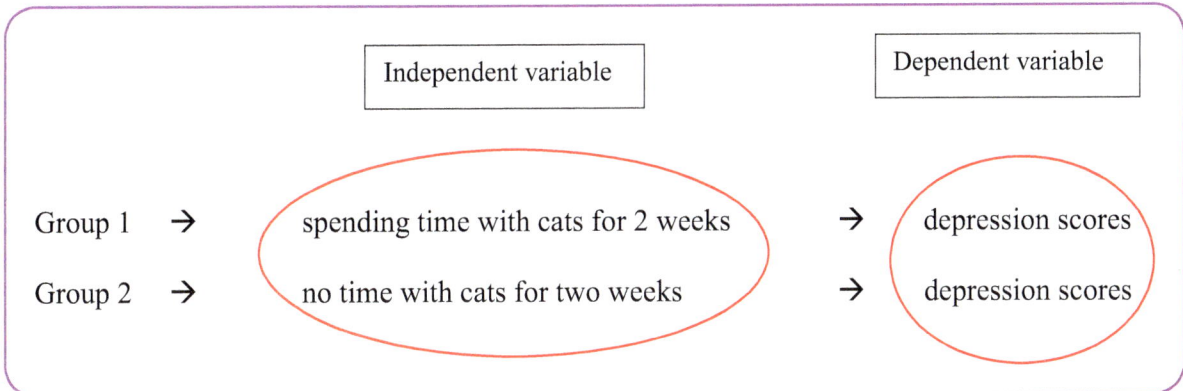

FIGURE 15-1. Independent and dependent variables.

who have mild depression. Now, because I want to determine what (if any) effect spending time with cats has on depression, *spending time with cats* will be my independent variable. I will set up my study so that one group of adults spends 2 hours a day with cats for 2 weeks, and the other group of adults spends 0 hours a day for 2 weeks with cats. At the end of the 2 weeks, I will determine if the group that spent time with cats scored differently on measures of depression compared to the group that did not spend time with cats. The **dependent variable** can be thought of as the outcome(s) of the experiment because it is dependent on the independent variable(s). So, in our example of depression in adults, the dependent variable would be the participants' depression scores after the 2 weeks of receiving the intervention (the independent variable).

Quantitative Research

Quantitative research provides us data in the form of numbers. This can include frequency counts of specific behaviors (e.g., how many times per week a person engages in exercise), measurements of physical characteristics (e.g., how tall a person is), test scores, and numeric information gleaned from surveys and rating scales. **Quantitative data** provides us with objective, fact-based information about *how much* and *how often* something occurs. There are (it is hoped and for the most part) no biased assumptions with quantitative data; the numbers (more or less) tell the story. In this type of research, data is collected to answer research questions and test hypotheses that have been posed by the researchers. Within quantitative research, there are two overarching categories depending on the research question: experimental research and nonexperimental research.

Experimental Research

When researchers randomly assign participants to groups and actively manipulate or have control over one or more variables, they are conducting **experimental research**. Experimental research ranges from highly structured and controlled designs to less controlled designs and includes between-subjects designs and within-subjects designs. **Between-subjects designs** compare two distinct groups, whereas **within-subjects designs** examine one group across time. The study design with the most control, and often referred to as the gold standard of research designs, is called a **randomized controlled trial** (RCT). In an RCT, the researchers randomly assign participants to a group, and this is usually either the intervention group (where participants receive the treatment or drug under investigation) or the control group (where the participants receive either a placebo drug or no treatment). Returning to our cat and depression study: In an RCT, the researchers would randomly decide who gets to spend time with cats and who does not. To help ensure that any changes in the outcome are in fact due to our independent variable (i.e., spending time with cats), we want to make sure that our two random groups look pretty much the same (i.e., are matched) in terms of factors such as age, gender, baseline depression scores, and, in this case, amenability to cats. If we do not ensure that our groups are matched, we will not know if our independent variable (i.e., spending time with cats) is what actually affected our outcome (i.e., post-depression scores) or if it was something else (e.g., maybe people in Group 1 were all people who liked cats and people in Group 2 were all people who did not like cats, which could have impacted the post-depression scores regardless of time spent with cats). A strength of an RCT is that because the groups were randomly assigned and there was tight control over the independent variables, the researchers can be more certain that any effects they find are in fact due to the independent variable and not to other factors. A slight complication with RCTs is that sometimes it is not possible or ethical to randomly assign participants to groups to receive an intervention or a control/placebo. For example, it may not be ethical to randomly assign a group of people to receive a life-saving treatment versus no treatment. In addition, when there is such tight control on the variables of interest, this may impact generalizability of the findings because the variables of interest may not be so tightly controlled in real-world settings. That is, if a researcher is interested in the effects of an intervention on children with autism but excludes children who have co-occurring attention-deficit/hyperactivity disorder (ADHD) to determine the effectiveness of the intervention on autism without ADHD, this may not translate to real-world populations because it is estimated that 70% of autistic individuals have some sort of co-occurring condition (Rosen et al., 2018). In addition, experimental research usually requires a somewhat large number of participants to detect significant and meaningful relationships between groups. Similar to an RCT, in a **randomized clinical trial**, participants are randomly assigned to an intervention group. This type of study compares various treatments to examine the effectiveness of a new intervention without the use of a control group.

Quasi-Experimental Research

Quasi-experimental research is similar to experimental research, with one major distinction: There is no random group assignment. This type of design is useful when it is not possible to randomly assign participants to groups. For example, imagine that you wanted to compare whether adding weekly pop quizzes increases undergraduate student engagement in the content they are learning. You design the study so that Instructor A adds weekly pop quizzes to her class and Instructor B does not add weekly pop quizzes to his class, and at the end of the semester you measure student engagement. You cannot randomly assign students to the groups because they are already registered for their courses. Like experimental research, a limitation of quasi-experimental research is that it is not always possible to manipulate the variable of interest that you wish to study or have enough participants for each group.

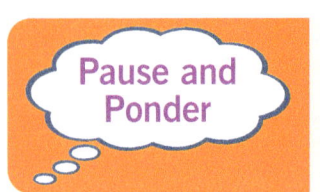

If an RCT is the gold standard, why or when would you choose to do a quasi-experimental study?

Nonexperimental Research

Sometimes it is not possible or ideal to have experimental control over certain variables you wish to study. When this happens, researchers turn to **nonexperimental research** designs or **descriptive research**, in which they examine relationships, patterns, or differences without manipulating any variables. Much of the research done in communication sciences and disorders relies on nonexperimental designs because it is often not possible to randomly assign participants to groups, especially when you are investigating differences between conditions (e.g., children with autism vs. children with Down syndrome). Although there are a variety of nonexperimental research designs, we briefly describe three main ones here: case–control designs, cohort designs, and survey studies.

One widely used method of investigation in speech-language pathology is the **case–control design**. This study design allows the researcher to compare a specific group of people with a condition (the *case*) to a group of people without the condition (the *control*) on specific variables of interest. For example, imagine you were interested in utterance length in preschoolers who use AAC compared to preschoolers who use verbal speech. To determine this, you would measure utterance length in both groups and compare the two groups (or cases). This type of study design allows researchers to make comparisons between naturally occurring groups as it pertains to variables of interest, which can be helpful in describing differences and similarities across groups of people. However, because participants are not randomly assigned to their groups, researchers cannot be certain that the differences between groups are in fact due to the conditions of interest and not some other **confounding variable**—an unmeasured variable that could potentially impact the results that has nothing to do with the variable you were investigating.

Cohort designs are particularly useful for gathering information about a group of people (i.e., a cohort) over time (longitudinally). These types of studies can provide us with information about how conditions look and change over time, including how many people are diagnosed with a specific condition in a certain time frame (e.g., 1 year) and the relationships between different variables in a group of people (e.g., literacy skills and AAC-use proficiency in children who are deaf). Because studies of this kind are nonexperimental, no variables are manipulated, and participants are not randomly assigned to a group. As such, researchers are unable to make claims about what is *causing* a particular behavior or phenomenon.

When it is not possible or feasible to gather groups of people to carry out the research, **survey studies** can come in handy. For this type of study, researchers send out a survey, often in the form of a questionnaire, to the group of individuals of interest, who then fill out the survey themselves. When collecting information from a survey, researchers are unable to manipulate any variables; they are simply asking questions to a broad audience in a systematic way. For example, Biggs et al. (2022) were interested in learning about speech-language pathologists' (SLPs) experiences providing services to students who used AAC when learning remotely during the COVID-19 pandemic. Researchers sent an online survey to SLPs asking open- and closed-ended questions about their experiences providing telehealth services to children who used AAC. Because this was a national survey and was accessible online through various platforms (e.g., websites, social media), the researchers were able to obtain information from large numbers of respondents (i.e., 331 SLPs). Researchers gained valuable insights about the successes and challenges providers had using AAC via telehealth and were thus able to discuss how teletherapy can continue to be used in the future as a potential option for services for individuals who use AAC. Note that although many SLPs completed the survey, not *all* SLPs who provided services during the pandemic filled out and returned the survey, and so the sample may not be totally representative of SLPs' experiences more broadly.

In addition to the nonexperimental study designs described above, we also want to bring your attention to correlational research. The term **correlation** basically means that there is a relationship between two or more variables. In correlational research, investigators determine the relationship (if any) between variables and *not* whether one variable caused a change in another variable. Because correlational research is nonexperimental, researchers do not manipulate variables, which is why we cannot say that the relationship between these variables is causal. One common phrase among researchers and those teaching research methods is that *correlation does not imply causation*.

Now that we have established this, let's talk about the different types of correlation: positive and negative. When two variables are positively correlated, this means that the variables are moving in the same direction. On the other hand, when two variables are negatively correlated, it means they are moving in the opposite direction. Let's consider some examples. Imagine that you are interested in the relationship between ice cream consumption and sunscreen sales in Canada. Throughout the year, you collect data on how much ice cream people are eating and how much sunscreen is being sold. You notice that when the stores are selling out of sunscreen, people are eating a lot more ice cream. Surely these things do not *cause* each other to happen. It is not that eating ice cream causes me to buy sunscreen, or buying sunscreen causes me to eat ice cream. But they are related. When it is hot enough outside to wear sunscreen in Canada, ice cream is usually a refreshing treat. So as sunscreen sales go up, so does the amount of ice cream consumed. This is a **positive correlation** because both variables are moving together in the same direction (and in this case, both are increasing). Similarly, when there are lower rates of sunscreen sales, there is less ice cream consumption. Although the rates of each are decreasing, this is still a positive correlation (because both variables are moving together in the same direction). Let's consider a **negative correlation** now. Imagine that you are interested in the relationship between wearing swimsuits and shoveling snow in Switzerland. You collect data throughout the year on the frequency of people wearing swimsuits and the frequency of people shoveling snow. You find that the more people opt to wear swimsuits, the less they seem to shovel snow. Now, there is no causal relationship here—wearing swimsuits is not what causes people to shovel snow less—but there is a correlation. As swimsuit wearing goes up, snow shoveling goes down (and vice versa). Can you see the connection? Because snow shoveling generally occurs when it is cold outside, not too many people wear swimsuits. This is a negative correlation because the variables are moving in opposite directions (Figure 15–2). In addition to the direction of the correlation (positive vs. negative), the relationships between variables range from weak to strong. That is, the relationship between some variables is stronger than the relationship between other variables.

Qualitative Research

Qualitative research provides us data in the form of words and subjective experiences. That is, **qualitative data** is collected and reported in the form of descriptive information often about participants' experiences, and it usually includes direct quotes about those experiences. This type of research examines the "thoughts, values, attitudes, perceptions, and intentions of individuals and groups of individuals that help explain the *reasons* for behavior or *how* an outcome occurs" (Orlikoff et al., 2015, p. 105). Unlike quantitative research, there are no hypotheses to test in qualitative research; the aim of the research is more exploratory, with an interest in **phenomenology**—a person's lived experiences. For that reason, qualitative investigations in communication sciences and disorders tend to be conducted through observations, semistructured interviews, and case studies.

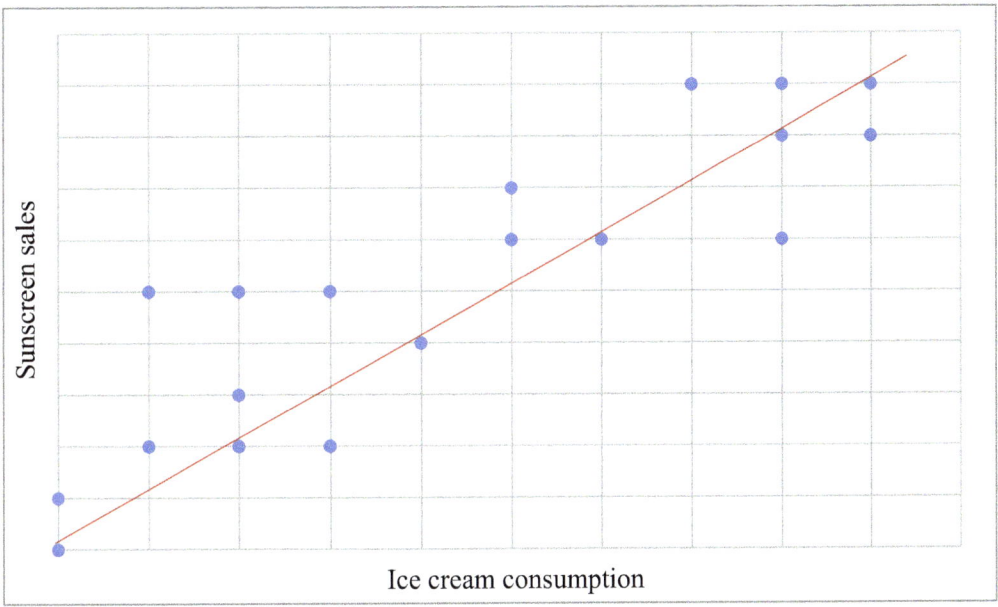

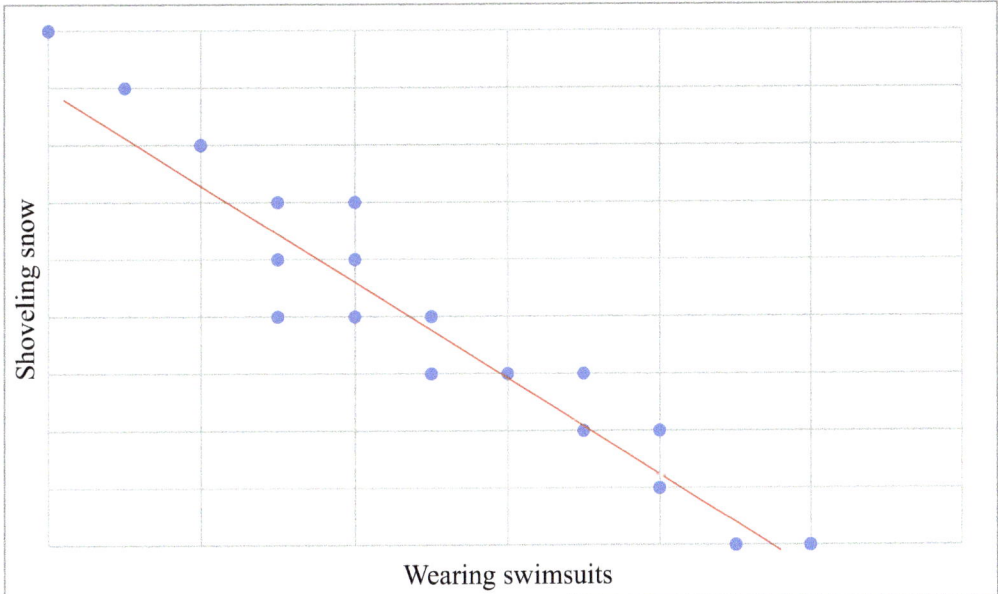

FIGURE 15-2. Examples of positive and negative correlations.

Although many qualitative researchers combine various methodologies to explore the topic of interest, we discuss each in turn. When a researcher wants to gain the most unobstructed, unbiased, and naturalistic information about a phenomenon, their best bet is to conduct an **observational study**. During an observational study, the researcher systematically records the behaviors or phenomenon of interest with or without it being known that the researcher is observing. That is, a researcher may wish to conceal their identity as a researcher or otherwise make their recording unknown to the individuals being studied (this is called **covert observation**). Or the researcher may choose to inform their subjects that they are being recorded, but that they should not let that influence their behaviors and they should act as they normally would (this is called **overt observation**). Researchers may also wish to conduct **semistructured interviews** as part of their qualitative methodology. During a semistructured interview, the researcher asks their participants a set of interview questions in a flexible manner. That is, when participants answer any given question, the researcher may ask follow-up questions that were not part of the interview script to glean a better understanding of the participants' experiences. For example, a researcher who is interested in gathering information about parents' perceptions of their children's memories asks the following interview question: "Does your child seem to remember certain events more easily than others?" If the parent describes a list of events that appear to be positive experiences, such as "He remembers when we went to Disney last year, his cousin's birthday party, the time we saw the cheetah at the zoo," the researcher might follow up with a probing question. The researcher may go off script (but purposefully) and say something like "It sounds like these events were positive experiences. Does your child ever remember negative experiences?"

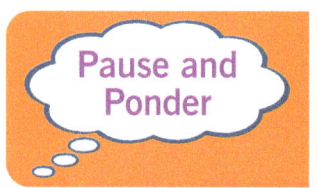

What is the value of covert versus overt observation? What is the value of overt versus covert observation? Under what circumstances would it be ideal to use each?

Case studies offer a deep descriptive dive into one or a few individual cases, where a "case" often refers to an individual person or an individual unit. Case studies are especially useful when not much is known about a particular condition. For example, imagine that a researcher is interested in learning more about autistic adults who also have deafblindness and use tactile communication. There is likely not much information about this specific population in the existing literature. To conduct a **case study**, the researcher would first get access to one or a few people who present with this condition. Then the researcher would collect various pieces of information about the people related to what the researcher is interested in learning. For example, if the researcher is interested in learning about an individual's communication profile, they may choose to collect descriptive information about how and with whom the person communicates, any barriers that prevent the person from communicating in certain environments, the communicative functions the person uses, and so on. Perhaps the researcher is interested in gathering information about a new type of AAC method for individuals who are deafblind to see how it may work with autistic deafblind individuals. The researcher may teach the autistic individual the new system and document the process, including challenges and barriers that the person faces, as well as benefits of the system. The case study may also include measuring the participant's communication skills (e.g., number of communicative functions, number of initiations, use of greetings) both prior to implementing the new AAC system and after its implementation to determine if the new AAC method had an impact on their skills. Although case studies can provide a launching point for future rigorous research studies, information gathered for them may not be generalizable to other cases. That is, the data gathered for the autistic deafblind individual who uses tactile communication cannot be assumed to be applicable for all autistic deafblind individuals who use tactile communication; everyone is unique in their experiences and is impacted by internal and external factors that are unique to them.

Importance of Research for Clinical Practice

We have established that there are various types of research and that each contributes unique knowledge and understanding of complex topics. We can take it one step further. Not only does scientific research exist to expand our understanding of clinical topics but also clinical research often complements and expands upon this scientific research. Clinical research can take the form of case studies (described previously), which often serve as preliminary to more rigorous research study designs. In this sense, clinicians can methodologically document their experiences with clients and contribute to the study of topics that may not be well understood. This type of study is useful in getting the ball rolling on how best to support these unique populations.

Clinicians not only conduct their own research but also base their clinical decisions on scientific findings. Researchers do not conduct research solely for their own benefit and interests; they often study topics that have relevance in the clinical world. Consider a researcher who is interested in studying interventions to support social learning in children who have autism. The researcher may recruit participants who have autism and implement Social Story (Gray, 2010) interventions to teach a social communicative skill such as greeting others. Assuming that the study and intervention are carried out with **fidelity** (i.e., as intended based on the established guidelines and procedures), the results of this study could guide clinicians in implementing Social Stories to teach using greetings to children with autism who have similar characteristics to those in the study. To thoughtfully and effectively carry out research in clinical practice, however, clinicians must have a solid understanding of the different types of research studies and their purposes, as well as the implications and limitations that are inherent in each type of research design and specific study.

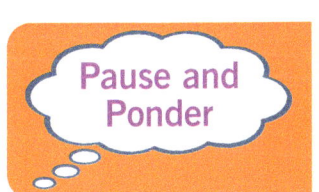 What are the advantages and disadvantages of each type of study design? How does each methodology contribute to clinical knowledge? What are the limitations for clinical application for each?

In addition to being knowledgeable about the strengths and weaknesses of the different types of study designs, it is beneficial to understand that there is no such thing as a perfect study and that all studies have limitations. A **study limitation** is a shortcoming or weakness of the study, which often involves the generalizability of the findings due to the type of study conducted, the participants who were able to participate (and how many of them there were), or the ways in which variables were measured or manipulated. Another way that we can think about limitations is if something inherent in the study has the potential to impact the findings or conclusions of the specific research (Ross & Bibler Zaidi, 2019). Limitations are optimal for thinking about how future research can address the challenges of a study to enhance generalizability of the findings and, in the field of communication sciences and disorders, better inform clinical practice. These are considered directions for future research. Researchers will often highlight one or two limitations (and directions for future research) of their study at the end of the research article; however, there are often many that go undisclosed. As a reader of the research who understands the different types of study designs and what the methodology means for the findings and conclusions, you are in a prime position to draw your own limitations about any study, and we encourage you to do just that.

Once you have read the research, thought about the advantages and disadvantages of the study design, and critically evaluated the study for its limitations, you are ready to translate research into clinical practice. Incorporating research findings into clinical practice is one component of evidence-based practice. **Evidence-based practice** (EBP) is the integration of three key components: evidence, clinical experience, and client perspectives (Figure 15–3). According to the American Speech-Language-Hearing Association (ASHA, 2023), "When all three components of EBP are considered together, clinicians can make informed, evidence-based decisions and provide high-quality services reflecting the interests, values, needs, and choices of individuals with communication disorders." This means that to provide good care, clinicians must understand both **external evidence**—evidence that is based on scientific findings—and **internal evidence**—data that is specific to the client receiving intervention. Clinicians then incorporate the evidence with their **clinical expertise**—the knowledge that they have gained through their professional experiences—while also considering the values and perspectives of their clients. If all the components of EBP are not considered in clinical practice, intervention may not be effective or even ethical. Consider, for example, an autistic adolescent who has social communication challenges, one of which is the inability to understand sarcasm. Perhaps you have read studies that have shown that the understanding of sarcasm can be taught through a specific training method (evidence), and you have used this training method successfully with other autistic individuals (clinical experience). If your client does not see the value in understanding sarcasm, and this is not a priority for intervention for them (client perspectives), then implementing an intervention to support understanding of sarcasm would not be EBP. Let's consider another example. You have a client who has a swallowing disorder and cannot swallow thin liquids. You find a study that states patients who are unable to swallow thin liquids should not be given thickened liquids (evidence); however, your clinical experience has shown that thickened liquids can be offered to these patients methodologically (clinical experience), and the client is wishing to try

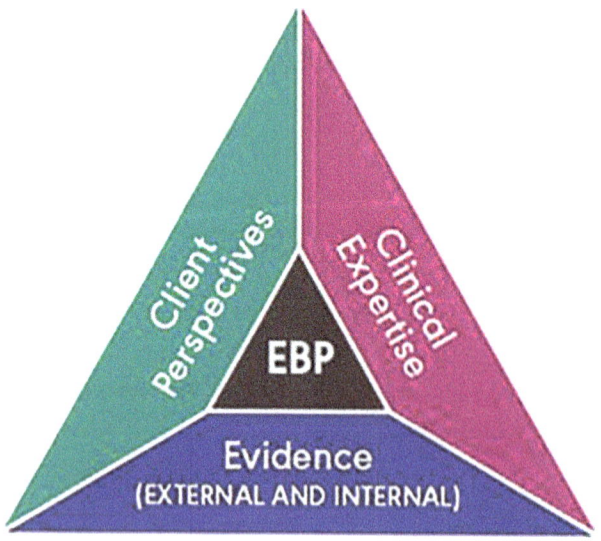

FIGURE 15–3. Evidence-based practice (EBP) triangle from ASHA. *Source:* Copyrighted by the American Speech-Language-Hearing Association (ASHA). Used with permission.

oral intake strategies before being given a feeding tube (client perspective). In this case, strictly adhering to the recommendations discussed in the empirical literature does not reflect EBP.

You might be thinking that two of the legs of the EBP triangle are relatively simple to acquire: internal evidence and clinician expertise. But what about external evidence? How do clinicians become familiar with scientific findings? Remember how we previously stated that research often seems like it is something done *over there*? Well as clinicians, we are responsible for keeping up to date in the field of SLP or audiology. This means that we are committed to maintaining an updated knowledge base that is applicable to the clients who we serve. In fact, this is required by our national governing organization, ASHA. External evidence comes in many forms, including attending conferences, participating in workshops, taking courses, as well as reading books and journal articles. It is important that the external evidence we incorporate into our clinical practice has been vetted by others; ideally peer-reviewed; and is not purely a reflection of the authors' opinions, beliefs, or anecdotal evidence. When a source has been **peer-reviewed**, this means that other experts in the field (other than the author of the journal, book, or workshop) have identified the research findings as having merit or somehow contributing to science. The peer-review process helps ensure that scientific methodology is upheld in the dissemination of research findings. We know what you might be thinking: Although it is important to read peer-reviewed research, and because this often comes in the form of journal articles, reading a research article can be time-consuming, overwhelming, and requires a lot of cognitive effort. This does not have to be the case! We offer a guide for reading scientific articles in Appendix 15–1.

You may already be beginning to see why research is important in clinical practice and why it matters to you as a student studying in communication sciences and disorders. To be competent clinicians who care about supporting the clients (and their families) with whom they work, clinicians must understand research and the methods that go into conducting it. Imagine a clinician who is working with an adult with a motor speech disorder, specifically spastic dysarthria. The clinician is interested in learning about a new communication treatment approach to try with the client, so the clinician reads through the literature and finds an article that examines the success of this new approach for a group of people who have spastic dysarthria. At face value, and without having a deeper understanding of the research methods involved in this study, the clinician may assume that this treatment approach will work for their client as well. Consider, however, that the study examined this new treatment approach in a group of individuals who have spastic dysarthria and who also have depression, are older than age 70 years, and live in Greenland. The results of this study may not generalize to the target client if he does not have depression, is younger than age 70 years, and does not live in Greenland.

Let's consider another way that understanding research can inform clinical practice. Imagine that a clinician is interested in assessing a child's personal narrative skills, so the clinician uses an assessment measure that is designed for gathering information about children's narrative abilities, including personal narratives. At face value, this seems like it could be the perfect test to use for this student, so the clinician administers the test. The clinician finds that according to the assessment, the child's personal narrative skills are above average, which does not seem to match with what the clinician and the child's caregivers are noticing. Upon further inspection of the assessment manual, the clinician discovers that the researchers who developed the test define personal narratives *differently* than how the clinician defines them and has come to understand them based on the literature. Perhaps the assessment tool did not capture the information that the clinician was interested in because it was not measuring the skill that the clinician was interested in. Without understanding how the researchers define personal narratives, and if it is the same construct that the clinician is interested in, the clinician is at risk for unnecessarily providing treatment or not providing intervention that would be beneficial to the client.

Here is another example. Consider an adult clinic setting for clients who have aphasia. One client, Trevor, has word-finding difficulties and is in need of treatment that targets word finding. Clinician A is skilled in providing one treatment for word finding (i.e., semantic feature analysis), and Clinician B is skilled in another (i.e., verb network strengthening treatment). Following an assessment of Trevor's skills, it is evident that he is a candidate for either treatment approach, so either clinician is fit to provide him services based on their current expertise. Here, all legs of the EBP triangle are considered. Now imagine that a new client, Fabiola, gets referred to the clinic. She also has word-finding challenges, but her intake assessment reveals that she is not a candidate for semantic feature analysis. When Fabiola becomes a client at this clinic, Clinician B (who has clinical expertise in verb network strengthening treatment) is on maternity leave and so Clinician A (who has knowledge of semantic feature analysis) must provide the intervention services. To ensure that Clinician A is using EBP, she is responsible for learning about the treatment approach that is appropriate for Fabiola (in this case, verb network strengthening treatment) instead of simply relying on her area of expertise. If Clinician A used semantic feature analysis with Fabiola, she would only be considering two legs of the EBP triangle: evidence and clinical experience. Learning about how to deliver an intervention that would be appropriate to Fabiola would ensure that the clinician is addressing the third leg of the triangle: client perspectives.

Chapter Summary

Research is often a topic that students are inclined to shy away from, and there has historically been a disconnect between what is done in the research lab and what is done in clinical practice. This could not be further from the truth! It is crucial that clinicians understand research methods because this will help them make informed clinical decisions. There are various research methodologies, and each has its own strengths and limitations. In this chapter, we described the difference between experimental and nonexperimental research and provided examples of different methodologies for each. We then discussed how all research has inherent limitations and that it is necessary for consumers of research to think critically about how a study's limitations have the potential to impact the generalizability of research findings in clinical practice. It is not just researchers in the lab who conduct research; practitioners in clinical settings must also conduct research. The integration of research evidence, clinical expertise, and client preferences and values makes up EBP, which is valuable in providing treatment for individuals receiving care provided by SLPs and audiologists.

Chapter Review Questions

1. If an RCT is the gold standard, why or when would you choose to do a quasi-experimental study?
2. What is the difference between experimental research and quasi-experimental research?
3. What is one advantage and one disadvantage of each type of research discussed in this chapter?
4. What is the difference between an independent variable and a dependent variable?
5. Describe what is meant by the phrase "correlation does not imply causation."

6. Why are limitations of a study important?
7. What are the three legs of ASHA's EBP triangle?
8. Give an example of each of the legs of the EBP triangle.

Learning Activities

1. You are a qualitative researcher for the day. Your job is to conduct observational research. Choose a behavior or a phenomenon of interest to you and spend at least 30 minutes observing this behavior covertly (i.e., without the participants knowing they are being observed). Record what you observe. Now choose another behavior and spend another 30 minutes observing this behavior overtly (i.e., the participants know they are being observed). Write up your findings for each study. Compare and contrast these observational styles. Was one easier or more difficult to conduct than the other? Do you believe you gained more information from one or the other? What type of information did you gain from each style?

2. Find a research article to read. Follow the steps in Appendix 15–1 as you read the article.
    a. Provide a summary of the study (about 1 page)
        i. Study design
        ii. Participant characteristics
        iii. Purpose of the study
        iv. Research question and/or hypothesis
    b. Discuss the significance of the study (about 1 page)
        i. Brief description of what the authors found (no need to report statistics)
        ii. Why these findings are significant (or not) in the field of communication sciences and disorders

3. Using the same article you used for the previous question, critically appraise the study.
    a. Methods section
        i. What are the dependent and independent variables?
        ii. What is one pro and one con of the chosen study design? Why is it a pro? Why is it a con?
        iii. What is one confounding variable in the study that you can think of?
    b. Results
        i. Are the results generalizable to the entire population that the authors are interested in?
    c. Discussion/conclusion
        i. What are two limitations of the study? (Please include one limitation the authors state and one you came up with on your own.)
        ii. What are two areas for future research based on this study? (Please include one future direction discussed by the authors and one that you came up with on your own.)

Suggested Reading

Aldemir, H., Solís-Campos, A., Saldaña, D., & Rodríguez-Ortiz, I. (2023). A systematic review and meta-analysis of vocabulary interventions for deaf/hard of hearing children and adolescents. *Journal of Speech, Language, and Hearing Research, 66*(8), 2831–2857.

This systematic review and meta-analysis evaluated the effectiveness of vocabulary interventions for deaf/hard of hearing children and adolescents by examining 25 group studies that reported on vocabulary interventions for children aged 2 to 18 years.

Biggs, E., Therrien, M., Douglas, S., & Snodgrass, M. (2022). Augmentative and alternative communication during the COVID-19 pandemic: A national survey of speech-language pathologists. *American Journal of Speech-Language Pathology, 31*, 303–321.

This study employed a survey design to collect data on SLPs' experiences providing AAC intervention services via telehealth to children and young adults (aged 3–21 years) during the COVID-19 pandemic.

Guiberson, M., & Ferris, K. (2023). Speech-language pathologists' preparation, practices, and perspectives on serving Indigenous families and children. *American Journal of Speech-Language Pathology, 6*, 2858–2870.

This study employed a survey design to collect data from 333 SLPs who provided services to Indigenous children in the United States. Researchers gathered information about the SLPs' clinical and professional practices around working with Indigenous children.

Hutchins, T., & Brien, A. (2016). Conversational topic moderates social attention in autism spectrum disorder: Talking about emotions is like driving in a snowstorm. *Research in Autism Spectrum Disorders, 26*, 99–110.

This quasi-experimental study compared the eye-gaze patterns of autistic children and neurotypical children when engaging in conversations about things that people do and how people feel.

Iacono, T., Torr, J., & Wong, H. (2010). Relationship amongst age, language and related skills in adults with Down syndrome. *Research in Developmental Disabilities, 31*(2), 568–576.

This correlational study examined the relationship between language skills and certain cognitive skills in adults with Down syndrome.

Kohmäscher, A., Primaßin, A., Heiler, S., Da Costa Avelar, P., Franken, M., & Heim, S. (2023). Effectiveness of stuttering modification treatment in school-age children who stutter: A randomized clinical trial. *Journal of Speech, Language, and Hearing Research, 66*(11), 4194–4205.

This randomized controlled trial examined the effectiveness of a stuttering modification intervention in children aged 7 to 11 years who received the intervention immediately compared to those who received the intervention 3 months later.

Persson, M., Opdahl, S., Risnes, K., Gross, R., Kajantie, E., Reichenberg, A., . . . Sandin, S. (2020). Gestational age and the risk of autism spectrum disorder in Sweden, Finland, and Norway: A cohort study. *PLoS Medicine, 17*(9), Article e1003207.

This cohort study examined population data from Sweden, Finland, and Norway to gather information on estimates of the likelihood of an autism diagnosis for children born preterm.

Pfeiffer, D., Feuerstein, J., & Landa, R. (2023). Speech-language pathologists' perceptions of language and literacy instruction for pre-K children with developmental language disorder. *Language, Speech, and Hearing Services in Schools, 54*(4), 1295–1307.

This study employed a semistructured interview to gather information on school-based SLPs' perspectives of early language and literacy instruction for preschool children with developmental language disorder.

McDonnell, C., Valentino, K., & Diehl., J. (2017). A developmental psychopathology perspective on autobiographical memory in autism spectrum disorder. *Developmental Review, 44*, 59–81.

This literature review provides an overview of the research on autobiographical memory in individuals with autism across the lifespan.

Quinn, E., Kurin, K., Atkins, K., & Cook, A. (2023). Identifying implementation strategies to increase augmentative and alternative communication adoption in early childhood classrooms: A qualitative study. *Language, Speech, and Hearing Services in Schools, 54*(4), 1136–1154.

This study employed a semistructured interview to gather information from SLPs and special education teachers about implementation strategies for AAC users in the school setting.

Swann, Z., Tesman, N., Rogalsky, C., & Honeycutt, C. (2023). Word repetition paired with startling stimuli decrease aphasia and apraxia severity in severe-to-moderate stroke: A stratified, single-blind, randomized, Phase 1 clinical trial. *American Journal of Speech-Language Pathology, 6*, 2630–2653.

This randomized controlled trial examined the effectiveness of Startle Adjuvant Rehabilitation Therapy (compared to a control intervention) on aphasia, apraxia of speech, and quality of life in adults with chronic stroke.

Van der Straeten, C., Verbeke, J., Alighieri, C., Bettens, K., Van Beveren, E., Bruneel, L., & Van Lierde, K. (2023). Treatment outcomes of interdisciplinary care on speech and health-related quality of life outcomes in adults with cleft palate. *American Journal of Speech-Language Pathology, 6*, 2654–2675.

This case–control study examined speech outcomes and quality of life of adults born with a cleft palate with or without a lip palate compared to adults born without a cleft/lip palate.

Walker, V., & Chung, Y. (2022). Augmentative and alternative communication in an elementary school setting: A case study. *Language, Speech, and Hearing Services in Schools, 53*, 167–180.

This case study examined how five students diagnosed with autism or intellectual disability used AAC throughout their school day.

References

American Speech-Language-Hearing Association. (2023). *Evidence-based practice (EBP)*. https://www.asha.org/research/ebp

Biggs, E., Therrien, M., Douglas, S., & Snodgrass, M. (2022). Augmentative and alternative communication during the COVID-19 pandemic: A national survey of speech-language pathologists. *American Journal of Speech-Language Pathology, 31*, 303–321.

Gray, C. (2010). *The new social story book.* Future Horizons.

Haynes, W., & Johnson, C. (2009). *Understanding research and evidence-based practice in communication disorders: A primer for students and practitioners.* Pearson.

Nelson, L., & Gilbert, J. (2021). *Research in communication sciences and disorders: Methods for systematic inquiry* (4th ed.). Plural Publishing.

Orlikoff, R., Schiavetti, N., & Metz, D. (2015). *Evaluating research in communication disorders* (7th ed.). Pearson.

Rosen, T., Mazefsky, C., Vasa, R., & Lerner, M. (2018). Co-occurring psychiatric conditions in autism spectrum disorder. *International Review of Psychiatry, 30*(1), 40–61.

Ross, P., & Bibler Zaidi, N. (2019). Limited by our limitations. *Perspectives on Medical Education, 8*, 261–264.

Walker, V., & Chung, Y. (2022). Augmentative and alternative communication in an elementary school setting: A case study. *Language, Speech, and Hearing Services in Schools, 53*, 167–180.

APPENDIX 15-1
Tips for Reading a Primary Source

Looking at a *primary source* (firsthand account of a topic from those who wrote it or had a direct connection with the information—article, textbook, etc.) can be intimidating, but this guide breaks down the most important elements and how to use them to increase your understanding. This may take you a few hours to complete, but be patient. If you find yourself distracted, take a break, and pick back up where you left off.

General Tips

These tips should be used throughout the document you are reading. An important part of reading a primary source is interacting, actively, with the material.

- Find an easy way to write on the primary source, be that on paper, a tablet, or a computer.
- Highlight or underline each section you read with a different color (e.g., introduction–yellow, methods–blue, results–green, discussion–purple).
- Write your questions down as you are reading. If you are confused, put a question mark and keep reading.

Abstract

The abstract contains what the authors believe is the most important parts of their work. Typically, this paragraph is great to look at to see if the paper has what you are looking for.

Tip 1

- Read this paragraph at least twice for your first read.
  - Once before starting the paper and once after finishing the paper.

Tip 2

- On your first read, underline or highlight what makes sense to you and mark what does not.
  - The information that does not make sense is what you will be looking to figure out by reading the paper.

Tip 3

- Look up words that you do not know, and keep the definitions on hand.

Tip 4

- If you see any abbreviations, write down what they stand for.
  - This makes it so you are not constantly flipping back and forth between pages.

Introduction

The introduction usually contains background information from other studies or papers. This is the first thing that should be read because it will give you context for the rest of the reading. It should build a case or rationale for the significance of the paper you are reading.

Tip 5

- As you read, mark what you find important or interesting because the authors most likely thought this as well.
- Important details will also come from others the authors cite.

Tip 6

- Identify the hypotheses of the paper and comment on what you think about them.
    - Does this line up with the background you read?
    - Are there any other hypotheses you might make from the background you read?

Discussion

For your first read, skip the methods and results sections for now. This allows you to try to understand the beginning and ending of the paper without being confused by the middle. You will then use your understanding from the introduction and discussion to make sense of the methods and results. Skim this section first, and then read for understanding on the second pass. This technique is highlighted below. If this section is still difficult to discern, try these strategies.

Skimmed Reading

Tip 7

- Mark any significant findings that are mentioned and analyzed.

Tip 8

- Mark the limitations mentioned in the study.
    - This could look like "We had a limited number of participants, so our results may not be accurate for the whole population" or "Going further we would change . . . "

Reading for Understanding

Tip 9

- Look for conclusions of the results and decide whether you agree or not.
    - It is okay to not agree with a paper.

Tip 10

- Try to re-explain the discussion in your own words.
  - Use the findings you underlined to facilitate this. Explain what these mean in terms of the hypothesis.

Tip 11

- Think about what further investigation you would like to see.
  - From anything such as "Is gender correlated with this statistic?" to "Would you see a similar but modified result if they underwent this experiment in a different condition with a different population, or with a different variable?"

Results

This is the next section to read. This section is all about the figures. Do not skip the figures! The figures can be the most important part of an entire paper. This is where you have to decide whether or not the authors came to the right conclusions from their data.

Figures

Tip 12

- Look at these before trying to read the section.

Tip 13

- Using your previous knowledge, write down what is happening in each figure and what data are significant.

Tip 14

- Sometimes the methods are diagramed in this section.
  - If this is the case, try to figure out what the researchers did.

Written

Tip 15

- Mark the statistics mentioned in this section and whether or not they are statistically significant.
  - If the results are not significant, they will usually be denoted with "*n.s.*" after the numbers. If the results are significant, they may be denoted with "$p < .05$."

Tip 16

- Do not get stuck on something if you do not know what it is.
  - If you understand the discussion, then you can understand what the paper is about enough to talk about it.

Methods

For most undergraduate students, the methods section can be intimidating. It is very detailed about what techniques are being used. This section is used by other researchers to replicate the experiment.

Tip 17

- If you do not know what something is, look it up. If you still do not understand, then move on.
  - In order to understand the paper, you do not need to understand every detail in the methods.

Tip 18

- Look for a description of the participants and the activities/tasks/measures in which they were engaged.
- Look for figures or tables that help explain what the researchers did in a different way. If there are no figures, then draw it out for yourself.
  - If you are not a fan of drawing, then you can use a flowchart or images or even a list to help.

Conclusion

This section ties all of the sections together. This section can be read at any point, but reading it at the end will allow you to pull the pieces together yourself.

Tip 19

- In the conclusion, you will find that information from other parts of the paper is restated. Try to use the same color scheme as the rest of the paper to highlight or underline each piece of related information with a specific color. If there is a tie to the background information, use the same color to highlight or underline that piece of information, such as yellow.
  - This is helpful for your second comprehensive read because your attention will be drawn to the ideas in the conclusion that you highlighted as you read each section.

After Reading Once

After you finish your read-through, go back to the abstract and your notes and see if you understand the content you were initially confused about and if you have any new conclusions of your own. Once you have marked the paper up with notes and questions, leave it for at least a few hours. When you come back to the paper, read through it again and then try to rewrite the abstract or conclusion in your own words. Once you have completed this, you have finished reading your paper.

Glossary

AAC abandonment: Discontinuation or rejection of AAC.

abduction: Movement that pulls the vocal folds apart.

ableism: Discrimination of disabled people; the belief that able-bodied people are superior.

ableist language: The use of words or phrases that devalue a person with a disability.

accent: The unique pronunciation of speech by people who speak the same language.

acceptance and commitment therapy: A stuttering intervention approach that helps the individual recognize their thoughts, without requiring changing those thoughts, and learn that negative thoughts do not necessarily determine a person's feelings.

access barriers: Barriers to accessing AAC that are internal to the person with complex communication needs, such as motor or visual challenges.

acoustic immittance testing: A common audiological evaluation using tympanometry which assesses middle ear function.

acoustic or auditory nerve: Also known as the **vestibulocochlear nerve**, it is the sensory nerve responsible for transmitting auditory information from the cochlea of the inner ear to the brain; it is cranial nerve VIII.

acoustic reflex testing: A procedure that uses headphones and a small probe placed in the ear canal through which various sound intensities are sent through the ear canal while recording the reflex responses.

active articulator: Articulators that move during the production of speech.

adduction: Bringing together of the vocal folds.

affricates: Phonemes made by producing a stop followed immediately by a fricative.

aging with disability: Individuals who have disabilities when they are younger and age as a part of life.

agrammatical: Having incorrect grammatical structure.

aided AAC: Augmentative systems used for communication that are external to the speaker, including picture boards, electronic communication devices, and typing system.

aided language stimulation: When a communication partner models language using an AAC system; also referred to as modeling.

air conduction: The process by which sound moves through the air in the outer ear, hits the eardrum, and is sent to the middle ear and then the cochlea of the inner ear.

alveolar: Place of articulation involving the bumpy ridge behind the teeth.

alveolar process: The lining of the tooth's socket; referred to as the alveolus.

alveolar ridge: The bony ridge that holds the sockets of the teeth.

alveolo-palatal: Place of articulation involving both the bumpy ridge behind the teeth and the palate.

Alzheimer disease: The most common type of dementia.

Americans With Disabilities Act (ADA): A law that provides disabled people with protection against discrimination in the workplace and in public spaces such as housing, transportation, education, health care, and voting.

amplitude: The strength of sound waves (transmitted vibrations), perceived as loudness or volume; it is measured in decibels (dB) or sound pressure level.

amyotrophic lateral sclerosis (ALS): A degenerative disease associated with muscle weakness.

anomia: Word-retrieval difficulties.

anomic aphasia: A fluent aphasia that occurs because of damage to the temporal and parietal lobes of the brain and is characterized by word-finding difficulties.

aphasia: A language disorder that typically presents with impairments in comprehending and/or producing written and spoken language.

aphonia: Loss of voice.

apraxia of speech: A disorder of the motor planning or programming of speech that usually results from damage in motor areas in the left hemisphere.

aprosodia: Deficits in comprehension and production of pitch and intonation to express emotional information.

articulation: The formation of sounds in speech.

articulation disorder: Difficulty with the accurate production of individual sounds.

articulators: Lips, tongue, teeth, soft palate, hard palate, alveolar ridge, and so on used to help create various sounds.

arytenoid cartilage: A pair of cartilages in the back of the larynx important in the production of voice.

aspiration: When food or liquid enters the lower part of the airway, below the vocal folds and into the larynx and sometimes even the lungs.

ataxic dysarthria: A motor speech disorder that is primarily concerned with the incoordination of muscles.

audiogram: A chart displaying hearing test results indicating how well a person can hear sounds at different frequencies from high- to low-pitched sounds with varying intensity or loudness.

auditory brainstem response (ABR) test: An assessment often used with children who cannot complete a typical hearing screening; it is typically used in newborn hearing screening programs to test how the brain responds to sounds.

auditory cortex: An area of the brain that is responsible for recognizing auditory information.

auditory evoked potential: A measurement of how long it takes for the brain to respond to sound.

auditory neuropathy: A condition in which the sound is detected by the ear but does not get transmitted to the brain.

augmentative and alternative communication (AAC): Any form of communication that supplements or replaces verbal speech.

autoimmune inner ear disease: A condition in which the immune system attacks the inner ear.

awareness: A stuttering intervention strategy designed to educate the person who stutters about the systems important to understanding communication (i.e., respiration, phonation, articulation, and resonance).

basilar membrane: The main mechanical component of the inner ear.

bedside swallow evaluation: An assessment that helps determine if a patient presents with signs and symptoms of dysphagia within the context of other variables, such as mealtime performance, feeding posture/positioning, and environmental conditions; also referred to as a clinical swallow evaluation.

Bell's palsy: Sudden weakness or paralysis that typically occurs on one side of the face.

Bernoulli effect: During speech, as air rushes through a very narrow opening between the vocal folds, it must accelerate to get through, creating a suction effect that brings the vocal folds together.

between-subjects design: An experimental study design with two or more groups; each group experiences different levels of the independent variable.

bilateral hearing loss: Hearing loss that affects both ears.

blocked practice: One stimulus is practiced repeatedly before moving on to the next stimulus.

bolus: The mixture of saliva and food that is created in the oral phase of swallowing.

bone conduction: The process by which vibrations are transmitted to the cochlea through the bones of the skull.

bone oscillator: A small square box on the end of a metal headband used in hearing testing to assess the type and severity of hearing loss through bone-conduction audiometry.

brainstem: A part of the brain that connects the brain and spinal cord and is how the brain and the rest of the body communicate.

Broca's aphasia: A nonfluent aphasia that results in damage to Broca's area and is characterized by slow and halted speech that is agrammatical.

Broca's area: An area in the frontal lobe of the brain that plays a role in language production.

case–control design: A nonexperimental study design that allows the researcher to compare a specific group of people with a condition (the *case*) to a group of people without the condition (the *control*) on specific variables of interest.

case study: A type of qualitative research that provides descriptive information about one or a few individuals or units.

celiac disease: An autoimmune disorder that causes damage to the small intestine when the individual consumes foods containing gluten.

central nervous system: A system made up of the brain and spinal cord; responsible for processing incoming sensory information and responding.

cerebellum: A part of the brain that sits under the cerebrum and is responsible for body positioning, maintaining balance, fine motor coordination, as well as various language abilities.

cerebral palsy: A group of neurological congenital conditions that occur as the fetus is developing in the womb, during birth, or shortly after birth (up to age 5 years) due to disruptions in brain development; often results in dysarthria.

cerebrum: The main part of the brain, which is divided into the left and right hemisphere and consists of four lobes.

cerumen: Ear wax.

CHARGE syndrome: A rare genetic condition resulting in *c*oloboma, *h*eart defects, *a*tresia choanae, growth *r*etardation, *g*enital abnormalities, and *e*ar abnormalities.

childhood apraxia of speech: A motor speech disorder diagnosed in children that is associated with motor programming and motor planning.

cholesteatoma: A rare condition causing conductive hearing loss that can be congenital but is usually the result of a chronic ear infection leading to an abnormal collection of skin cells inside the ear.

chorea: A movement disorder resulting in rapid and unpredictable movements.

cleft lip/palate: Congenital conditions characterized by a split in the upper lip (cleft lip) and/or the roof of the mouth (cleft palate) that occur during fetal development.

clinical expertise: Knowledge that clinicians have gained through their professional experiences.

clinical swallow evaluation: An assessment that helps determine if a patient presents with signs and symptoms of dysphagia within the context of other variables, such as mealtime performance, feeding posture/positioning, and environmental conditions; also referred to as a bedside swallow evaluation.

closed syllables: Syllables that end with a consonant.

cluster reduction: A phonological process in which a consonant from a cluster of consonants in a word is dropped, such as saying "pay" for "play."

cochlea: The spiral-like portion of the inner ear that includes the organ of Corti and is responsible for the transduction of sound waves into electrical impulses that the brain interprets as individual sound frequencies.

cochlear implant: A small, complex electronic device that helps provide a sense of sound to those who are deaf or hard of hearing; one part of the implant sits behind the ear and the other is surgically placed beneath the skin.

cochlear synaptopathy: Hidden hearing loss that indicates nerve damage between the cochlea and the vestibulocochlear nerve; not typically detected through pure-tone testing.

cognitive–behavioral therapy: A stuttering intervention approach that helps limit an individual's negative thoughts about their stuttering by identifying those thoughts, obtaining evidence that those thoughts are unwarranted, and substituting more helpful thoughts.

cognitive communication training: Intervention that supports the cognitive processes that are important to communication.

cognitive referencing: A practice comparing language and IQ scores to determine if a person is eligible for speech-language services.

cohort design: A type of nonexperimental research that gathers information about a group of people over time, particularly relating to how conditions look and change over time, how many people are diagnosed with a specific condition in a certain time frame (e.g., a year), and the relationships between different variables in a group of people.

communication difference: A variation of a symbol system used by a group and determined by the social, cultural, and regional norms of that group.

communication disorder: An impairment in the ability to receive and send messages, as well as understand concepts, including verbal, nonverbal and graphic symbols.

communication partner training: Teaching those who frequently communicate with the AAC user how to use the system, what to expect from the AAC user, and how to model language.

communicative efficiency: The rate at which a speaker conveys intelligible and/or comprehensible information to their listener.

compensatory strategies: An approach to intervention that involves teaching the client strategies to help compensate for any resulting deficits.

comprehensibility: The extent to which a listener can understand the message a speaker is trying to communicate using the auditory speech signal generated by the speaker as well as all other information relevant to the communicative exchange (setting, nonverbal cues, context, listener familiarity, etc.).

conditioned play audiometry: Used to test the hearing of very young children in which the infant or toddler is taught to respond to sounds by putting a block in a box or looking in the direction of a stuffed animal, noisemaker, or other toy when a sound is delivered from that direction.

conduction aphasia: A fluent aphasia that is characterized by mild language comprehension with more severe impaired repetition, particularly repetition of multisyllabic and complex words.

confounding variable: An unmeasured variable that can potentially impact the relationship between the independent and dependent variables.

continuous phonation: Voicing throughout an utterance.

convenience sampling: Recruiting participants in research studies who are readily available to the researchers and who are not necessarily representative of the general population of interest.

core vocabulary: High-frequency words that are used across people and settings and include frequently used pronouns, verbs, prepositions, and articles.

corpus callosum: The white matter tract that connects the two hemispheres of the brain.

correlation: A relationship between two or more variables.

covert observation: When the participants being observed are unaware that they are being observed.

covert stuttering behaviors: Behaviors used to mask or hide a person's stuttering, such as finding ways to avoid speaking situations.

cranial nerves: Pairs of nerves that are important to the muscle movements associated with various aspects of speech production.

Creutzfeldt–Jakob disease: A progressive neurodegenerative disorder that leads to brain damage, dementia, and death.

cricoarytenoid joint: The joint that connects the arytenoid cartilage with the cricoid cartilage, which allows for sliding and circular movements; it is important for facilitating the opening and closing movements of the vocal folds during voicing.

cricoid cartilage: The top of the ring of the trachea that is linked with the thyroid and arytenoid cartilages.

cricothyroid muscle: A muscle attached to the cricoid and thyroid cartilages that is responsible for lengthening (thinning) and tensing (thickening) the vocal folds.

criterion-reference measure: A measure that evaluates a student's learning against a predetermined set of criteria without comparing the student's performance to that of others.

cul-de-sac resonance: When sound resonates and is stuck in the throat or nose with no outlet, making speech sound muffled.

curb cut phenomenon: When physical structures or systems are modified so that they are accessible to disabled people, which results in benefits for nondisabled people as well.

decibel (dB): A unit of measurement for sound pressure level.

deglutition: The act of transporting food from the oral cavity to the stomach; also referred to as swallowing.

deinstitutionalization movement: A project of the disability rights movement aimed at exposing institutions housing disabled people to the public.

dementia: A progressive neurocognitive disorder that results in significant decline in complex attention, executive ability, learning and memory, language, and social cognition and interferes with daily functioning and independence.

dental: Place of articulation involving the teeth.

dependent variable: The outcome variable, which is dependent on other variables (namely, the independent variable).

descriptive research: Nonexperimental research examining relationships, patterns, or differences without the manipulate.

desensitization: A stuttering intervention approach that limits the negative personal reactions to stuttering through gradual exposure to uncomfortable stimuli.

dialect: A rule-governed language system that reflects the regional and social background of a speaker.

differential exposure hypothesis: A theory that states that women (compared to men) are exposed to more risk factors and have access to fewer resources that protect against certain disabilities.

differential vulnerability hypothesis: A theory that states that women have similar exposure to the risk factors as men, yet women present with greater challenges and disabilities as a result.

dignity of risk: The feeling of empowerment to make one's own choices in life, assume personal responsibility for one's actions, and consequently succeed or fail.

direct activation pathway: The path on which messages get sent from the cortex to the muscles regarding the initiation of complex and voluntary muscle movements; also called the pyramidal tract.

disability: A complex and multifaceted concept that describes the interactions of physical, psychological, intellectual, and socioeconomic differences that affect a person's ability to function and participate in society.

disability–poverty cycle: The idea that poverty impacts disability, and disability impacts poverty.

disability rights movement: A movement created to fight for equal rights for those with disabilities.

disability with aging: Individuals who develop disabilities due to older age.

discourse: The exchange of ideas through verbal or written means.

distributed practice: The child practices various skills (e.g., several syllable shapes) in a single session.

Down syndrome: A genetic condition in which an individual has a full or partial copy of chromosome 21 that impacts cognitive, motor, and speech and language development.

dynamic assessment: a method of assessment that focuses on the learning process and a child's capacity for learning with scaffolded support using modeling, cueing, and prompting.

dynamic temporal and tactile cueing (DTTC): A motor-based intervention approach used with children who have childhood apraxia of speech; DTTC uses auditory and visual models, slowed rate, fading of cues, and feedback about speech production to support accurate production.

dysarthria: Motor speech disorders in which the muscles and movements (in terms of speed, strength, range of motion, tone, and accuracy) that are required for the processes associated with speech production (i.e., respiration, phonation, resonance, articulation, and prosody) are impacted.

dyscalculia: A learning disorder associated with mathematics, including difficulty understanding numbers and math facts, completing math calculations, and processing numerical information.

dysgraphia: A learning disorder associated with difficulty with writing.

dyslexia: A learning disorder associated with reading; difficulty decoding and spelling words with inaccurate recognition of words when reading.

dysphagia: A swallowing disorder.

dysphonia: Loss of phonatory control usually characterized by a breathy voice in which a person seems to lose their voice and other times the voice seems appropriate.

dysphoria: Unease or discontent about an aspect of life; in voice disorders, voice dysphoria suggests a disparity between how someone views themselves and how they communicate or how their voice sounds.

dyspnea: The feeling of running out of air and not being able to breathe during physical activity.

dystonia: Slow, involuntary movements that are abnormal in their posture.

easy onset: A fluency technique that involves gradual voicing of initial vowels.

edema: Swelling.

edentulous: Without teeth.

effortful control: A component of temperament that facilitates self-regulation.

electromagnetic articulography (EMA): A technique using an electromagnetic field created around the head to track sensors placed on different articulators, such as the lips, tongue, and jaw, to measure the position and movement of these structures during speech.

electromyography (EMG): A technique used to measure electrical activity generated in skeletal muscle by inserting electrodes through the skin into the muscle.

empirical research: Research resulting from the collection of new data.

enhanced milieu teaching: A naturalistic intervention that incorporates behavioral strategies to help shape functional language in children who are in an early language development stage.

enlarged vestibular aqueduct syndrome: Inner ear malformation causing both hearing loss and vestibular problems.

eosinophilic esophagitis: An immune disease in the esophagus resulting from a buildup of white blood cells.

epiglottis: The flap of cartilage that is located at the base of the tongue in the pharynx that closes over the trachea during swallowing, which prevents food and liquid from entering into the airway.

epistaxis: Nose bleeding.

esophageal dysphagia: A swallowing disorder in which food cannot move through the esophagus.

ethnographic interviewing: An assessment technique where the clinician gathers in-depth and descriptive information from a child, their family, and teachers to better understand what the child's language abilities looks like in different contexts and with different people.

eustachian tube: The passage that leads from the pharynx to the middle ear and is important for equalizing pressure on each side of the tympanic membrane.

evidence-based practice: The integration of current research evidence, clinical experience, and client perspectives when approaching treatment.

executive functions: Cognitive functions that include attention, memory, planning, and inhibition.

exercise-induced laryngeal obstruction (EILO): Obstruction occurs during exercise; vocal cords adduct, involuntarily and intermittently restricting one's airway when inhaling and exhaling.

experimental research: Research in which there is random group assignment and the researchers have control over one or more variables.

expiratory pressure device: A small handheld device typically used to move mucous out of the lungs.

expressive language: The output of language to communicate a message using verbal (e.g., spoken and/or written) or nonverbal (e.g., gestures) language.

external auditory meatus: External ear canal

external evidence: Evidence that is based on scientific findings.

extrapyramidal tract: The path on which the brainstem sends involuntary muscle movements and reflexes that support movement and motor control to the spinal cord; also known as the indirect activation pathway.

extrinsic feedback: Feedback provided by others.

facial nerve: The seventh pair of cranial nerves that control facial movements, hyoid elevation, salivation, and taste.

fast mapping: The ability to learn new words or concepts after minimal exposure.

features of an alternative response: A principle in functional communication training (FCT) that considers the response match, success, efficiency, acceptability, recognizability, and the social environment.

feeding: The process of eating food.

feeding disorder: A disorder in which an individual (usually an infant or child) has trouble eating food often based on textures of certain food groups.

fiberoptic endoscopic evaluation of swallowing (FEES): A type of instrumental swallowing assessment that uses a flexible endoscope to visualize the larynx and pharynx.

fidelity: Research or intervention is carried out as intended based on the established guidelines and procedures.

final consonant deletion: A phonological process in which the final consonant is dropped at the end of words, such as saying "do" for "dog."

flaccid dysarthria: A motor speech disorder that includes hypernasality, breathiness, abnormalities with speech–breath coordination, and reduced vocal quality with vocal use.

fluency: The effort, rate, and smoothness of one's speech.

fluency disorder: A communication disorder where there is disruption to the flow of one's speech, including hesitations; sound, syllable, and word repetitions; and significant tension when speaking.

focused stimulation: A language intervention technique that uses predetermined vocabulary in a highly concentrated way to support vocabulary development.

fragile X: A genetic condition caused by changes in the fragile X messenger ribonucleoprotein gene leading to delays in cognitive, motor, and speech and language development, as well as social and behavioral problems and learning disabilities.

frequency: The number of times a vibration cycle repeats itself in 1 second, commonly referred to as pitch.

fricatives: Sounds made when the articulators are not quite closed or touching so the air escapes as if to create a hissing or friction-like sound; the most common fricatives are sibilant sounds such as the [s] in "sip" or the z in "zoo."

Friedreich's ataxia: A progressive neurodegenerative disorder that impacts movement, including posture, challenges with walking, and increased fatigue.

fringe vocabulary: Primarily nouns that are used less frequently and are usually specific to certain contexts, environments, or topics.

frontal lobe: A lobe of the brain located in the front of the brain that houses the prefrontal cortex and motor cortex; important for executive functions.

fronting: A phonological process in which a sound that occurs in the back of the mouth (e.g., [k]) is substituted with a sound that occurs in the front of the mouth (e.g., [t]), such as saying "tat" for "cat."

frontotemporal dementia: One type of dementia that occurs because of damage to neurons in the frontal and temporal lobes.

functional communication training: A type of intervention that focuses on teaching communication that is most personally relevant to the individual communicator.

functional equivalence: A principle of FCT in which a behavior is replaced by another behavior if the new behavior serves the same function and is more efficient at gaining the desired reinforcers.

functional magnetic resonance imaging (fMRI): A noninvasive and safe technique for mapping and measuring brain activity.

functional speech sound disorders: Speech disorders with no known cause.

functional voice disorder: A voice disorder in which there are no differences in the physical mechanism used to speak, but there is inefficient use of the vocal mechanism.

fundamental frequency: The rate at which the vocal folds vibrate when voiced speech sounds are made.

gastroesophageal reflux disease (GERD): Chronic acid reflux that contributes to heartburn or other pain.

gender-affirming voice therapy: A new area of study and intervention used to support gender-diverse individuals who are undergoing gender transition.

gender dysphoria: A mismatch with gender identity and desired voice.

gestalt: An organized and synthesized whole that is not just the sum of its parts; the "bigger picture."

gestalt imagery: Use of language to help us think about what we see, hear, and feel.

global aphasia: A nonfluent aphasia that results from damage to much of the left hemisphere and is characterized by widespread receptive and expressive language difficulties.

glottal: Sounds made at the very back of the windpipe, such as [h] in "hello."

glottal stop: Rapid closure of the vocal folds during speech and then a quick release of air to make a sound.

glottic stenosis: A narrowing of the larynx at the vocal folds due to scarring, webbing, and so on.

glottis: The space between the vocal folds that varies according to the actions of the vocal folds.

graphic organizers: Organizational tools that visually arrange key words or concepts.

gray matter: A type of brain and spinal cord tissue that is important to day-to-day functioning; it is where sensation, voluntary movement, learning, speech, and cognition take place.

Guillain–Barré: A neurodegenerative autoimmune disorder that results in weakness in the arms and legs and can lead to paralysis.

hair cells: Located in the cochlea of the inner ear, these are the sensory receptor cells that are responsible for transferring sound-induced vibrations into electrical signals which are sent to the brain.

hard palate: The bony part of the roof of the mouth behind the gum ridge that separates the oral cavity from the nasal cavity.

healthy disabled: Disabled individuals whose abilities and limitations are relatively stable and predictable

hearing or auditory threshold: The level at which humans can first detect sound (often approximately 50% of the time).

hemorrhagic stroke: A stroke that occurs when arteries or blood vessels burst, which causes bleeding on the exterior of the brain or inside of the brain tissues.

hertz (Hz): The physical measure of sound frequency determined by the number of vibrations that occur per second; what is perceived perceptually as pitch.

hiatal hernia: A condition in which part of the stomach pushes into an opening in the diaphragm and into the chest.

high-tech systems: AAC systems that come in the form of computers or tablets and have voice output.

human papilloma virus: A viral infection that causes skin or mucous membrane growths (warts).

Huntington's disease: A progressive neurodegenerative disease that impacts a person's cognitive, physical, and mental abilities over time.

hyoid bone: A small U-shaped bone situated in the neck between the chin and the thyroid cartilage that is important for swallowing function and speech production.

hyperadduction: Too much tension in the vocal folds.

hyperkinetic dysarthria: A motor speech disorder associated with involuntary and abnormal muscular movements of the muscles necessary for respiration, phonation, articulation, resonance, and prosody.

hypernasality: Too much resonance in the nasal cavity due to sound being channeled through the nose.

hypoglossal nerve: The 12th pair of cranial nerves that is important for movement of the tongue.

hypokinetic dysarthria: A motor speech disorder associated with rigidity of movement or a reduced range of motion.

hyponasality: Occurs when there is reduced resonance in the nasal cavity, causing a person's speech to sound stuffed up or congested.

hypothesis: A prediction about the outcome of the study or the relationship between the variables being studied.

identity-first language: Language used where the person's disability is mentioned before the individual (e.g., disabled person, autistic adult) to signify their disability.

impairment: A loss of function or some difference in structure that impedes behavior.

impairment-based approaches: Intervention approaches that focus on improving skills that have been negatively affected; also called restorative approaches.

incidence: The number of identified new cases with a specific condition.

incus: A bone in the middle ear also called the anvil; one of the three small bones in the ossicular chain.

independent living movement: A movement that supports disabled people by providing them independence to begin making their own decisions about medical care separate from the institutions.

independent variable: The variable that the researcher wants to study that is manipulated or varied and does not depend on any other variable.

indirect activation pathway: The path along which the brainstem sends involuntary muscle movements and reflexes that support movement and motor control to the spinal cord; also known as the extrapyramidal tract.

Individuals With Disabilities Education Act (IDEA): A law ensuring that all children in the United States have access to free and appropriate education.

initial consonant deletion: A phonological process in which the initial consonant in a word is dropped, such as "at" for "cat."

initiation of joint attention: Intentionally directing another person's attention for social purposes, as in sharing an experience rather than requesting an action or object; a child may demonstrate this by raising an object toward a caregiver's face while making eye contact and showing the object.

intelligibility: Clarity of an individual's speech and the amount of their speech that a listener can understand.

intensity: Loudness.

intercostal muscles: Many different muscle groups that run between the ribs that help form and move the chest wall; these muscles are involved in breathing by helping expand and shrink the size of the chest cavity.

interdental (frontal) lisp: Occurs when the tongue sticks out between the front teeth during production, usually occurring as substituting a "th" sound for /s/ or /z/ (e.g., saying "thity" for "city").

internal evidence: Data that is specific to the client receiving intervention.

International Classification of Functioning, Disability and Health model: A functional model of disability that considers how the person's health condition interacts with the environment to either support or hinder participation in various life activities.

interprofessional education: Learning with and from other disciplines with the goal of collaborating to improve a patient's or client's quality of care.

interprofessional practice: A practice in which professionals from different disciplines learn about, from, and with one another to provide care to their clients.

intraoral pressure: Pressure created by movement of the tongue to the pharyngeal wall.

intrinsic feedback: Awareness of the sensory information associated with speech production to monitor one's own production of speech

ischemic stroke: A stroke that occurs when blood flow to the brain is disrupted due to a complete or partial block in the artery.

labial: Lips.

labial-dental: Consonant sounds made when the top teeth contact the bottom lip.

language scaffolding: Incorporating segments of a child's utterance into an adult response that adds new information, such as new vocabulary or more complex grammar.

laryngeal cleft: A rare condition resulting in an opening between the larynx and the esophagus accompanied by hoarseness, stridor, dysphagia, and coughing.

laryngeal nerve: A nerve that branches from cranial nerve X (i.e., the vagus nerve) and provides innervation to the intrinsic laryngeal muscles except for the cricothyroid muscles.

laryngeal webbing: Tissue that connects the vocal folds which can block the airway; frequently occurs in infancies during weeks 4 to 10 of gestation.

laryngomalacia: A congenital laryngeal condition that is a frequent cause of stridor in infants.

laryngoscopy: A procedure in which an endoscope (i.e., a medical instrument attached to a light source) is used to examine the larynx and other surrounding structures in the throat.

laryngospasm: Spasming of the vocal folds.

lateral cricoarytenoid muscle: One of two muscles that helps bring the vocal folds together (adduction).

lateral lisp: Where air is forced over the sides of the tongue for sounds such as /s/, /z/, and "sh" instead of out the front, resulting in a "slushy" speech quality; also called a lateral /s/ or palatal lisp.

learning disability: A term that was initially used to describe individuals with learning disorders or specific learning disorders related to challenges in reading, writing, and math.

Lewy body dementia: A type of dementia that occurs when protein deposits develop in the brain.

liquid: A consonant sound in which the tongue produces a partial closure in the mouth, resulting in a resonant, vowel-like consonant (e.g., l and r in English).

literature review: A comprehensive summary of existing research on a topic.

loudness: The human perception of sound intensity.

lower motor neuron system: Part of the peripheral nervous system that is composed of the cranial nerves and spinal nerves.

malleus: The first of three small bones in the middle ear that is attached to the eardrum or tympanic membrane.

mandible: The lower part of the jaw.

manner: The way in which speech sounds are produced.

masking: Introducing noise to a non-test ear during audiological testing to ensure that the ear being tested hears the presented tone.

mastication: Chewing.

maxilla (or maxillae—plural): The upper part of the jaw.

maxilla bone: The bone structure that houses the upper teeth and forms a portion of the jaw; important for chewing and speaking.

medical model of disability: A model of disability that describes disability as occurring from a health condition or disease.

medulla oblongata: The connection between the brainstem and the spinal cord; composed of the cardiovascular–respiratory regulation system and motor and sensory tracts. It is the origin of four cranial nerves (CNs): the glossopharyngeal nerve (CN IX), the vagus nerve (CN X), the accessory nerve (CN XI), and the hypoglossal nerve (CN XII).

melodic intonation therapy: An intervention approach that targets verbal expression; often used with individuals with motor speech disorders or aphasia.

Ménière's disease: Inner ear disease causing vertigo, tinnitus, and fluctuating hearing loss.

meta-analysis: A statistical analysis that combines the results of various studies that attempt to answer a specific research question.

metacognitive skills: The ability to think about one's thoughts, which is helpful for learning.

metalinguistic skill: The awareness of language and of one's own thinking about language.

mindfulness: A stuttering intervention strategy that involves learning ways to increase awareness and respond to mental processes that create emotional distress and atypical behavior.

minority group model: A model in line with the social model of disability which states that people are disabled by the barriers constructed by society and thus society should be held responsible for providing resources to disabled people.

modeling: When a communication partner models language using an AAC system.

modified barium swallow study (MBS): A type of instrumental swallowing assessment that provides speech-language pathologists with a direct view of the oral, pharyngeal, and esophageal phases of swallowing; also referred to as the videofluoroscopic swallowing study (VFSS).

morphemes: The smallest units of language that cannot be divided into smaller units

morphology: A component of language that deals with the structure of words (e.g., words are made of smaller meaningful unit or parts).

motor speech disorder: A group of disorders associated with neurological conditions that impact a person's muscle movements and/or motor planning necessary for speech production.

multiple sclerosis: A progressive central nervous system condition that causes communication problems between the brain and the rest of the body.

myasthenia gravis: An autoimmune disorder resulting in muscle weakness and difficulties with speech production and swallowing.

myoelastic–aerodynamic theory: A theory of phonation that suggests that vocal fold movement is determined by interactions between aerodynamic stresses.

nasal regurgitation: When liquid or solid bolus is expelled from the nose.

nasoendoscopy: A procedure in which a thin, flexible endoscope is inserted through the nose and passed into the throat to examine structures of the nose and throat, including the larynx.

nasometry: An instrument used to quantify nasal air escape during speech; this tool is particularly valuable in the assessment and treatment of individuals who have difficulties closing off their velopharyngeal port.

nasopharynx: The upper part of the throat behind the nose.

natural communities of reinforcement: A principle in FCT that uses communication as a replacement behavior to help obtain desired reinforcers.

naturalness (of speech): Speech that sounds typical to the listener.

negative correlation: When two or more variables are related and move in opposite directions.

negative reinforcement: A component of operant conditioning that involves the removal of an aversive stimuli when a specific behavior is performed.

neologisms: Novel, invented words.

neurodevelopmental disorder: A condition affecting how the brain functions that ranges from mild impairments to severe disorders; examples include attention-deficit/hyperactivity disorder, autism, and speech and language disorders.

neurogenic voice disorders: Voice disorders that result from problems in the nervous system that affect vocal mechanism functioning.

nonempirical research: Research that makes use of data that have already been collected, analyzed, and interpreted.

nonexperimental research: Research examining relationships, patterns, or differences without the manipulation of any variables. See **descriptive research**.

nonsyllabic: A speech sound that does not stand alone as a syllable.

norm-referenced measure: A measure that compares an individual's score to the performance of others.

no-tech systems: AAC systems that do not require any technology, and therefore do not have a voice output (e.g., picture boards, alphabet boards, communication books).

observational study: A type of nonexperimental research, usually qualitative, in which the researcher systematically records the behaviors or phenomenon of interest with or without it being known that the researcher is observing.

occipital lobe: An area of the brain located in the back, above the cerebellum, and houses the visual cortex.

occipital–temporal: Area of the brain that stores the recognition and meaning of words that supports reading fluency.

open syllables: Syllables that end with a vowel.

operant conditioning: A behavioral modification strategy in which behaviors are shaped based on positive and negative reinforcement and punishments.

opportunity barriers: Ways in which the environment limits the person's ability to participate using AAC.

oral dysphagia: A swallowing disorder that occurs in the oral phase of the swallow and usually involves challenges with the tongue and lips.

orbicularis oris muscle: A complex, multilayered muscle attached to the dermis of the upper lip and lower lip; attachment site for several facial muscles in the oral region.

organ of Corti: Part of the inner ear responsible for producing nerve impulses as a response to vibrations of sound.

organic speech sound disorders: Speech disorders resulting from an underlying neurological, structural, motor, or perceptual problem.

organic voice disorders: Voice disorders that occur due to changes in the mechanisms used to speak, whether it is the laryngeal area, the vocal tract, or the respiratory function.

oropharynx: The middle part of the throat that is behind the mouth; it includes the soft palate, side and back walls of the throat, the tonsils, and the back one-third of the tongue.

ossicular chain: Part of the middle ear consisting of three bones—the malleus, incus, and stapes—comprising the main sound conduction mechanism to transmit sound vibrations from the eardrum to the oval window in the cochlea.

otitis media with effusion (OME): Collection of non-infected fluid in the middle ear; also known as serous or secretory otitis media (SOM).

otoacoustic emissions (OAE): Sounds generated from the cochlea transmitted through the middle to the external ear canal, where they can be recorded and help detect hearing loss.

otoscopy: A procedure that examines the ear structure, specifically the external auditory canal and tympanic membrane.

oval window: The opening from the middle ear to the cochlea of the inner ear.

overextensions: A language error in which an individual uses words with similar features, but does not differentiate multiple features of the word, such as saying "cow" for both a "cow" and a "pig."

overt observation: When the participants being observed are aware that they are being observed.

overt stuttering behaviors: Aspects of stuttering that are observable, such as sound prolongations, syllable or word repetitions, and blocking on words.

palatal lift: A prosthetic device with a posterior projection to help keep the velum in a raised position.

palatine bone or process: A paired, L-shaped facial bone that comprises a portion of the nasal cavity and palate.

papilloma: A benign wart-like growth on the voice box caused by human papillomavirus.

paradoxical vocal fold movement (PVFM): A voice disorder in which the vocal folds come together when a person inhales significantly impacting breathing.

parallel talk: Commenting on what a child is doing while they are doing it.

parietal lobe: A lobe of the brain that is located behind the frontal lobe and includes the somatosensory cortex; processes sensory and visuospatial information.

parietal–temporal: An area of the brain that facilitates word analysis and sounding out words.

Parkinson's disease: A progressive neurodegenerative disease that often results in tremors, stiffness, and slow movement as well as soft and slurred speech.

passive articulators: Articulators that do not move during the production of speech.

peer-reviewed: When a piece of scientific work (e.g., book, article, presentation) has been reviewed by others in the field who have expertise on the topic and has been identified as having merit or contributing to science.

Pendred syndrome: A rare genetic condition in children characterized by bilateral hearing loss at birth and a goiter (enlarged thyroid gland in the neck) that usually appears during the teenage years.

penetration: When the bolus enters the top of the airway, above the vocal folds.

peripheral nervous system: Consists of nerves and ganglia outside of the brain and spinal cord; responsible for transmitting information between the brain and the body.

peristalsis: When the muscles of the esophagus contract, causing the bolus to move into the stomach.

person-first language: Language used in which the person is mentioned before the disability (e.g., person with a disability, child with autism).

pharyngeal or oropharyngeal dysphagia: A swallowing disorder that occurs in the pharyngeal phase of the swallow and usually involves challenges with passing food through the throat.

pharynx: The muscular tube that connects the mouth and nasal cavity to the esophagus; also known as the throat.

phenomenology: The study of a person's lived experiences.

phonemes: Distinct sound units that distinguish one word from another.

phonemic awareness: Understanding that the sounds of spoken language or phonemes work together to make words.

phonics: A technique to teach reading that focuses on the relationship between phonemes (the sounds in spoken language) and graphemes (the letters used to represent the sounds in written language).

phonological awareness: The awareness of the structures of sounds and syllables and how sounds make up syllables and syllables make up words.

phonological disorder: A speech sound disorder that occurs when a child makes speech sound errors that follow a particular pattern (e.g., deletes the final consonants in words).

phonological processes: Error patterns in speech sound development.

phonology: The patterns of speech sounds and speech sound systems in language and across languages.

pitch: The perception of how high or low a tone is.

pinna: The visible portion of the outer ear; also known as the auricle.

place: Where the articulators make contact with the vocal tract for the production of sound.

positive correlation: When two or more variables are related and move together in the same direction.

positive reinforcement: A component of operant conditioning in which desired behaviors are reinforced.

positron emission tomography (PET): A functional imaging technique that uses radioactive tracers to assess metabolic and physiologic activity in bodily organs such as the brain.

postural changes: A behavioral strategy used in dysphagia management in which the person makes changes in their posture to help with swallowing.

pragmatic difficulties: Challenges with the use of language for social purposes.

pragmatics: The use of language in social situations; also referred to as social communication.

prelinguistic milieu teaching: A play-based natural language intervention.

presbycusis: Hearing loss associated with aging.

presbyphonia: Aging voice.

prevalence: The number of individuals who are living with a specific condition.

primary progressive aphasia: A neurodegenerative condition that is not caused by a specific event or brain injury and is associated with deficits that are solely language-based, beginning with mild word-finding difficulties and progressing to more severe difficulties in word retrieval and comprehension.

print awareness: Knowledge that print carries a message and that there are print conventions (i.e., reading from left to right and from the top to bottom, knowing some words are capitalized and other are not, and that there are different forms of punctuation).

progressive bulbar palsy: A motor neuron disorder involving the lower motor neurons that results in muscle weakness and impacts speech production and swallowing.

Prompts for Restructuring Oral Muscular Phonetic Targets (PROMPT) system: A tactile-kinesthetic approach that uses touch cues to manually guide patients' articulators (e.g., tongue, lips) through production of a targeted word, phrase, or sentence.

pseudobulbar palsy: A condition that leads to dysarthria, dysphagia, and weakness in the face and tongue.

pseudohypacusis: Exaggerated or false hearing loss.

psychogenic conversion aphonia/dysphonia: A condition in which a person experiences sudden loss of voice or phonatory control due to psychological or emotional distress.

psychogenic voice disorder: A condition that affects a person's voice quality but has no structural or neurogenic explanation; often caused by psychological factors.

puberphonia: A functional voice condition usually affecting adolescent males following their voice changes during puberty in which they maintain a high-pitched voice.

pyramidal tract: The path along which messages get sent from the cortex to the muscles regarding the initiation of complex and voluntary muscle movements; also called the direct activation pathway.

qualitative data: Data that are collected and reported in the form of descriptive information often about participants' experiences, and usually include direct quotes about those experiences.

quantitative data: Numerical-based data that offer information about how much and how often something occurs.

quasi-experimental research: Research in which the researchers have control over one or more variables but groups are not randomly assigned.

random practice: Mixed stimuli are practiced throughout a session.

randomized clinical trial: An experimental study in which participants are randomly assigned to receive some sort of intervention to examine the effectiveness of a new treatment.

randomized controlled trial: An experimental study design in which participants are randomly assigned to the intervention or control group.

rapid syllable transition (ReST): A motor learning intervention used with children who have apraxia of speech to improve accuracy of speech production by targeting the transitions between sounds and words.

reading comprehension: Understanding the meaning of what is read, including both decoding (ability to translate text into speech) and language comprehension (ability to understand words and sentences).

reading fluency: The ability to read text accurately, automatically, and with expression, while also understanding what is being read.

recasting: Repeating what a child says and expanding on their utterance to include accurate and new semantic and syntactic information.

receptive language: What a person understands in oral and written communication.

reduplicated babbles: Strings of identical consonant–vowel syllables that are repeated.

reliability: The degree to which test results can be relied on as accurate.

research question: A specific question the researchers are attempting to answer.

response to joint attention: An early developmental skill that requires the child to be able to "read" the direction of their communication partner's eye gaze; the child may demonstrate this by turning their head and/or pointing to an object that a communication partner is attending to.

restorative approaches: Approaches to intervention that focuses on improving skills that have been negatively impacted; also called impairment-based approaches.

retrocochlear pathology: A difficult condition to diagnose that impacts the vestibulocochlear nerve or other components of the central auditory system, leading to hearing loss that often is the result of infections, multiple sclerosis, acoustic neuromas, or auditory neuropathy.

right hemisphere disorder: A cognitive communication disorder that results from damage to the right hemisphere and is associated with deficits in nonverbal communication and social communicative skills.

sarcopenia: Muscle atrophy that occurs with aging.

secondary behaviors: Body movements, facial grimaces, and/or eye blinks that occur during moments of stuttering.

Section 504 of the Rehabilitation Act: An act which states that people with disabilities cannot be denied benefits or face discrimination under any program or activity that has federal financial assistance.

self-disclosure: A stuttering intervention strategy in which the individual who stutters tells others about their stuttering.

self-feeding: When a child engages in the act of feeding themself.

semantic clustering: A technique of groupiing items into semantic categories such as food, clothing, and animals.

semantics: Word meaning and word relationships.

semicircular canals: Three small ones filled with fluid that support balance; located in the inner ear.

semistructured interview: A method of data collection used in qualitative research in which the researcher asks participants interview questions in a semistructured and flexible way.

sensitivity: The ability of a test to determine that a person has a disorder.

sequential bilingualism: Acquiring a second language.

siblants: Fricative consonants made by directing a stream of air with the tongue moving toward the teeth.

signal-to-noise ratio (SNR): A measure comparing the level of a desired signal to that of the background noise signal (e.g., signal at 55 dB SPL and noise at 45 dB SPL equals +10 SNR).

silent aspiration: When swallowed material enters the airway but no behavioral response such as a cough or throat clear is elicited due to decreased sensation in the upper respiratory tract.

simultaneous bilingualism: Learning two languages simultaneously.

social model of disability: A model of disability that describes a person as being disabled not because of their impairments but, rather, because the environment is not accessible.

social referencing: Referencing others in our environments to learn about the world and understand how we are supposed to react to certain (often novel) stimuli.

soft palate: A continuation of the hard palate, comprising the posterior third of the palate and consisting of muscle fibers and connective tissue covered by a mucous membrane.

somatosensory cortex: An area of the brain that receives and processes sensory information; located in the parietal lobe.

sound pressure level (SPL): A logarithmic scale measured in decibels (dB) and is the result of pressure variations in the air achieved by sound waves. The lowest sound pressure humans hear is known as hearing threshold, and the highest sound pressure humans can tolerate is known as pain threshold. A sound level meter is used to measure SPL.

spasmodic dysphonia: A voice disorder that occurs when there are involuntary movements of one or more laryngeal muscles; frequently found most often in females aged 30 to 50 years.

spastic dysarthria: A motor speech disorder characterized by spasticity, which can be described as resistance to passive stretch.

specificity: The ability of a test to determine that a person does not have a disorder.

speech intelligibility: The degree to which a listener can understand the auditory speech signal produced by the speaker.

spinal nerves: Nerves that are important for supporting the respiration functions that are associated with speech production.

spirometry: A breathing test that measures the amount and speed of air that a person can inhale into and exhale out of their lungs.

spontaneous novel utterance generation (SNUG): An approach used within AAC that supports infinitely generative communication across settings.

stapes: The last of the three bones in the middle ear that make up the ossicular chain; it fits into the oval window of the cochlea.

sterilization: Preventing the sexual reproduction of an individual.

sternum: Breastbone; a bone in the middle of the chest.

stimulability: The ability to correctly imitate a sound previously misarticulated when the clinician provides an accurate model for the sound.

stimulability testing: A diagnostic intervention approach in which the individual is asked to decrease their rate of speech or to increase their pausing to reduce symptoms of cluttering.

stridor: A high-pitched or noisy sound made when breathing, which may indicate the upper airway is partially blocked.

stroke: A condition that occurs when the blood supply to the brain is cut off or interrupted, preventing oxygen from getting to brain tissue.

structural voice disorders: Voice disorders resulting from physical changes in the vocal mechanism.

study limitation: A shortcoming or weakness of the study that may impact the results or conclusions.

subglottal air pressure: Air that builds up below the vocal folds.

submucous cleft palate: A congenital defect of the palate in which the cleft is under the mucous membrane forming the roof of the mouth.

support: A strategy frequently used to facilitate self-confidence and decrease isolation and may include group therapy and self-help groups.

survey study: A nonexperimental study design in which a researcher collects self-reported information from participants in the form of a survey.

swallowing: The act of transporting food from the oral cavity to the stomach; also referred to as deglutition.

swallowing disorder: A disorder that occurs when there are physical/anatomical (or psychological) concerns that impact a person's ability to successfully complete the swallow cycle; also referred to as dysphagia.

swallowing efficiency: The ability to move food from the oral cavity to the esophagus without leaving any residual material in the oral and/or pharyngeal cavities after the swallow.

swallowing maneuvers: Compensatory strategies in dysphagia management that aim to bring certain involuntary aspects of the swallow under the patient's voluntary control.

swallowing safety: The ability to swallow material safely without penetrating or aspirating.

syllabic: (pertaining to syllabic consonant) A consonant that forms its own syllable, such as the sounds [m, n, l] in the words "bottom," "mutton," and '"rattle."

syncope: Fainting.

syntax: How words are put together to create sentences that follow a set of rules in a language.

systematic review: A review of existing literature that attempts to answer a specific research question through systematic methodology, critical appraisal of existing studies, and interpretation of these findings.

temporal bones: A pair of symmetrical bones on each side of the head that are part of the base of the skull; they protect the temporal lobes of the brain as well as cranial nerves, in addition to the inner and middle ear.

temporal lobe: A lobe of the brain that is located on the side and bottom of the cerebrum and contains the auditory cortex and Wernicke's area.

temporomandibular joint: Two joints that connect the lower jaw to the skull; these joints slide and rotate in front of each ear and consist of the mandible and the temporal bone.

thinking maps: Visual patterns used to map out content to define, classify, describe, sequence, and compare information that supports critical thinking and problem-solving.

thorax: The area of the body between the neck and abdomen; also known as the chest.

thyroarytenoid muscle: The dense part of the vocal fold that is attached to the thyroid and arytenoid cartilages; also known as the vocalis muscle.

thyroid cartilage: A flexible tissue forming the front part of the larynx or voice box that supports and protects the vocal cords and helps create voice; it forms the Adam's apple, often appearing as a lump on the front of the neck.

tics: Rapid patterned movements that are not always involuntary; includes motor and vocal tics.

tinnitus: A ringing or buzzing sound in the ears when there is no actual source of the sound.

Tourette syndrome: A condition of the nervous system that causes people to have "tics" or sudden and repeated sounds, twitches, or movements.

tracheostomy: A medical procedure that helps air and oxygen reach the lungs by creating an opening into the windpipe or trachea from outside the neck; a person breathes through a tracheostomy tube placed in the opening of the trachea.

training specificity: The idea that communication training should be specific to the targeted skills required for the activity being practiced.

transcortical motor aphasia: A nonfluent aphasia that results from damage to the frontal lobe and is characterized by challenges initiating speech spontaneously, resulting in reduced verbal output.

transcortical sensory aphasia: A fluent aphasia that results in deficits in comprehension of speech, but intact repetition skills.

traumatic brain injury: A brain injury that results from an external force to the head, such as a fall or an assault.

tremors: Involuntary movements associated with rhythmic movements; includes musculature and vocal tremors.

trigeminal nerve: The fifth pair of cranial nerves that are responsible for sending sensory information from the face, mouth, and jaw to the brain.

tympanic membrane: The tissue that separates the outer ear from the middle ear; also known as the eardrum.

tympanometry: A test of tympanic membrane movement.

unaided AAC: Any mode of communication that a person uses that does not rely on an external tool; includes facial expressions, gestures, and pointing.

underextensions: A developmental language phenomenon where a child restricts the usage of a word. For example, they may say "cat" in response to a pet at home but may not use the word when they see a "cat" in a picture book.

unhealthy disabled: Individuals with disabilities who have chronic illnesses that cannot be reliably cured and persist over time or acute diseases that result in death.

unilateral hearing loss: Hearing loss that affects only one ear.

unilateral upper motor neuron dysarthria: A motor speech disorder associated with damage to the upper motor neuron system, resulting in weakness to one side of the lower face and tongue.

unilateral vocal fold paralysis: One of the two vocal folds are paralyzed.

universal model: A model in line with the social model of disability that brings attention to the fact that all people are at risk for becoming disabled at any point in time and that the environment should be structured in a way that is accessible to all.

upper esophageal sphincter (UES): Part of the upper digestive tract that separates the esophagus from the pharynx.

upper motor neuron system: Composed of the extrapyramidal and pyramidal tracts.

Usher syndrome: An inherited condition involving hearing (mild to deaf) and vision loss.

uvula: A small cone-shaped tip of the velum or soft palate.

vagus nerve: The 10th pair of cranial nerves that are responsible for digestion, heart rate, respiration, as well as pharyngeal, palatal, and laryngeal movement.

validity: The degree to which a test or evaluation tool measures what it was intended to measure.

valleculae: Small mucosa-lined depressions located at the base of the tongue just between the folds of the throat on either side of the median glossoepiglottic fold.

variegated syllables: When the consonants and/or vowels are varied across syllables (e.g., "wata," "daddy").

velopharyngeal closure: The closure of the velopharyngeal valve (soft palate and pharyngeal walls); air and sound are directed into the mouth and blocked from entering the nasal cavity during the production of most sounds.

velopharyngeal (VP) mechanism: A muscular valve that controls the amount of nasal acoustic energy and oral pressure for speech production through opening and closing.

velum: The soft palate.

ventricular phonation: When the false vocal folds compress over the true vocal folds with insufficient capacity to vibrate enough to make a loud sound.

vertebral column: Bones, muscles, tendons, and other tissues that reach from the base of the skull to the tailbone and that enclose the spinal cord and fluid surrounding the cord; also known as the backbone or spinal column.

vestibulocochlear nerve: The 8th cranial nerve that transfers auditory information from the cochlea to the brain; also known as the acoustic nerve

videoendoscopy: A procedure used to visually examine the upper digestive system, including the esophagus.

videofluoroscopic swallowing study (VFSS): A type of instrumental swallowing assessment that provides speech-language pathologists with a direct view of the oral, pharyngeal, and esophageal phases of swallowing; also referred to as the modified barium swallow study (MBS).

videofluoroscopy: A dynamic X-ray examination that involves a contrast material such as barium to visualize the anatomy and physiology of structures involved in speech and swallowing.

videostroboscopy: A technique involving an endoscope, microphone, video camera, and strobe light to examine vocal cord function and vocal cord vibration; an important tool used in voice assessments to visualize vocal fold vibration.

visual cortex: An area of the brain that decodes incoming visual stimuli.

visual scene display: A type of AAC that uses contextualized photographs with embedded messages or text.

vocabulary development: Knowledge about the pronunciation, meaning, and use of words.

vocal cord paralysis: A condition in which an individual cannot control the movement of the muscles of the vocal cords.

vocal cords or vocal folds: The elastic-like bands that vibrate to make sound and open and close to direct airflow.

vocal cyst: Benign growth on the vocal cord.

vocal fatigue: Experienced when one uses their voice a lot or has engaged in rigorous physical activity.

vocal nodules: Small and benign callouses on the vocal folds due to vocal overuse or misuse.

vocal polyps: Lesions on only one vocal cord due to vocal misuse.

voiced: Sounds produced with the vocal folds vibrating.

voiceless: Sounds produced without the vocal folds vibrating.

voicing: Whether the vocal folds vibrate to produce the sound.

Waardenburg syndrome: An inherited condition that results in deafness.

Wernicke's aphasia: A fluent aphasia that results from damage to Wernicke's area of the brain and is characterized by impaired comprehension and speech that is smooth and effortless but contains neologism and jargon.

Wernicke's area: An area of the brain that is important for understanding language.

white matter: A large network of nerves in the brain that allows for the exchange of information and communication between areas of the brain.

within-subjects design: An experimental study design with one group that gets compared to itself over time; this one group experiences all levels of the independent variable.

zone of proximal development: The area between what a child can do completely unaided and what they cannot do even with adult support.

Index

Note: Page numbers in **bold** reference non-text material.

A

AAC (Augmentative and alternative communication), 127, 388
  abandonment, 399
  access to, 391
  assessment, 394–396
  bilingual users, 400
  characteristics of, 388–393
  considerations for, 398–401
  importance of, 393–394
  intervention, 396–398
  multimodal communication, 399–400
  myths of, 400–401
  scanning selection method, **392**
  symbols, 393
  teaching, 397–398
  users, 394
  vocabulary, 393
AAE (African American English), 90
ABCD (Arizona Battery for Communication Disorders), 90, 239
Abducens nerve, **112**
Abducted, defined, 74
Able-bodied
  cultural view of, 21
  women, disabled and, 30
Ableism
  accessibility and, 27–28
  defined, 27
  described, 22
  internalized, 28
Ableist
  language, 262
  thinking, 28
ABR (Auditory brainstem response) testing, 361
Academic skills, 355
  children with hearing loss, 355
  learning disorders and, 188

Accents, speech and, 89–90
Acceptance therapy, for stuttering, 269
Access barriers, 399
Accessibility, ableism and, 27–28
Accessory nerve, **112**
Acid reflux, dysphagia and, 319
Acoustic
  assessment, voice disorders and, 291
  immittance testing, 357
  methods, speech signal display, 120
  nerve, 348
  neuroma, sensorineural hearing loss and, 352
  reflex testing, 358
  samples, voice disorders and, 291
Acquired communication disorders, AAC (Augmentative and alternative communication) and, 388
Acquired conditions, AAC intervention for, 397–398
Acquired disorders, 3
Active articulators, 77
  tongue, 78
AD (Alzheimer disease), 7, 235
ADA (Americans With Disabilities Act), 19
Adapted Kagan Scales, 238
Adducted, defined, 74
ADHD (Attention deficit/ hyperactivity disorder), 263
  cluttering and, 264
Adolescents
  hearing loss and, incidence/prevalence of, 355
  language disorders, intervention for, 167–168
  NVLD (Nonverbal learning disability) and, 195
  speech sound disorders and, incidence/ prevalence of, 88
Adults
  with cerebral palsy, 117
  dysphagia, 317
  hearing loss, 356

Adults *(continued)*
  intervention options for, 362–365
  speech sound disorders and, incidence/prevalence of, 88
  swallowing and
    assessment of, 321–324
    treatment approaches, 325–328
Aerodynamic
  approaches, 120
    tracking air flow, 120
  assessment, voice disorders and, 291
Affricatives, age of acquisition of, **49**
African American English (AAE), 90
African Americans
  black as a disability, 30
  evidence-based program for, 264
Age, disability and, 32
Agrammatical, defined, 228
Aided
  AAC, 388, 389
  language stimulation, AAC (Augmentative and alternative communication) and, 397–398
AIDS (Assessment of Intelligibility in Dysarthric Speech), 120
  movement, 35
Air pressure
  subglottal, 74
  vocal folds and, 76
Albert Einstein School of Medicine, studies at, 11
Alerting device, 364
ALS (Amyotrophic lateral sclerosis), 114, 115
  AAC (Augmentative and alternative communication) and, 388
  loss of speech function in, **114**
  swallowing and, 317
Alveolar
  articulator, 48
  process, 78
  ridge, 77
Alveolo-palatal, articulator, 48
Alzheimer disease (AD), 7, 235
American Psychological Association (APA), disability defined by, 19
American Speech-Language-Hearing Association (ASHA), 388
  State-by-State requirements, 9
  Voice Disorders Practice Portal, 288
Americans With Disabilities Act (ADA), 19
Amplification, voice therapy, **295**
Amplitude, loudness and, 77

Amyotrophic lateral sclerosis (ALS), 114
  AAC (Augmentative and alternative communication) and, 388
  dysarthria and, 115
  loss of speech function in, **114**
  swallowing and, 317
Analytic vocabulary instruction, 200
Anchored word instruction, 200
Angelman syndrome, 151, 153, **154–155**
  AAC (Augmentative and alternative communication) and, 388
  described, 155
Anomic aphasia, 227
Anxiety
  caregiver, 118
  disorders, NVLD (Nonverbal learning disability) and, 195
  vocal fatigue, 289
AoS (Apraxia of speech), 115
  AAC (Augmentative and alternative communication) and, 394
  articulation and, **124**
  characteristics of, childhood, **123**
  childhood, differential diagnosis of, 121–122
APA (American Psychological Association), disability defined by, 19
Aphasia, 226–230
  adjustment to, 230
  anomic, 227
  assessment of, 237
  Broca's, 228
  causes of, 229
  conduction, 227–228
  defined, 11
  fluent, 227–228
  global, 228
  impact of, 229–230
  intervention for, 240–241
  nonfluent, 228–229
  PPA (primary progressive), 229
  transcortical, sensory, 228
Aphonia, **288**
  defined, 287
  psychogenic, 287
Approximants, age of acquisition of, **49**
Apraxia Battery for Adults, MSD (Motor speech disorders), 119
Apraxia of speech (AoS), 115
  AAC (Augmentative and alternative communication) and, 388, 394

characteristics of, childhood, **123**
childhood, differential diagnosis of, 121–122
Aprosodia, RHD (Right hemisphere disorder) and, 231
AR (Auditory rehabilitation), 362–363
Arizona Battery for Communication Disorders–Second Edition (ABCD), 239
Arm movements, excessive, 260
Articles, **57**
Articulation
    acoustic samples and, 291
    AoS (Apraxia of speech) and, **124**
    defined, 3, 86
    description/examples of, **45**
    disorders, 86–87
Articulators, 77
    fricatives and, 48
Articulatory
    impairments, clear speech and, 127
    kinematic, AoS treatment and, 125
    system, 77–78
Arytenoid cartilage, 74
ASHA (American Speech-Language-Hearing Association)
    State-by-State requirements, 9
    Voice Disorders Practice Portal, 288
Asian/Pacific Islander, autism and, 152
Aspiration, 315–316
    imaging and, 325
    silent, 321–322
Assessment, 60–61
    AAC (Augmentative and alternative communication) and, 394–396
    acoustic, voice disorders and, 291
    aerodynamic, 291
    aphasia, 237
    components of, 236–237
    comprehensive, 163
    curriculum-based, **162**, 163
    dynamic, 60–61, **161**
    hearing, 357–362
        in children, 361–362
        importance of, 356–357
        procedures, 357–361
    of intelligibility, 93
    of language, **161–162**
    language disorders, 159
        approaches, 160, 162
    of learning disorders, 196–197
    self, voice disorders and, 291

speech sound
    disorders, 91–93
    outcomes, 94
standardized, 160, **161**
steps in, 61
of stimulability, 93–94
swallowing
    adult population, 321–324
    pediatric population, 324–325
voice, 291
    disorders, 291–293
Assessment Battery for Communication (ABaCo), 238
Assessment of Intelligibility in Dysarthric Speech (AIDS), 120
Asthenia voice quality, **288**
Ataxic
    cerebral palsy, 116, **117**
    dysarthria, 113
Attention
    deficit/ hyperactivity disorder (ADHD)
        cluttering and, 263, 264
        NVLD (Nonverbal learning disability) and, 195
        RHD (Right hemisphere disorder) and, 231
    tinnitus and, 346
Atypical
    voice quality
        loudness, **288**
        pitch, **288**
        resonance, **288**
Audiogram, 359
    bone conduction, **360**
Audiological rehabilitation, cochlear implants and, 263–264
Audiologists, 5–6
    career pathways for, 9
    health care settings, 6
Audiology assistants, responsibilities of, 10
Audiometry
    bone conduction, 360
    conditioned play, 362
    speech, 360
Auditory
    cortex, 226
    evoked potentials, 361
    masking, voice therapy, **295**
    meatus, external, 347
    nerve, 348, 352
    neuropathy, **353–354**
        incidence/prevalence of, 355

Auditory *(continued)*
  perceptual analysis, 120
  processing disorder, **353**
    described, 354
  training exercises, 10–11
Auditory brainstem response (ABR) testing, 361
  MSD (Motor speech disorders), 119
Auditory rehabilitation (AR), elements of, 362–363
Augmentative and alternative communication (AAC), 127
  abandonment, 399
  access to, 391
  assessment, 394–396
  bilingual users, 400
  characteristics of, 388–393
  considerations for, 398–401
  described, 388
  importance of, 393–394
  intervention, 396–398
  multimodal communication, 399–400
  myths of, 400–401
  scanning selection method, **392**
  symptoms, 393
  teaching, 397–398
  users, 394
  vocabulary, 393
Aural
  atresia, hearing loss and, 354
  intervention plan, 362
Autism, 3, 152–153
  AAC (Augmentative and alternative communication) and, 394
  cluttering and, 264
  diagnostic criteria, 152
  NVLD (Nonverbal learning disability) and, 195
  social communication disorders and, 152
  stuttering, 262
Autism Center of Excellence, Boston University, 11
Autoimmune disease, sensorineural hearing loss and, 352
Autosomal dominant hearing loss, 356
Awareness, 269

B

Babbling, canonical, stage of, **51**
Bagenstos, Samuel, *Law and the Contradictions of the Disability Rights Movement*, 35
Barbarin, Imani, disability defined by, 20
Barriers, individuals with disabilities and, 29
BDAE (Boston Diagnostic Aphasia Examination), 237
Bedside swallow evaluation, 321
Behavioral
  feeding interventions, 329
  management, 127
  problems, 366
  strategies, swallowing disorders and, 325
Behaviors
  associated with language, 223
  secondary, 260
  self-determined, cerebral palsy and, 117
Bell's palsy, 112
Bernoulli effect, 76
Bilateral hearing loss, 345
  prevalence of, 345
Bilingual
  children
    cultural considerations of, 94
    stuttering and, 263
  speakers, AAC (Augmentative and alternative communication) and, 400
Bilingualism
  sequential, 163
  simultaneous, 163
Biofeedback
  providing, 96
  voice therapy, **295**
Birth
  defects, sensorineural hearing loss and, 352
  learning disorders and, 191
  premature, speech sound disorders and, 88
Birthweight, speech sound disorders and, 88
Black adults
  evidence-based program for, 364
  prevalence of hearing loss, 345
Black children
  autism and, 152
  cerebral palsy and, 116
  communication disorders and, 4
  learning disorders incidence/prevalence and, 189
Black people
  black as a disability, 30
  disabled, 30
Blade of tongue, 78
Blindness, cultural view of, 21
Blinking, eye, 260

Index

Blocked practice, 125, 129
Blocks, 260
Body, of tongue, 78
Bolus, 314
Bone
   breast, 73
   conduction
      audiogram, **360**
      audiometry, 360
      testing with, 359
      vibrator, 360
   hyoid, 74
   mastoid, 360
   oscillators, 360
   temporal, 78, 347
   vibratory conduction, 360
Boston Diagnostic Aphasia Examination (BDAE), 237
Boston University
   Autism Center of Excellence, 11
   studies at, 11
Brain, 223
   closed/open-head injuries and, 232
   damage, aphasia and, 226
   described, 109
   development, learning disorders and, 191
   hemispheres, 224
      disorder of right, 230–232
   injury, aphasia and, 229
   lobes of, 225
   reading and, 192, **192**
   stuttering, 264
   tumors
      dysarthria and, 115
      swallowing and, 317
Brainiac, defined, 223
Brainstem, 223
Brazil, learning disorders incidence/prevalence and, 189
Breastbone, 73
Breastfeeding, mother–child skin-to-skin contact, 329
Breath, rate, 73
Breathing, diaphragmatic, 126
Breathy voice quality, **288**, 294
Broca's area, 225, 226
   aphasia, 226, 228
Buck v. Bell, Supreme Court, 22
Bulbar palsy, progressive, 112

C

Canada, receptive language disorder, median prevalence, 150
Cancer, laryngeal, intervention for, 294–296
Canonical babbling, stage of, **51**
Carbon dioxide, 73
Caregivers
   AAC abandonment, 399
   dysphagia, 320, 330
   of individuals with dysarthria, 118
   mealtime and, 317
   social communication training, 317
   Spanish speaking, 367
   support of, 339
   training of, 338
Caregivers Optimizing Achievement of Children With Hearing Loss (COACH), 367
Carter-Long, Lawrence, disability defined by, 19
Cartilages, thyroid and, 74
CAS (Childhood apraxia of speech), 115
   characteristics of, **123–124**
   speech/language and, 118
   treatment approaches, 129
Case
   history, includes, 93
   studies, 422
Case Western Reserve University, studies at, 12
CBT (Cognitive–behavioral therapy), for stuttering, 269
CCNs (Complex communication needs), 388
Center for Health Statistics, childhood speech sound disorders and, 88
Central nervous system (CNS), 109
   responsibilities of, 73
Cerebellum, 223
Cerebral palsy (CP), 115–116
   AAC (Augmentative and alternative communication) and, 388, 394
   types of, **117**
Cerebrovascular accident. *See* Stroke
Cerebrum, 223–224
Cerumen, 347
CHARGE syndrome, 352, 356
Cheerleaders, vocal fold changes and, 286
Child report measures, **162**
Childhood
   DLDs (Developmental language disorders), 147
   hearing loss, 345, 352–356

Childhood *(continued)*
    speech sound disorders and, incidence/
        prevalence of, 88
Childhood apraxia of speech (CAS), 115
    characteristics of, **123–124**
    speech/language and, 118
    treatment approaches, 129
Childhood language disorders
    autism, 152–153
    causes of, 150–151
    cultural considerations of, 163–164
    genetic syndromes, 153–158
    incidence/prevalence of, 150
    intellectual developmental disorder and, 153
    intervention for, 164–168
        preschoolers, 165–167
    knowledge about, 146–158
    learning disorders and, 152
    signs/symptoms of, 148–150
    social communication disorders and, 151–152
    swallowing and, treatment approaches,
        328–329
Children
    bilingual, cultural considerations of, 94
    communication disorders and, 4
    deaf and hard of hearing (DHH), 354–355, 365
        cultural/linguistic considerations, 367
        vocabulary development, 372
    dysphonia and, 285
    hearing disorders and, prevalence of, 345
    hearing loss, 352–356
        effects of, 355
        literacy challenge, 366
    intervention options for, 365–367
    MSD (Motor speech disorders), diagnosis, 121
    NVLD (Nonverbal learning disability) and, 195
    school-age, audiologists and, 6
    speech sound disorders and, intervention for,
        94–97
    stuttering, stop, 260–261
    swallowing and, treatment approaches,
        328–329
Chin tuck against resistance (CTAR), 327
Cholesteatoma
    described, 354–355
    hearing loss and, 354
Chorea, defined, 113
Chronic illnesses, 20
CIs (Cochlear implants)
    audiological rehabilitation, 263–264

    auditory neuropathy and, 355
    components of, **263**
    hearing aids and, 355
    recommended age for, 366
City University of New York (CUNY), translating
    research to practice and, 12
Classroom observation, 162
Clear speech, described, 127
Cleft
    laryngeal, 290
    palate, 3
        otitis media and, 354
        submucous, 91
        view of, **81**
Clinical swallow evaluation (CSE), adult
        population, 321–322
Closed
    captions, **28**
    syllables, 48
Closed-head injuries, 232
CLQT (Cognitive Linguistic Quick Test), 239
Cluster reduction, 89
Cluttering
    causes of, 263–264
    characteristics of, **264**
    defined, 263
    intervention for, 270
CNS (Central nervous system), 109
    of central nervous system (CNS), 73
COACH (Caregivers Optimizing Achievement of
        Children With Hearing Loss), 367
Coaches, vocal fold changes and, 286
Cochlea, hearing loss and, 352
Cochlear
    hair cells, 348
        damage to, 352
    synaptopathy, 356
Cochlear implants (CIs)
    audiological rehabilitation, 263–264
    auditory neuropathy and, 355
    components of, **263**
    hearing aids and, 355
    recommended age for, 366
Cochleovestibular nerve, **112**
Cognitive, 7
    affective therapy, 241
    behavioral therapy (CBT), for stuttering, 269
    communication
        disorders and, assessment of, 236
        training, 243

decline, hearing loss and, 356
deficits
   children and, 128
      therapy, stuttering and, 269
      tinnitus and, 346
   disorders, cerebral palsy and, 117
   impairments, RHD (Right hemisphere disorder) and, 231
   processing problem, co-occurring language disorder, 150
Cognitive Linguistic Quick Test (CLQT), 239
Cohort designs, 419
Colleges
   audiologists and, 6
   SLPs and, 9
Coma, **233**
Communication
   challenges, addressing, 159–170
   defined, 1
   difference, described, 4
   disorders, 20
      AAC (Augmentative and alternative communication) and, 388
      cultural considerations, 4
      cultural considerations of, 239
      described, 3–4
      frequency of, 3
      gender and, 4
      intervention for, 239–240
      research innovations in, 10–12
   improving efficiency, stuttering and, 268
   intentional, 52
   partner training, 398–399
   RHD (Right hemisphere disorder) and, 231
   sciences, research innovations in, 10–12
   voice disorders and, 287
Communicative efficiency, defined, 120
Compensation, children with hearing loss, 355
Compensatory strategies, 240
Complex communication needs (CCNs), 388
Complexity approach, **97**
Comprehensibility, defined, 120
Comprehension, reading, 199
Comprehensive assessment, 163
Concerts, hearing loss and, 356
Conditioned play audiometry, 362
Conduction aphasia, 227–228
Conductive hearing loss, 351–352, **353**
Confounding variable, 419
Congenital disorders, 3

   hearing loss, 345, 354, 368
Consistent practice, 125
Consonants
   age of acquisition of, **49**
   cluster, reduction, **90**
   final deletion of, 89, **90**
   fricative, 48
   initial deletion of, 89
   liquid sound, 48
   place, manner, voicing for English, **96**
   speech development and, 47
Contextual utilization, **97**
Contractible
   auxiliary, **57**
   copula, **57**
Convenience sampling, 244
Conversation training therapy, **295**
Conversations
   autism and, 152
   discourse, 230–231
   social communication disorders and, 152
Co-occurring language deficits, 128, 150, 191
Cooing, stage of, **51**
Core
   vocabulary, 393
      approach, **97**
   words, 393
Corpus callosum, 224
Correlation
   defined, 420
   negative, 420, **421**
   positive, **421**
Coughing, voice disruption, 289
Council for Exceptional Children, Division for Early Childhood, 61
Council on Academic Accreditation for Speech-Language Pathology, 7
Counseling, intervention and, 264
Covert
   observation, 422
   stuttering
      behaviors, 262
      impacts of, 262–263
CP (Cerebral palsy),
   AAC (Augmentative and alternative communication) and, 388, 394
   types of, **117**
Cranial nerves, 109, **112**
   posterior view, **111**
Creutzfeldt–Jakob disease, dysarthria and, 115

Cricoarytenoid
  joint, 74
  muscles, 74
Cricoid cartilage, 74
  cricothyroid muscle and, 74
Cricothyroid muscle, 74
Criterion-referenced tests, 61
CSE (Clinical swallow evaluation), adult population, 321–322
CTAR (Chin tuck against resistance), 327
Cul-de-sac resonance, 292
Cultural considerations
  childhood language disorders, 163–164
  communication disorders and, 4
  diverse populations, 97
  of intervention, 244
  MSD (Motor speech disorders), 118
  reading disorders, 193
  speech production, 89–91
CUNY (City University of New York), translating research to practice and, 12
Curb cut phenomenon, 28
Curb cuts/ramps, **28**
Curriculum-based
  assessment, **162**, 163
  writing process, 205
Cyclical strategy, 97
Cysts, defined, 289

D

Data
  qualitative, 420
  quantitative, 417
DB (Decibel), defined, 344–345
DCT (Discourse Comprehension Test), 238
Deaf and hard of hearing (DHH)
  children, 354–355, 365
    cultural/linguistic considerations, 367
    vocabulary development, 372
  vocabulary development, 355, 372
Deaf movement, 35
Deafness, cultural view of, 21
Decibel (DB), defined, 344–345
Declarative sentences, 56
Deglutition, defined, 313
Deinstitutionalization movement, 35
Delivery options, service, 97
Dementia, 7, 234–236
  Alzheimer disease, 7, 235
  assessment of, 239
  causes of, 235
  defined, 234–235
  impact of, 236
  intervention for, 243–244
Demyelinating diseases, dysarthria and, 115
Dental
  articulator, 48
  fricative, 48
Dependent variables, 417
Depression
  caregiver, 118
  hearing loss and, 356
  vocal fatigue, 289
Descriptive
  research, 419
  sentences, 56
Desensitization, for stuttering, 269
Designs, cohort, 419
Developmental disabilities, 20
Developmental language disorders (DLDs), 128
  AAC intervention for, 396–397
  assessment of, 60
  causes of, 150
  childhood, 147
  risks for, 147
DHH (Deaf and hard of hearing), 372
  children, 354–355, 365
    cultural/linguistic considerations, 367
    vocabulary development, 355, 372
Diagnostic and Statistical Manual of Mental Disorders, 86
Dialects, described, 90
Diaphragm, 73
Diaphragmatic breathing, 126
Difference, 3
Differential
  diagnosis, 121–122
  exposure hypothesis, 31
  vulnerability hypothesis, 31
Differentiated instruction, 200
Diminutization, **90**
Diplegia, 116
Direct
  instruction, 200
  activation pathway, 109
  treatment, for stuttering, 268
Disability
  adaptations designed for, **28**
  advocacy, 27

age and, 32
barriers/disadvantages and, 29
defined, 3–4, 19–20
gender and, 30–32
history of, 20–23
illness and, 27
intersectionalities of, 28–29
medical versus social models of, 24
models of, 23–25
   medical, 23
   social, 23
poverty cycle, 33
race and, 29–30
rights
   in the United States, 34–36
     movement, 34–35
social model of, 23, 36
socioeconomic status and, 32–34
types of, 20
ugly laws and, 21
Disabled
   Black people, 30
   healthy, defined, 27
   unhealthy, defined, 27
   women, disabled and, 30
Disadvantages, individuals with disabilities and, 29
Discourse, described, 230–231
Discourse Comprehension Test (DCT), 238
Diseases, spread of, 21
Disorder, defined, 3
Distinctive feature approach, **97**
Distributed practice, 129
Diverse populations, intervention considerations, 97
DLDs (Developmental language disorders), 128
   AAC intervention for, 396–397
   assessment of, 60
   causes of, 150
   childhood, 147
   risks for, 147
Dorsum of tongue, 78
Doubling, **90**
Down syndrome, 3, 29, 151, 153, **154–155**
   AAC (Augmentative and alternative communication) and, 388, 394
   co-occurring language disorder, 150
   described, 155
   ICF framework for, 23–24
   otitis media and, 354
   stuttering, 262

Drooling, 314
DTTC (Dynamic temporal and tactile cueing), 129
Dwarfism, Lavinia Warren and, 21
Dynamic assessment, 60–61, 160, **161**
Dynamic temporal and tactile cueing (DTTC), 129
Dysarthria, 110–112
   ataxic, 113
   causes of, 115
   cerebral palsy and, 116
   described, 126
   differential diagnosis of, 121–122
   flaccid, 112
   hyperkinetic, 113
   mixed, 114
   RHD (Right hemisphere disorder) and, 231
   spastic, 112–113
   treatment for, 127
   unilateral upper motor neuron, 113
Dyscalculia, defined, 189
Dysgraphia, defined, 189
Dyskinetic, cerebral palsy, 116, **117**
Dyslexia, described, 188
Dysphagia, 7, 313
   adult, 317
   characteristics of, 316–319
   impact of, 320
   neurological etiologies, 317–318
   pediatric, 316–317, 329
   RHD (Right hemisphere disorder) and, 231
Dysphonia
   described, 288
   psychogenic, 287
   spasmodic, 286, 289
   vocal nodules and, 285
   voice disorders and, functional, 285
Dyspnea, 287
Dystonia, defined, 113

E

Ear
   anatomy of, **347**
   bones of, 347
   external canal, 347
   infection, Cholesteatoma and, 354
   inner, hair cells, 10
Early
   intervention, 8
     audiologists and, 6
     delays in, 61

Early *(continued)*
　language development, 50–53
　speech development, 47–48, **48–49**
　vocalizations, stages of, **51**
Early Learning in Mathematics program, 206
EAT (Eating Assessment Tool), 321
Eating, cross-cultural information, 320
Eating Assessment Tool (EAT), 321
EBP (Evidence-based practice), components of, 424–426
Edema
　defined, 289
　vocal fold changes and, 286
Edentulous, 327
Education, intervention and, 264
EF (Executive function) difficulties
　DLDs (Developmental language disorders), 147
　frontal lobe and, 225
　second language challenges, 234
Effortful swallow, 327
EILO (Exercise-induced laryngeal obstruction), 287, 293
　intervention for, 296–297
Elasticity
　vocal folds, 76
　　fundamental frequency and, 77
Electromagnetic articulography (EMA), 120
Electromyography (EMG), 120
Elementary schools, intervention and, 8
Elevators, **28**
EMA (Electromagnetic articulography), 120
EMG (Electromyography), 120
Empirical research, 415
EmPOWER writing strategy, 205
　outline of, **205**
EMST (Expiratory muscle strength training), **295**, 327–328
English, phonological processes in development of, **90**
Enlarged vestibular aqueduct syndrome, sensorineural hearing loss and, 352
Epenthesis, **90**
Epiglottis, swallowing and, 315
Epilepsy, cerebral palsy and, 116
Epistaxis, 324
Esophageal
　dysphagia, 7
　phase of swallowing, 316
Ethnographic interviewing, 160–161, **161**
Eustachian tube, 347

Evidence-based practice (EBP), components of, 424–426
Executive function (EF)
　difficulties, DLDs (Developmental language disorders), 147
　frontal lobe and, 225
　second language challenges, 234
Exercise-induced laryngeal obstruction (EILO), 287, 293
　intervention for, 296–297
Exercises, swallowing, 327–328
Exhalation, 73
Experimental research, 417–418
Expiratory muscle strength training (EMST), **295**, 327–328
Expressive
　disorders, 7, 8
　language, 53–57, 223
　　delays, 58
　vocabularies, early language development of, 54
External
　cues, 127
　evidence, 424
Extrapyramidal tract, 109
Extrinsic feedback, 129
Eye
　blinking, 260
　contact, autism and, 152

F

Face-to-face therapy, aphasia and, 241
Facial
　musculature, 78
　nerve, **112**
Fainting, 324
False
　hearing loss, 360
　ribs, 73
Family Check-Up for Children Who Are Deaf and Hard of Hearing (FCU-DHH), 366–367
Family history, speech sound disorders and, 88
Fast mapping, defined, 149
Fatigue, vocal, 286–287
FCT (Functional communication training), 169, 240
FCU-DHH (Family Check-Up for Children Who Are Deaf and Hard of Hearing), 366
FDA (Frenchay Dysarthria Assessment), 120
　MSD (Motor speech disorders), 119

Feedback, 125
  motor-based approaches and, 129
Feeding
  behavioral interventions for, 329
  defined, 313
  disorder, defined, 313
  tube, placement of, **323**
FEES (Fiberoptic endoscopic evaluation of swallowing), 322–323
  swallow symptoms, 325
Fetal alcohol syndrome, 151. *see also* Intellectual disability
  described, 155–156
Fiberoptic endoscopic evaluation of swallowing (FEES), 322–323
  swallow symptoms, 325
Final consonant deletion, 89
Finger tapping, 127
Flaccid dysarthria, 112
FLCI (Functional Linguistic Communication Inventory), 239
Floating ribs, 73
Flowcharts, 202, **203**
Fluctuating hearing loss, Ménière disease and, 352
Fluency
  cultural/linguistic considerations of, 266–267
  defined, 260
  description/examples of, **45**
  disorders, 188
    addressing, 267
    assessment & results, 264–266
    defined, 260
    reading, 199
FM (Frequency modulation) system, 364, 365
fMRI (Functional magnetic resonance imaging), 120
Focused stimulation, **166**
Food spillage, 314
Fragile X syndrome, 151, 153, **154–155**
  described, 157
  stuttering, 262
Freak shoes, 21
Frenchay Dysarthria Assessment (FDA), 120
  MSD (Motor speech disorders), 119
Frequency modulation (FM) system, 364, 365
Fricative consonant, 48
Fricatives, age of acquisition of, **49**
Friedreich's ataxia, dysarthria and, 115
Fringe vocabulary, 393
Frontal lobe, 224

EF (Executive function) and, 225
Fronting, described, 89
Functional
  dysphonia, 286
    voice disorders and, 285
  speech sound disorders, 87
    risk factors for, 88
  voice disorders, 286–287
Functional communication training (FCT), 169, 240
Functional Linguistic Communication Inventory (FLCI), 239
Functional magnetic resonance imaging (fMRI), 120
Fundamental frequency, 77

G

Gastroesophageal reflux disease (GERD), dysphagia and, 319
Gender
  affirming voice
    services, 7
    voice therapy, 297–298
  cerebral palsy and, 116
  communication disorders and, 4
  disability and, 30–32
  dysphonia, 297–298
  learning disorders and, 189
  speech sound disorders and, incidence/prevalence of, 88
  voice disorders and, 285
Gene variations, co-occurring language disorder, 150
Genetic
  disorders, stuttering, 262
  syndromes, 153–158, 356
    auditory neuropathy and, 355
GERD (Gastroesophageal reflux disease), dysphagia and, 319
Gestalt imagery, 206
Gestures, autism and, 152
Girls, disabled, violence and, 31
Gliding, **90**
Global aphasia, 228
Glossopharyngeal nerve, **112**
Glottal
  attacks, 294
  stop, 286
Glottic stenosis, defined, 289
Glottis, 74

Grammar, 55
　late talkers and, 59
　learning disorders and, 188
Grammatical morphemes, acquisition of 14, **57**
Graphic organizers, 201–202
Gray matter, stuttering and, 264
Group therapy, aphasia and, 241
Guillain–Barré, dysarthria and, 115
Gurgly voice quality, **288**

H

Hair cells
　damage to, 352
　ear, 348
Hand tapping, 127
Hard palate, 79
　tongue hitting, 62
Harvard University, Medical School, studies at, 11–12
Haskins Laboratories, translating research to practice and, 12
HATS (Hearing assistive technologies systems), 264
Head
　life exercise, 327
　rotation posture, swallowing disorders and, 326
　tilt posture, swallowing disorders and, 326
　trauma, hearing loss and, 352
Healthy disabled, defined, 27
Hearing
　aids, 346, 364
　　cochlear implants (CIs) and, 355
　　tinnitus and, 365
　anatomy of, 346–348
　assessment of, 357–362
　　importance of, 356–357
　　procedures, 357–361
　impairment, 351–356
　longitudinal study of, Medical University of South Carolina, 10
　loss
　　adult, 356
　　bilateral, 345
　　childhood, 345, 352–356
　　congenital, 354, 368
　　degree/range of, **352**
　　false, 360
　　fluctuating, 352
　　prevalence of, 345, **346**
　　stuttering, 262
　　treatment planning/management/options, 362–367
　　types/description of, **353–354**
　　unilateral, 345
　normal development of, 348–351
　prevalence of, 345, **346**
　sensory disabilities, 20
　stuttering, 262
　symptoms of, 351
　thresholds, 359
　treatment planning/management/options, 362–367
　types/description of, **353–354**
　unilateral, 345
Hearing disorders
　cultural/linguistic considerations, 367–368
　prevalence of, 344
　tinnitus, 345–346
　　impact of, 346
Heart, rib cage and, 73
Hemiplegia, spastic, 116
Hemorrhagic strokes, aphasia and, 229
Hereditary traits, good/bad, 22
Hiatal hernia, 332
High schools, intervention and, 8
High-tech AAC, 390–391
Hispanics
　autism and, 152
　communication disorders and, 4
　learning disorders incidence/prevalence and, 189
Hoarse voice sounds, 286
Holmes, Oliver Wendell, *Buck v. Bell* and, 22
Horizontal strategy, 97
Human papillomavirus, 289
Huntington's disease, 113
　dysarthria and, 115
　swallowing and, 317
Hyoid bone, 74
　swallowing and, 315
Hyperadduction, individuals with, 126
Hyperkinetic dysarthria, 113
Hypernasality, 127, 292
Hypoglossal nerve, **112**
Hyponasality, 292
Hypothesis, defined, 415

I

ICF *(International Classification of Functioning, Disability and Health)*, 23–24, 92, 131, 236, 245, 330

augmentative/alternative communication and, 25
    model example, **331**
IDD (Intellectual developmental disorder). *See* Intellectual disability
IDEA (Individuals With Disabilities Education Act), 30, 35, 196, 446
Identification, delays in, 61
Identity-first language, 19
Illness, disability and, 27
Impairment
    based approaches, intervention, 240
    defined, 3
Implicit word learning, 166
Incus, 347
Independent
    living movement, 35
    variable, 416–417
Indigenous peoples, 20–21
    signing by, 21
Indirect
    activation pathway, 109
    treatment, for stuttering, 268
Individuals With Disabilities Education Act (IDEA), 30, 35, 197, 446
Induction loop system, 364
Infants
    assessment of, 60
    audiologists and, 6
    communication and, 51–53
Infant-toddler programs, intervention and, 8
Infections
    ear, cholesteatoma and, 354
    speech sound disorders and, 88
Infectious diseases, dysarthria and, 115
Inflammation, voice disorders and, 285
Inflammatory diseases, dysarthria and, 115
Information, sharing, social communication disorders and, 152
Infrared system, 364
Inhalation, 73
    phonation, voice therapy, **296**
Initial consonant deletion, 89
Initiation of joint attention, 52, 53
Inner ear
    autoimmune disease, sensorineural hearing loss and, 352
    hair cells, 10
    malformation, sensorineural hearing loss and, 352
    oval window of, 347
    temporal bone of, 347

Inspiration, **76**
Integral stimulation
    AoS treatment and, 125
    protocol, 126
Integrated treatment, for stuttering, 268
Intellectual developmental disorder (IDD), described, 153
Intellectual disability
    cerebral palsy and, 116
    described, 153
    social communication disorders and, 152
Intelligibility
    assessment of, 93
    drills, 127
    speech development and, 48
Intensity, 351
    loudness and, 77
    sound, 351
Intentional communication, 52
Interarytenoid muscle, 74
Intercostal muscles, 73
Interdental lisp, 89
Internal
    evidence, 424
    thyroarytenoid muscles, 74
Internalized ableism, 28
International Classification of Functioning, Disability and Health (ICF), 23–24, 92, 131, 236, 245, 330
    augmentative/alternative communication and, 25
    model example, **331**
Interprofessional education (IPE), 61
Interprofessional practice (IPP), 61
Intervention, 61–62
    AAC (Augmentative and alternative communication) and, 396
        for acquired conditions, 397–398
        for developmental conditions, 396–397
    aphasia, 240–241
    approaches, **97–98**
    cultural considerations of, 244
    dementia, 243–244
    exercised-induced laryngeal obstruction, 296–297
    goals, 362
    impairment-based approaches, 240
    language disorders
        adolescents, 167–168
        cultural groups, 168
        preschoolers, 165–167
        school-age children, 167

Intervention *(continued)*
   learning disorders, 198–199
   narrative, 169
   options for
      adults, 362–365
      children, 365–367
   parent
      directed, 329
      mediated, 170
   restorative approaches to, 240
   RHD (Right hemisphere disorder) and, 241
   speech sound disorders and, in children, 94–97
   for stuttering, 268
   supporting techniques/strategies, 95–97
   TBI (Traumatic brain injury), 242–243
   vocal
      cord paralysis, 297
      fatigue, 298
   voice disorders, 293–298
      physiologic techniques, 294
      principles of, 293
      symptomatic techniques, 294
Interviewing
   ethnographic, 160–161, **161**
   semistructured, 422
Intraoral pressure, swallowing and, 315
Intrinsic
   feedback, 129
   laryngeal muscles, **75**
IPE (Interprofessional education), 61
iPods, hearing loss and, 356
IPP (Interprofessional practice), 61
Irregular
   past tense, **57**
   third person, **57**
Ischemic strokes, aphasia and, 229

J

Jargon, stage of, **51**
Jaw
   lower, 78
   oral exercises, 327
Johns Hopkins University, studies at, 11–12
Joint attention, 52
   initiation of, 52, 53
   response to, 52

K

Kansas, University of, studies at, 11

Kinematic tracking systems, 120
   speech signal and, 120
Knowledge outcomes, expected, **8**

L

La Trobe Communication Questionnaire, 238
Labial sounds, 62
Labiodental fricative, 48
Ladau, Ellen, disability defined by, 19
Language
   assessment of, **161–162**
   behaviors associated with, 223
   boosting, 199
   breakdowns in, **149**
   casual model of, **151**
   cerebral palsy and, 116
   child's capacity, synergistic relationship, 151
   deficits, co-occurring, 128
   defined, 1–2, 3
   early development of, 50–53
   expressive, 53–57, 223
   identity-first, 19
   impairment, reading and, 192
   importance of development of, 62–63
   intervention for
      adolescents, 167–168
      cultural groups, 168
      preschoolers, 165–167
      school-age children, 167
   model of, **223**
   person-first, 18
   receptive, 53–57
   sampling, 160, **161**
   scaffolding, **166**
   secondary challenges, 234
   sign, Indigenous peoples and, 21
Language disorder
   assessment of, 236–239
   co-occurring, 150
   intervention for, 164–168
      preschoolers, 165–167
      school-age children, 167
   cultural considerations of, 163–164
   receptive, median prevalence, 150
   SLPs and, 7
   written, 193–194
Laryngeal
   cancer, intervention for, 294–296
   cleft, 290
   imaging, 291

Index

muscles
  intrinsic, **75**
  speech production and, 72
nerve, 289
obstruction, intervention for, 296–297
penetration, imaging and, 325
webbing, defined, 289–290
Laryngomalacia, defined, 289
Laryngoscopy, 120
Laryngospasm, 324
Larynx
  described, 74
  oral exercises, 327
  phonatory system and, 74
Late talkers, 58–60
  predicting outcomes for, 58–59
  red flags for, **59**
  vocabulary and, 58
Lateral
  cricoarytenoid muscle, 74
  lisp, 89
Laterals, age of acquisition of, **49**
Law and the Contradictions of the Disability Rights Movement, 35
Learning
  disability, 187
  disorders, 3
    academic skills and, 188
    areas of impairment, **188**
    assessment of, 196–197
    boosting language/literacy, 199
    causes of, 191
    childhood language disorders and, 152
    co-occurring disorders, 191
    cultural considerations of, 193
    described, 187
    diagnosis, 187
    incidence/prevalence of, 189–190
    intervention, 198–199
    math, 194
    motor, principles of, 125
    nonverbal, 194–196
    reading and, 188, 191–193
    severity levels of, **189**
    signs/symptoms of, 190
    specific, interventions, **199**
    stuttering and, 262
    symptoms of, 187
    written language, 193–194
Lee Silverman Voice Treatment (LSVT), 126, 294, **295**

Left-side neglect, 231
Letter identification, 191
Liebowitz, Cara, disability defined by, 19
Life Participation Approach to Aphasia, 241
Lingual, muscle, 77–78
Linguistic
  achievement, hearing loss and, 355
  approaches, motor speech disorders, 129
  challenges, cerebral palsy and, 117
Lips, 78
  oral exercises, 327
Liquid consonant sound, 48
Lisp, 89
Listening, tinnitus and, 346
Literacy
  boosting, 199
  children with hearing loss, 366
Literature review, 415
Loneliness, hearing loss and, 356
Longitudinal study of hearing, Medical University of South Carolina, 10
Lou Gehrig's disease, 114
Loud talking, vocal folds and, 286
Loudness
  level
    acoustic samples and, 291
    dysphonia and, 288
  vocal folds and, 77
  voice, 76–77
Low birthweight, speech sound disorders and, 88
Lower
  airway, 73
  jaw, 78
  motor neuron system, 109
Low-tech AAC, 389–390
LSVT (Lee Silverman Voice Treatment), 126, 294, **295**
  LOUD, 128
Lungs
  diaphragm and, 73
  rib cage and, 73
  trachea and, 74

M

Malleus, 347
Mandible, 78
Maps, thinking, 206
Masako exercise, 327
Masking noise, 360
Mass, vocal folds, fundamental frequency and, 77

Massachusetts Institute of Technology (MIT), studies at, 11
Massed practice, 129
Mastication, described, 314
Mastoid, bone conduction vibrator and, 360
Math
   gender and, 189
   learning disorders and, 188, 194
   NVLD (Nonverbal learning disability) and, 195
   reading and, 188
   supporting understanding of, 205–207
MBS (Modified barium swallow study), 322
MCT (Milieu communication theory), 169
Meals, sharing, cross-cultural information, 320
Measures
   child report, **162**
   patient report, **162**
   teacher report, **162**
MEC (Montreal Evaluation of Communication), 238
Medical
   model of disability, 23
   versus social models of disability, 24
Medical University of South Carolina, longitudinal study of hearing, 10
Medulla oblongata, carbon dioxide and, 73
Melodic intonation therapy, 129
Mendelsohn maneuver, 326, 327
Ménière disease, 352
Meningitis, sensorineural hearing loss and, 352
Mental health disorders, 20
Meta-analysis, 415
Metacognitive skills, developing, 206
Metalinguistic skill, defined, 148
Metaphon approach, **97**
Metronome, 127
Middle ear
   bones of, 347
   composed of, 347
   ear wax and, 347
   fluid in, 88
   key structures of, **348**
   tympanogram of function of
      abnormal, **359**
      normal, **358**
   tympanometry and, 358
Milieu communication theory (MCT), 169
Mindfulness, 269
Minimally conscious state, **233**
Minority group model, 36

MIT (Massachusetts Institute of Technology), studies at, 11
Mitochondrial genetic condition, auditory neuropathy and, 355
Mixed
   cerebral palsy, **117**
   dysarthria, 114
   hearing loss, 352, **353**
MLG (Motor learning guided) intervention, 125–126
   AoS treatment and, 125–126
Modeling
   AAC (Augmentative and alternative communication) and, 397–398
   video, 170
Modification of speech, for stuttering, 268
Modified barium swallow study (MBS), 322–323
Montreal Evaluation of Communication (MEC), 238
Morphemes, 55
   acquisition of 14
   grammatical, **57**
Morphology, 3, 55, 148
   description/examples of, **45**
   difficulties in, 148
Mother–child skin-to-skin contact, 329
Motor
   based approaches, 129
   cortex, 109
   functioning, cerebral palsy and, 117
   learning, principles of, 125
   neuron system, 109
   skills, NVLD (Nonverbal learning disability) and, 195
Motor learning guided (MLG) intervention, AoS treatment and, 125–126
Motor speech disorders (MSD), 73, 109–118
   assessment
      adult population, 119–120
      cross-cultural, 122–124
      pediatric population, 120–121
   cerebral palsy and, 115–116, **117**
   cross-cultural information, 118
   diagnosis, in children, 121
   dysarthria, 110–112
      ataxic, 113
      causes, 115
      flaccid, 112
      hyperkinetic, 113
      mixed, 114

spastic, 112–113
    unilateral upper motor neuron, 113
  linguistic approaches to, 129
  multimodal communication approaches, 129
  pediatric population and, 128
  treatment
    adult population, 125–128
    pediatric population, 128–130
Motor Speech Disorders Severity Rating Scale, 120
Motoric-imitative treatment, 241
Mouth, upper airway and, 73
Movie theaters, hearing loss and, 356
MSD (Motor speech disorders), 73, 109–118
  assessment
    adult population, 119–120
      cross-cultural, 122–124
      pediatric population, 120–121
  cerebral palsy and, 115–116, **117**
  cross-cultural information, 118
  diagnosis, in children, 121
  dysarthria
    causes, 115
    flaccid, 112
    hyperkinetic, 113
    mixed, 114
    spastic, 112–113
    unilateral upper motor neuron, 113
  linguistic approaches to, 129
  multimodal communication approaches, 129
  pediatric population and, 128
Multimodal communication approaches, MSD (Motor speech disorders), 129
Multiple sclerosis, 289
  dysarthria and, 115
Musculoskeletal problems, cerebral palsy and, 116
Myasthenia gravis, 112
Myoelastic–aerodynamic theory, 76
Myths, AAC (Augmentative and alternative communication) and, 400–401

N

Narrative interventions, 169
Nasal
  cavities, 72
  regurgitation, 315
  sounds, speech development and, 47–48
Nasals, age of acquisition of, **49**
Nasoendoscopy, 120
Nasometry, 120

Nasopharynx, 79, 347
National Assessment of Educational Progress, 205
National Association of Young People Who Stutter, 270
National Institutes of Health (NIH), 198
National Reading Panel, 199
National Stuttering Association, 270
Natural communities of reinforcement, 169
Naturalistic speech intelligibility approach, **97**
Nebraska, University of, studies at, 11
Neck, extension posture, swallowing disorders and, 325–326
Negative
  correlation, 420, **421**
  positive, 420
  reducing negative, for stuttering, 269
  reinforcement, 329
  responses, reducing, for stuttering, 268
Neglect, left-sided, 231
Neologisms, 227
Nerves
  acoustic, 348
  auditory, 348, 352
  cranial, 73
  spinal, 73
Nervous system
  central, 109
  peripheral, 109
Neurobiological disorders, cluttering and, 264
Neurodevelopmental disorders, 147
  cluttering and, 264
Neurodiverse, 3
Neurogenic vocal nodules, 286
Neuroimaging, speech signal and, 120
Neurological disabilities, 20
New York University, translating research to practice and, 12
Nielsen, Kim, history and, 20
Nightclubs, hearing loss and, 356
NIH (National Institutes of Health), 198
Nodules vocal, voice, 286
  disorders and, 285
  disruption and, 289
Noise
  hearing loss and, 352, 356
  masking, 360
Nonempirical research, 415
Nonexperimental research, 419
Nonnutritive sucking, 329
Nonspeech oral motor exercises, 129

Nonsyllabic consonant, 48
Nonverbal learning disability (NVLD), 194–196
   neuropsychological assets/challenges, **195**
   support strategies, 206
Norm-referenced
   measure, 61
   tests, 61
Normal, defined, 21
Normalcy, 21
   impacts of concept, 22
Normality, described, 21
North America, NVLD (Nonverbal learning disability) and, 195
Northeastern University, studies at, 11
Northern Ireland, learning disorders incidence/prevalence and, 189
Northwestern University, studies at, 11
Nose
   bleeding, 324
   upper airway and, 73
No-tech AAC, 389–390
Numerical scale, speech sound disorders and, 93
NVLD (Nonverbal learning disability), 194–196
   neuropsychological assets/challenges, **195**
   support strategies, 206

O

OAE (Otoacoustic emissions), testing, 359
Observation
   classroom, 162
   covert, 422
   overt, 422
   systematic, **161**
Observational study, 421–422
Obstruction, laryngeal, intervention for, 296–297
Occipital
   lobe, 224, 226
   temporal area, sounding out words and, 192
Oculomotor nerve, **112**
Office of Special Education Programs, on special education services, 30
Olfactory nerve, **112**
OME (Oral mechanism examination), 119
Open
   head injuries, 232
   syllables, speech development and, 48
Operant
   conditioning, 329
   treatment, for stuttering, 268

Opportunity barriers, 399
Optic nerve, **112**
Oral
   cavity, 72
      mechanism examination, 93, 291
   desensitization, 329
   motor exercises, 327
      nonspeech, 129
   preparatory phase, swallowing and, 314
Oral mechanism examination (OME), 119
Orbicularis oris muscle, 78
Organ of Corti, 348
Organic dysphonia, 286
Oropharyngeal dysphagia, 7
Oropharynx, 79
Oscillators, bone, 360
Otitis media, 345
   hearing loss and, 354
   with effusion, **88**
Otoacoustic emissions (OAE), testing, 359
Otoscopy, 357–360
Ototoxic drugs, hearing loss and, 352
Oval window, ear, 347
Overextension, early language development and, 54
Overt
   observation, 422
   stuttering behaviors, 262
Oxygen, 73

P

Pacing boards, 127
Palatal lift, 127
Palsy, pseudobulbar, 289
Papilloma, recurrent respiratory, defined, 289
Paradoxical vocal fold movement (PVFM), 287
Parallel talk, **166**
Paralysis, vocal cord, intervention for, 297
Parent
   directed intervention, 329
   mediated interventions, 170
   report measures, **162**
Parietal
   lobe, 224–225
      function of, 226
   temporal area, word analysis and, 192
Parkinson's disease, 289
   dysarthria and, 115
   swallowing and, 317
Passive articulators, 77

Past tense
    irregular, 57
    regular -ed, 57
PCC (Percentage of consonants correct), speech sound disorders and, 93
Pediatric, 328–329
    dysphagia, 316–317, 329
    populations, motor skills disorders and, 121
    swallowing, assessment of, 324–325
Pendred syndrome, 352
Penetration
    laryngeal, imaging and, 325
    swallowing and, 315
Percentage of consonants correct (PCC), speech sound disorders and, 93
Perinatal difficulties, speech sound disorders and, 88
Peripheral nervous system, 109
Peristalsis, 316
Personal amplification system, 364
Person-first language, 18
PET (Positron emission tomography), 120
Pharyngeal
    dysphagia, 7
    phase of swallowing, 315–316
    residue, imaging and, 325
Pharynx, 72
Phenomenology, 420
Phonating, defined, 285
Phonation, **76**
    acoustic samples and, 291
    AoS (Apraxia of speech) and, childhood, **123**
    breaks, **288**
    described, 74
    ventricular, 289
Phonation Resistance Training Exercises (PhoRTE), 126, 294, **295**
Phonatory system, 74–76
Phonemes, described, 53
Phonemic awareness instruction, 199
Phonics, 199
    systematic, 200
Phonological
    awareness, 148, 191
        reading and, 192
    contrast approach, **97–98**
    disorders, 86–87
    processes, 89
        in English development, **90**
Phonology, 3, 53, 148

description/examples of, **45**
PhoRTE (Phonation Resistance Training Exercises), 126, 294, **295**
Physical
    disabilities, 20
        cultural view of, 21
    tension reduction, stuttering and, 268
Physiologic methods
    speech signal and, 120
    voice disorders and, 294
Pitch, 76–77
    acoustic samples and, 291
    dysphonia and, 288
Pivotal response treatment (PRT), 170
Plosive sounds, speech development and, 47–48
Plosives, age of acquisition of, **49**
Polyps, defined, 289
Populations, diverse, intervention considerations, 97
Positive
    correlation, 420, **421**
    reinforcement, 329
Positron emission tomography (PET), 120
Possessive -s, **57**
Posterior cricoarytenoid muscle, 74
Post-traumatic confusional state, **233**
Postural changes, swallowing disorders and, 325–326
PPA (Primary progressive aphasia), 229
Practice
    blocked, 129
    distributed, 129
    massed, 129
    options of, 125
    random, 125, 129
Pragmatics, 3, 56, 150
    description/examples of, **45**
Pregnancy
    learning disorders and, 191
    speech sound disorders and, 88
Premature infants
    cerebral palsy and, 116–117
    speech sound disorders and, 88
    voice disorders and, infants, 285
Prenatal difficulties, speech sound disorders and, 88
Preoral phase, swallowing, 314
Presbycusis, 352
    adult population and, 356
Presbyphonia, 285

Preschoolers
  intervention and, 8
  language disorders, intervention for, 165–167
Present progressive -ing, **57**
Preventive Services Task Force, 91
Primary motor cortex, 109
Primary progressive aphasia (PPA), 229
Private practice
  audiologists and, 6
  SLPs and, 9
Problem-solving, cerebral palsy and, 117
Progressive bulbar palsy, 112
Prolongations, stuttering, 262
PROMPT (Prompts for Restructuring Oral Muscular Phonetic Targets) system, 129
Prompts for Restructuring Oral Muscular Phonetic Targets (PROMPT) system, 129
Prosody, AoS (Apraxia of speech) and, childhood, **123**
PRT (Pivotal response treatment), 170
Pseudobulbar palsy, 289
Pseudohypacusis, 360
Psychogenic
  conversion, aphonia/dysphonia, 287
  voice disorders, 287
Psychogenic causes, vocal fatigue, 289
Puberphonia, defined, 290
Pulmonary system, 73
Pulsed voice quality, **288**
Punctuation, learning disorders and, 188
Purdue University, study of stuttering at, 12
Pure-tone thresholds, 359
PVFM (Paradoxical vocal fold movement), 287
Pyramidal tract, 109

Q

Quadriplegia, spastic, 116
Qualitative research, 415, 421–422
Quality of life, tinnitus and, 346
Quantitative, 415
  data, 417
  research, 417
Quasi-experimental research, 418
Questionnaires, voice disorders intervention and, 293

R

Race
  cerebral palsy and, 116
  communication disorders and, 4

Ramps, **28**
Random practice, 125, 129
Randomized controlled trial (RCT), 417–418
Rapid syllable transition (ReST), 129
RCT (Randomized controlled trial), 417–418
Reading
  brain and, 192
  comprehension, 199
  disorders, 191–193
    cultural considerations of, 193
    language, 192
  fluency, 199
  gender and, 189
  learning disorders and, 188
Recasting, **166**
Receptive, 150
  disorders, 7, 8
  language, 53–57
    late talkers and, 58
    disorder, median prevalence, 150
Recreational noise, hearing loss and, 356
Reduction, cluster, 89
Reduplication, **90**
Reflex, testing acoustic, 358
Reflexive vocalizations, **51**
Reflux
  acid, dysphagia and, 319
  voice disorders and, 285
Regular
  past tense -ed, **57**
  plural -s, **57**
  third person -s, **57**
Regurgitation, nasal, 315
Rehabilitation Act, Section 504 of, 35
Reinforcement
  negative, 329
  positive, 329
Relaxation, voice therapy, **296**
Research
  between-subjects designs, 417
  descriptive, 419
  experimental, 417–418
  importance of, 423–426
  innovations, 10–12
  nonexperimental, 419
  qualitative, 421–422
  quantitative, 417
  quasi-experimental, 418
  question, 415
  subject-designs, 417
  types of, 415–422

Index

within-subject designs, 417
Research in Communication Sciences and Disorders: Methods for Systematic Inquiry, 415
Resonance
    acoustic samples and, 291
    AoS (Apraxia of speech) and, childhood, **123**
    cul-de-sac, 292
    physiologic impairments in, 127
    vocal, assessment of, 292
Resonant voice therapy, 294, **295**
Respiration, AoS (Apraxia of speech) and, childhood, **123**
Respiratory
    cycle, 73
    muscles, 73
    system, described, 73
Response to intervention (RTI), 197
Response to joint attention, 52
ReST (Rapid syllable transition), 129
Restorative approaches, to intervention, 240
Retrieval practice (RP), 166
Retrocochlear pathology, 358
RHD (Right hemisphere disorder), 230–232
    assessment of, 238
    causes of, 232
    impact of, 232
    intervention and, 241
Rhythm approaches, AoS treatment and, 125
Rib cage, 73
Ribs, 73
    false, 73
Rich vocabulary instruction (RVI)., 166
RIDE approach, 206
Right hemisphere disorder (RHD), 230–232
    assessment of, 238
    causes of, 232
    impact of, 232
    Intervention and, 241
Root of tongue, 78
Rough voice quality, **288**
RP (Retrieval practice), 166
RTI (Response to intervention), 197
Rubella, sensorineural hearing loss and, 352
RVI (Rich vocabulary instruction), 166

S

Sampling
    convenience, 244
    language, 160, **161**
Sarcopenia, defined, 289
Scaffolding, language, **166**
Scanning
    AAC (Augmentative and alternative communication) and, 391
    selection methods, **392**
Scarlet fever, Indigenous peoples and, 21
School-age children, audiologists and, 6
Scope of Practice for Speech-Language Pathology, 264
Screaming
    language disorders, 159
    vocal folds and, 286
    voice disruption, 289
Secondary behaviors, 260
Section 504, of Rehabilitation Act, 35
Seizure disorders, dysarthria and, 115
Self
    assessment, voice disorders and, 291
    determined behaviors, cerebral palsy and, 117
    disclosure, stuttering, 269
    feeding interventions, 329
    learning, 125
Self-regulated strategy development (SRSD), stages, 198–199
Semantics, 3, 53
    description/examples of, **45**
    feature analysis, 202, **204**
    language content and, 149
    relationships, toddlers and, **56**
    webs, 202
Semicircular canals, 348
Semistructured interviews, 422
Sensorineural hearing loss, 351–352, **353**
Sensory disabilities, 20
Sentences, complex, children with hearing loss, 355
Sequential bilingualism, 163
Service delivery options, 97, 170
Shaker exercise, 327
Shrill voice quality, **288**
SIB (Severe Impairment Battery–Language Scale), 239
Sibilants, 48
Sickle cell anemia, 352
Sign language, Indigenous peoples and, 21
Signal to noise ratio, SIN (Speech-in-noise) testing and, 361
Silent aspiration, 321–322
Simultaneous bilingualism, 163
SIN (Speech-in-noise) testing, 360
    testing acoustic, 361

Singers, vocal fold changes and, 286
SIT (Speech Intelligibility Test), 120
Sleep, tinnitus and, 346
SLPs (Speech-language pathologists), 7–9
   career pathways for, 9
   expected knowledge outcomes, **8**
   health care settings, 8
   roles of, 158
   services of, 7
Smallpox, Indigenous peoples and, 21
Smartphones, hearing loss and, 356
SNUG (Spontaneous novel utterance generation), 390–391
Social
   communication, 56
     autism and, 152
     disorders, childhood language disorders and, 151–152
   emotional reciprocity, autism and, 152
   interaction, autism and, 152
   isolation, hearing loss and, 356
   model of disability, 23, 36
   pragmatic language disorders, 7
   referencing, 25–26
   skills, NVLD (Nonverbal learning disability) and, 195
Socioeconomic status, disability and, 32–34
Soft palate, 79
Somatosensory cortex, 225
Sound
   acquisition of speech, **50**
   prolongations, 260
   pressure level (SPL), 344–345
     of environmental sounds, **351**
   supporting production of, 97
Sound production treatment (SPT), AoS treatment and, 125
South Carolina, University of, longitudinal hearing study at, 10
Spasmodic dysphonia, 286, 289
Spastic
   cerebral palsy, 116, **117**
   dysarthria, 112–113
   hemiplegia, 116
   quadriplegia, 116
Spasticity, cerebral palsy and, 116
Special education services, school-age children, 189–190
Specific learning disorder. *See* Learning disorders
Spectrogram, speech signal display, 120

Speech
   apraxia of, 115
   audiometry, 360
   cerebral palsy and, 116
   defined, 3
   detection threshold, 360
   early development, 47–48, **48–49**
   elements/examples, description of, **45**
   importance of development of, 62–63
   intelligibility, 120
     defined, 120
   otitis media and, 354
   production, 72, 73
     breath support and, 126
     cultural considerations in, 89–91
   rate
     acoustic samples and, 291
     AoS (Apraxia of speech) and, **123**
   signal
     acoustic display methods, 120
     physiologic methods, 120
   sound, 87, 92–93
     acquisition of, **50**
     assessment, 91–92, 94
   sound perception training, **98**
   tinnitus and, 346
Speech sound disorders (SSDs), 87
   Case Western Reserve University study of, 12
   characteristics of, 89
   children, **87**
     intervention for, 94–97
   choosing target sounds, 95
   family history and, 88
   functional, 87
     risk factors for, 88
   incidence/prevalence of, childhood, 88
   intervention, supporting techniques/strategies, 95–97
   non-motor-based speech, 122
   SLPs and, 7
Speech Intelligibility Test (SIT), 120
Speech Systems Intelligibility Treatment (SSIT), 128
Speech-in-noise (SIN) testing, 360
Speech-language pathologists (SLPs)
   assistants, responsibilities of
   career pathways for, 9
   colleges/universities and, 9
   expected knowledge outcomes, **8**
   health care settings, 8
   roles of, 158

services of, 7
Speech-to-text, using, 96
Spelling
   gender and, 189
   learning disorders and, 188
Spinal nerves, 73
Spirometry, 120
SPL (Sound pressure level), 344–345
Spontaneous novel utterance generation (SNUG), 390–391
Sporting events, hearing loss and, 356
SPT (Sound production treatment), AoS treatment and, 125
SRSD (Self-regulated strategy development), stages to a, 198–199
SSDs (Speech sound disorders), 87
   Case Western Reserve University study of, 12
   characteristics of, 89
   children, **87**
      intervention for, 94–97
   choosing target sounds, 95
   family history and, 88
   functional, 87
      risk factors for, 88
   incidence/prevalence of, childhood, 88
   intervention, supporting techniques/strategies, 95–97
   non-motor-based speech, 122
   SLPs and, 7
SSIT (Speech Systems Intelligibility Treatment), 128
Standardized assessments, 160, **161**
Stapes, 347
STAR model, 200
State-by-State requirements, 9
Sterilization, good/bad traits and, 22
Sternum, 73
Stigmas
   defined, 25
   determined by, 25
Stimulability
   assessment of, 93–94
   testing, 265
Stimulation, focused, **166**
Stopping, **90**
Strained voice quality, **288**
Strangled voice quality, **288**
Stress
   caregiver, 118
   vocal fatigue, 289

Stridor, laryngomalacia and, 289
Stroke
   AAC (Augmentative and alternative communication) and, 388
   aphasia and, 226
      hemorrhagic, 229
      ischemic, 229
   awareness of, 229
   recovery from, SLPs and, 11
   swallowing and, 317
Structural voice disorders, 286
Study limitations, 423
Stuttering, 12
   behaviors, primary/secondary, 262
   causes of, 263–264
   characteristics of, 262–263
   children, stop, 260–261
   covert
      behaviors, 262
      impacts of, 262–263
   cultural/linguistic considerations of, 271
   described, 260
   incidence/prevalence of, 261–262
   indicators, positive change, 290
   interventions for, 267–270
   overt behaviors, 262
   persistent, effects of, 261
   secondary behaviors, 260
Stuttering Association for the Young, 270
Subglottal air pressure, 74
Submucous cleft palate, 91
Sucking, nonnutritive, 329
Super-supraglottic swallow, 326
Supraglottic swallow, 326
Supreme Court, *Buck v. Bell*, 22
Swallowing
   assessment of
      adult population, 321–324
      pediatric population, 324–325
   cycle, 313
   defined, 313
   disorders, 7, 313
      compensatory strategies, 325–327
      impact of, 319–320
   efficiency, 322
   exercises, 327–328
   hard, 328
   maneuvers, 326
   phases of, **313**, **318**
      esophageal, 316

Swallowing *(continued)*
  phases of *(continued)*
    oral preparatory, 314
    pharyngeal, 315–316
    preoral, 314
  safety, 322
  screening, 321
  structural etiologies of, 318–319
  treatment approaches
    adult population, 325–328
    pediatric population, 328–329
  voice disruption, 289
Swallowing Quality of Life (SWAL-QOL), 321
SWAL-QOL (Swallowing Quality of Life), 321
Swelling, vocal fold changes and, 286
Syllabic consonant, 48
Syllables
  closed, 48
  repetitions, stuttering, 262
  unstressed deletion, **90**
Symptomatic methods, voice disorders and, 294
Syncope, 324
Syntax, 55, 148
  defined, 3
  description/examples of, **45**
  difficulties in, 148
Systematic
  observation, **161**
  review, 415
Systematic phonics, 200

T

Taking turns, social communication disorders and, 152
Talk, parallel, **166**
Talking, loud, vocal folds and, 286
Target
  implementing, 96
  sounds, amplifying, 95
TBI (Traumatic brain injury), 3, 232–234
  AAC (Augmentative and alternative communication) and, 388
  assessment of, 238
  causes of, 234
  co-occurring language disorder, 150
  impact of, 234
  intervention for, 242–243
  levels of consciousness, 232
  swallowing and, 317

Teacher report measures, **162**
Teachers, vocal fold changes and, 286
Telephone amplifier, 364
Television assistive device/accessories, 364
Telling stories, social communication disorders and, 152
Temporal
  bone, 78, 347
  lobe, 224, 226
Temporomandibular joint, 78
Tension
  reduction of physical, stuttering and, 268
  vocal folds, fundamental frequency and, 77
Test–teach–retest framework, assessment and, 60–61
Text telephone (TTD), 364
Texting, **28**
Theaters, hearing loss and, 356
Thinking
  ableist, 28
  maps, 206
Third person
  irregular, **57**
  regular, **57**
Thoracic cage, 73
Thorax, 73
Throat
  clearing, vocal folds and, 286
  upper airway and, 73
Thyroarytenoid muscles, 74
Thyroid cartilage, 74
  cricothyroid muscle and, 74
Tics, defined, 113
Tinnitus, 345–346
  attention and, 346
  hearing aids and, 365
  impact of, 346
  Ménière disease and, 352
  sound and, 346
Tip of tongue, 78
Toddlers
  assessment of, 60
  audiologists and, 6
  semantic relationships, **56**
Tongue
  described, 77–78
  hold maneuver, 327
  oral exercises, 327
Tourette syndrome, cluttering and, 263, 264
Toxic diseases, dysarthria and, 115

Toxin exposure, learning disorders and, 191
Trachea
   larynx and, 74
   lower airway and, 73
   swallowing and, 74
Training specific states, 125
Transcortical
   motor aphasia, 228
   sensory aphasia, 228
Trauma, dysarthria and, 115
Traumatic brain injury (TBI), 3, 232–234
   AAC (Augmentative and alternative communication) and, 388
   assessment of, 238
   causes of, 234
   co-occurring language disorder, 150
   impact of, 234
   intervention for, 242–243
   swallowing and, 317
Tremorous voice quality, **288**
Tremors, defined, 113
Trigeminala nerve, **112**
Trochlear nerve, **112**
TTD (Text telephone), 364
TTY (Text telephone), 364
Tube, feeding, placement of, **323**
Tutoring, individual, 200
Tympanic membrane, 347
Tympanogram
   middle ear
      normal function, **358**
      function, **358**
Tympanometry, 358

U

UES (Upper esophageal sphincter), 326
   head life exercise and, 327
Ugly laws, 21
Ultrasound imaging, 95
Unaided AAC, 388, 389
Uncontractible
   auxiliary, **57**
   copular, **57**
Underextension, early language development and, 54
Understanding Research and Evidence-Based Practice in Communication Disorders: A Primer for Students and Practitioners, 415

Unhealthy disabled, defined, 27
Unilateral
   hearing loss, 345
   upper motor neuron, dysarthria, 113
United Kingdom, receptive language disorder, median prevalence, 150
United States
   disability rights in, 34–36
   disorders
      hearing and, 344
      learning incidence/prevalence and, 189
   receptive language disorder, median prevalence, 150
Universal
   model, 36
   newborn hearing screening, 345
Universities
   audiologists and, 6
   SLPs and, 9
University of Cincinnati, translating research to practice and, 12
University of Kansas, studies at, 11
University of Nebraska, studies at, 11
University of Syracuse, translating research to practice and, 12
University of Washington
   auditory training exercises and, 10–11
   Virginia Merrill Bloedel Hearing Research Center, 10–12
University of Wisconsin–Madison, studies at, 11
Upper airway, 73
Upper esophageal sphincter (UES), 326
Upper motor neuron system, 109, **110**
U.S. Preventive Services Task Force, 91
Usher syndrome, 356
Uvula, 79

V

Vagus nerve, **112**
Variable practice, 125
Variables, 416–417
   confounding, 419
Vascular diseases, dysarthria and, 115
Vegetative state, **233**
Velocardiofacial syndrome, 151, 153, **154–155**
   described, 158
Velum, 79
Venn diagrams, 202, **204**
Ventricular phonation, 289

Verbal
  apraxia, 115
  behaviors, autism and, 152
Vertebral column, 73
Vertebrobasilar insufficiency, 352
Vertigo, Ménière disease and, 352
Vestibular, aqueduct syndrome, sensorineural hearing loss and, 352
Vestibulocochlear nerve, 352
  cochlear synaptopathy and, 356
VFSS (Videofluoroscopic swallowing study), 322–323
  swallow symptoms, 325
Vibration, vocal folds, 76–77
Vibrator, bone conduction, 360
Video modeling, 170
Videoendoscopy, 291
Videofluoroscopic swallowing study (VFSS), 322–323
  swallow symptoms, 325
Videofluoroscopy, 120
Videostroboscopy, 120, 291
Violence, disabled women/girls and, 31
Virginia Merrill Bloedel Hearing Research Center, 10–12
Vision
  loss, cultural view of, 21
  sensory disabilities, 20
Visual
  cortex, 226
  cueing, 95
  patterns, 206
  spatial abilities, 194–195
Visual executive function, NVLD (Nonverbal learning disability) and, 195
Vocabulary
  acquisition of, 53–54
  analytic instruction, 200
  children with hearing loss, 355
  core, 393
  fringe, 393
  late talkers and, 58, 59
  teaching, 200
Vocal
  cord
    paralysis, intervention for, 297
    voice disorders and, 285
  exercises, voice disorders and, 285
  fatigue, 286–287, 289
    intervention for, 298
  folds, 73, 76
    described, 286
    paralysis, 286
    phonation/inspiration of, **76**
    spasm of, 324
    vibration and, 76–77
    weakness, 126
  hygiene, 286
  nodules, 286
    voice disorders and, 285
    voice disruption, 289
  play, stage of, **51**
  quality, dysphonia and, 288
  resonance, assessment of, 292
Vocalis muscle, 74
Vocalizations, **90**
  early stages of, **51**
Voice
  assessment, 291
  box, phonatory system and, 74
  carryover telephone, 364
  changes in older adults, 285
  description/examples of, **45**
  disruption, 288–289
    causes of, 289–290
  production, pitch/loudness, 76–77
  quality, symptoms of, **288**
  therapies, **295–296**
  therapy, gender-affirming, 297–298
Voice disorders
  addressing, 290
  assessment of, 291–293
  communication and, 287
  functional, 286–287
    causes of, 289
  identification of, 286–287
  intervention for, 293–298
    physiologic techniques, 294
    symptomatic techniques, 294
  organic, 286
  prevalence of, 285
  principles of, 293
  psychogenic, 287
  voice disruption in, 288–289
Voice Disorders Practice Portal, 288
Voiced sounds, 48
Voiceless sounds, 48
Vowels, speech development and, 47

W

Waardenburg syndrome, 352
WAB-R (Western Aphasia Battery–Revised), 237

"Wait and see" approach, late talkers and, **59**
Warren, Lavinia, 21
Washington University of
  auditory training exercises and, 10–11
  hair cells study, 10
Waveform, speech signal display, 120
Weintraub, Liz, disability defined by, 20
Wernicke's area, aphasia and, 226, 227
Western Aphasia Battery–Revised (WAB-R), 237
White adults, prevalence of hearing loss, 345
White children
  autism and, 152
  cerebral palsy and, 116
  communication disorders and, 4
  learning disorders incidence/prevalence and, 189
White matter, stuttering and, 264
WHO (World Health Organization)
  International Classification of Functioning, Disability, and Health (ICF), 92
  prevalence of disability, gender and, 31
Williams syndromes, 151, 153, **154–155**
  described, 157
Wisconsin-Madison, University of, studies at, 11
Women
  disabled, violence and, 31
    vs able-bodied, 30
Word
  analysis, parietal-temporal area, 192
  blocking on, 262
  knowledge, 200
    anchored, 200
    STAR model, 200

learning, implicit, 166
problems, RIDE approach, 206
recognition testing, 360
repetitions, stuttering, 262
Words
  core, 393
  sounding out, Occipital-temporal area and, 192
World Health Organization (WHO)
  International Classification of Functioning, Disability, and Health (ICF), 92
  prevalence of disability, gender and, 31
Writing
  EmPOWER strategy, 205
  lab approach, 205
  learning disorders and, 188
Written language
  disorders, 193–194
  facilitating, 201–205

X

X-linked hearing loss, 356

Y

Yale Swallow Protocol, 321
Yelling, voice disruption, 289

Z

Zone of proximal development (ZPD), 160
ZPD (Zone of proximal development), 160